A Strategic Approach to Knee Arthritis Treatment

Seung-Suk Seo
Editor

A Strategic Approach to Knee Arthritis Treatment

From Non-Pharmacologic Management to Surgery

Springer

Editor
Seung-Suk Seo
Department of Orthopedics
Haeundae Bumin Hospital
Busan
South Korea

ISBN 978-981-16-4216-6 ISBN 978-981-16-4217-3 (eBook)
https://doi.org/10.1007/978-981-16-4217-3

This Springer imprint is published by the registered company Springer Nature Singapore Pte Ltd.
The registered company address is: 152 Beach Road, #21-01/04 Gateway East, Singapore 189721, Singapore

Dedicated to those I cherish the most, my wife Da-Hyun, my mother Hu-Bun, and two my sons.

Foreword

It is a great challenge and hard to write a book in English for Korean scholars. I sincerely congratulate Dr. Seung-Suk Seo on the publication of this book through continuous research and efforts with a passion for academics, even in the midst of being busy treating patients.

The knee joint is one of the most studied and mentioned topics in orthopedic surgery. The knee joint is a specialized structure that supports repetitive loads and enables joint movement by reducing friction. It is built by the physiological conditions of articular cartilage and cellular matrix. Also, the knee joint is a complex and complicated structure, and is the structure with the most to do.

This book deals with osteoarthritis of the knee joint that is one of the most common and important knee joint disease. Due to the gradual aging of the population, osteoarthritis of the knee joint is more frequent, especially in developed countries. Therefore, proper diagnosis and treatment of knee osteoarthritis is an important responsibility for general physicians, rheumatologists, and orthopedic surgeons. Many books on knee arthritis have already been published. This book contains all the basic and practical, up-to-date knowledge of knee osteoarthritis, from the basics of the knee, such as the anatomy and biomechanics of the knee, the structure and function of articular cartilage and meniscus, to the diagnosis and various treatments of arthritis. In particular, a number of visual illustrations were added appropriately to complement the text and enhance understanding. In addition, in order to provide the evidence-based and most modern view on knee arthritis, the author's opinion and many influential references have been reviewed.

This book was made with continuous inspection and efforts for many days, with the dedication of well-versed authorities and competent young doctors in the field of knee joints. Thanks to all the doctors who have contributed to this book. Their dedication will be a good guide for the numerous trainees, clinicians studying, and treating knee osteoarthritis. Special thanks to Dr. Seung-Suk Seo for collecting and revising all the texts. He is one of the best, most delicate, and academically outstanding doctors of many orthopedic surgeons I have ever seen. His leadership has undoubtedly led to the publication of a great book.

The medicine is advancing day by day. The knee joint is no exception. I am sure this book will be a good guide to treating osteoarthritis in the knee and will be a stable and lasting reference for the next few years. I hope this book will be of great help to all doctors who treat knee arthritis.

Finally, if the book does not flow like water, it rots and disappears. Do not settle for this. I hope that a more complete revision comes out by supplementing any missing or updated parts.

Jin Hwan Ahn, MD, PhD
Department of Orthopedics, Sae Um Hospital
Seoul, South Korea

Department of Orthopedics, College of Medicine
Sungkyunkwan University
Seoul, South Korea

Foreword

The diagnosis and treatment of arthritis of the knee has various treatment methods as well as a long history. Now, when the world's knowledge is connected through the Internet, many of these treatment methods are introduced through papers or books. The pace of development of treatment has accelerated over time, and a vast amount of research is being updated even now. Knowledge of these treatment methods is also open to patients, so patients who search for a treatment for their disease ask a doctor for the treatment they searched for or ask more deeply about the treatment. Mastering all of the new treatments is practically difficult and the selection of treatment is hard. In order to choose the right treatment, it is necessary to understand the pathology and progression of degenerative arthritis of the knee and to classify the mechanisms and effects of various treatment methods.

The editor of this book, whom I have known for a long time, is an orthopedic specialist who has been treating patients with knee joint disease for more than 30 years while actively conducting academic activities such as serving as president of the Korean Knee Society. He is probably one of those who can explain the diagnosis and treatment of degenerative knee arthritis well. This book goes beyond simply recording the author's experiences and observations and is the result of organizing them on a theoretical basis concretely and systematically. This book provides comprehensive information about knee arthritis as well as the latest knowledge on the effects of each of the non-surgical and various surgical treatments. Along with this latest knowledge, the pros and cons of the technique based on the editor's extensive clinical experience are clearly described. In addition, detailed illustrations help to understand the anatomy of the knee, the pathology of osteoarthritis, and its exacerbation process.

Knee osteoarthritis has been studied for a long time with various treatments; however, there is still a need for improvement of more effective treatments and basic research. Even treatments within the same category have varying results depending on the dose, technique, and approach, and adverse events have been reported that cannot be ignored. These unorganized variable results may rather confuse doctors trying to treat patients. In this respect, this book, which summarizes the existing knowledge of knee arthritis that is comprehensive and up-to-date, is a very valuable resource for improving the diagnosis and treatment of knee arthritis. In addition, it is believed that various knee treatment mechanisms, techniques, and tips are organized in an easy-to-understand manner in this book, helping doctors who do not major in knee but want to access knee disease treatment to broaden their understanding of knee arthritis. I do not doubt that this book will make it easier for many patients suffering from knee arthritis and doctors who treat it, and wish the editors great success.

Dae Kyung Bae, MD, PhD
Department of Orthopedics, Seoul Sacred Heart Hospital
Seoul, South Korea

Department of Orthopaedics, College of Medicine
Kyung Hee University
Seoul, South Korea

Preface

Osteoarthritis is one of the most common diseases that occur in humans. In particular, knee osteoarthritis exacts a tremendous socioeconomic burden upon those who suffer from it due to the hardship it places upon an individual's personal and professional activities. As a young man, while completing my medical studies and residency I understood osteoarthritis to be a disease of articular cartilage that progressed naturally through daily "wear and tear." However, as medical knowledge has advanced over the last several decades, many breakthroughs have been made with regard to the etiology, pathogenesis, diagnosis, and treatment of osteoarthritis. My knowledge too has grown right alongside these advances as I have been an orthopedic surgeon specializing in knee joint surgery for the past 30 years.

In my practice, I have encountered countless patients with knee osteoarthritis who have been referred to my clinic for surgery. However, only a few of the patients I treat are provided with surgical treatment and most patients are treated non-surgically. My thoughts, as a practicing surgeon, while varied, have often focused on my belief that many healthcare providers, including myself, have failed to provide appropriate medical care to patients with knee osteoarthritis. Despite many academic societies and government regulators having drafted therapeutic guidelines for osteoarthritis, in my opinion, in practice, many patients have not been properly treated with the established guidelines in clinics. While varied, reasons for this include social and environmental factors, including the healthcare systems in many countries, the education provided to healthcare providers, and various patient-related factors. Among the issues I have outlined here, I believe the education provided to healthcare providers is of critical importance. One of the key reasons, I believe that educational practices are lacking, is that despite the abundance of knowledge regarding osteoarthritis that has been introduced in textbooks, journals, and web-based articles, it is difficult to find texts specific to knee osteoarthritis. Additionally, of the texts that exist focused on knee osteoarthritis, most focus almost exclusively on surgical techniques. Knee osteoarthritis is treated not only by orthopedic surgeons, but also by rheumatologists, general physicians, and family medical doctors, so I believe it requires a textbook that provides integrated knowledge with a focus on both non-surgical treatment and surgery-specific knowledge. Osteoarthritis is caused by a variety of etiologies and is characterized by gradual destruction of the joints that progresses through a variety of disease stages. Osteoarthritis has a variety of causes and disease progressions, so treatment of knee osteoarthritis should not be insisted on in one way. Instead, the treatment of knee osteoarthritis requires personalized and strategic approaches for each patient. Therefore, this book aims to provide integrated knowledge of knee osteoarthritis to various healthcare providers with the knowledge base they need to provide a personalized and strategic treatment solution.

This book is divided into three main parts. The first part describes basic knowledge with respect to the anatomy and biomechanics of the knee joint and the histology and biochemical composition of the articular cartilage to develop an understanding of the structure and role of the knee joint. The second section describes the etiologies, pathogenesis, and diagnosis of osteoarthritis. Globally, due to an overall increase in socioeconomic status, an increasing number of individuals are participating in athletics. Accordingly, many patients are curious about the relationship that exists between sports activities and knee osteoarthritis. This section, specifically Chap. 4, will delve into these relationships. It clearly describes the relationship between sports and osteoarthritis. The third section describes the treatment of osteoarthritis, including nonpharmacologic, pharmacologic, and surgical treatment. Nonpharmacologic treatment is known for its cost-effectiveness. However, although numerous nonpharmacological treatments have been introduced, the efficacy of these treatments is controversial. One chapter in particular, Chap. 8, introduces various nonpharmacologic treatments used to treat knee osteoarthritis and describes the efficacy of each treatment. Chapter 11 deals with injection therapy for symptomatic knee osteoarthritis. As it is widely used, the chapter details the pharmacokinetics and intra-articular injection techniques most commonly used and describes the efficacy of intra-articular injections currently in use. Furthermore, it also explains the various types and corresponding effectiveness of intra-articular injection treatments with biologic agents that have recently seen increased use. This is to help readers expand their knowledge of the latest treatments. Surgical treatment is a subspecialty in orthopedics. This book accordingly describes the surgical treatment of knee osteoarthritis, including common indicators of problems that may exist. The reason for doing so is to provide healthcare workers, other than orthopedic surgeons, with a basic understanding of surgical treatment to help treat patients with knee osteoarthritis. Orthopedic surgeons who want to know more about various surgical techniques should refer to the corresponding textbooks that describe the surgical methods in more detail. Knee osteoarthritis is caused by a variety of etiologies and symptoms vary at different stages of the disease, so treatment also requires a varied approach. Chapter 15 uses a step-wise and algorithmic guideline to describe how the previously described treatments for knee osteoarthritis are applied to clinical practices. They are also intended to provide guidelines on how to provide more personalized medical treatment to patients by identifying patients with knee osteoarthritis as clinical phenotype and providing appropriate treatment.

Finally, I truly hope this textbook will be an invaluable resource that helps those suffering from knee osteoarthritis improve, in some way, the quality of their lives.

Standing on the Shoulders of Giants

It was not just myself and my fellow contributors that led to the publishing of this book. As with all developments, the achievements, instructions, and support of a great many people were all a part of this text. These individuals include the outstanding doctors, researchers, and teachers from the past without whom academic progress would not exist. Specifically, I would like to express my gratitude to everyone who helped me with the creation of this textbook. In 1987, at the end of my mandatory military service, I had to choose a residency course as a military officer. I would like to thank Professor Kyung-Taek Kim as well as President and Dr. Jong-Ho Park for helping me choose the orthopedic residency program at that time as I was fortunate to be accepted for residency at Inje University's Busan Paik Hospital. I would also like to thank the outstanding clinicians and teachers who have taught me through the years: Drs. Young-Goo Lee, Jang-Seok Choi, Jae-Gong Park, Jung-Hwan Son, and Young-Chang Kim. In particular, I would like to thank Professor and Dr. Jang-Seok Choi for instructing me with regard to the basic knowledge I required as an orthopedic surgeon. His valuable lessons included how to conduct physical examinations, how to diagnose, and how to treat my patients. After my orthopedic residency, I had a particular interest in knee surgery. Dr. Jang-Seok Choi kindly introduced me to two outstanding knee surgeon, Drs. Jin-Hwan Ahn and Dae-Kyung Bae. As a visiting fellow at Kyung-Hee medical center, I was privileged to work with them. In my time there, Professor and Dr. Jin-Hwan Ahn left me with invaluable knowledge regarding knee sports medicine and arthroscopic surgery. Professor and Dr. Dae-Kyung Bae also greatly influenced me and left me with a deep understanding of knee reconstructive surgery, including HTO and arthroplasty. Both Dr. Jin-Hwan Ahn and Dae-Kyung Bae also left me with a deeper understanding with regard to physicians who do their best at all times with their patients. These lessons included the importance of a thorough preoperative preparation and finding a passion for perfection in surgery. I am still trying to follow these teachings, and I am grateful to them for teaching me to the best of their respective abilities at that time. While serving as a member of the Korean Knee Society, I also met several excellent doctors. Among them, I consider myself very lucky to have met Professor and Dr. Sung-Il Bin. He became a mentor to me academically and personally and helped me extensively over the years. I am also grateful to Drs. Hyun-Oh Jo, Jung-Tak Suh, Kyung-Taek Kim, Sung-Do Jo, and Jong-Hu Park. They helped and stimulated me to achieve academic progress as a member of the regional Knee Society. Especially, I would like to thank Professor and Dr. Jung-Tak Suh for giving me a lot of guidance in my experiences with the Korean Knee Society. Additionally, I am especially grateful to President and Dr. Hung-Tae Jung. He provided with a stable and supportive environment that has allowed me to complete this text.

Finally, I would like to thank all the contributors to this book, the illustrator, and the publishers including Saanthi Shankharaman for their participation.

Busan, South Korea — Seung-Suk Seo, MD, PhD

Contents

1 Anatomy and Biomechanics 1
Seung-Suk Seo, Gi-Hun Lee, and Kyung-Jae Seo

2 Structure, Function, and Healing Response of Articular Cartilage and Meniscus 35
Seung-Suk Seo, In-Seung Lee, and Young-Chae Seo

3 Etiology and Risk Factors 55
Ok Gul Kim and Seung-Suk Seo

4 Knee Osteoarthritis and Sports 63
Chang-Rack Lee

5 Epidemiology and Pathogenesis 79
Young Choi

6 Radiographic Findings of the Knee Osteoarthritis 91
Sun Joo Lee

7 Diagnosis and Differential Diagnosis 111
Sang-Min Lee

8 Non-Pharmacologic Management 123
Soung-Kyun Hong and Seung-Suk Seo

9 Pharmacologic Treatment 143
Ki-Bong Park

10 Intra-articular Injection Therapy and Biologic Treatment 171
Seung-Suk Seo, In-Seung Lee, and Gi-Hun Lee

11 Arthroscopic Treatment 213
Lih Wang and HyunHo Kim

12 Osteotomy Around Knee 225
Sang Won Moon and Young-Kyoung Min

13 Unicompartmental Knee Arthroplasty 251
SeungJoon Rhee

14 Total Knee Arthroplasty 273
Chang-Wan Kim, Chang-Rack Lee, Young-Chae Seo, and Seung-Suk Seo

15 How to Make a Strategy for Knee Arthritis Treatment 365
Seung-Suk Seo and Sang-Myung Roh

Index 393

1 Anatomy and Biomechanics

Seung-Suk Seo, Gi-Hun Lee, and Kyung-Jae Seo

Abstract

The bony structures of knee joint are composed of femur, tibia, fibula, and patella. The bony structures are connected with surrounding soft tissues, such as ligaments, tendons, and capsular structures. The quadriceps and patella tendon are located in the anterior aspect of the knee joint. In the posteromedial aspect of the knee the medial hamstring tendons are observed. The iliotibial tract and biceps femoris are placed in the posterolateral aspect of the knee joint. The medial collateral ligament is a flat band-like structure attached to the medial epicondyle of the knee and to the medial metaphysis of the proximal tibia. The lateral collateral ligament is a cord like structure connecting the lateral femoral epicondyle to the fibula head. The menisci are a crescent shaped fibrocartilaginous structures placed between the distal femur and the tibial plateau. The cruciate ligaments are intraarticular, extrasynovial structures connecting the femur and the tibia. The knee joint is supplied blood from branches of the femoral and the popliteal artery. The nerve distribution to the knee joint is made by the branches of the femoral nerve, tibial nerve, common peroneal nerve, and obturator nerve. The knee joint is a modified hinge joint and can be moved in 6 directions, but the main movement is a flexion-extension. A combination of rolling and gliding movement of the femur against the tibial articular surface enables a maximum flexion of the knee joint. The tibia is externally rotated about 15 degrees during full extension of the knee joint. This rotational motion is called a screw-home movement. In the patellofemoral joint movement, the patella contacts the trochlea in a 30 degrees flexion, and the contact surface moves proximal as the flexion progresses.

Keywords

Femur · Tibia · Patella · Medial collateral ligament · Lateral collateral ligament Rolling and gliding movement · Screw-home movement

1.1 Anatomy of the Knee

1.1.1 Bony Structure

1.1.1.1 Distal Femur

The distal femur consists of medial and lateral femoral condyle, trochlear groove, and intercondylar notch. The femoral condyle is divided into

S.-S. Seo (✉) · G.-H. Lee
Department of Orthopedics, Haeundae Bumin Hospital, Busan, South Korea
e-mail: seoss@bumin.co.kr

K.-J. Seo
Inje University Busan Paik Hospital, Busan, South Korea

S.-S. Seo (ed.), *A Strategic Approach to Knee Arthritis Treatment*,
https://doi.org/10.1007/978-981-16-4217-3_1

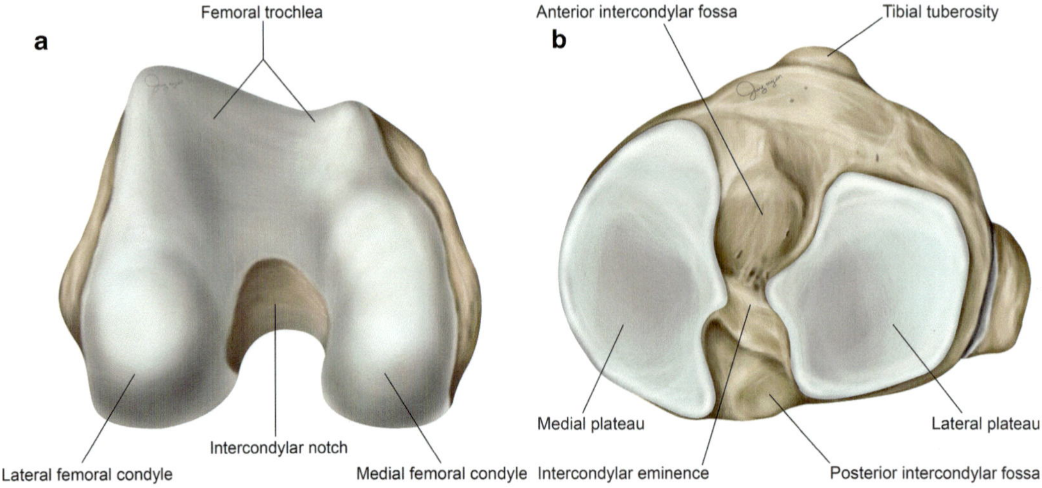

Fig. 1.1 (**a**) Axial view of distal femur. The length of the articular surface of the medial condyle is longer and the width of the articular surface of the lateral condyle is wider at the level of the intercondylar notch (**b**) Axial view of tibial plateau. The articular surface of the medial side is flat or concave, and that of the lateral side is convex. The anterior intercondylar fossa is located in front of the intercondylar eminences

medial and lateral condyle by a trochlear groove anteriorly and an intercondylar notch posteriorly (Fig. 1.1a). The shape and size of medial and lateral femoral condyle are different. The medial condyle has a longer and symmetrical curve in anteroposterior axis. The lateral condyle is the more prominent distally and is the broader both in its anteroposterior and transverse axis (Fig. 1.1b, c). The length of the articular surface of the medial condyle is longer. The width of the articular surface of the lateral condyle is wider at the level of the intercondylar notch. The long axis of the lateral condyle is almost identical to the sagittal plane of the body, and the long axis of the medial condyle is about 22 degrees inclined to the sagittal plane. Therefore, the shape of distal femur is trapezoidal from the axial view. The posterior part of the femoral condyle is divided by intercondylar notch. The width of the intercondylar notch is a narrow distally and widens proximally. On the other hand, the height of the intercondylar notch is the highest in the middle and lower in the proximal to distal part. The anterior cruciate ligament and the posterior cruciate ligament are attached to the intercondylar notch. There are the medial epicondyle and the lateral epicondyle on the inner and outer sides of the femoral condyle, respectively, attached by the medial collateral ligament and the lateral collateral ligament. The medial epicondyle is a large convex eminence and the lateral epicondyle, smaller and more prominent than the medial. The medial epicondyle consists of a C-shaped ridge and a sulcus at the center, and the medial collateral ligature is attached to the sulcus. There is a groove on the distal surface of the lateral epicondyle, with a popliteus muscle attached to the front, which is located directly at the proximal part of the lateral articular cartilage (Fig. 1.2).

1.1.1.2 Proximal Tibia

The articular surface of the tibial plateau has a varus slope of about 3–5 degrees to the coronal plane and a posterior slope of about 7–10 degrees to the long axis of the tibia to the sagittal plane. The articular surface of the tibial plateau is divided into the medial and lateral plateau by intercondylar eminence. The medial tibial plateau is larger than the lateral tibial plateau. The articular surface of the medial side is flat or concave, and that of the lateral side is convex (Fig. 1.1b). There is the anterior intercondylar fossa located in front of the intercondylar eminences. The anterior horn of the medial meniscus, the anterior cruciate ligament (ACL), the anterior horn of lateral meniscus, the posterior

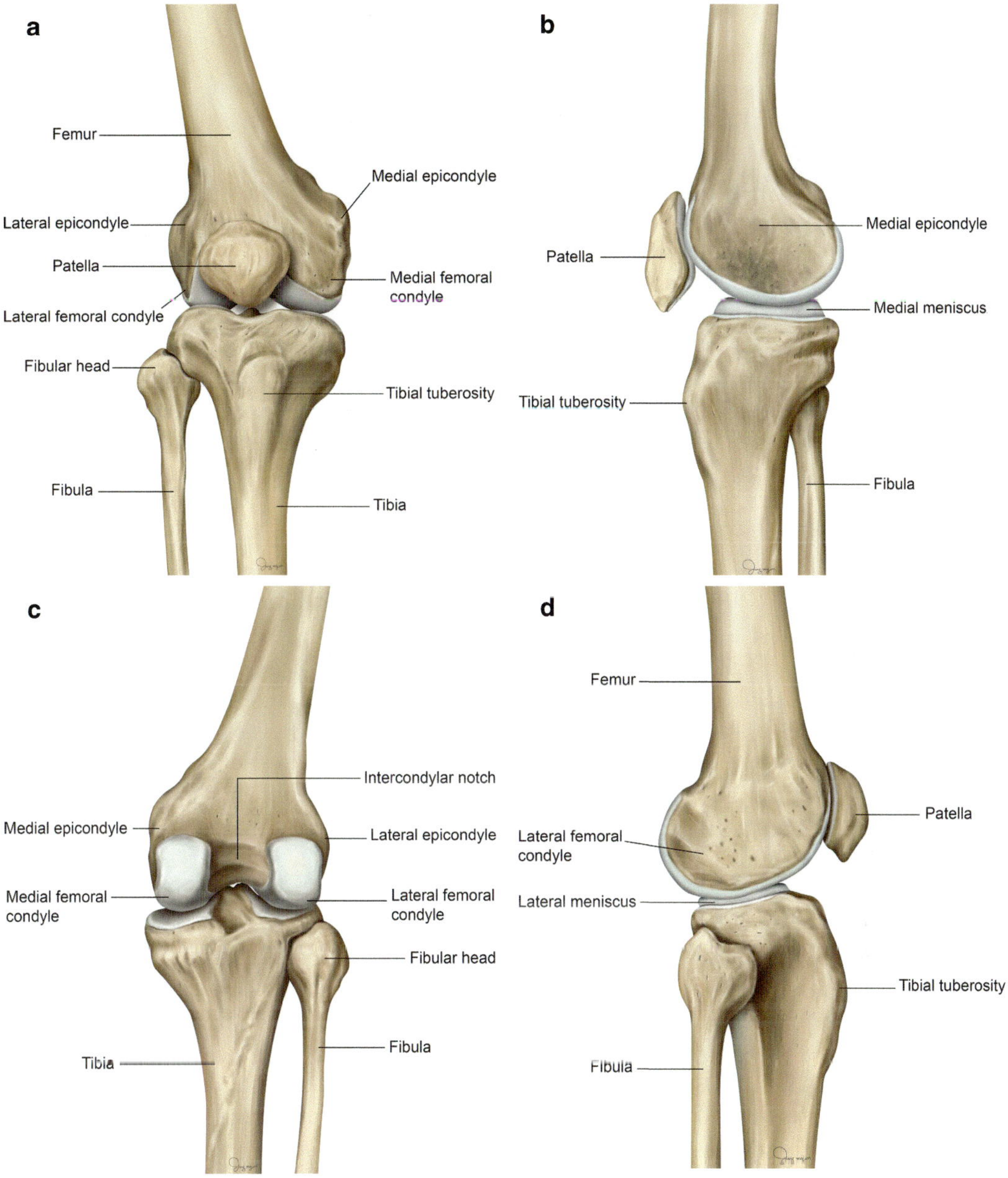

Fig. 1.2 Bony structures of the knee joint (right side). (**a**) Anterior aspect, (**b**) medial aspect, (**c**) posterior aspect, (**d**) lateral aspect

horn of lateral meniscus, the posterior horn of medial meniscus, and the posterior cruciate ligament (PCL) are located in order from anterior to posterior in the median portion of the tibial plateau. There is the intercondylar eminence consisting of the medial tibial spine and the lateral tibial spine behind the attachment of the anterior horn of the lateral meniscus. The medial tibia spine is more prominent upwards and is located more forward than the lateral spine. As an extraarticular anatomical bony structure, there is the tibial tuberosity attached by the patella tendon on the anterior part of the proximal tibia, and there is Gerdy's tubercle attached by the iliotibial band about 2–3 cm laterally from the tibial tuberosity.

1.1.1.3 Fibula

The fibula head articulates with the proximal tibia and forms the proximal tibiofibula joint. Anatomical structures that are important for the stability of the lateral and posterolateral side of the knee joint attach to the fibula head (Fig. 1.2). The popliteofibular ligament (PFL) inserts to the apex of the fibula styloid. The fabellofibular ligament inserts on the posterolateral edge of the fibula styloid just distal and lateral surface of the PFL insertion. The lateral collateral ligament (LCL) inserts proximally about 28 mm distal to the fibula styloid and about 8 mm from the anterior cortex of the fibula head. Tendon of the biceps femoris inserts to the anterior and lateral aspect of the fibula head between PFL and LCL insertion (Fig. 1.10).

1.1.1.4 Patella

The patella is the largest sesamoid bone in the body, which articulated with the distal femur. The patella protects the anterior surface of the knee joint, and increases the lever arm of the extensor mechanism to facilitate the knee joint extension. The articular surface of the patella is elliptical and is divided into the lateral and medial facet by the vertical median bridge in the center. The lateral facet is wider and longer than the medial facet, accounting for about two-thirds of the total articular surface of the patella, and the cartilage in the lateral facet is thicker than the medial facet. The cartilage in the medial facet is slightly convex or flat, while the cartilage in the lateral facet forms a concave shape. There are two transverse ridges, where the articular surface of each facet is divided into three parts: proximal, middle, and distal. There is another small longitudinal ridge near the medial border of the patella which separates the medial facet from a thin strip of articular surface known as the odd facet. The odd facet contacts the femoral condyle only when the knee joint is deeply bent. Including this, there are seven facets in the articular surface of the patella (Fig. 1.3a, b, c).

1.1.2 Anterior Aspect

1.1.2.1 Surface Anatomy

Most prominent structure in the anterior aspect of the knee is the patella that lies in the center of the joint and the whole margin of the patella can be easily palpated. The tendon of the quadriceps femoris can be observed on the superior margin of the patella. The vastus medialis is located on the medial side of the quadriceps tendon, its muscular portion is observed on the more distal part of the quadriceps tendon and inserts to the superomedial border of the patella. The vastus lateralis is placed on the lateral side of the quadriceps tendon and its muscular portion is observed on more proximal aspect and forms a tendinous portion about 3 cm above the patella and inserts to the superolateral margin of the patella. The second prominent bony structure in the anterior aspect is the tibial tuberosity that is located between the medial and lateral condyle of the proximal tibia. The patella tendon runs distally from the distal border of the patella to the tibial tuberosity, and it is easily visible and palpable (Fig. 1.4a).

1.1.2.2 Quadriceps

The quadriceps composed of the rectus femoris, the vastus lateralis, the vastus medialis, and the vastus intermedius, and converge distally to form a quadriceps tendon that passes through the anterior surface of the patella and turn into a patella tendon. The rectus femoris forms a superficial layer, the vastus medialis and lateralis form a middle layer, and the vastus intermedius forms a deep layer. The rectus femoris and vastus intermedius insert almost vertically to the superior pole of the patella. On the other hand, the vastus medialis and lateralis attach obliquely to the patella at 55 degrees (28–70 degrees) and 14 degrees (6–45 degrees) on average, respectively [1–3] (Fig. 1.4b, c).

Rectus Femoris The rectus femoris has a fusiform shape, accounting for about 15% of the quadriceps cross-section. The muscular portion of the rectus

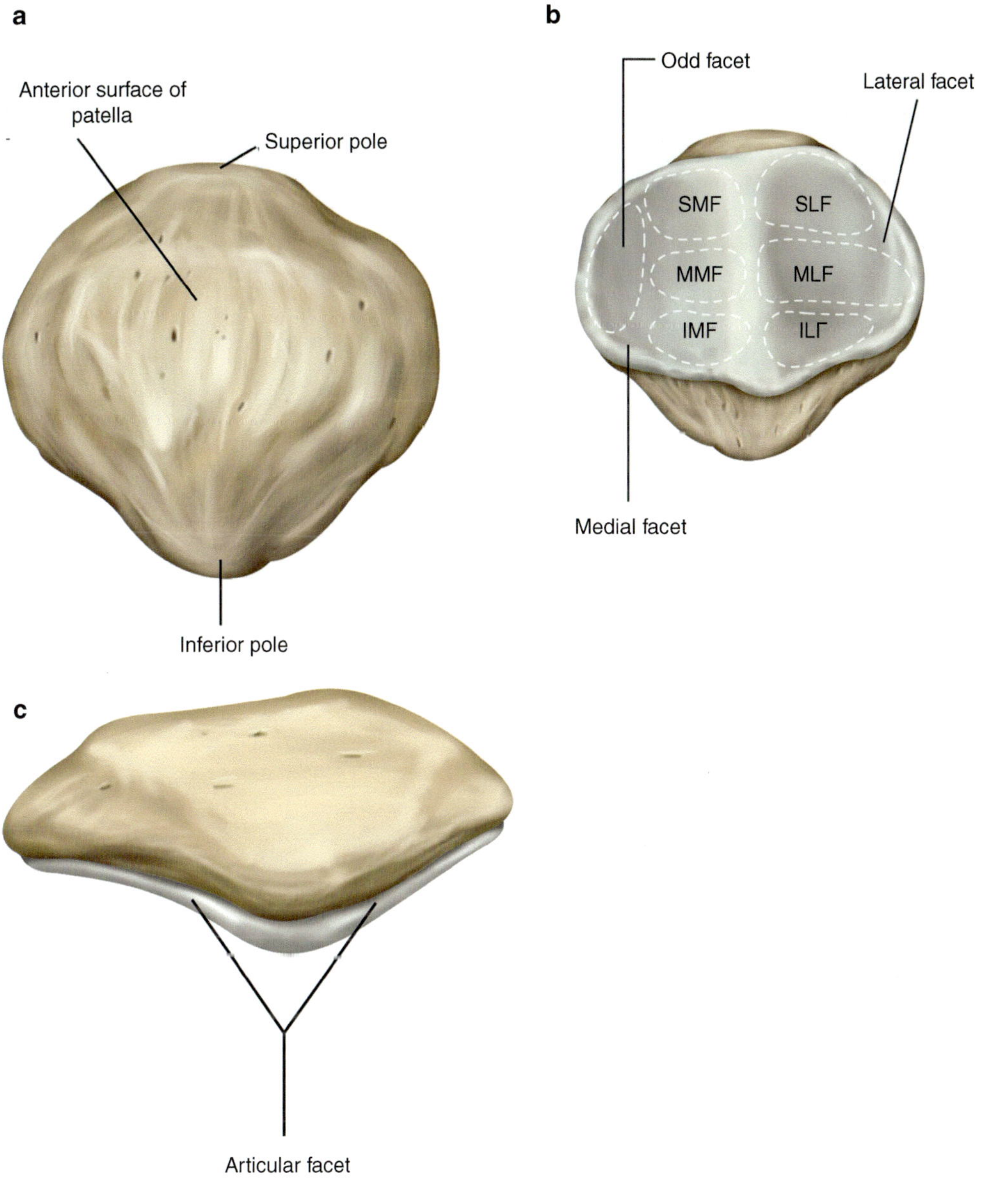

Fig. 1.3 Patella. (**a**) Anterior surface, (**b**) the articular surface is divided into the lateral and medial facet by the vertical median bridge in the center and divided into three parts such as proximal, middle, and distal facet by two transverse ridges, (**c**) axial view

femoris is changed to a narrow tendinous structure at 5–8 cm proximal part of the superior pole of the patella, and gradually widens in the distal part. Located at the superficial and middle of a quadriceps mechanism in cross-section, some fibers insert to the superior pole of the patella and most fibers passing through the anterior surface of the patella proceed distally and become the patella tendon.

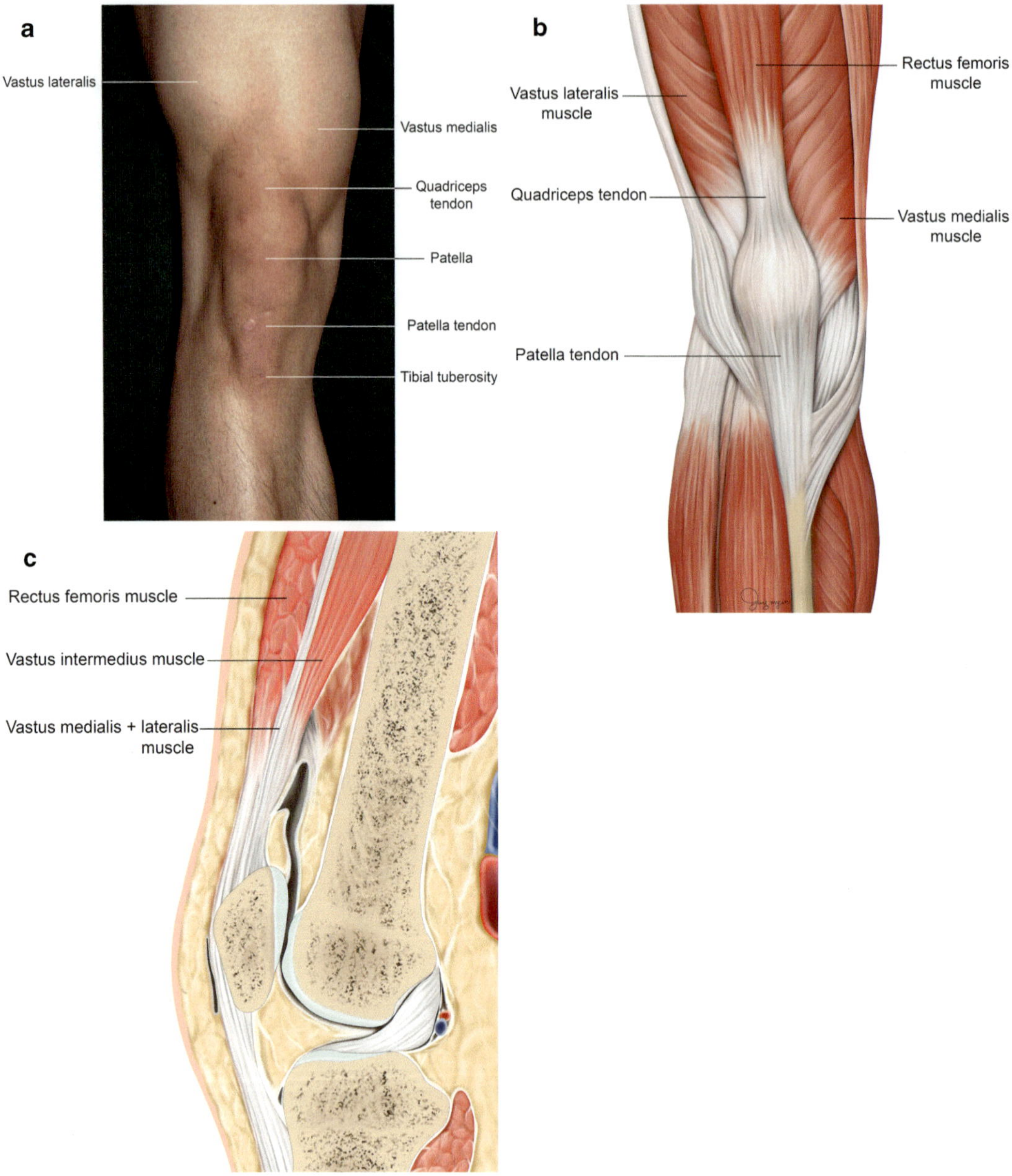

Fig. 1.4 Anterior aspect of the knee joint. (**a**) Surface anatomy, (**b**) the quadriceps muscle composed of the rectus femoris, the vastus lateralis, the vastus medialis, and the vastus intermedius. The patella tendon connects the patella and the tibial tuberosity, (**c**) lateral view. Most fibers of the rectus femoris passing through the anterior surface of the patella proceed distally and become the patella tendon

Vastus Medialis The vastus medialis is divided into two types depending on the direction of muscle fibers attached to the patella. The muscle fiber that runs parallel to the rectus femoris in the proximal region is called vastus medialis longus (VML), and originates from the femur and inserts perpendicularly to the superomedial area of the patella. The muscle fiber in the distal region of the vastus medialis that runs obliquely in relation to the rectus femoris is called the vastus medialis obliqus (VMO). The VMO is originated from the adductor longus tendon proximal to the adductor tubercle and the medial intermuscular septum and inserted in an oblique direction of about 55–70 degrees to the upper 1/2 and superomedial part of the patella. Unlike rectus femoris, VMO muscle fibers change to tendinous fibers in close proximity to the patella. The VMO has a fibrous extension in the distal region, which is continuous with the medial retinaculum [4].

Vastus Lateralis The vastus lateralis is divided into a longus and obliquus muscle fibers. The fibers of the vastus lateralis run more parallel to the rectus femoris than the vastus medialis. Muscle fibers convert to tendinous fibers at 3 cm above the patella and attached to the superolateral pole of the patella, and distally connected and contributed to the lateral retinaculum [5].

Vastus Intermedius The vastus intermedius is located in the deepest of the quadriceps and inserts into the superior pole of the patella. The fibers of the vastus intermedius blend with fibers in the vastus medialis and lateralis.

1.1.2.3 Patella Tendon

The patella tendon is a strong, flat ligament with about 35–55 mm length, which runs from the inferior pole of the patella to the tibial tuberosity. The patella tendon composed mainly of the fibers of rectus femoris.

1.1.3 Medial Aspect

1.1.3.1 Surface Anatomy

The pes anserinus tendon that composed of the sartorius, gracilis, and semitendinosus can be palpated on the medial aspect of the tibia, medial, and posterior location from the tibial tuberosity. The most superficial structure is the sartorius muscle that is hardly palpable. However, deep to the sartorius muscle, the cordlike tendons of the gracilis and semitendinosus muscles can be easily palpated. The medial femoral and tibial condyles can be palpated easily with the knee in 90 degrees of flexion. The medial collateral ligament (MCL) runs distally from the medial epicondyle of the femur to the medial tibial condyle, and is hardly seen or palpated because it is a flat structure except the very thin body (Fig. 1.5a).

1.1.3.2 Medial Layers

The medial structure of the knee joint can be divided into three layers. The three layers can be best distinguished in the area of the superficial medial collateral ligaments (SMCL), one of the structures forming the layer 2. Layer 1 composed of the deep fascia including sartorial fascia. Between 1 and 2 layers, there are the gracilis tendon and the semitendinosus tendon. Layer 2 includes the SMCL, the medial patellofemoral ligament (MPFL), and medial retinaculum. Layer 3 consists of the deep medial collateral ligament (DMCL) and the knee joint capsule [6] (Fig. 1.5b).

Layer 1 Layer 1 is the first visible deep fascia when skin incision is made on the medial side of the knee joint, which extends proximally to cover the quadriceps, posteriorly to overly the two heads of the gastrocnemius and the popliteal fossa, and distally to invest the sartorius muscle and sartorial fascia.

Layer 2 Most prominent structure in the layer 2 is the SMCL. From about 1 cm anteriorly of SMCL, it is difficult to distinguish between the layer 1 and 2. Although it is known to be attached to the depression of the medial epicondyle (ME) approximately 4.8 mm posterior and 3.2 mm proximal to the ME, it is difficult to identify the exact insertion site because it has a broad attachment site. The tibial attachment of SMCL has two insertion sites [7]. Proximal insertion is located to near the medial tibial articular margin. Distal insertion is located onto the medial tibial metaphysis an average 61.2 mm from the medial joint line underlying the pes anserinus. The SMCL has two kinds of fiber direction which are vertical fibers in the anterior portion and the oblique fibers in the posterior part (Fig. 1.6c). The pes anserinus is the conjoined tendon of the sartorius, gracilis, and semitendinosus that attach to the proximal medial metaphysis of the tibia

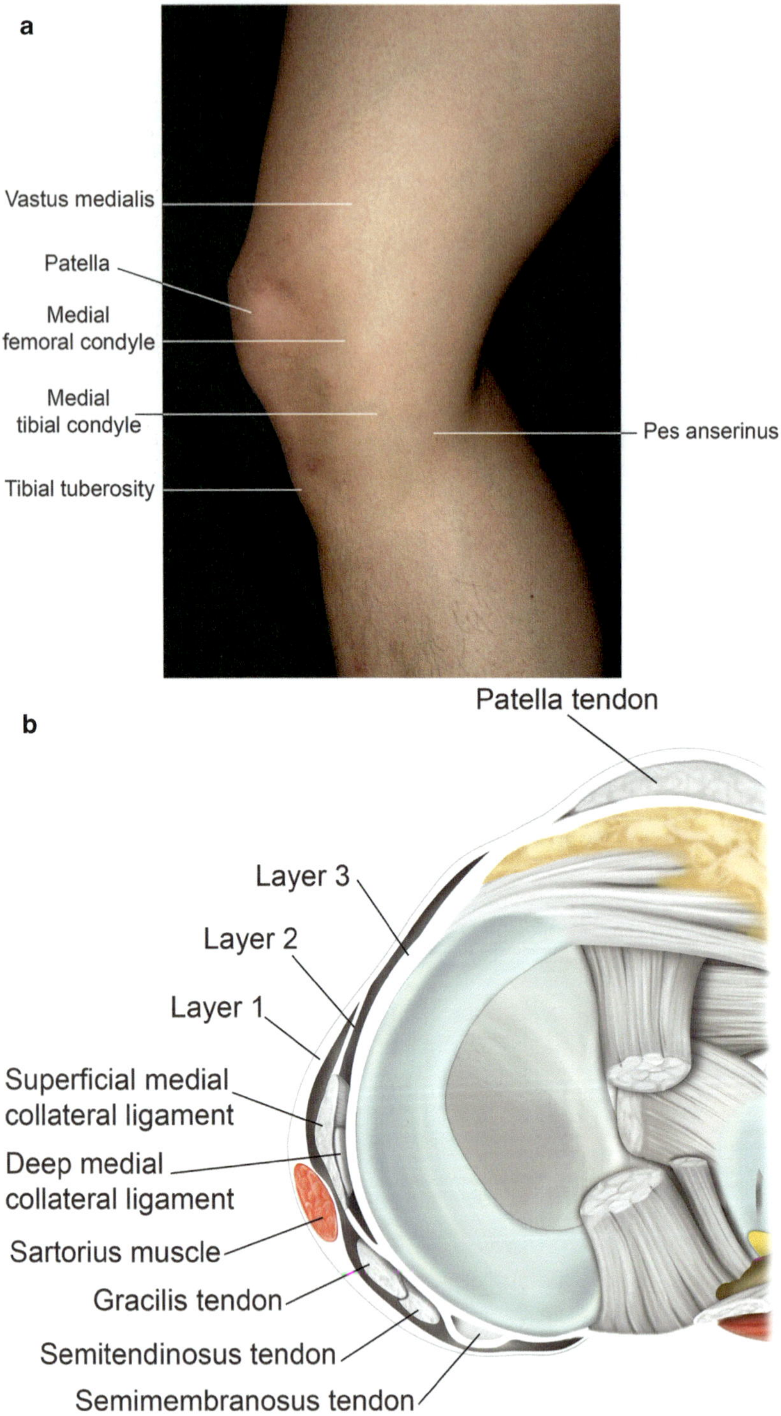

Fig. 1.5 Medial aspect of the knee joint. (**a**) Surface anatomy, (**b**) medial layers. The medial structure of the knee joint can be divided into three layers that can be best distinguished in the area of the superficial medial collateral ligaments (SMCL)

[8]. The gracilis originates by the inferior pubic ramus and runs distally along the medial side of the thigh. At 1/3 of the distal thigh, the muscle fiber of the gracilis attaches to the medial tendon of the semitendinosus (Fig. 1.6a). The medial patellofemoral ligament (MPFL) is the flat, pan-shaped structure that primarily resists the lateral displacement of the patella between 0 and 30

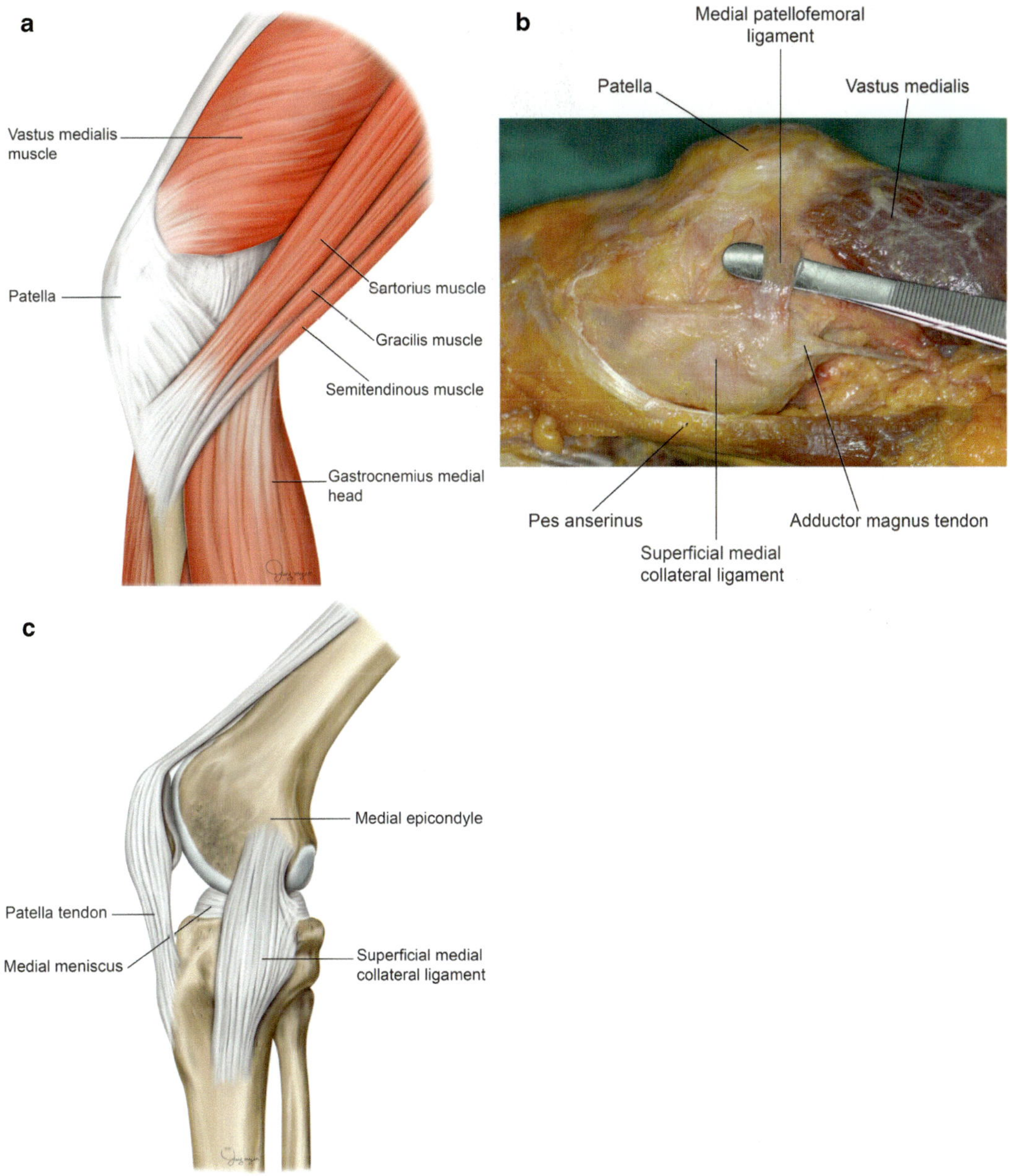

Fig. 1.6 Layer 2 of medial structures. (**a**) The pes anserinus is the conjoined tendon of the sartorius, gracilis, and semitendinosus, (**b**) the medial patellofemoral ligament (MPFL) is a flat, pan-shaped structures connecting the patella and the medial condyle of the distal femur, (**c**) the superficial medial collateral ligament (SMCL) is a flat band-like structure attached to the medial epicondyle of the femur and to the medial metaphysis of the proximal tibia

degrees of the knee joint motion and is classified as layer 2. The average length is about 56 mm and is an hourglass shaped with a wider patella attachment than the middle part. The femoral side is attached to the triangular area formed by the adductor tubercle, medial epicondyle, and gastrocnemius tubercle, and the patella side is attached to the proximal two third of the medial margin of the patella [9] (Fig. 1.6b). It is also attached to the VMO and the vastus intermedius. The posterior oblique ligaments (POL) extend from the posterior border of SMCL to the inser-

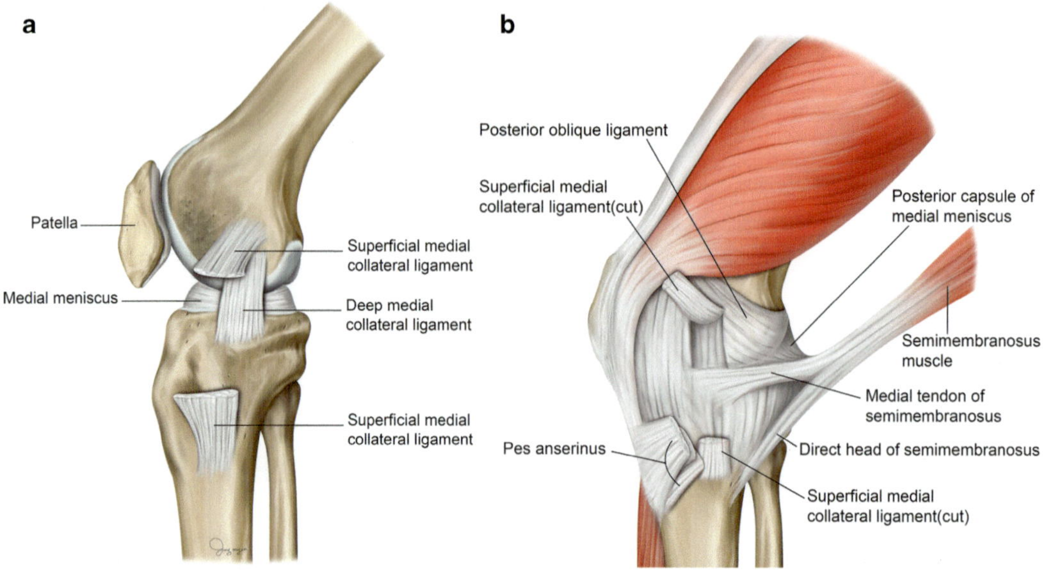

Fig. 1.7 Layer 3 of medial structures. (**a**) The deep medial collateral ligament (DMCL) is a thickened, vertically oriented fibers located in the middle one third of the medial joint capsule, (**b**) the semimembranosus tendon has a complex insertions in the posteromedial corner of the knee joint

tion of the semimembranosus. This is a structure in which layer 2 and layer 3 merge in the posteromedial aspect of the knee joint (Fig. 1.7b). The POL divides into superficial, central, and articular arm, of which the central arm is the largest, the thickest, and forms most of the femoral attachment. The distal portion of the central arm attaches to the posteromedial portion of the medial meniscus, the meniscotibial portion of the joint capsule, and the posteromedial corner of the tibia [10].

Layer 3 The layer 3 consists of the joint capsule. The middle one third of medial joint capsule forms the deep medial collateral ligament (DMCL), which composes of a thickened, vertically oriented fibers under the SMCL. The DMCL spreads from the femur to the midportion of the peripheral margin of the medial meniscus and to the articular margin of the tibia. Anteriorly, the DMCL is clearly distinguished from the SMCL with the interposing bursa, but posteriorly, it is difficult to distinguish because meniscofemoral portion of the DMCL merges with overlying the SMCL (Fig. 1.7a). On the other hand, in the tibia, it becomes a structure called the coronary ligament and can be distinguished from the SMCL [11].

Semimembranosus The semimembranosus tendon inserts to the posteromedial corner of the knee joint as direct and anterior insertion (Fig. 1.7b). Direct insertion attaches to a bony prominence approximately 1 cm below the posteromedial joint line of the tibia. Anterior insertion attaches to the tibial periosteum just distal to the joint capsule under the SMCL. Both insertions do not contribute to any of the 3 layers. The semimembranosus tendon sheath sends to multiple fibrous expansions upward and downward into layer 2. The most distinguishable expansion is the oblique popliteal ligament (OPL) which is a lateral expansion off the tendon sheath and courses laterally and proximally across the posterior capsule to the attachment of the lateral head of gastrocnemius. The capsular expansion attaches it to the posterior horn of the medial meniscus and joint capsule along the superior border of OPL. The distal expansion runs distally and merges into the peritoneum of the medial tibial in the form of fibrous expansion over the popliteus [12, 13].

1.1.4 Lateral Aspect

1.1.4.1 Surface Anatomy

The lateral femoral and tibial condyles can be palpated with the knee in 90 degrees of flexion. The fibular head is located onto distal to the lateral condyle of the tibia and can be easily palpated in the lateral aspect of the knee joint. The lateral collateral ligament (LCL), a cordlike structure that runs from the fibular head to the lateral condyle of the femur, is easily palpable or visible with the 90 degrees knee flexion in varus force. Gerdy's tubercle is observed on the lateral and proximal site to the tibial tuberosity, which is the insert site for the iliotibial tract (Fig. 1.8a).

1.1.4.2 Lateral Layers

The lateral side of the knee joint is composed of three layers (layers 1, 2, 3). The layer 1 consists of the fascia lata, the iliotibial band, and the biceps femoris with an aponeurotic expansion (Fig. 1.8b). The layer 2 contains the quadriceps retinaculum anteriorly and it becomes an incomplete structure including patellofemoral and two patellomeniscal ligaments posteriorly. The layer 3 is composed of joint capsule of which posterior part is divided into the deep and superficial lamina. The deep lamina forms the coronary ligament and the arcuate ligament. The superficial lamina consists of the lateral collateral ligament and the fabellofibular ligament [14] (Fig. 1.8c).

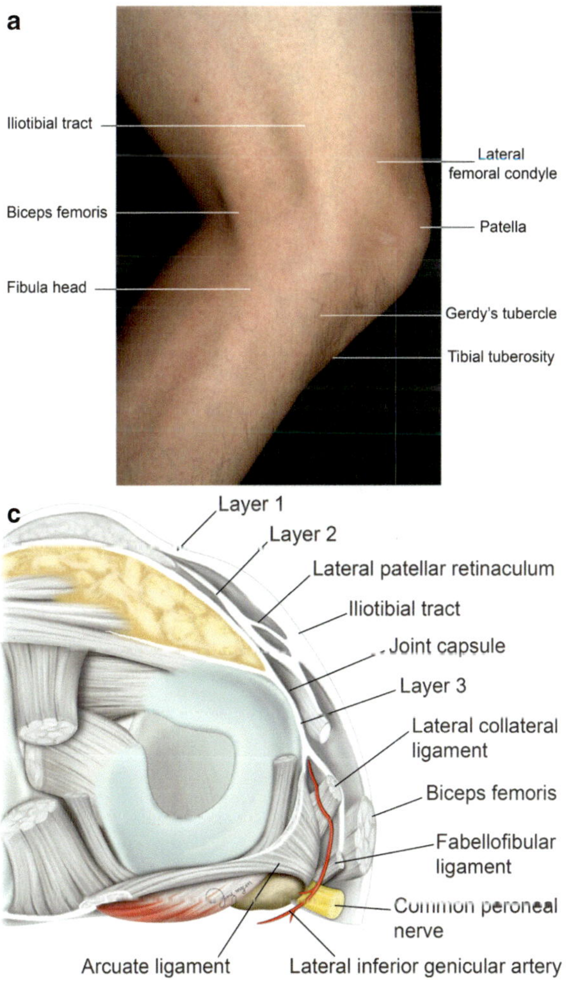

Fig. 1.8 Lateral aspect of the knee joint. (**a**) Surface anatomy, (**b**) layer 1 consists of the fascia lata, the iliotibial band, and the biceps femoris with an aponeurotic expansion, (**c**) lateral layers is less discernable than medial layers

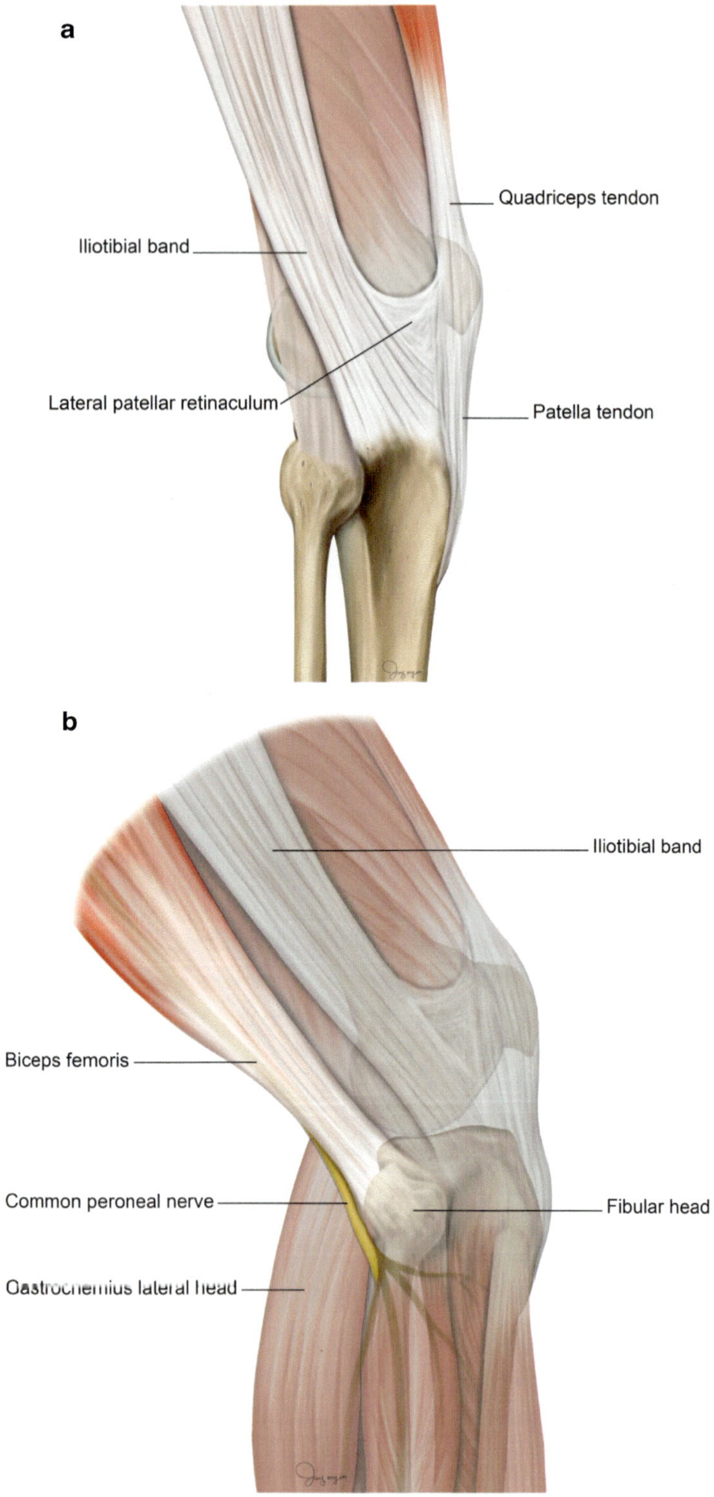

Fig. 1.9 (**a**) The iliotibial band is divided into three separate layers; superficial, deep, and capsulo-osseous layer around the knee joint and has a broad insertional areas, (**b**) the biceps femoris attaches to the posterolateral side of the knee joint in a complex mode. The direct arm attaches to the posterolateral border of the fibula head

Iliotibial Band The iliotibial band (ITB) originates on the anterior-superior iliac spine and runs distally along the lateral aspect of the thigh and around the knee joint, is divided into three separate layers; superficial, deep, and capsulo-osseous layer (Fig. 1.9a). A part of the superficial layer is a structure called the iliopatellar band that extends to the lateral aspect of the patella, and most of superficial layer attaches to Gerdy's tubercle. The iliopatellar band prevents an excessive medial glide of the patella and plays an important role in a patellofemoral tracking. The deep layer extends from the medial part of the superficial layer to the lateral intermuscular septum of the distal femur. The distal part of the deep layer attaches to the posterior surface of the lateral femoral condyle. The capsulo-osseous layer extends to the medial and distal to the deep layer and is mixed with fibers from the short head of the biceps femoris. The capsulo-osseous layer extends more distally, making a sling to the posterior to the lateral femoral condyle and inserts to the posterosuperior aspect of Gerdy's tubercle [15].

Biceps Femoris The biceps femoris is a fusiform muscle consisting of two head: long and short. The two heads of the biceps femoris around the knee joint is located just behind the ITB. The biceps femoris attaches to the posterolateral side of the knee joint in a complex mode (Fig. 1.9b). Among the insertions of the long head of biceps femoris, the direct arm, the anterior arm, and the lateral aponeurotic expansion are a major part. The direct arm attaches to the posterolateral border of the fibula head. The anterior arm inserts onto the lateral fibula head and lateral collateral ligament. The short head of biceps femoris has six distal attachments. Among them, the capsular arm, the direct arm, and the anterior arm are important attachments. The capsular arm inserts onto the posterolateral aspect of the joint capsule, the fabella, and fabellofibula ligament. The direct arm is attached to the fibula head just behind and above of the direct arm of the biceps long head. The anterior arm inserts onto the superolateral tibia 1 cm posterior to Gerdy's tubercle that is the attachment site of the mid third knee joint capsule [16, 17].

Lateral Collateral Ligament The lateral collateral ligament (LCL) is a cord like ligament that extends from the lateral femoral epicondyle to the anterolateral aspect of the fibula head (Fig. 1.10a). Comparing with its surrounding structures, the femoral attachment of the LCL is approximately 14 mm anterior and slightly distal to the origin of the lateral head of the gastrocnemius and is located about 1.4 mm proximal and 3.1 mm posterior to the lateral femoral epicondyle. The femoral insert of the LCL is located at an average of 18.5 mm away from where the popliteus tendon is attached. The LCL courses distally to insert approximately 8 mm posterior to the anterior border of the fibula head and about 28 mm distal to the tip of the fibula styloid process [18].

Popliteus The popliteus muscle inserts onto the posterior aspect of the tibia, the immediate proximal part of the soleal line. The popliteus muscle has three origins; the popliteus tendon from the lateral femoral condyle, the popliteofibula ligament, and the posterior horn of the lateral meniscus (Fig. 1.10b). The popliteus tendon has three attachments to the lateral meniscus, which are the anteroinferior, posterosuperior, and posteroinferior fascicles [19]. The popliteus tendon attaches to approximately 18 mm anterior and distal to the insertion site of the lateral collateral ligament. The popliteofibula ligament originates at the musculotendinous junction of the popliteus muscle and inserts onto the medial border of the fibular head underlying the fabellofibula ligament (Fig. 1.10b). The arcuate ligament is the Y-shaped structure composed of the femoral and fibula origin of the popliteus muscle. It is not a separate ligament but condensation of the fibers of the popliteus (Fig. 1.11a). The inferior lateral genicular artery courses between the fabellofibula ligament and the popliteofibula ligament [20].

Fabellofibular Ligament The fabellofibular ligament originates from the lateral aspect of the fabella and inserts to the posterolateral margin of the fibular styloid process which is the posterolateral site to the PFL insertion (Fig. 1.11b). If there is no fabella, it begins at the posterior aspect of the supracondylar process of the distal femur. The presence of these ligaments has been reported in a variety of ways up to 40–68 percent of the specimens.

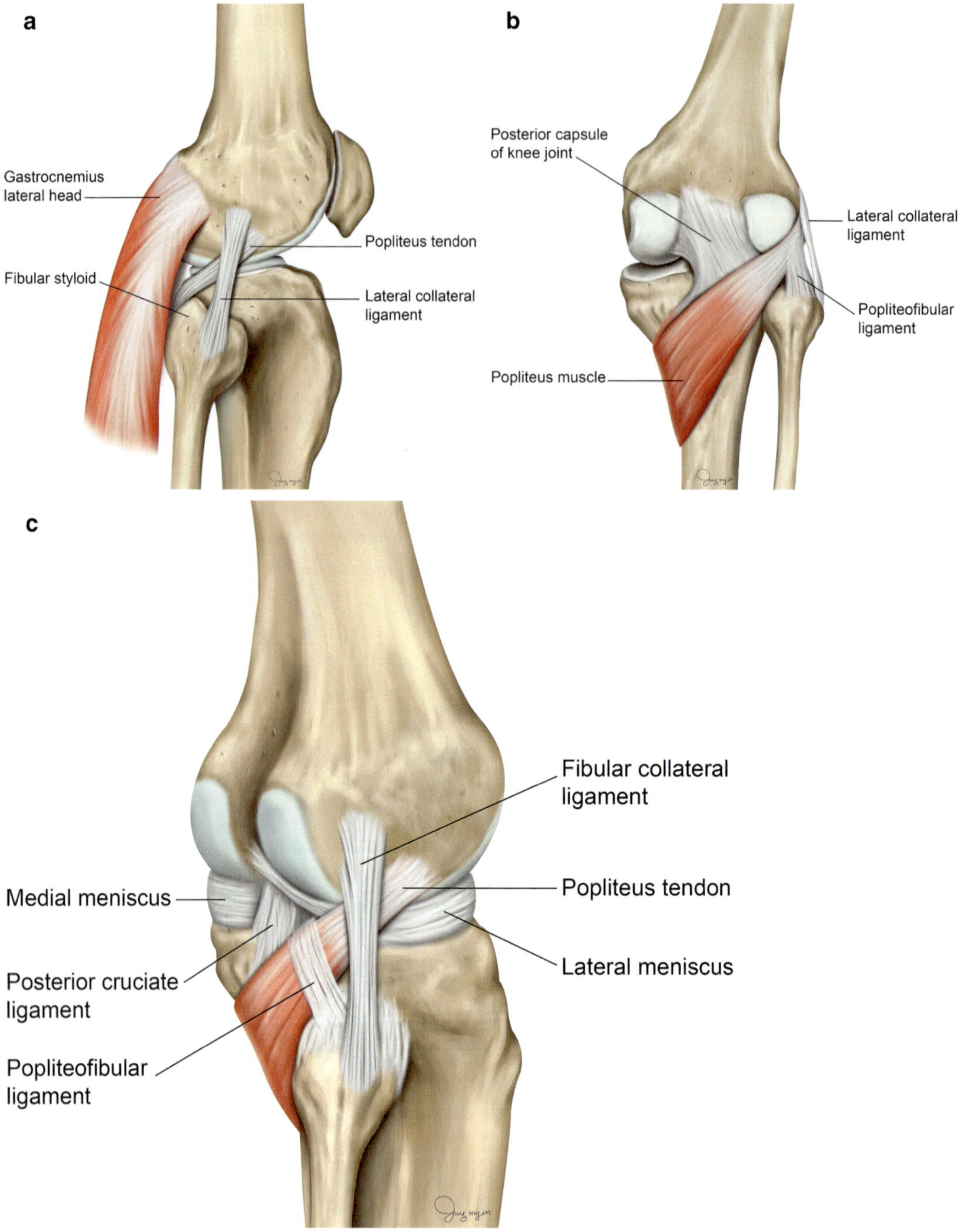

Fig. 1.10 Lateral aspect of the knee joint. (**a**) Lateral collateral ligament, (**b**), (**c**) popliteus muscle and popliteofibular ligament

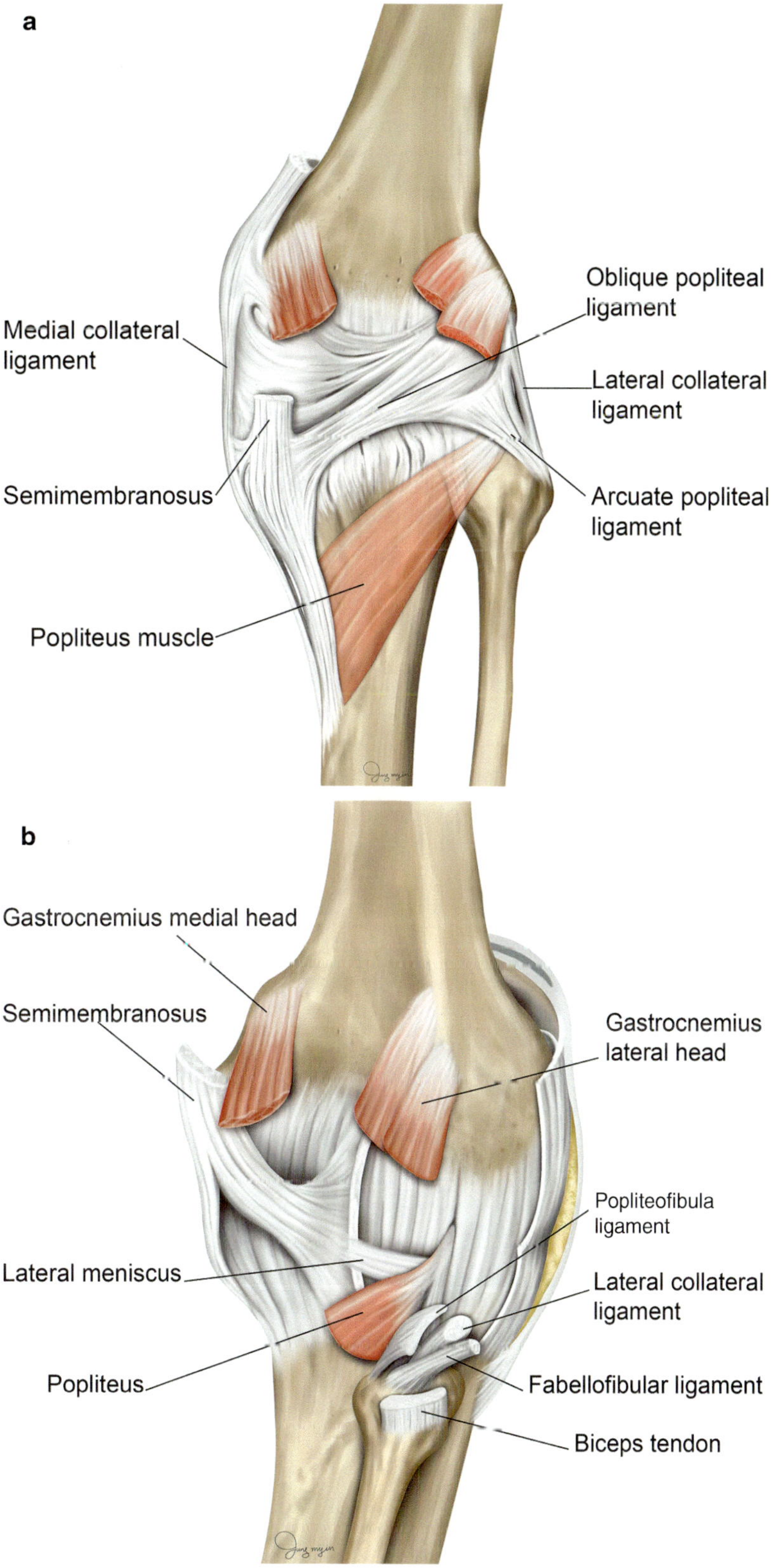

Fig. 1.11 Posterior and posterolateral corner of the knee joint. (**a**) The arcuate ligament is the Y-shaped structure composed of the femoral and fibula origin of the popliteus muscle, (**b**) the fabellofibular ligament and the popliteofibular ligament

1.1.5 Posterior Aspect

The popliteus fossa is the rhomboid shaped space observed on the posterior aspect of the knee joint. In the middle of the popliteal fossa a horizontal line is traversed, that corresponds to the flexion crease of the knee (Fig. 1.12a). The superomedial border composed of the tendons of the semitendinosus superficially and the semimembranosus deeply. The semitendinosus arises from the lower and medial impression on the ischial tuberosity. The semimembranosus arises from the proximal and lateral sides of the ischial tuberosity and runs inward in the deep site comparing to the course of the semitendinosus. The semimembranosus and semitendinosus insert to the medial and posterior condyle of the tibia. The superolateral border corresponds to the tendon of the biceps femoris that is located at the posterior aspect of the iliotibial band. The medial and lateral inferior borders of the popliteal fossa correspond to the medial and lateral head of the gastrocnemius muscle, respectively, which are divergent at their origin but converge distally. The gastrocnemius originates as two heads from the distal femur. The medial head originates from the popliteal surface of the distal femur and the posterior aspect of the medial condyle. The lateral head originates from a facet on the upper lateral surface of the lateral femoral condyle. The two heads are merged to form a common tendon with the soleus. There are several neurovascular structures such as the tibial nerve, the common peroneal nerve, and the popliteal artery in the popliteal fossa. The tibial nerve courses down in the centromedial region of the popliteal fossa and can be palpated as a cordlike structure. The common peroneal nerve runs distally along with the biceps femoris tendon in the superolateral border of the fossa. The popliteal artery is located medial to the tibial nerve and is easily detected by palpation of its pulse [21] (Fig. 1.12b).

1.1.6 Intraarticular Structure

1.1.6.1 Meniscus

The structure and function of the medial and lateral meniscus are described in the Chap. 2.

1.1.6.2 Anterior Cruciate Ligament

The anterior cruciate ligament (ACL) resists the anterior displacement and internal rotation of the tibia. The ACL originates from medial aspect of the lateral femoral condyle and inserts onto the anterior intercondylar fossa between the anterior horn of medial meniscus and lateral meniscus. The length of the ACL is approximately 31–35 mm and the width of the midsubstance is an average of 11 mm (7–13 mm). The width of the femoral and tibial insertion area is wider than the middle portion of the midsubstance. The femoral insertion area is an elliptical shape with an average length of 18 mm (12–20 mm) and a width of 10 mm (5–13 mm) on average. That is located in immediately behind the lateral intercondylar bridge called the resident's ridge and parallel to the anterior margin of the posterior condylar articular surface. The tibial insertional area has a roughly oval to triangular shape with an average length of 18 mm (15–20 mm), the width of 10 mm on average, mainly inserted to the lateral slope of the medial tibial spine [22] (Fig. 1.13a). The tibial insertional area is wider and stronger than the femoral side. Although the ACL is structurally difficult to discriminate into two or three bundles, it is functionally divided into anteromedial and a posterolateral bundle depending on the location of the femoral and tibial attachment. In the femoral attachment, the anteromedial bundle inserts to the posterosuperior area and the posterolateral bundle to the anteroinferior area based on the lateral bifurcate ridge. The anteromedial bundle becomes tense when the knee joint flexes to 90 degrees, and the posterolateral bundle becomes tense when the knee joint extends [23] (Fig. 1.13b). According to a recent anatomical study, the femoral insertion of the ACL has a direct insertion attached to the lateral intercondylar posterior ridge which is an

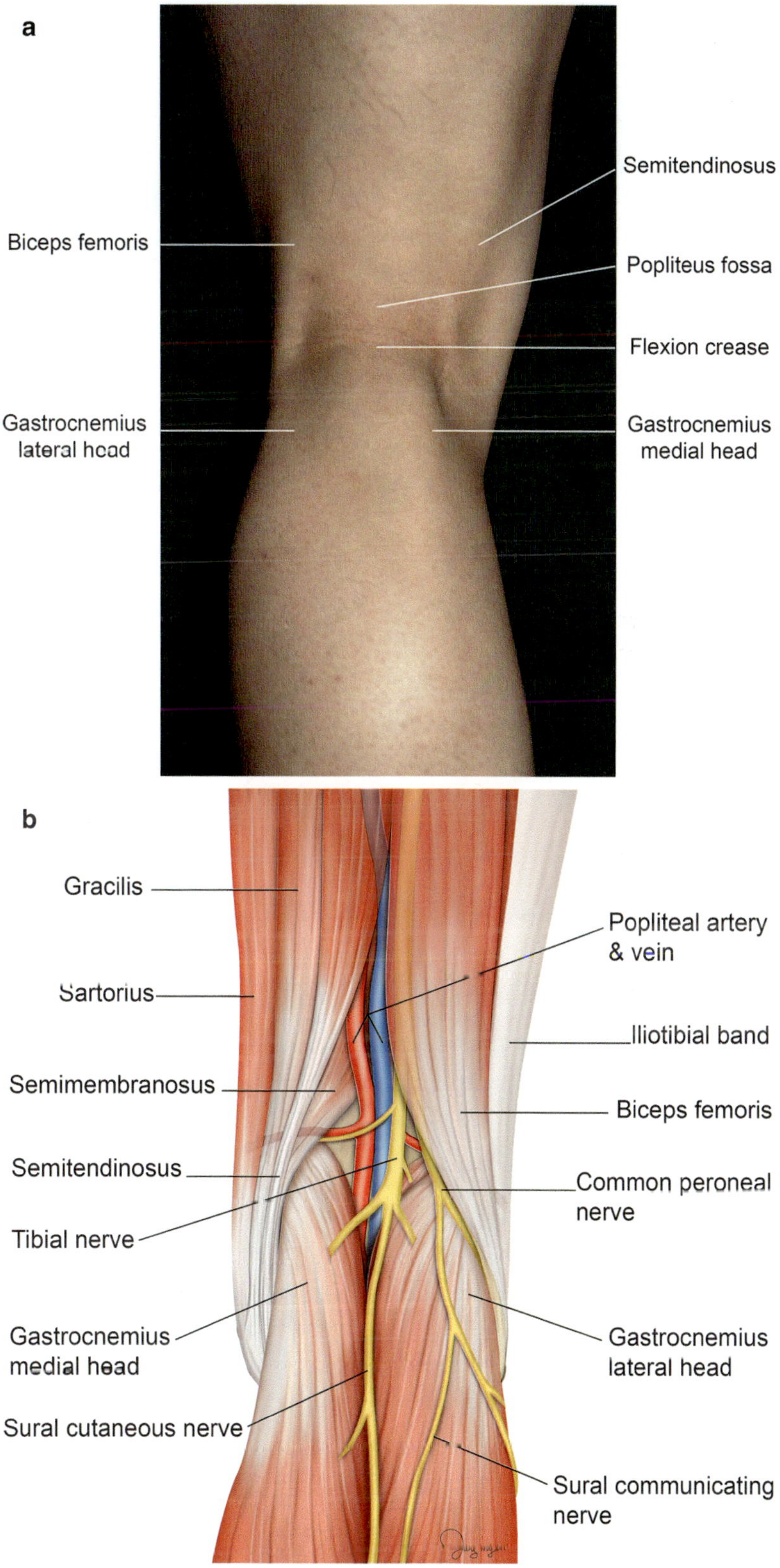

Fig. 1.12 Posterior aspect of the knee joint. (**a**) Surface anatomy. The popliteus fossa is a rhomboid shaped space that bounded with hamstrings and gastrocnemius muscles, (**b**) boundary of the popliteal fossa and its contained neurovascular structures

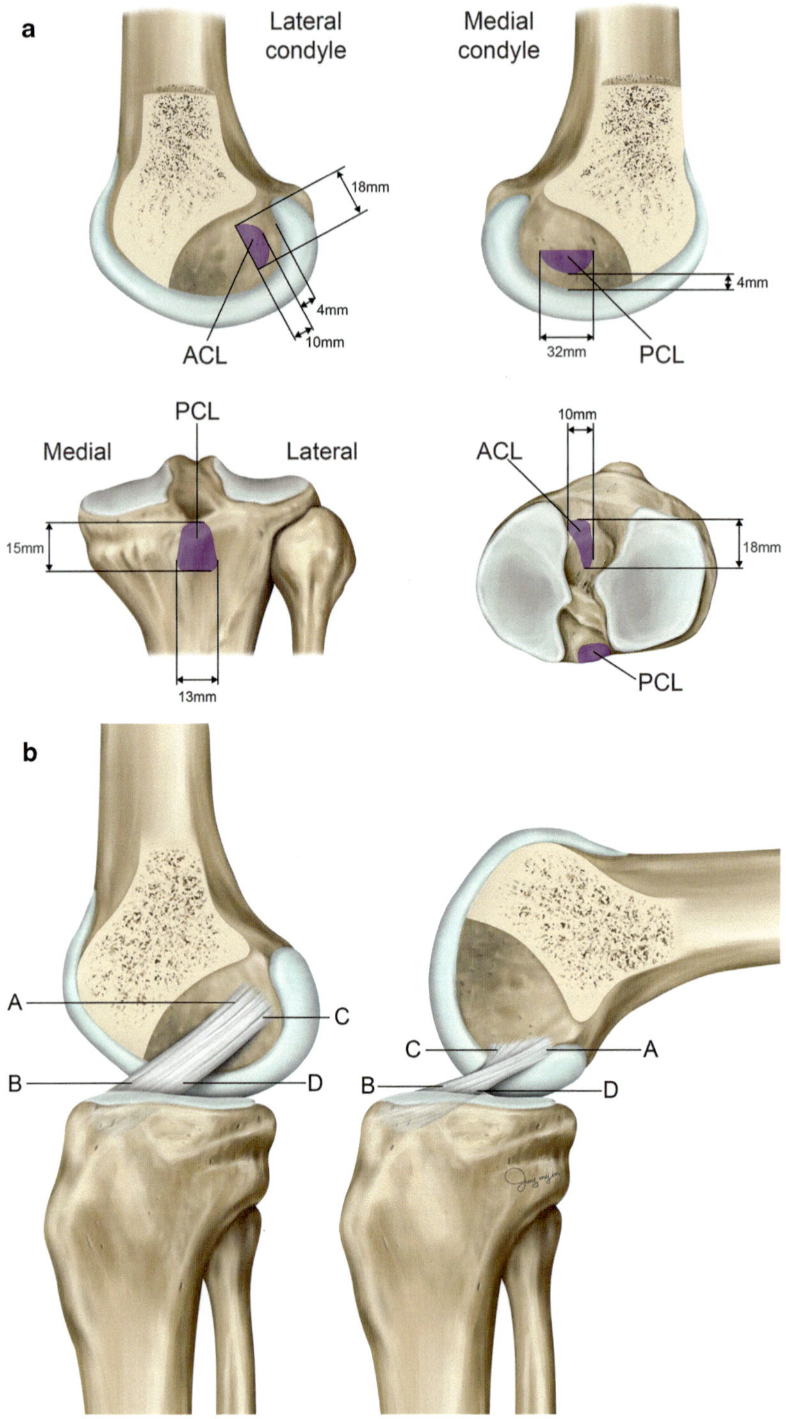

Fig. 1.13 Cruciate ligaments. (**a**) The dimension of bony insertion site of the anterior (ACL) and posterior (PCL) cruciate ligament, (**b**) ACL in extension and flexion. In extension position, posterolateral bundle (C–D) is taut. In flexion position, anteromedial bundle (A–B) becomes tight, (**c**) PCL in extension and flexion. In extension position, anterolateral bundle (C–D) becomes loose. In flexion position, anterolateral bundle (C–D) becomes tight

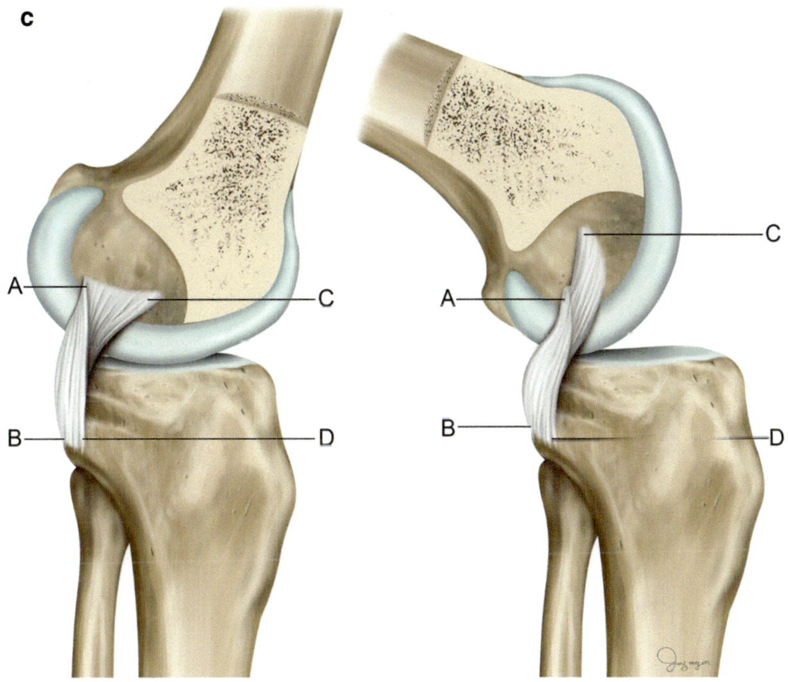

Fig. 1.13 (continued)

extension of the posterior cortical line of the femur shaft and indirect insertions attached thinly to the behind of the direct insertion [24]. Direct insertion attaches firmly and is more important for the anterior stability of the knee joint. The ACL from the femoral attachment to the midportion is not a round cylinderical shape, but a thin, flat ribbon like appearance [25].

1.1.6.3 Posterior Cruciate Ligament

The posterior cruciate ligament (PCL) is a primary restraint to posterior displacement of the knee joint. The PCL originates the lateral aspect of the medial femoral condyle which runs distally toward the tibia. The length of the PCL is about 32–38 mm and the width of the middle part is about 13 mm. The cross-sectional area of the PCL femoral insertion is about three times wider than the middle part. The femoral attachment is semi-lunar shaped and is located clockwise between 12:00 and 5:00 p.m. (right knee) and the anterior boundary is located approximately 3–5 mm backward of the articular margin (Fig. 1.12b). The length of the anteroposterior axis of the femoral attachment is about 32 mm, and the cross-sectional area varies from about 125–200 mm^2. The tibial attachment of the PCL has rectangular or trapezoidal shape. The PCL inserts to posterior intercondylar fossa located 1–1.5 cm below the posterior articular margin. The anteroposterior dimension has a length of about 14–16 mm and a mediolateral dimension has about 10–16 mm in length [22] (Fig. 1.13a). The fibers of the PCL located on the medial side of the tibial attachment insert to the posterior aspect of the femoral origin, and the lateral fibers of the tibial attachment insert to the anterior aspect. Depending on this arrangement, the PCL is functionally divided into an anterolateral and posteromedial bundle (Fig. 1.13c).

1.1.7 Blood Supply

Blood supply to the knee joint is from the arteries branching out from the femoral and the popliteal artery (Fig. 1.14a). The descending

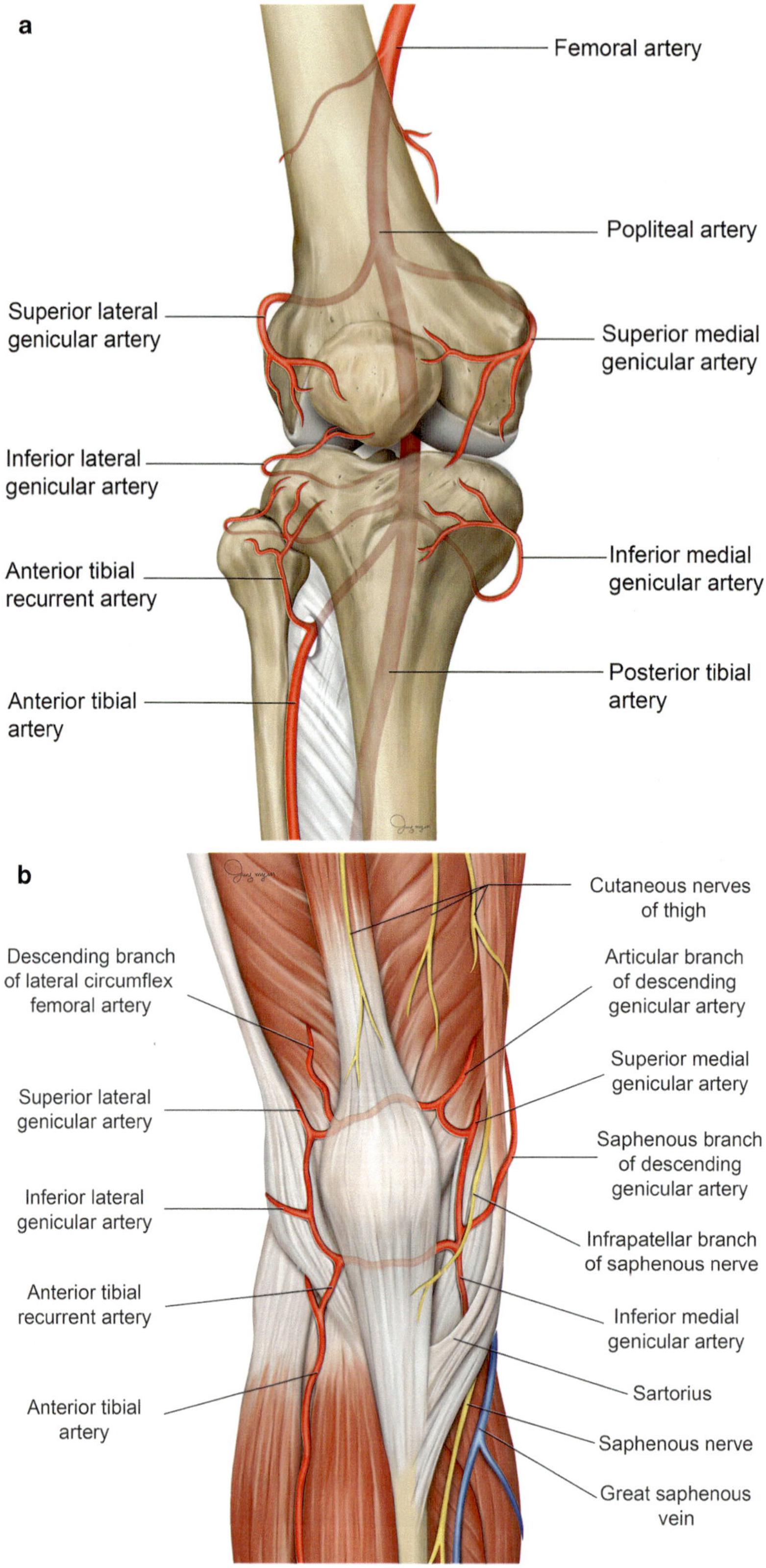

Fig. 1.14 Blood supply of the knee joint. (**a**) Branches of the popliteal artery, (**b**) peripatellar arterial networks, (**c**) middle genicular artery supplies to the intraarticular structures

c

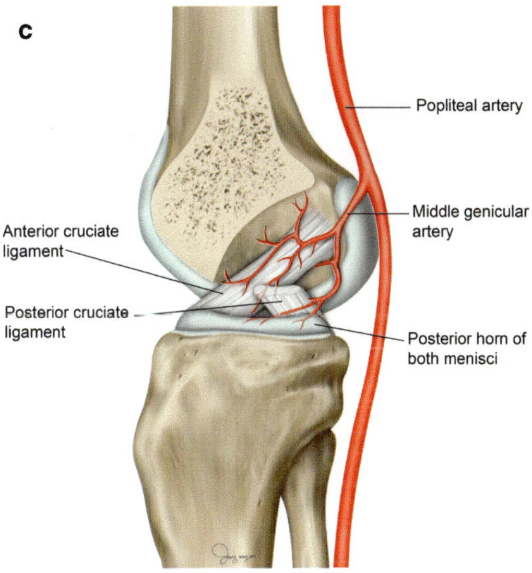

Fig. 1.14 (continued)

genicular artery is branched from the femoral artery in the proximal part of the adductor canal and gives off the saphenous branch, the articular branch, and the deep oblique branch [26]. The saphenous branch travels distally with the saphenous nerve and veins and passes over the sartorius and anastomoses with the inferior medial genicular artery in the medial aspect of the patella tendon. The articular branch travels distally through the vastus medialis and anastomoses with the lateral superior genicular artery to form a peripatellar network (Fig. 1.14b). The popliteal artery exits from Hunter's canals and enters the popliteal fossa and is divided into the anterior and posterior tibial arteries in the lower part of the popliteal fossa. The popliteal artery gives off numerous muscle branches and five articular branches (the superior lateral and medial genicular arteries, the middle genicular artery, the inferior lateral and medial genicular arteries). The middle genicular artery branches off at the front of the popliteal artery and enters the joint through the posterior joint capsule and the posterior oblique ligament (Fig. 1.14c). The middle genicular artery supplies in the intraarticular structures such as the ACL, the PCL, the posterior horn of both menisci, and the synovial membrane [27]. The anterior arterial anastomosis of the knee joint compose of the superior and inferior genicular artery, branches of the descending genicular artery, descending branch of the lateral femoral circumflex artery and recurrent branch of the anterior tibial artery. This anastomosis forms a vascular loop around the patella, and more than 10 nutrient arteries arise at the lower pole of the patella, penetrate and run forward through the anterior surface of the patella [28]. The medial retinaculum is mainly supplied by the descending genicular artery and the lateral retinaculum is supplied by the lateral anastomosis formed by the superior and inferior lateral genicular arteries. The blood supply of the patella tendon is from the medial anastomosis formed by the inferior medial genicular artery and the descending genicular artery on the medial side, whereas on the lateral side, the lateral genicular arteries and the recurrent branch of the anterior tibial artery supplies.

1.1.8 Nerve Innervation

The anterior aspect of the knee joint is innervated by the articular branches of the femoral nerve, the common peroneal nerve, and the saphenous nerve [29]. The posterior aspect of the knee joint is innervated by the articular branch of the tibial nerve and the posterior articular branch of the obturator nerve. The nerve that innervates the ligaments and the joint capsule in anterior aspect of the proximal knee joint is branched from the nerves that innervate the quadriceps. The largest nerve branch is branched from the nerves that supply the vastus medialis, and it innervates the anteromedial joint capsule [30] (Fig. 1.15a). In the anterolateral area, branches from the nerves supplied in the vastus lateralis innervate the superolateral capsule. The saphenous nerve is branched from the posterior division of the femoral nerve and divides into the sartorial branch and the infrapatellar branch at the distal end of the adductor canal [31]. In particular, the infrapatella branch traverses the sartorius and superficially penetrates the deep fascia of the medial knee joint between the sartorius and the gracilis muscle to form a patella plexus (Fig. 1.15b). It innervates

Fig. 1.15 Nerve innervation of the knee joint. (**a**) Superficial nerve innervation in the anterior aspect of the knee joint, (**b**) saphenous nerve and its infrapatellar branch, (**c**) common peroneal nerve and its branch, (**d**) tibial and common peroneal nerve

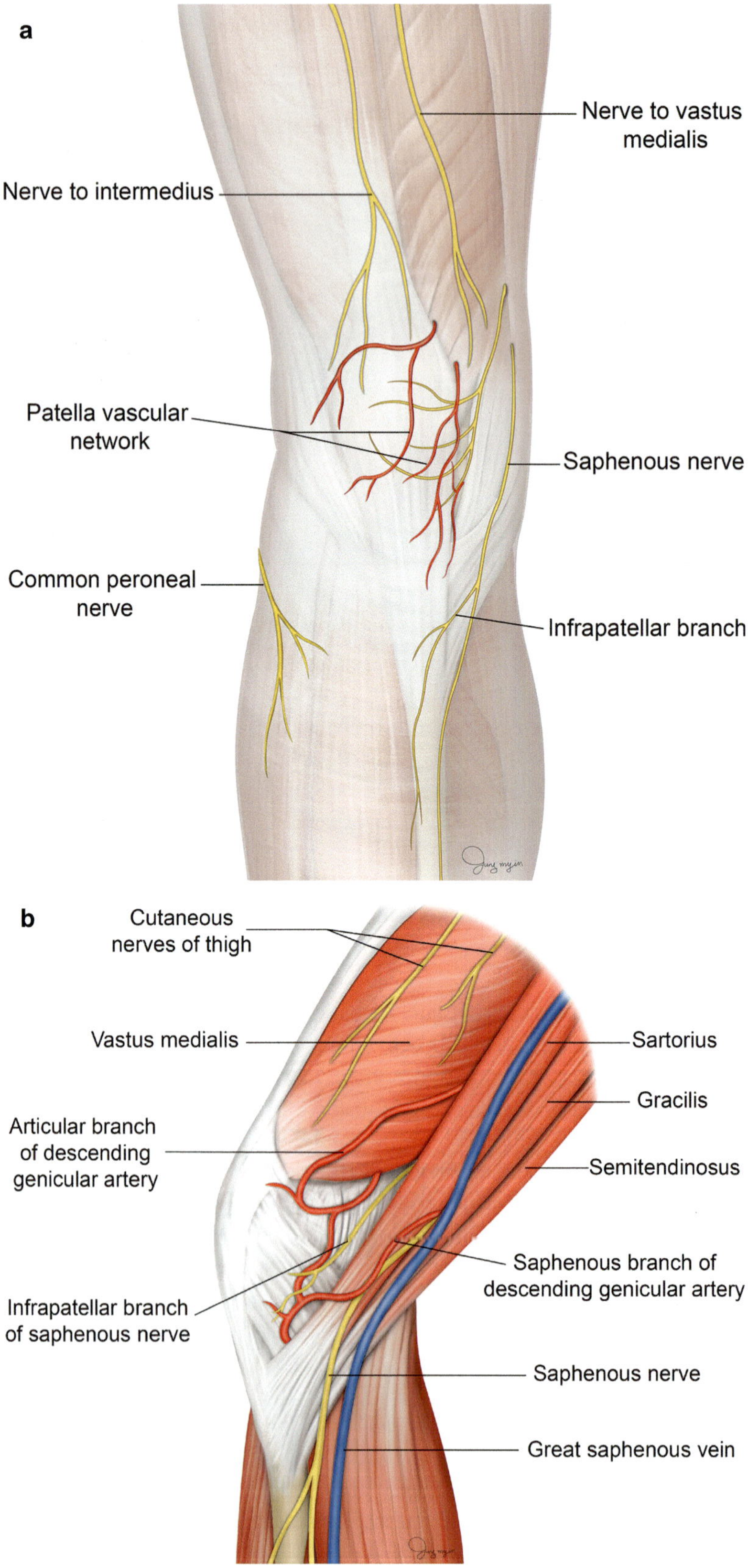

Fig. 1.15 (continued)

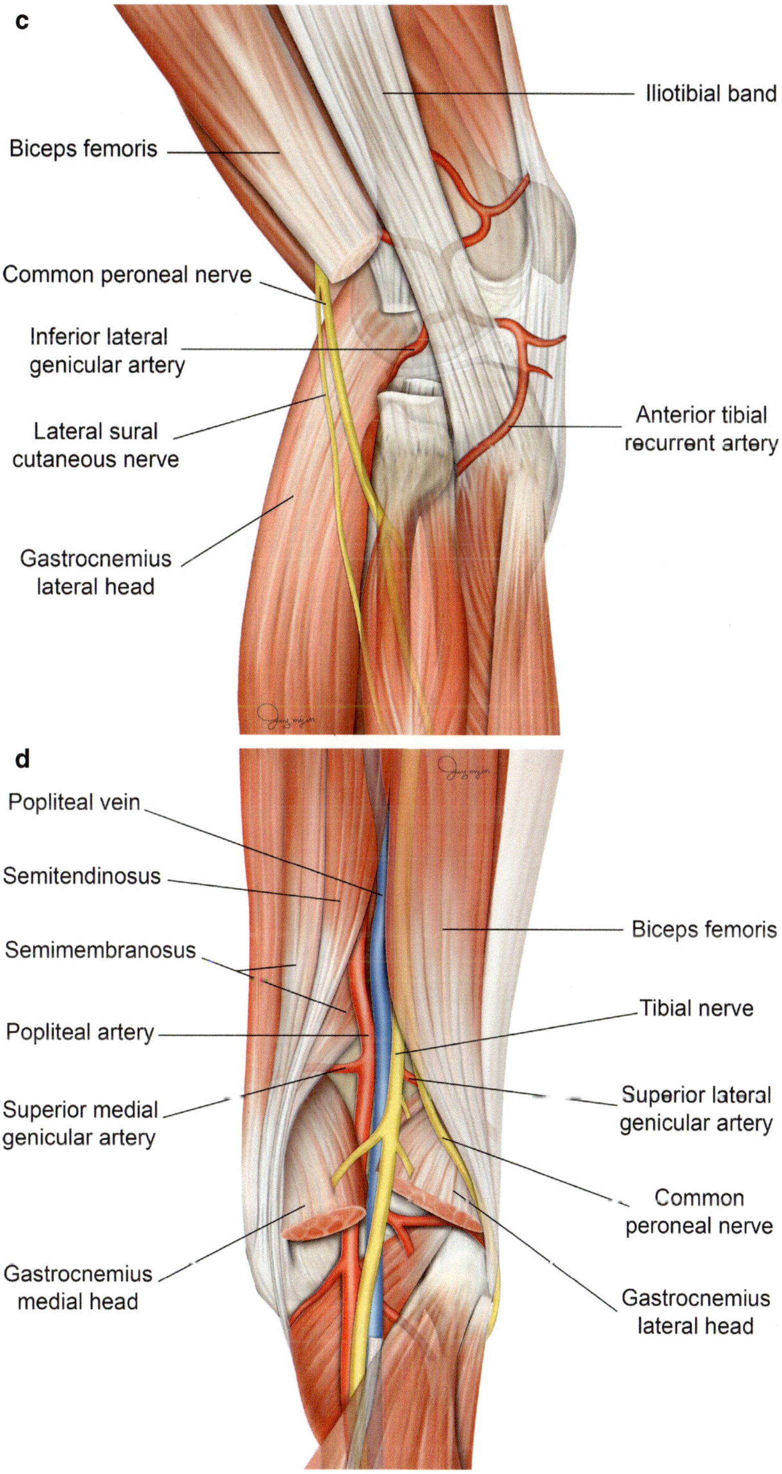

to the anteromedial capsule, the patella tendon, and skin anteromedially. The common peroneal nerve runs distally along the inner side of the biceps femoris tendon in the popliteal fossa and passes between the biceps femoris tendon and the lateral head of the gastrocnemius and continues distally posterior to the fibula head. It winds superficially over the lateral side of the fibula neck before penetrating the peroneus longus and then divides into the superficial peroneal nerve and the deep peroneal nerve (Fig. 1.15c). The superficial peroneal nerve branches off the lateral sural cutaneous nerve and the small branch that innervates to the skin over the anterolateral aspect of the proximal part of the lower leg. The deep peroneal nerve branches off two articular branches, which are the lateral articular nerve and the recurrent peroneal nerve [32]. The lateral articular nerve arising at the level of the joint line innervates the inferior lateral capsule and the LCL. The recurrent peroneal nerve arising from more distal area ascends the anterior aspect of the tibia and innervates the anterolateral side of the joint. The tibial nerve arises from the sciatic nerve and lies in the fat tissue beneath the deep fascia in the popliteal fossa and runs distally between the two heads of the gastrocnemius (Fig. 1.15d). Muscular branches innervate the both heads of the gastrocnemius, the plantaris, the soleus, and the popliteus muscles. The cutaneous branch runs distally on the surface of the gastrocnemius as medial sural cutaneous nerve. The tibial nerve has several joint branches. Among them, the largest and most consistent branch is the posterior articular nerve which courses laterally and winds around the popliteal vessels to form the popliteal plexus. This nerve innervates in the posterior and perimeniscal capsule and the synovial covering of the cruciate ligaments. The terminal branch of the posterior division of the obturator nerve follows the course of the femoral artery into popliteal fossa and forms the popliteal plexus and innervates to the posterior capsule and menisci.

1.2 Alignment and Biomechanics of the Knee Joint

1.2.1 Normal Knee Alignment

The alignment status of the knee joint can be evaluated with the full-length radiograph of the lower extremity taken with the patella facing forward. The ideal alignment of the lower limbs is that the load-bearing axis is located at the center of the knee joint. When viewed from the front, the deviation of the weight-bearing axis from the center of the knee joint to the medial or lateral side is referred to as a varus or valgus deformity, respectively (Fig. 1.16). Similarly, when viewed from the lateral side, if it deviates to the anterior or posterior side, flexion deformity or recurvatum deformity occurs, respectively. These malalignments may have no symptoms in children, but in older people, the joints are overloaded and the joint surface wears out due to excessive friction, leading to the development of arthritis.

The hip–knee–ankle (HKA) angle is used to describe the coronal alignment between the femoral and tibial mechanical axis. In the neutral position, the HKA angle is 0 degrees, and when the value is negative, it means varus, and if positive, it means valgus deformity. The evaluation of the patellar alignment can be done with a Q angle, which is measured in the supine position with the knees in full extension. On normal knees, the Q angle is about 11 degrees on average for men and 14 degrees on average for women [33] (Fig. 1.17). The posterior slope of the tibial plateau and the posterior offset of the tibia and femoral condyles allow the knee to flex up to 160 degrees. The central axis of flexion and extension movement of the knee joint is known to be similar to the transepicondylar axis (TEA). During the movement, the tibia rotates about 30 degrees around the posteromedial portion of the tibial plateau, and the patella rotates almost parallel to the TEA [34].

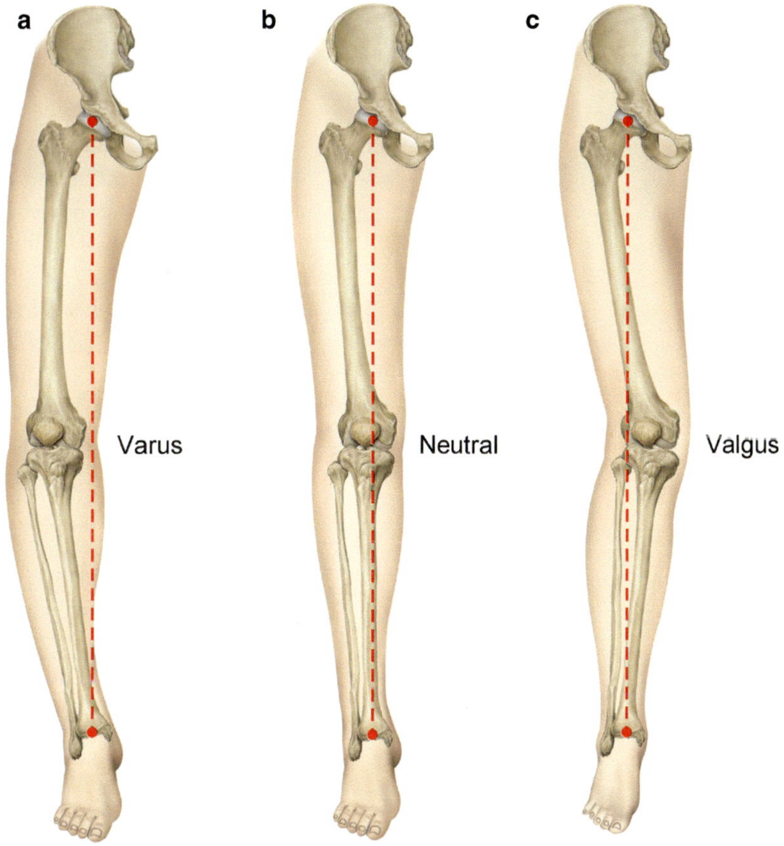

Fig. 1.16 Alignment of the lower limb. (**a**) Varus, (**b**) neutral, (**c**) valgus

1.2.1.1 Alignment in Coronal Plane

Alignment in the coronal plane is mainly assessed using weight-bearing radiographs. The line connecting the center of the femur head to the center of the ankle joint is called the axis of the weight bearing. The mechanical axis of the femur is the line connecting the center of the femur head and the center of the knee joint, and the mechanical axis of the tibia is the line connecting the center of the tibial spine and the center of the talus. Neutral alignment refers to the mechanical axis of the femur and tibia appearing as a single line. However, even in asymptomatic adults, the HKA angle shows mild negative degrees. According to the report, in normal Koreans, the HKA angle is about 3 degrees varus state, the angle between the tibial joint surface and the mechanical axis is about 4 degrees, and the angle between the femoral joint surface and the mechanical axis is about 3 degrees valgus state [35]. These coronal angles of lower limb alignment are reported differently depending on gender, age, and presence of joint disease.

A line connecting the mid diaphyseal point at proximal one-third and two-thirds of the femoral shaft is called the anatomical axis of the femur, and a line connecting the mid-diaphyseal point at proximal one-third and two-thirds of the tibial shaft is called the anatomical axis of the tibia. In the femur, the angle between the mechanical axis and the anatomical axis is about 6 degrees (4–7 degrees). However, the mechanical axis of the tibia coincides with the anatomical axis. In the "at attention" standing position, the angle between the midline of the body and the mechanical axis of the lower extremity is form an angle

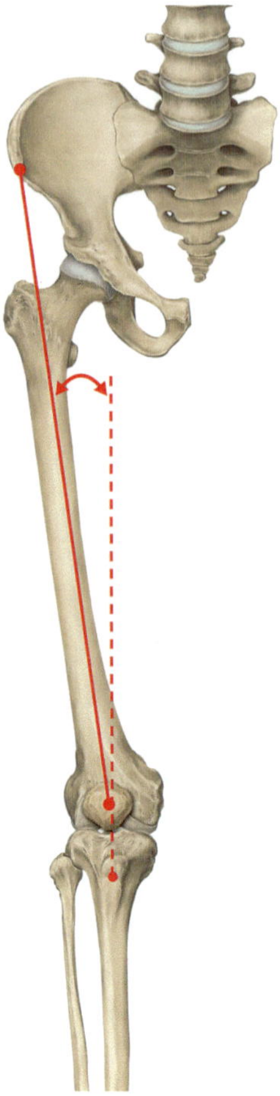

Fig. 1.17 Q-angle is measured by drawing a line between the center of the patella and the anterior-superior iliac spine and a second line between the center of the patella and the center of the tibial tubercle

about 3 degrees. As a result, the angle between the axis of the body weight and the anatomical axis of the femur is 7–10 degrees [36, 37]. Meanwhile, since the tibial plateau is 3 degrees varus to the mechanical axis, the axis of body weight is perpendicular to the tibial plateau.

1.2.1.2 Alignment in Sagittal Plane

The mechanical axis in the sagittal plane is the line passing from the center of the femoral head to the center of the ankle joint. The criterion for distal femur alignment on the sagittal plane cannot be clearly defined because the distal femur consists of a round condyle. However, there are two methods to measure the angle between the femoral condyle and the anatomical axis of the femur on the sagittal plane. The first method is to measure the posterior distal femoral angle (PDFA), an angle between the femoral anatomical axis and the femoral articular marginal line which connecting the anterior and posterior margins of the condyle, which is reported to be approximately 83 degrees. The second method is to measure the angle between the Blumensaat's line and the anatomical axis of the distal femur, and this angle has been reported on average about 37.5 degrees [38]. The sagittal alignment of the tibia is defined as the angle formed by the articular surface of tibial plateau and the tibial mechanical axis, which inclined backward about 8.4 degrees [39].

1.2.1.3 Alignment of the Patella

The patellar alignment is defined as the Q angle, the angle formed by the action line of the quadriceps muscle and the patellar tendon. This is the acute angle formed by the line connecting the ASIS to the center of the patella and the line connecting the center of the patella to the tibial tuberosity. One of the causes of the patellar malalignment is due to the various locations of the tibial tuberosity, which can show an average 9 ± 4 degrees lateral deviation in the median plane of the tibia. The Q angle increases in the valgus knee, and the sum of forces directs the patella outward. On the other hand, in the varus state, the Q angle becomes smaller and the patella is directed inward.

Patellar axial radiograph, computed tomography, and magnetic resonance imaging are mainly used for evaluation of the patellar rotational alignment. Since patellar axial radiographs do not have a reference line, it is recommended to evaluate the rotational alignment of the patella based on TEA in computer tomography or magnetic resonance imaging [40].

1.2.1.4 Malalignment

If the knee alignment described above is not within the normal range, it is called the malalignment, which causes pain of the knee joint and the arthritic changes. In normal knees, the medial compartment of the knee is responsible for 60%

of the weight load, and the rest in the lateral compartment. The varus alignment causes overload of the medial compartment, whereas the valgus alignment causes overload of the lateral compartment. And this overload accelerates the deformity of the compartment. In patients with the varus deformity, the medial femoral and the tibial condyle can be expected to reduce the amount of cartilage and increase bone denuding. Therefore, when a surgical treatment is considered in patients with the cartilage damage of the knee joint, the alignment status of the knee joint should be evaluated first, and realignment osteotomy should be considered together with the cartilage restoration procedures.

1.2.2 Biomechanics

The tibiofemoral joint of the knee is a modified hinged joint, capable of three translational (medial-lateral, anterior-posterior, proximal-distal) and three rotational motions (flexion-extension, internal rotation-external rotation, varus-valgus) by the anatomical structures such as the joint capsule, surrounding muscles, and ligaments. The stability of the knee joint changes its mechanism according to the posture. When the knee is fully extended, the collateral ligaments and the cruciate ligaments are taut, and the anterior portion of the meniscus is locked between the tibia and the femoral condyle to maintain stability. At the beginning of the flexion, the contraction of the popliteus muscle makes the external rotation of the femur, and the internal rotation of the tibia (approximately 15 degrees) is unlocking the knee joint [41]. The meniscus is locked on the articular surface during full extension, but it is moved backward during flexion, which is more prominent in the lateral meniscus than in the medial meniscus [42]. The rollback movement of the femur to the tibia occurs mainly during the first 20 degrees of flexion, after which the sliding occurs mainly. And during flexion, the femoral condylar rolling movement is mostly occurred in the lateral side.

The medial femoral condyle has an anatomical characteristic that the anterior-posterior length of the articular surface is longer than the lateral femoral condyle. So, when the knee joint extends from the flexion position, even if the lateral femoral condyle and tibial joint surface reach the full extension position, the anterior joint surface of the medial femoral condyle does not reach the full extension position and remain slightly more likely to exercise. Therefore, at 20 degrees before the medial compartment is fully extended, the tibia has an external rotational motion compared to the lateral femoral condyle. This rotational movement is called a screw-home movement, which occurs about 15 degrees during full extension [43].

The contact point of the articular surface of the patellofemoral joint is complex and dynamic. In the extended state, the patella and the trochlear groove do not have a contact surface. As the flexion progresses, the contact surface moves from distal to the proximal part of the patella, and when the 120-degree flexion reaches, the contact area of the patella is the far medial and lateral side of the joint surface. At full flexion, the odd facet is the only articulating contact between the patella and the medial femoral condyle [44].

1.2.2.1 Femur-Tibia Joint Biomechanics

To understand the movement of the tibiofemoral joint, the shape of the bone should be considered first. On the articular surface of the femur, the medial condyle is longer than the lateral condyle, whereas the lateral condyle is wider than the medial condyle. On flexion 90 degrees, when viewed from the front, the long axis of the lateral condyle is almost parallel to the anterior–posterior axis, but the long axis of the medial condyle is approximately 22 degrees incline. Therefore, the lateral condyle appears longer on the lateral radiograph. When viewed from the side, the medial femoral condyle has a curve of round shape with a similar radius length at the anterior and posterior, while the lateral femoral condyle has a curve of increasing radius toward the posterior.

The knee joint is a kind of hinge joint, but the movement is not only a simple flexion–extension movement, but also a combined movement accompanied by a rotation of the tibia against the femur. The basic mechanism of flexion–extension movement of the knee joint is a combination of rolling and sliding movements of the femur against the tibial joint surface (Fig. 1.18). Rolling is the same movement as a hoop rolls a plane, and the transverse axis of the rotation moves horizontally. Sliding, on the other hand, is the movement in which the hoop rotates while constantly contacting a fixed point of the plane, and the horizontal axis of the rotation is fixed. If rolling occurs only, the femoral condyle can roll-off from the tibial plateau before the maximum flexion of the knee joint occurs, and if only sliding occurs, the femoral condyle may bump into the tibia. Therefore, the maximum flexion of the knee joint is possible only when rolling and sliding are combined. The flexion–extension movement of the normal knee joint usually involves rolling at the first 20 degrees of flexion, but then at the next 20 to 90 degrees of flexion, sliding occurs mainly. Rolling and sliding occur at a ratio of 1:2 in the beginning of flexion, and at a ratio of 1:4 in the end of flexion. Thus, the transverse axis of the flexion–extension (the center of rotation) is not fixed but moves constantly to draw a "J"-shaped curve (Fig. 1.19).

The screw-home movement rotates the tibia externally in a knee extension, resulting in tighter anterior and posterior cruciate ligament, contributing to the stability of the knee joint (Fig. 1.20). The opposite rotational motion occurs when starting flexion at the fully extended position. The internal rotational movement of the tibia during the initial flexion is achieved by the contraction of the popliteus muscle. When the knee joint flexes 0 to 120 degrees, the tibia rotates averages 29.2 degrees based on the femur. Also, while the knee joint is flexed, the center of rotation moves from the distal condyle of the femur to the posterior condyle, and especially, the movement of this center is evident in the lateral compartment of the knee.

The movement of the center during the flexion of the knee joint occurs in harmony with the anatomical structure of the tibial plateau. The lateral side of the plateau is the shape of a convex horse saddle, while the medial side is the shape of a concave dish. This results in less anterior–posterior translation in the medial compartment than the lateral compartment. Therefore, during normal knee flexion from 0 to 120 degrees, posterior femoral rollback occurs mainly on the lateral side and rarely on the medial side. This medial pivot movement results in an asymmetric femoral posterior translation. When flexion over 120 degrees, the femoral posterior translation causes flexion on the lateral side without the condylar contact. And at over 150 degrees, the lateral femoral condyle becomes subluxation toward the posterior side of the tibia. Although there is no such femoral posterior translation from the medial side, the offset of the posterior femoral condyle helps the deep knee flexion [45].

1.2.2.2 Patellofemoral Joint Biomechanics

The quadriceps is attached to the proximal part of the patella and serves to transmit the force around the femur to the patellar tendon and the tibial tubercle without friction. The most important function of the patella is the role of the pulley mechanism that increases the efficiency of the quadriceps by increasing the lever arm of the extensor mechanism. Since the patellar tendon is positioned more forward than the tibiofemoral joint as much as the thickness of the patellar bone, the efficiency of the extensor mechanism of the knee joint can be increased by lengthening the lever arm of the quadriceps.

In order to explain the dynamics of the patellofemoral joint, it is necessary to understand the direction of force of the quadriceps muscle, the direction of the patellar tendon movement, and the patellofemoral joint reaction force. Q angle is

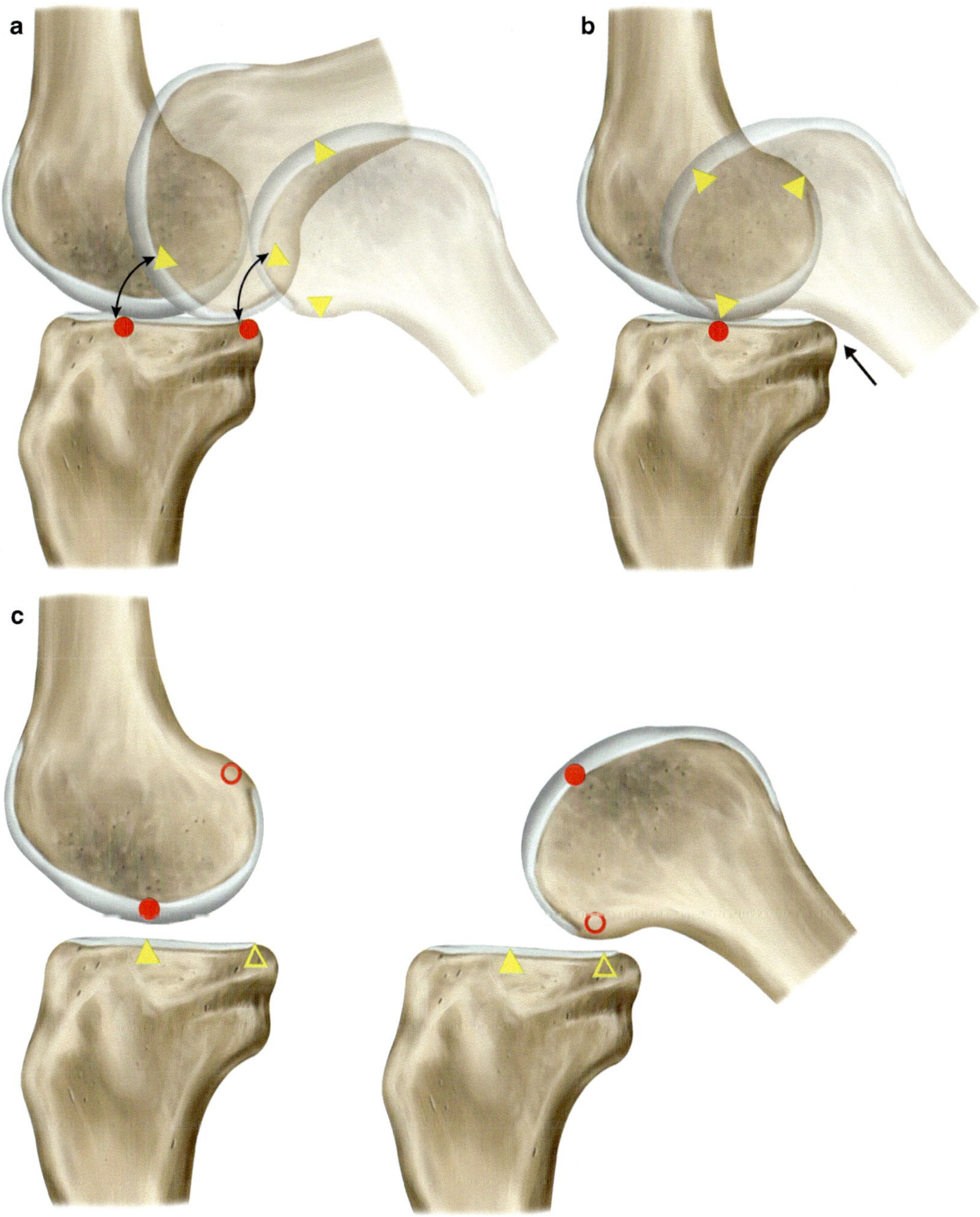

Fig. 1.18 Rolling and gliding movement. (**a**) Rolling occurs only, (**b**) gliding occurs only, (**c**) when rolling and gliding are combined

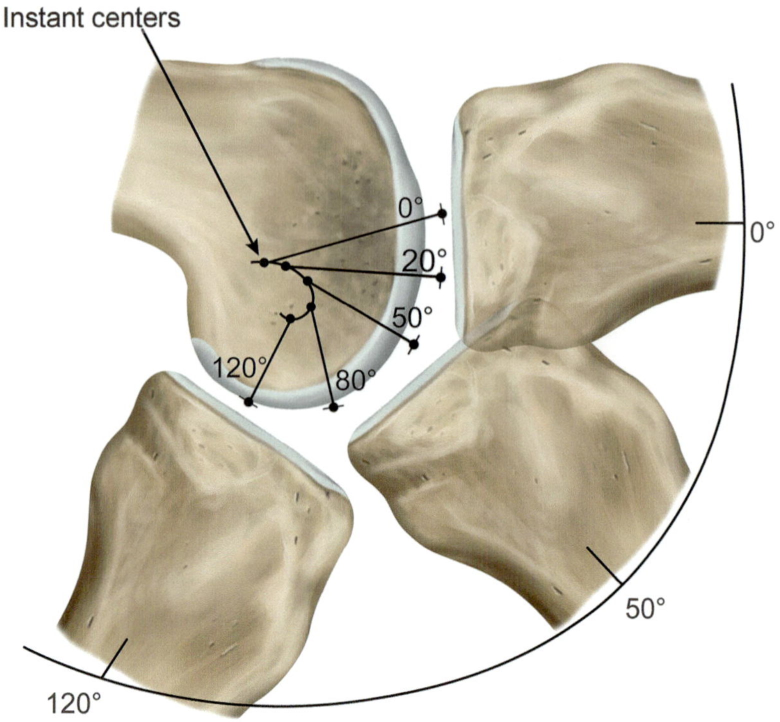

Fig. 1.19 Instant centers of rotation draw "J" shape during flexion–extension movement

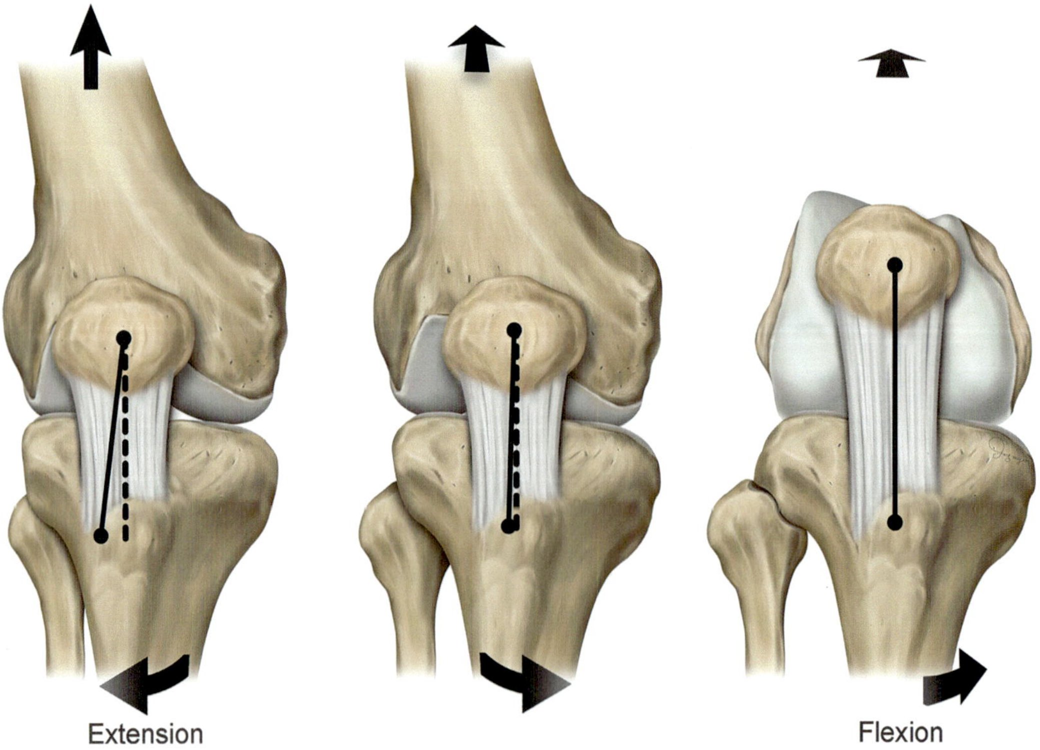

Fig. 1.20 Screw-home movement. The tibia rotates externally in the terminal extension of the knee joint. As the result, the tibial tubercle locates lateral to the center of the patella in full extension position

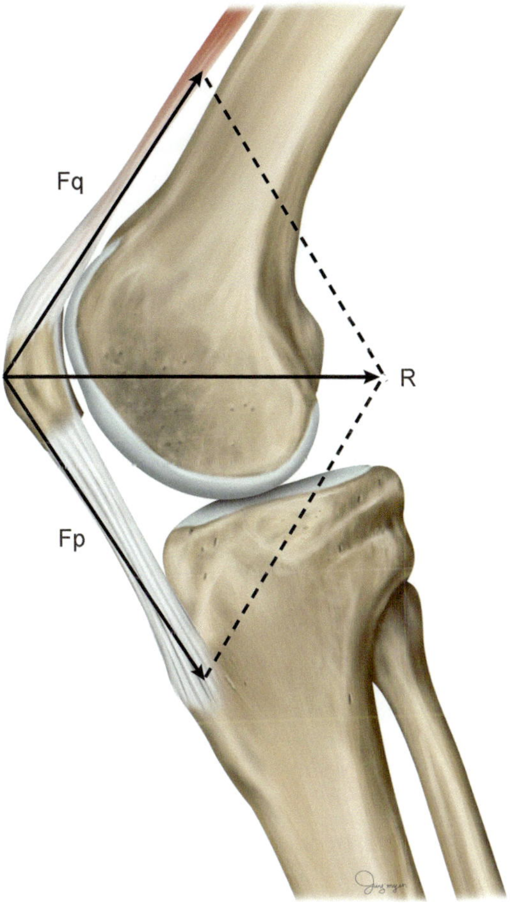

Fig. 1.21 The patellofemoral joint reaction force (R) is vector sum of the quadriceps force (Fq) and the patellar tendon force (Fp)

the angle formed by the longitudinal axis of the quadriceps and the longitudinal axis of the patellar tendon. When a force is applied by the extensor mechanism (the quadriceps femoris, the patellar tendon), the Q angle creates a valgus force on the patellofemoral joint. These valgus forces generate a compressive force of the patella against the femoral condyle, and the pressure increases as the flexion angle of the knee joint increases.

The patellofemoral joint reaction force (PFJRF) is expressed as a vector sum of the quadriceps force (Fq) and the patellar tendon force (Fp) (Fig. 1.21). When the knee joint flexes, the flexion moment arm increases, and the angle formed by the direction of each force of the quadriceps and the patellar tendon decreases, so the PFJRF increases. The PFJRF at rest is 1.5 times the weight in the 30-degree flexion of the knee joint and 6 times the weight in the 90-degree flexion. The PFJRF when walking on a flat land is 0.5 times the weight, 3.3 times the weight when walking up and down stairs, and 7.8 times the weight when squatting [46]. A strong quadriceps force is required for full extension because the moment arm sharply decreased in the 20-degree flexion from full extension [47]. Therefore, in the case of patients with anterior knee pain due to the patellofemoral joint problem, the knee extension exercise against resistance or the terminal extension exercise should be restricted. In addition, a straight leg raise exercise or short-arc isotonic exercise is recommended for quadriceps rehabilitation, which does not exacerbate symptoms.

The patella does not contact the trochlear groove in the fully extended state of the knee joint, and when the 30 degrees flexion, the distal portion of the patella begins to contact the proximal portion of the trochlear groove. As the knee joint flexes, the contact portion of the patella surface moves from the proximal to distal patella, and until 90 degrees, the contact surface is constantly increased to help lower the patellofemoral contact pressure (Fig. 1.22). Knee flexion over 90 degrees causes the quadriceps tendon to contact with the femoral condyle and the tendo-femoral contact surface is formed to lower the patellofemoral contact pressure. The average patellofemoral contact pressure was 2.0 MPa at 20-degree flexion, 2.4 MPa at 30-degree flexion, 4.1 MPa at 60-degree flexion, and 4.4 MPa at 90-degree flexion, and decreased to 3.5 MPa at 120-degree flexion [48].

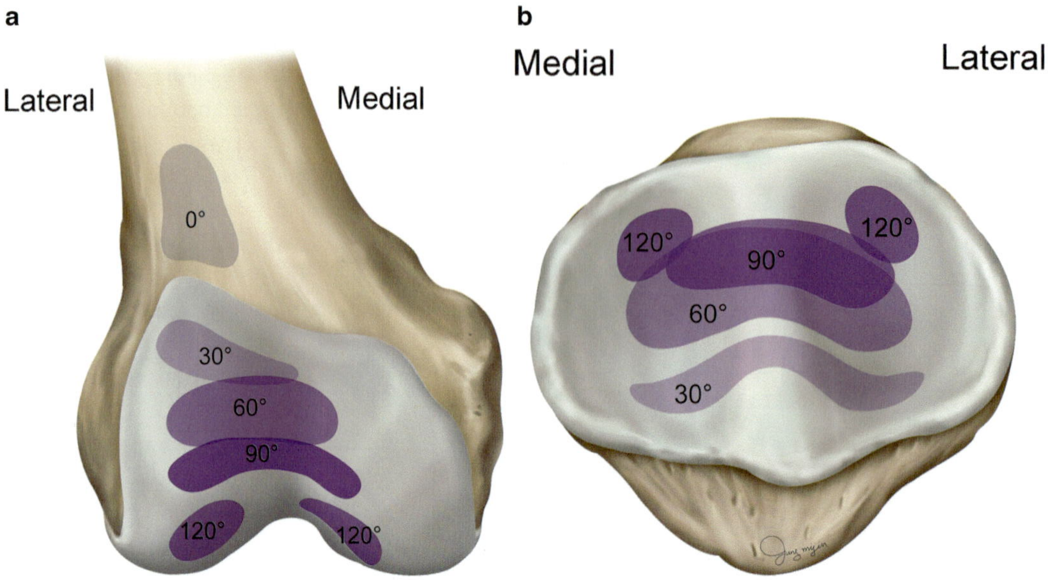

Fig. 1.22 Contact area of the patellofemoral joint. (**a**) Articular surface of the trochlea, (**b**) articular surface of the patella

References

1. Andrikoula S, Tokis A, Vasiliadis HS, Georgoulis A. The extensor mechanism of the knee joint: an anatomical study. Knee Surg Sports Traumatol Arthrosc. 2006;14(3):214–20.
2. Lieb FJ, Perry J. Quadriceps function: an anatomical and mechanical study using amputated limbs. J Bone Joint Surg Am. 1968;50(8):1535–48.
3. Hayes CW, Conway WF. Normal anatomy and magnetic resonance appearance of the knee. Top Magn Reson Imaging. 1993;5(4):207–27.
4. Conlan T, Garth WP Jr, Lemons JE. Evaluation of the medial soft-tissue restraints of the extensor mechanism of the knee. J Bone Joint Surg Am. 1993;75(5):682–93.
5. Hallisey MJ, Doherty N, Bennett WF, Fulkerson JP. Anatomy of the junction of the vastus lateralis tendon and the patella. J Bone Joint Surg Am. 1987;69(4):545–9.
6. Warren LF, Marshall JL. The supporting structures and layers on the medial side of the knee: an anatomical analysis. J Bone Joint Surg Am. 1979;61(1):56–62.
7. LaPrade RF, Engebretsen AH, Ly TV, Johansen S, Wentorf FA, Engebretsen L. The anatomy of the medial part of the knee. J Bone Joint Surg Am. 2007;89(9):2000–10.
8. Mochizuki T, Akita K, Muneta T, Sato T. Pes anserinus: layered supportive structure on the medial side of the knee. Clin Anat (New York, NY). 2004;17(1):50–4.
9. Baldwin JL. The anatomy of the medial patellofemoral ligament. Am J Sports Med. 2009;37(12):2355–61.
10. Hughston JC, Eilers AF. The role of the posterior oblique ligament in repairs of acute medial (collateral) ligament tears of the knee. J Bone Joint Surg Am. 1973;55(5):923–40.
11. Liu F, Yue B, Gadikota HR, Kozanek M, Liu W, Gill TJ, et al. Morphology of the medial collateral ligament of the knee. J Orthop Surg Res. 2010;5:69.
12. Beltran J, Matityahu A, Hwang K, Jbara M, Maimon R, Padron M, et al. The distal semimembranosus complex: normal MR anatomy, variants, biomechanics and pathology. Skelet Radiol. 2003;32(8):435–45.
13. Benninger B, Delamarter T. Distal semimembranosus muscle-tendon-unit review: morphology, accurate terminology, and clinical relevance. Folia Morphol (Warsz). 2013;72(1):1–9.
14. Seebacher JR, Inglis AE, Marshall JL, Warren RF. The structure of the posterolateral aspect of the knee. J Bone Joint Surg Am. 1982;64(4):536–41.
15. Terry GC, Hughston JC, Norwood LA. The anatomy of the iliopatellar band and iliotibial tract. Am J Sports Med. 1986;14(1):39–45.
16. Terry GC, LaPrade RF. The biceps femoris muscle complex at the knee. Its anatomy and injury patterns associated with acute anterolateral-anteromedial rotatory instability. Am J Sports Med. 1996;24(1):2–8.
17. Vieira EL, Vieira EA, da Silva RT, Berlfein PA, Abdalla RJ, Cohen M. An anatomic study of the iliotibial tract. Arthroscopy. 2007;23(3):269–74.
18. Yan J, Takeda S, Fujino K, Tajima G, Hitomi J. Anatomical reconsideration of the lateral collateral ligament in the human knee: anatomical observation and literature review. Surg Sci. 2012;3(10):484.
19. Stäubli HU, Birrer S. The popliteus tendon and its fascicles at the popliteal hiatus: gross anatomy and functional arthroscopic evaluation with and without anterior cruciate ligament deficiency. Arthroscopy. 1990;6(3):209–20.

20. LaPrade RF, Ly TV, Wentorf FA, Engebretsen L. The posterolateral attachments of the knee: a qualitative and quantitative morphologic analysis of the fibular collateral ligament, popliteus tendon, popliteofibular ligament, and lateral gastrocnemius tendon. Am J Sports Med. 2003;31(6):854–60.
21. LaPrade RF, Morgan PM, Wentorf FA, Johansen S, Engebretsen L. The anatomy of the posterior aspect of the knee. An anatomic study. J Bone Joint Surg Am. 2007;89(4):758–64.
22. Girgis FG, Marshall JL, Monajem A. The cruciate ligaments of the knee joint. Anatomical, functional and experimental analysis. Clin Orthop Relat Res. 1975;106:216–31.
23. Zantop T, Petersen W, Sekiya JK, Musahl V, Fu FH. Anterior cruciate ligament anatomy and function relating to anatomical reconstruction. Knee Surg Sports Traumatol Arthrosc. 2006;14(10):982–92.
24. Iwahashi T, Shino K, Nakata K, Otsubo H, Suzuki T, Amano H, et al. Direct anterior cruciate ligament insertion to the femur assessed by histology and 3-dimensional volume-rendered computed tomography. Arthroscopy. 2010;26(9 Suppl):S13–20.
25. Śmigielski R, Zdanowicz U, Drwięga M, Ciszek B, Ciszkowska-Łysoń B, Siebold R. Ribbon like appearance of the midsubstance fibres of the anterior cruciate ligament close to its femoral insertion site: a cadaveric study including 111 knees. Knee Surg Sports Traumatol Arthrosc. 2015;23(11):3143–50.
26. Kawarai Y, Nakamura J, Suzuki T, Hagiwara S, Miura M, Ohtori S. Anatomical features of the descending genicular artery to facilitate surgical exposure for the subvastus approach-a cadaveric study. J Arthroplast. 2018;33(8):2647–51.
27. Salaria H, Atkinson R. Anatomic study of the middle genicular artery. J Orthop Surg (Hong Kong). 2008;16(1):47–9.
28. Lazaro LE, Cross MB, Lorich DG. Vascular anatomy of the patella: implications for total knee arthroplasty surgical approaches. Knee. 2014;21(3):655–60.
29. Horner G, Dellon AL. Innervation of the human knee joint and implications for surgery. Clin Orthop Relat Res. 1994;301:221–6.
30. Tran J, Peng PW, Lam K, Baig E, Agur AM, Gofeld M. Anatomical study of the innervation of anterior knee joint capsule: implication for image-guided intervention. Reg Anesth Pain Med. 2018;43(4):407–14.
31. Dunaway DJ, Steensen RN, Wiand W, Dopirak RM. The sartorial branch of the saphenous nerve: its anatomy at the joint line of the knee. Arthroscopy. 2005;21(5):547–51.
32. Kennedy JC, Alexander IJ, Hayes KC. Nerve supply of the human knee and its functional importance. Am J Sports Med. 1982;10(6):329–35.
33. Herrington L, Nester C. Q-angle undervalued? The relationship between Q-angle and medio-lateral position of the patella. Clin Biomech. 2004;19(10):1070–3.
34. Churchill DL, Incavo SJ, Johnson CC, Beynnon BD. The transepicondylar axis approximates the optimal flexion axis of the knee. Clin Orthop Relat Res. 1998;356:111–8.
35. Lee E, Youngbok J, Teckjin A. Radiographic analysis of the axial alignment of the lower extremity. Knee Surg Relat Res. 1989;1(2):140–4.
36. Luo C-F. Reference axes for reconstruction of the knee. Knee. 2004;11(4):251–7.
37. Yoshioka Y, Siu D, Cooke T. The anatomy and functional axes of the femur. J Bone Joint Surg Am. 1987;69(6):873–80.
38. Iwasaki K, Inoue M, Kasahara Y, Tsukuda K, Kawahara H, Yokota I, et al. Inclination of Blumensaat's line influences on the accuracy of the quadrant method in evaluation for anterior cruciate ligament reconstruction. Knee Surg Sports Traumatol Arthrosc. 2019:1–9.
39. de Boer JJ, Blankevoort L, Kingma I, Vorster W. In vitro study of inter-individual variation in posterior slope in the knee joint. Clin Biomech. 2009;24(6):488–92.
40. van der Linden-van der Zwaag HMJ, Valstar ER, van der Molen AJ, Nelissen RGHH. Transepicondylar axis accuracy in computer assisted knee surgery: a comparison of the CT-based measured axis versus the CAS-determined axis. Comput Aided Surg. 2008;13(4):200–6.
41. Logan MC, Williams A, Lavelle J, Gedroyc W, Freeman M. What really happens during the Lachman test? A dynamic MRI analysis of tibiofemoral motion. Am J Sports Med. 2004;32(2):369–75.
42. Smith PN, Refshauge KM, Scarvell JM. Development of the concepts of knee kinematics. Arch Phys Med Rehabil. 2003;84(12):1895–902.
43. Kim HY, Kim KJ, Yang DS, Jeung SW, Choi HG, Choy WS. Screw-home movement of the tibiofemoral joint during normal gait: three-dimensional analysis. Clin Orthop Surg. 2015;7(3):303–9.
44. Lengsfeld M, Ahlers J, Ritter G. Kinematics of the patellofemoral joint. Arch Orthop Trauma Surg. 1990;109(5):280–3.
45. Bellemans J, Banks S, Victor J, Vandenneucker H, Moemans A. Fluoroscopic analysis of the kinematics of deep flexion in total knee arthroplasty: influence of posterior condylar offset. J Bone Joint Surg Br. 2002;84(1):50–3.
46. Seering WP, Piziali RL, Nagel DA, Schurman DJ. The function of the primary ligaments of the knee in varus-valgus and axial rotation. J Biomech. 1980;13(9):785–94.
47. Grood E, Noyes F, Butler D, Suntay W. Ligamentous and capsular restraints preventing straight medial and lateral laxity in intact human cadaver knees. J Bone Joint Surg Am. 1981;63(8):1257–69.
48. Huberti HH, Hayes WC. Patellofemoral contact pressures. The influence of q-angle and tendofemoral contact. J Bone Joint Surg Am. 1984;66(5):715–24.

Structure, Function, and Healing Response of Articular Cartilage and Meniscus

2

Seung-Suk Seo, In-Seung Lee, and Young-Chae Seo

Abstract

Articular cartilage is a tissue that forms the surface of the joint, which reduces friction during the lifetime and enables the synovial joint to perform the painless joint movement. Articular cartilage consists of a rich matrix and specially differentiated chondrocytes sparsely distributed between them. The articular cartilage matrix protects chondrocytes from damage that may occur due to normal joint movement, provides elasticity to the joints, provides a lubrication system for low-friction movements between the synovial fluid and the cartilage, and regulates the movement of matrix macromolecules throughout life. However, with age, chondrocytes gradually lose their ability, and given repeated damage, cartilage dysfunction eventually leads to osteoarthritis. The meniscus is two crescent-shaped fibrocartilage structures between the femoral condyle and tibial plateau. The meniscus is the primary stabilizing structure of the knee joint having important functions such as load transmission, absorb shock, joint stability and lubrication. The inner two-third of the meniscus is a relatively avascular structure and is not well recover when torn. Since only the peripheral part of the meniscus has the ability to heal, the location of the tear is the most important factor in restoring the torn meniscus. However, in order to overcome this, several studies are being conducted that can improve the healing potential in the torn meniscus.

Keywords

Articular cartilage · Chondrocyte · Synovial fluid · Lubrication · Matrix macromolecules Meniscus · Fibrocartilage · Load transmission Absorb shock

2.1 Articular Cartilage

2.1.1 Structure and Composition

Articular cartilage, unlike most other tissues, is a tissue without blood vessels, nerves, and lymph nodes. The color is white pearlescent, glossy, and elastic, 2–4 mm thick on average and has a flat surface. Articular cartilage consists of sparsely distributed, highly specialized chondrocytes and a broadly distributed extracellular matrix. The extracellular matrix consists mainly of water,

S. S. Seo (✉) · I.-S. Lee
Department of Orthopedics, Haeundae Bumin Hospital, Busan, South Korea
e-mail: seoss@bumin.co.kr

Y.-C. Seo
Department of Orthopedics, Inje University Busan Paik Hospital, Busan, South Korea

S.-S. Seo (ed.), *A Strategic Approach to Knee Arthritis Treatment*,
https://doi.org/10.1007/978-981-16-4217-3_2

proteoglycans, collagens, non-collagenous proteins and glycoproteins, which provide the physical and mechanical properties of articular cartilage. These components have a unique and complex structure, which gives the articular cartilage-specific mechanical properties.

2.1.1.1 Chondrocytes

Chondrocytes are derived from mesenchymal stem cells and occupy about 1% of adult articular cartilage [1]. Although size, shape, and metabolic activity vary depending on the type or zone in which chondrocytes are located, all chondrocytes have organelles such as endoplasmic retinaculum and Golgi apparatus, which are essential for matrix synthesis [2]. It also has the intracytoplasmic filaments, glycogen, lipid, and secretory vesicles needed to maintain the matrix structure [3]. Synthesis of proteoglycan occurs in ribosomes and Golgi bodies, but collagen synthesis mainly occurs in the rough endoplasmic reticulum. Chondrocytes in the superficial zone are thin and elongated in shape similar to fibroblasts, while cells in the middle zone are rounded and have metabolic activity, and cells in the deep zone show a radial pattern, and cells under the tidemark become smaller and less functional [4]. Chondrocytes are responsible for creating and maintaining articular cartilage. Chondrocytes increase the amount of matrix during the growth phase and maintain the amount of matrix after growth. That is, chondrocytes are responsible for the maintenance and structural competence of collagen and proteoglycan by synthesizing and substituting appropriate amounts of macromolecules and combining them with a highly ordered macromolecular framework [3]. Aging significantly changes the function of the chondrocyte. As aging progresses, the ability to synthesize proteoglycans, the ability of cells to proliferate, and the degree of response to anabolic stimuli decrease [5–7]. These changes eventually lead to degenerative changes in the articular cartilage.

2.1.1.2 Extracellular Matrix

The extracellular matrix consists mainly of tissue fluid and structural macromolecules, with varying contents and distributions depending on joint area and age [8, 9]. The interaction of these two components determines the mechanical properties such as stiffness and resilience. The most common component of a normal articular cartilage matrix is water, which accounts for 65–80% of the total weight of articular cartilage [10]. One-third of the water component in the cartilage is in the cell, and the rest is attached to the protein in the extracellular matrix. When a load is applied to the joint, water moves out of the tissue and acts as a lubrication system on the joint surface. In order to maintain the concentration of water and electrolyte in the tissue, the interaction of macromolecules, especially aggregating proteoglycan, and water is important. Because macromolecules have negative charges, they increase the concentration of cations such as sodium and decrease the concentration of anions such as chloride. Eventually, an increase in total inorganic ions concentration increases tissue osmotic pressure [3].

2.1.1.3 Structural Macromolecules

The rest of the matrix, except water, is a macromolecular framework consisting mainly of collagens, proteoglycans, and non-collagenous proteins. It accounts for about 20–40% of the total weight of cartilage and has different contributions to tissue properties [11]. That is, collagen fibrillar meshwork provides the cartilage with its form, tensile strength and shear force and also maintains the physical location of chondrocytes. Proteoglycans and non-collagenous proteins are either bound to the collagen fibrillar meshwork or are mechanically entrapped, and water fills the rest of the framework. Some of the non-collagenous proteins stabilize the macromolecular framework, while some help chondrocytes bind to matrix macromolecules [3].

Collagens

Collagen is the main fibrous protein component of articular cartilage, accounting for approximately 60% of the dry weight of articular cartilage, and is relatively evenly distributed over all zones except for the collagen-rich superficial zone. Articular cartilage contains several genetically different collagen types, including types II, VI, IX, X, and XI [12]. Type II collagen is the main component of articular cartilage, accounting for 90–95% of the collagen that makes up the articular cartilage, and makes the main component of the cross-banded fibrils. Type VI collagen surrounds chondrocytes around the lacunae, forms an important part of the pericellular matrix, and serves to attach chondrocytes to the matrix [13]. Type IX collagen molecules are covalently bonded to the superficial zone of the cross-banded fibrils source by type II collagen and hydroxypyridinium, or they are introduced into the matrix to covalently bond with other type IX collagen molecules to form a collagen network, contributing to the stability of articular cartilage. Type XI collagen molecules makeup 3% of the articular cartilage collagen and are covalently bound to type II collagen molecules, forming part of the internal structure of the cross-banded fibrils. Type X collagen is only found in the calcified cartilage zone of the articular cartilage and the hypertrophic zone of the growth plate, so it is believed to has a role in the calcification of cartilage [14].

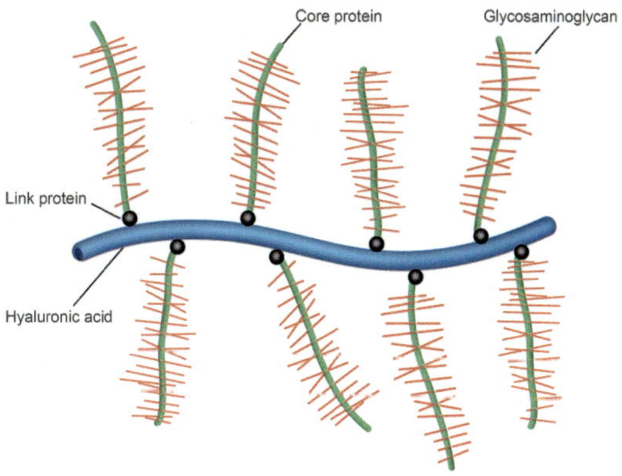

Fig. 2.1 Diagrammatic representation of the proteoglycan. Proteoglycan is a structure in which several glycosaminoglycans are attached to a core protein of a line, and glycosaminoglycan has a negative charge, so it has an affinity for cations

Proteoglycans

Proteoglycan accounts for about 25–35% of the amount of dry weight of articular cartilage and functions to resist pressure and distribute loads. Proteoglycan is a structure in which several glycosaminoglycans are attached to a core protein of a line, and glycosaminoglycan has a negative charge, so it has an affinity for cations (Fig. 2.1) [15]. Representative glycosaminoglycans include hyaluronic acid, chondroitin 4-sulfate, chondroitin 6-sulfate, keratin sulfate, heparan sulfate and dermatan sulfate and each concentration varies depending on the site, age, cartilage damage, and disease [16]. Chondroitin sulfate is the most common glycosaminoglycan in articular cartilage, chondroitin 6-sulfate has a higher concentration in mature cartilage, and chondroitin 4-sulfate is more in immature cartilage. Keratan sulfate is more found in mature cartilage.

The main proteoglycans found in articular cartilage include aggrecan, biglycan, decorin, and fibromodulin. Type IX collagen has a glycosaminoglycan component and is therefore considered a proteoglycan. Aggrecan is composed of a core protein, more than 100 chondroitin sulfate chains, and 20–50 keratan sulfate chains and serves to resist strain caused by loads in articular cartilage. Decorin, biglycan and fibromodulin have one, two, and several dermatan sulfate chains, respectively [15]. Aggrecan molecules occupy most of the space between the fibrous sources of cartilage matrix, accounting for about 90% of proteoglycan mass, whereas large nonaggregated proteoglycan accounts for less than about 10% and small nonaggregated proteoglycan occupies about 3%.

The link protein stabilizes the linkage between hyaluronic acid and aggrecan [17]. The anchor proteoglycan helps to form aggregates in the matrix and prevents displacement when the tissue is deformed. By forming this complex structure, the proteoglycan cannot move freely within the articular cartilage matrix.

The small nonaggregated proteoglycan has a shorter core protein than aggrecan, and unlike aggrecan, it neither fills the part of the tissue nor directly engages in the mechanical properties of the tissue. Instead, it may combine with other macromolecules to affect cell function. Decorin and fibromodulin combine with type II collagen to stabilize and organize the type II collagen meshwork. Biglycans are concentrated in the pericellular matrix and are known to interact with type VI collagen. Lubricin, a lubricating glycoprotein on the surface of articular cartilage, contributes to low-friction properties and boundary lubrication of cartilage. Chondrocalcin has an affinity for hydroxyapatite and may be involved in the calcification of the articular cartilage matrix. In addition, these small proteoglycans can combine with the transforming growth factor-ß to limit the healing of cartilage and regulate the production of degrading enzymes.

Non-Collagenous Proteins and Glycoproteins

Non-collagenous proteins do not contribute to the mechanical properties of cartilage tissue and are known to affect cell function by attaching to other molecules. Some of these may help maintain and organize the macromolecular structure of the cartilage matrix. The collagen-binding chondrocyte surface protein, anchorin CII is thought to be a receptor that secures chondrocyte to matrix collagen fibrils and transmits pressure signals to chondrocytes. Cartilage oligomeric protein is mainly distributed in the territorial matrix and has the ability to bind to chondrocytes. Other non-collagenous proteins, such as fibronectin and tenascin, also appear in cartilage, but their functions are not yet known.

2.1.2 Zones of Articular Cartilage

Depending on its depth and the shape of the chondrocyte and matrix, the articular cartilage is be divided into four zones from the articular surface to the subchondral bone: superficial zone, middle zone, deep zone and calcified cartilage zone (Fig. 2.2a, b). Although the boundary of each zone cannot be clearly distinguished, the shape and amount of chondrocytes in each zone, the diameter and arrangement of collagen fibrils, and the content of proteoglycan and water are different. In addition, the metabolic and biosynthetic activity is also different for each zone.

2.1.2.1 Superficial Zone

The superficial zone has the thinnest thickness of the articular cartilage and has special mechanical and biological properties due to its unique structure and composition. This zone is made up of two collagen layers. The outermost layer covering the joint surface is a sheet of fine fibrils, with few polysaccharides and no cells. Beneath this outer layer, there are chondrocytes of a flat ellipsoid shape similar to fibroblasts, arranged parallel to the joint surface. Chondrocytes synthesize a matrix rich in collagen and low in proteoglycan relative to other cartilage zones. The collagen fibrils make "cartilage skin," limiting the influx of harmful substances and the outflow of important components. Dense mats made of collagen fibrils arranged parallel to the joint surface are known to not only increase tensile stiffness and strength but also act to resist the compressive forces generated by joint motion. Alteration of tissues denatures the mechanical properties of the tissues and contributes to the development of osteoarthritis [18]. The injury of the superficial zone releases substances that stimulate the immune or inflammatory response by denaturing the mechanical properties along with the structure of the articular cartilage.

2.1.2.2 Middle or Transitional Zone

The shape and matrix composition of middle zone are intermediate between the superficial zone and the deep zone. In general, the volume is several times larger than the superficial zone, and chondrocytes contain higher concentrations of biosynthetic organelles than the superficial zone. Chondrocytes have a more spheroidal shape, contain less water and collagen and contain more proteoglycan than the superficial zone matrix, and synthesize large-diameter collagen fibrils.

2.1.2.3 Deep or Radial Zone

Chondrocytes in the deep zone have a spheroidal shape and are mostly arranged in columns, and the cell volume is the lowest. Compared to other zones, the proteoglycan content is high, the water content is lowest, and the collagen fibrils have the largest diameter. Collagen fibrils pass through the tidemark and are also known to resist shear stress because they are arranged perpendicular to the joint surface. When observed with an optical microscope, a blue thin line of wave-shaped basophilic is observed between the deep zone and the

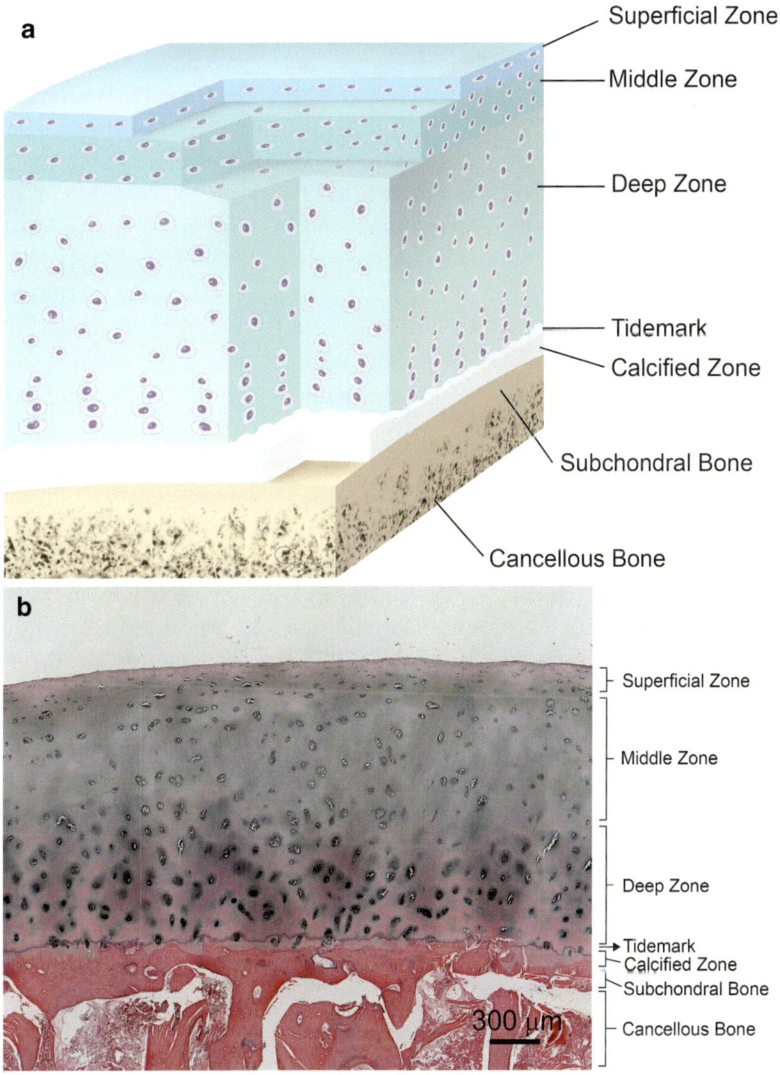

Fig. 2.2 General structure of articular cartilage. Depending on its depth and the shape of the chondrocyte and matrix, the articular cartilage is be divided into four zones from the articular surface to the subchondral bone: superficial zone, middle zone, deep zone and calcified cartilage zone (**a**) schematic, cross-sectional diagram. (**b**) histologic section (H & E staining ×300) Photograph courtesy from Professor Yang YI

calcified cartilage layer, which is called the tidemark, which corresponds to the boundary between the non-calcified cartilage and the calcified cartilage, and the number of tidemark increases with age. The small gaps in the tidemark probably provide a pathway for the passage of nutrients [19].

2.1.2.4 Calcified Cartilage Zone

The calcified cartilage zone is located between the subchondral bone and the deep zone of the articular cartilage and is known to have low metabolic activity and little function. However, another study suggests that it affects the development of osteoarthritis [20].

2.1.2.5 Matrix Regions

Depending on the distance from chondrocytes, the matrix regions can be divided into three regions, consisting of a pericellular matrix, a territorial matrix, and an interterritorial matrix from the side close to the cell [11]. In each region, the content of collagen, proteoglycan, and other substances constituting the matrix is different, and the diameter and composition of collagen fibrils are different. The pericellular matrix is a thin area that surrounds chondrocytes, consisting mainly of non-collagenous proteins such as proteoglycan and anchorin CII, with little collagen found. The territorial matrix is the area surrounding the pericellular matrix, where thin collagen forms a cross-network. The pericellular matrix and territorial matrix attach the macromolecules of the matrix to chondrocytes, prevent damage to chondrocytes when a load is applied to the cartilage tissue, and also act to transmit mechanical signals to chondrocytes when the matrix is deformed. The interterritorial matrix refers to the area between the territorial matrices, has large collagens and a large amount of proteoglycans, and is responsible for most of the mechanical properties of cartilage tissue.

2.1.3 Metabolism

Chondrocytes produce collagen fibrils, hyaluronic acid and proteoglycans, and at the same time release proteases and protease inhibitors to maintain articular cartilage and maintain homeostasis of the matrix. Chondrocytes are affected by changes in growth factors, cytokine and mechanical load, and cartilage growth factors such as IGF-1 (insulin-like growth factor-1), TGF-β (transforming growth factor-β), and bFGF (basic fibroblast growth factor) stimulate matrix production to form aggrecan and collagen fibrils to maintain normal joints [21]. IGF-1 is a substance that stimulates mitosis of chondrocyte and matrix production. As age increases, plasma concentrations decrease, and the response of IGF-1 to chondrocyte decreases, leading to a decrease in the ability to maintain articular cartilage. TGF-β inhibits the degeneration of the matrix by promoting the production of proteoglycans and collagen fibrils, antagonizing the catabolic effect of IL-1 (interleukin-1), and increasing the expression of TIMPs (tissue inhibitor of metalloproteinases) in chondrocytes. In addition, bFGF induces mitosis in chondrocytes and acts in the early stages of recovery in the event of damage to the superficial zone of cartilage. Degeneration of proteoglycan is caused by mononuclear cells in the synovial membrane or the formation of collagenase, protease, and PGE2 (Prostaglandin E2) by IL-1 produced by chondrocytes [5]. MMPs (Matrix metalloproteinases) are enzymes involved in the degeneration of matrix macromolecules in articular cartilage, including collagenase, stromelysin, and gelatinase. MMPs are substances produced by chondrocytes, synovial fibroblasts, and infiltrated leukocytes in response to inflammatory mediators, and their action is inhibited by TIMPs in vivo (Fig. 2.3). Proinflammatory cytokines affecting articular cartilage include IL-1, TNF-α (tumor necrosis factor-alpha), and TNF-β (tumor necrosis factor-beta), and they degrade the matrix through various pathways. In chondrocytes, IL-1 mainly stimulates collagenase and stromelysin to inhibit the production of type II collagen fibrils and proteoglycans. Collagenase degrades native helical collagen fibrils, and stromelysin degrades the protein core of aggrecan. IL-1 is inhibited by TIMPs induced by TGF-β and TIMPs prevent matrix degradation. In addition, IL-1 inhibits the growth stimulation effect of TGF-β and also stimulates the production of PGE 2. TNF-α is a proinflammatory cytokine that has a matrix-degrading effect similar to IL-1 but has less effect on articular cartilage cells than IL-1. TNF-α and TNF-β induce collagenase and PGE2 in synovial cells. On the other hand, IL-4 inhibits the production of TNF-α and IL-1 and PGE2, and the IL-6 group (IL-6, IL-11, and leukemia inhibitor factor) is known as an anti-inflammatory cytokines that protect cartilage by promoting the synthesis of TIMPs.

In normal joints, the degradation and synthesis of cartilage matrix by chondrocytes is well coordinated by cytokines, growth factors and mechanical stimulation. If the balance of degradation and synthesis of the matrix is broken and anabolic activity is less than the catabolic activity, the local recovery response becomes insufficient, resulting in gradual loss of articular cartilage, eventually leading to degenerative arthritis.

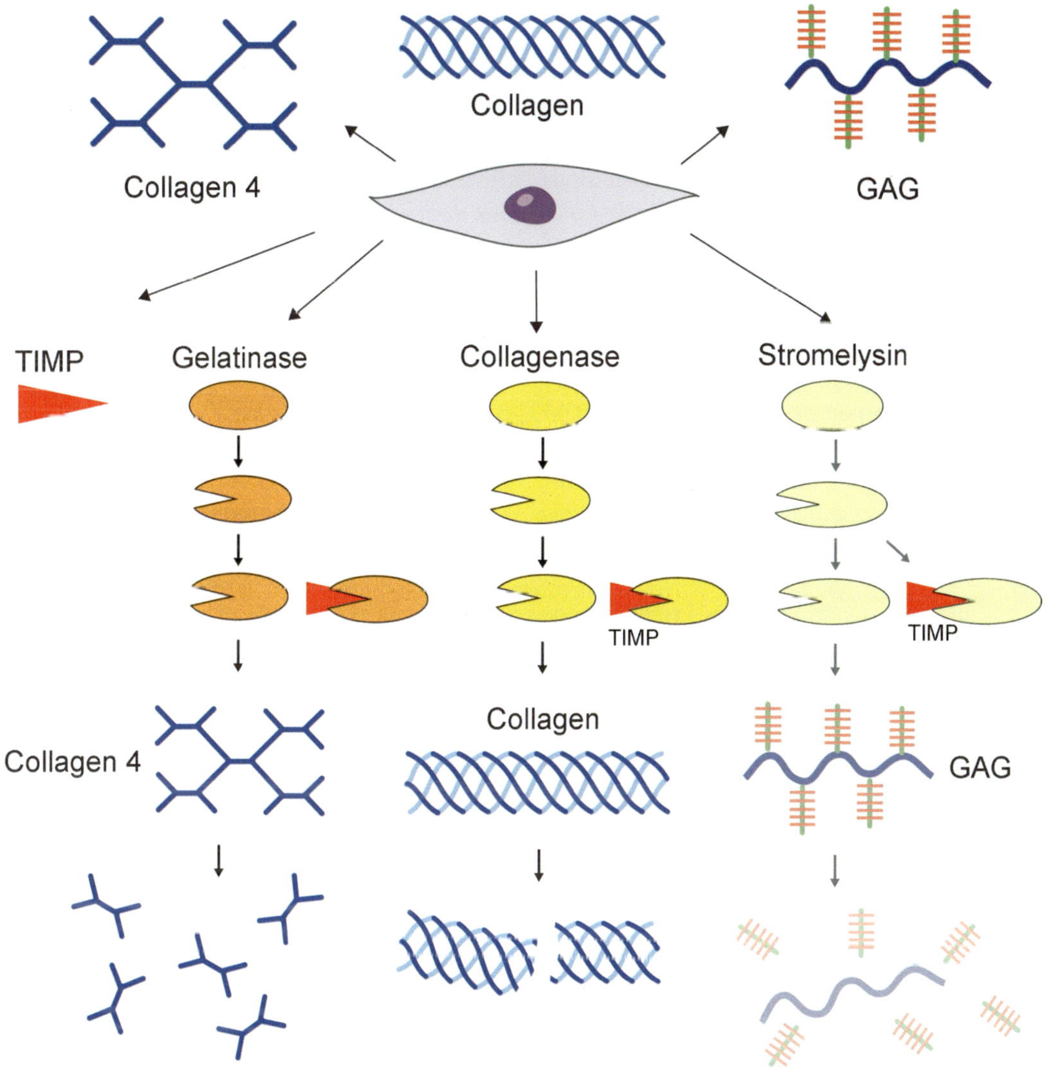

Fig. 2.3 Matrix metalloproteinases, including collagenase, stromelysin, and gelatinase, are involved in the degeneration of matrix macromolecules in articular cartilage. *TIMP* tissue inhibitor metalloproteinase, *GAG* glycosaminoglycan

2.1.4 Biomechanical Function

Articular cartilage is subject to repetitive and periodic loads. Cartilage has a relatively large deformation and fatigue strength and also has high elasticity, so the resistance to the tensile force applied to the cartilage is mainly obtained by collagen, while the resistance to the compressive force is a proteoglycan that regulates the amount and flow of water in the matrix. The superficial zone at the outermost part of the articular cartilage is resistant to shearing force.

The cartilage reacts differently depending on the speed of the load applied. If the load is applied to the joint for only a short time, the articular cartilage reacts like an elastic solid, returning to its original shape, and deformed for a while until the load disappears, and then returns to its original shape. On the other hand, if the load is slowly applied to the joint for a long time, the articular cartilage reacts like a viscoelastic solid and compresses as the extracellular matrix slowly deforms (creep phenomenon), and at this time, the water in the gap in the matrix escapes into the joint cavity. That is, the biomechanical properties of articular cartilage are biphasic and consist of a solid phase and a fluid phase. In addition, articular cartilage has a viscoelastic property and shows biphasic creep response and biphasic stress relaxation response [22]. During this process, the charge density of the proteoglycans in the cartilage increases and adheres to each other, at this time, the charges inherent in the proteoglycans push each other away, and this force contributes to the cartilage returning to its original shape after the load on the cartilage disappears. During the load, the squeezed liquid was filtered by the collagenous network and contained little proteoglycan. That is, the water in the synovial fluid enters the interstices of the cartilage matrix again and is rehydrated to recover the shape of the cartilage. During this process, various nutrients in synovial fluid are introduced into the cartilage, and waste products in the cartilage matrix are discharged into the synovial fluid, thereby providing the nutrient supply of chondrocytes.

The friction coefficient of articular cartilage is very low, 0.002 to 0.01, which is significantly lower than that of any artificial joint. Mechanisms that can lower the friction coefficient of cartilage include boundary lubrication and fluid film lubrication. Boundary lubrication is the sliding of the cartilage surface by coating the cartilage surface with a micromolecular layer, involving chemicals in low shear strength joints such as lubricin and hyaluronate-protein complex, especially lubricin is a low-molecular glycoprotein that contains hyaluronic acid and glycoproteins and has a very important lubricating action [23].

The elasticity of cartilage is very high, and the modulus of elasticity is 10^8–10^6 dyne/cm^2. The elastic modulus of the articular cartilage increases when the load is instantaneously applied in a short period of time but decreases when the load is slowly applied over a long period of time. In some cases, cartilage may completely lose elasticity. That is, when a periodic load is applied or a constant load is continuously applied for a long time, the cartilage gradually damaged. Due to the different physical properties in response to various loads, cartilage wear due to the compressive force and shear force generated during weight-bearing load can be reduced, and the joints can be preserved for a long time.

The tension depends on the location from the surface of the articular cartilage and is the strongest in the superficial zone. The mechanical load has an important effect on the metabolism of chondrocytes. When joint motion is achieved under normal load, the production of matrix proteoglycan is promoted. However, when the load is reduced, or the joint is fixed, the production of proteoglycan is reduced, and catabolism is promoted and causes the chondromalacia. On the other hand, when subjected to an excessive load, chondrocytes stop producing matrix and undergo degenerative changes.

2.1.5 Articular Cartilage Degeneration and Osteoarthritis

In the event of degenerative changes or injuries to the cartilage tissue, intrinsic restoration reactions, such as increased matrix synthesis and proliferation of chondrocytes, are observed but are so insignificant that even a very small damage is insufficient to heal. Chondrocytes perform anabolic and catabolic effects simultaneously and maintain the homeostasis of the extracellular matrix in the cartilage. Osteoarthritis is the case when the homeostasis is destroyed for any reason, and catabolic activity occurs more than anabolic activity. In osteoarthritis, there are several theories about changes in chondrocytes. There are theories that chondrocytes are dedifferentiated and that chondrocytes further differentiate and turn into thickened chondrocytes similar to chondrocytes in the growth plate. There is also the theory that chondrocytes dedifferentiate into chondroprogenitor cells, but no theory is certain.

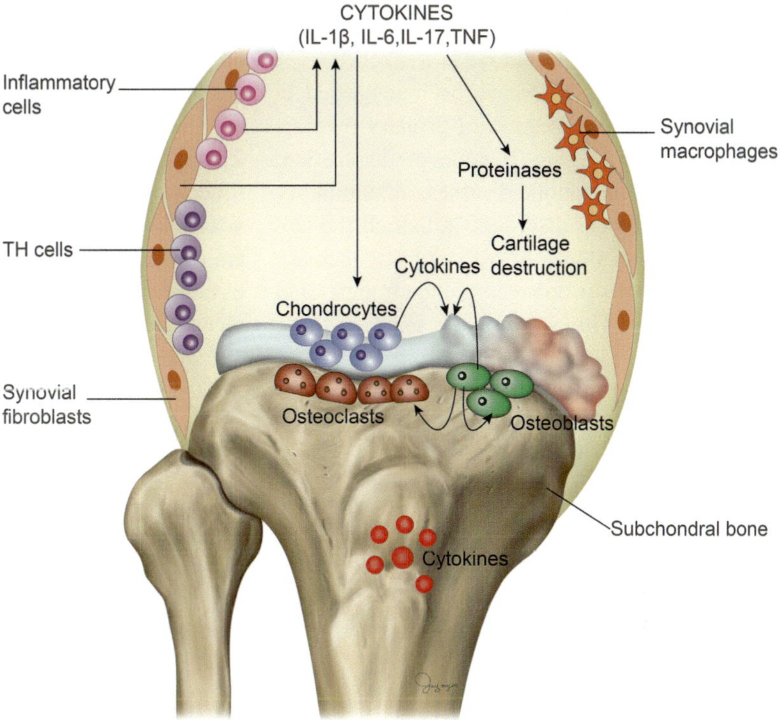

Fig. 2.4 Cells and various factors involved in the degradation of the matrix. As osteoarthritis progresses, the response of chondrocytes decreases and degradative enzymes are continuously released, leading to the destruction of the extracellular matrix. *IL* interleukin, *TNF* tumor necrosis factor, *TH* T helper

In the early stage osteoarthritis, chondrocytes are activated, increasing the type II collagen synthesis rate and proteoglycan, and consequently the extracellular matrix water. In addition, as the synthesis of most extracellular matrix molecules increases, the synthesis of degradative enzymes also increases, and cells are stimulated to divide. As osteoarthritis progresses, the response of chondrocytes decreases and degradative enzymes are continuously released, leading to the destruction of the extracellular matrix (Fig. 2.4). In osteoarthritis, various anabolic cytokines such as TGF, bone morphogenetic protein, and IGF-1 stimulate synthesis, and catabolism by inflammatory cytokines such as TNF-α and IL-1 occurs together. In the early stages of osteoarthritis, both synthesis and modification increase, and the synthesis of catabolic and anabolic cytokines activates chondrocytes, but as osteoarthritis progresses, the balance of matrix synthesis and destruction is disrupted, and the loss of extracellular matrix gradually increases. TNF-α and IL-1 are mainly involved in the catabolism of the extracellular matrix, which strongly increases the expression of metalloproteinase to promote protein degradation and inhibit the biosynthesis of the cartilage matrix. Collagen degradative enzymes MMP13 and stromelysin are known to play important roles in the degradation of collagen in osteoarthritis [24].

A significant amount of nitric oxide and nitric oxide synthase are synthesized in activated chondrocytes. The role of nitric oxide in osteoarthritis is not yet fully understood, but it is known to inhibit the synthesis of proteoglycan and is also involved in cell death. These growth factors and cytokines are produced by synovial cells, chondrocytes, and osteocytes that form joints. That is, osteoarthritis is an organ disease involving not only cartilage but also synovial and subchondral bones. In osteoarthritis, the balance between collagen and aggrecan synthesis is broken because collagen type II synthesis is significantly increased compared to normal cartilage. In addition, type X collagen not found in normal adult cartilage is found in osteoarthritis. As a result, cartilage wear increases on the surface of the cartilage, and the tidemark rises due to the increase in ossification in the deep zone, and the thickness of the cartilage gradually decreases. Elasticity decreases in the cartilage itself, and the force withstanding the physical load is weakened.

A number of factors have been suggested in relation to the pathogenesis of primary osteoarthritis, including aging, genetic predisposition, endocrine, and metabolic diseases, inflammatory and immunological disorders. Although the frequency and prevalence of osteoarthritis increase rapidly after age 40, changes in chondrocytes and matrix due to aging are not the same as those caused by osteoarthritis. However, if the ability of chondrocytes to maintain and recover tissue is lost due to aging, the risk of joint degeneration increases. Recent studies strongly support the opinion that inflammatory active factors, mainly of the interleukin, are active substances that cause cartilage injury [25]. The cause of inflammation of the synovial membrane in osteoarthritis is not clear, but it is presumed to occur in substances secreted from injured cartilage.

2.1.6 Injury and Healing Response

The injury to the articular surface can be divided into contusion, articular cartilage injury, and osteochondral injury according to the type of injured tissue and the healing response.

2.1.6.1 Contusion

Excessive trauma or repetitive load of a single impact that does not cause any visual damage to the articular surface results in an abnormality of the cartilage matrix resulting in a decrease in proteoglycan, an increase in water content, and destruction of the collagenous network [26]. In addition, the contusion of the joint surface causes cell death of the chondrocyte and thickens the tidemark. The chondrocytes recover the matrix even if limited by synthesizing new substances in response to changes in the surrounding cartilage matrix. However, if there is a lot of loss of the matrix, the elasticity of the matrix will be weakened, making joint damage easily caused by continuous loads. In addition, when the tidemark is thickened, the calcified cartilage zone is thickened, which increases the stiffness of the contact surface of the cartilage and bone and gradually precipitates degenerative changes in the articular cartilage.

2.1.6.2 Articular Cartilage Injury

Since cartilage tissue has no distribution of blood vessels and the ability of chondrocytes to regenerate is limited, there is little recovery of cartilage tissue if there is gross damage to the articular surfaces confined to the cartilage, and ultimately, articular cartilage injury can proceed to the calcified cartilage zone. Chondrocytes proliferate in response to injury to the cartilage matrix and increase the synthesis of the cartilage matrix. However, it is not enough to fill the damaged parts [27]. In addition, chondrocytes are almost impossible to move on their own because they are trapped in a solid extracellular matrix, and since there are no blood vessels or lymphatic tissues, they cannot move to the injured site and compensate for the cell deficit. The superficial zone of the cartilage is a very dense tissue that protects the cartilage matrix from inflammatory cells and enzymes in the joint. However, when a damaged cartilage fragment comes off, the cartilage is exposed to a deeper area, exacerbating the damage to the cartilage matrix. It causes an inflammatory reaction of the synovial membrane, causing degenerative changes in the joint surface.

2.1.6.3 Osteochondral Injury

When an injury to the joint surface is applied to the bone and bleeding occurs in the subchondral bone, a fibrin clot is formed, and regeneration is caused by an inflammatory reaction. Immediately after injury, blood from the subchondral bone creates a hematoma and temporarily fills the damaged area, forming fibrin clots within the hematoma and freeing vasoactive mediators, growth factors, or cytokine from platelets [28]. These growth factors are known to promote the proliferation of blood vessels to the site of injury, induce undifferentiated cells into fibrin clots, and affect cell proliferation and synthesis. After about 6 to 8 weeks after injury, cells similar to chondrocytes are observed at the site of cartilage damage, a matrix composed of type II collagen and proteoglycan, and immature bone and fibrous tissue are observed at the site of bone damage. The regenerated cartilage tissue shows an intermediate form of hyaline cartilage and fibrous cartilage and does not show the structure of normal articular cartilage. In most of the regenerated tissue, the amount of proteoglycan decreases throughout the year, collagen increases, and cells similar to chondrocytes gradually disappear. These changes reduce the physical strength and increase the permeability of cartilage tissue, causing degenerative changes of cartilage by repeated loads.

2.1.7 Summary

Articular cartilage consists of highly specialized connective tissue. The main function of the articular cartilage is to provide a lubricated surface for smoothing the joints and to facilitate the transfer of loads with low coefficients of friction. Chondrocytes form a matrix macromolecular framework composed of collagens, proteoglycans, and non-collagenous proteins. The matrix protects chondrocytes from damage caused by normal joint movement and determines the shape and concentration of molecules that move into the cells. The mechanical properties of articular cartilage depend on the interaction of these fluids and solid components. Aging causes changes in matrix composition and chondrocyte activity. These changes increase the likelihood of cartilage degeneration. The unique and complex structure of articular cartilage makes the treatment and recovery of cartilage challenge.

2.2 Meniscus

2.2.1 Gross Anatomy

The meniscus is a C-shaped or semi-circular fibrous cartilage structure located between the femoral condyle and tibial plateau and attached to the anterior and posterior area of the tibial plateau, covering the outer 1/3–1/2 of the tibial articular surface. The length of each meniscus is about 110 mm, and the thickness of the meniscus becomes thinner and thinner toward the center. The meniscus has important functions such as weight transfer, load distribution, cartilage protection, joint stability and lubrication.

2.2.1.1 Medial Meniscus

The medial meniscus is a 'C' type with a larger radius than the lateral one, and the width of the posterior horn is larger than that of the anterior horn (Fig. 2.5). The attachment of the anterior horn of the medial meniscus varies, which is classified into four types through anatomical studies [29]. Even though 14% of the cadaveric knees show no bony attachments, however, the anterior horn of the medial meniscus attaches firmly to the bone in most cases. The anterior horn of the medial meniscus is connected to the anterior horn of the lateral meniscus through the anterior intermeniscal ligament. The posterior horn of the medial meniscus is attached to the area between the medial tibial spine and the tibial insertion of the posterior cruciate ligament. The anterior horn of the medial meniscus had the widest area (61.4 mm^2), and the posterior horn of the lateral meniscus had the narrowest area (28.5 mm^2) [30]. Except for the bony attachment of the medial meniscus, the rest part strongly attaches to the joint capsule and the deep medial collateral ligament. The attachment of the tibial side of the medial meniscus is called the coronary ligament.

2.2.1.2 Lateral Meniscus

The lateral meniscus has almost a semi-circular shape. The proportion of the lateral meniscus in the tibial surface area is greater than that of the medial meniscus. The distance between the anterior and posterior horn of the lateral meniscus is much closer than the medial meniscus. The attachment of the anterior horn of the lateral meniscus is close to the tibial insertion of the anterior cruciate ligament, serving as a landmark in the reconstruction of the anterior cruciate ligament. The popliteus tendon passes through the popliteal hiatus in the lateral meniscus (Fig. 2.6). The popliteal hiatus does not have a capsular

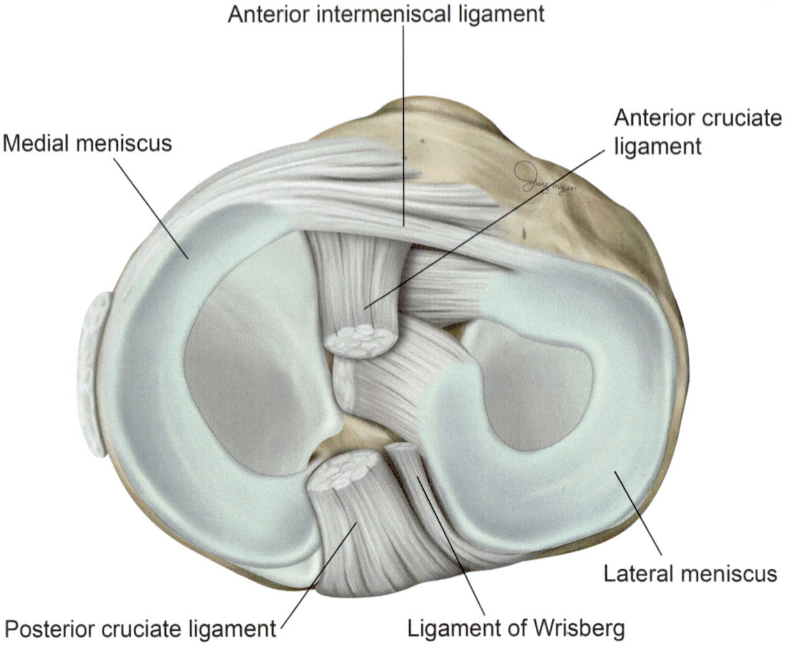

Fig. 2.5 Axial view of the left tibial plateau. The medial meniscus is a "C" type with a larger radius than the lateral one, and the lateral meniscus has almost a semi-circular shape

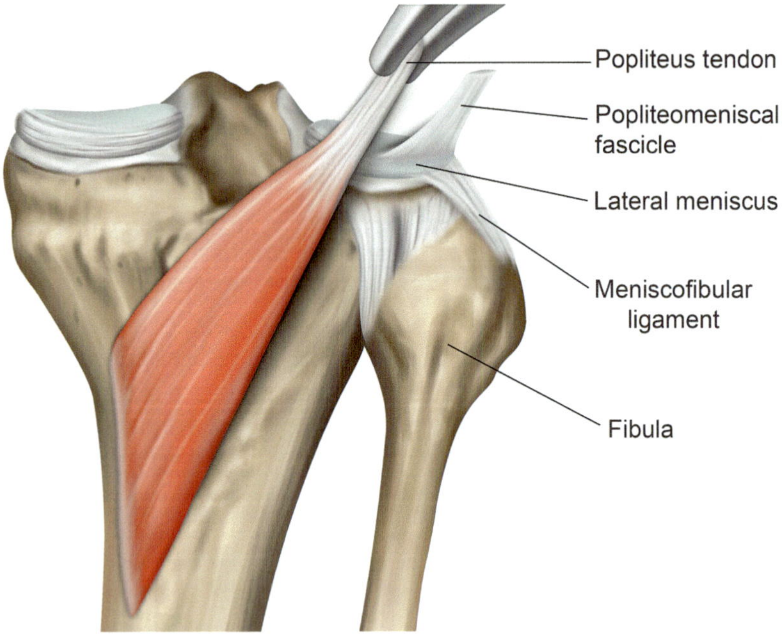

Fig. 2.6 Structure of posterolateral knee joint. The popliteomeniscal fascicle that holds the posterior horn of the LM in place plays an important role in the stability of the lateral meniscus

attachment, so the healing of the lateral meniscus is hardly achieved in this area. The popliteomeniscal fascicle plays an important role in the stability of the lateral meniscus. A damage to the popliteomeniscal fascicles increases the movement in the popliteal hiatus, causing excessive movement of the posterior horn of the lateral meniscus [31].

2.2.1.3 Discoid Meniscus

The congenital anomaly of the meniscus is the discoid meniscus. This anomaly had been known as a result of the failure of the discoid meniscus to evolve into semi-circular structure during the fetal period. It is very difficult to determine the prevalence of discoid meniscus. According to Western literature, the prevalence rate of the discoid lateral meniscus is reported from 2.5% to 7% and is the mostly incomplete type [32]. The discoid meniscus is more common on the lateral than on the medial side, and both sides of the discoid meniscus at the same knee is very rarely observed. In the far eastern countries, the prevalence rate is known to be higher.

2.2.1.4 Tibial Insertional Ligaments

The circumferential collagen fiber in the body of the meniscus becomes the anterior and posterior attachment ligaments connected to the subchondral bone of the tibia (Fig. 2.7). The anterior attachment ligament of the medial meniscus is fan-shaped and attaches to the intercondylar fossa [30]. This is about 6–7 mm anterior of the tibial insertion of the anterior cruciate ligament. The posterior horn of the medial meniscus attaches to the intercondylar fossa between the posterior attachment of the lateral meniscus and the tibial insertion of the posterior cruciate ligament. The anterior attachment ligament of the lateral meniscus inserts to the anterior intercondylar fossa of the tibia between the anterior horn of the medial meniscus and the tibial insertion of the anterior cruciate ligament. The posterior attachment ligament of the lateral meniscus is located between the lateral tibial eminence and the posterior attachment of the medial meniscus. The attachment ligament has fibrocartilagenic transition zones that allow for changes in stiffness between ligaments and osseous tissues. This can reduce the concentration of stress and reduce the risk of fatigue failure during knee exercises. The functional importance of the attachment ligaments was confirmed through the study of rabbits. The anterior or posterior attachment ligament of the rabbit meniscus was cut and was observed six and twelve weeks later. As a result, changes in bone and cartilage similar to those changes observed after total meniscectomy were shown [33].

2.2.1.5 Intermeniscal Ligaments

The anterior intermeniscal ligament are well known as the transverse geniculate ligament that connect the anterior horn of the medial and lat-

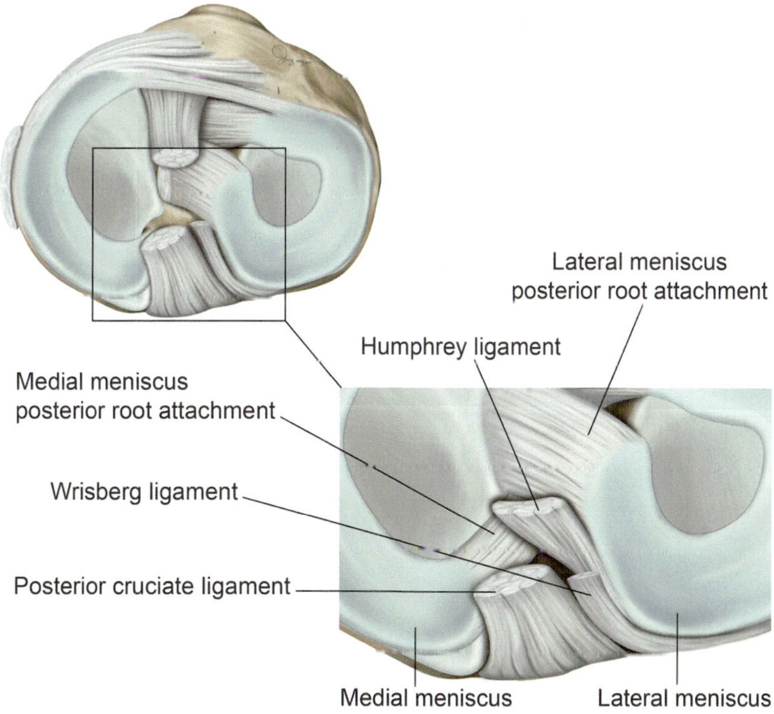

Fig. 2.7 Close look into the area of the meniscal posterior root. There are two ligaments connecting from the posterior horn of the lateral meniscus to the lateral surface of the medial femoral condyle, passing through the intercondylar notch. The Humphrey ligament passes in front of the posterior cruciate ligament, and the Wrisberg ligament passes behind the posterior cruciate ligament

eral meniscus (Fig. 2.5). The incidence of the ligament was about 64%–94% of the cadaveric knees [34]. The dimension of the anterior intermeniscal ligament is 33 mm length, 3.3 mm thickness for middle parts, and classified into three types. Type 1 (46%) is the form of a direct connection between the medial and the lateral meniscus that is a true intermeniscal ligament, and Type 2 (26%) is the form of the anterior horn of the medial meniscus that passes through the joint capsule and connects to the that of the lateral meniscus. Type 3 (12%) is when the major ligaments are attached only to the anterior joint capsule [34]. The functional relevance of ligaments has not been well studied, but it is thought to play a role in the movement of the meniscus during internal and external rotation of the tibia.

2.2.1.6 Meniscofemoral Ligaments

There are two ligaments connecting from the posterior horn of the lateral meniscus to the lateral surface of the medial femoral condyle, passing through the intercondylar notch. This is called the meniscofemoral ligament (Fig. 2.8). The anterior meniscofemoral ligament passes in front of the posterior cruciate ligament and is called the Humphrey ligament. The posterior meniscofemoral ligament passes behind the posterior cruciate ligament and is called the Wrisberg ligament. The Humphrey ligament was found in 50% and the Wrisberg ligament in 76% of the 92 cadaveric knees [35]. The size of the Humphrey ligament and the Wrisberg ligament was one-third, one-half of the posterior cruciate ligament, respectively. These have a mechanical property comparable to the posterior bundle of the posterior cruciate ligament and serve as secondary restraints preventing the posterior translation of the tibia [36]. The anterior meniscofemoral ligament has also been identified, a structure that connects the anterior horn of the medial or lateral meniscus in the intercondylar notch anterior to the anterior cruciate ligament. The anteromedial meniscofemoral ligament begins at the anterior horn of the medial meniscus, and the anterolateral meniscofemoral ligament starts at the anterior horn of the lateral meniscus, which was found in 15% of the 60 cadaveric knee joint [37].

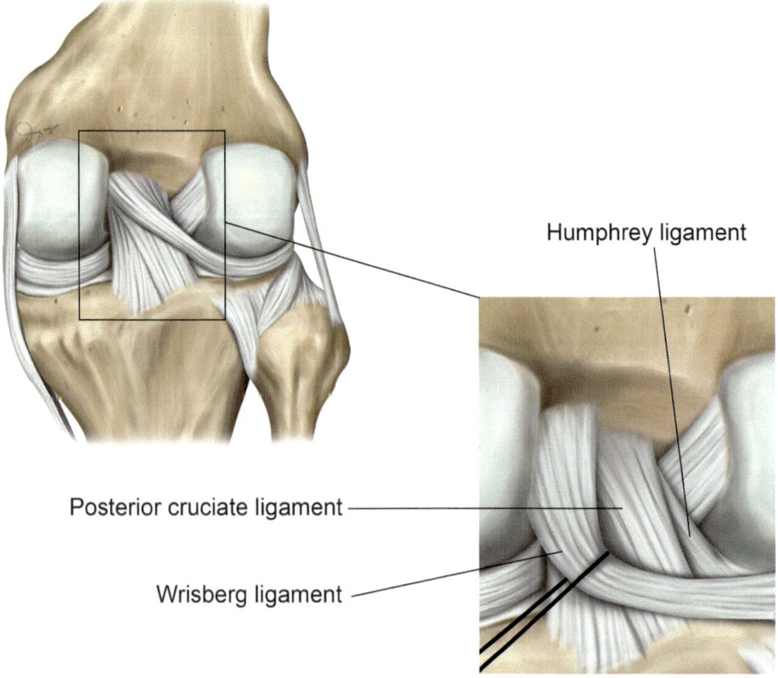

Fig. 2.8 Close look into the posterior aspect of the right knee joint. The size of the Humphrey ligament and the Wrisberg ligament was one-third, one-half of the posterior cruciate ligament, respectively

2.2.2 Biochemical Composition

The normal meniscus consists of 72% water, 22% collagen, 0.8% glycosaminoglycan, and 0.12% DNA. When dried, the meniscus of normal adults consists of 78% collagen, 8% non-collagen protein and 1% hexosamine [38]. Histologically, the meniscus is fibrous cartilage, consisting primarily of intertwined networks of collagen fibers connecting cells with the extracellular substrate of proteoglycan and glycoprotein. Ninety percent of collagen in the meniscus is of type I, with the remainder being of type II, III, and IV [39]. The ratio of collagen differs depending on the location of the meniscus in the cow. Except for Type 3 and Type 5 in small quantities, peripheral 2/3 of the meniscus was mostly composed of Type 1 collagen, and central 1/3 composed of Type 2, 60% and Type 1, 40% [40].

2.2.3 Micro-Anatomy

The orientation of collagen fibers in the meniscus is directly related to the function (Fig. 2.9). The direction of the collagen fibers in the meniscus is mainly circumferential to withstand tension, and that collagen fibrils located on the surface and the mid-substance of the meniscus have radial orientation [41]. Circumferential fiber makes the compressive force withhold, and radial fiber holds the circumferential fiber to help prevent the longitudinal tear of the meniscus. Surface fibers have a more dense mesh or irregular shape and are thought to be important for the transmission of shear stress. The meniscus is divided into two differentiated zones: central 2/3 and peripheral 1/3 of the meniscus. The collagen bundles in the central zone primarily have radial orientation, which is parallel to the articular surface, and larger bundles are formed at the peripheral zone, and circumferential orientation [42]. These structural differences make a difference in function, the central zone is optimized for conveying a compressive axial load from the femur to the tibia, and the circumferential fibers of the peripheral zone are suitable for resisting tensile force. Surface collagen fibers have directional properties that are irregularly similar to the hyaline cartilage. The cells of the meniscus are called fibrochondrocytes, because they make a fibrocartilaginous substrate. The fibrochondrocytes are in two forms, the cells on the surface are elliptical or fusiform, and the cells in the deep tissue are

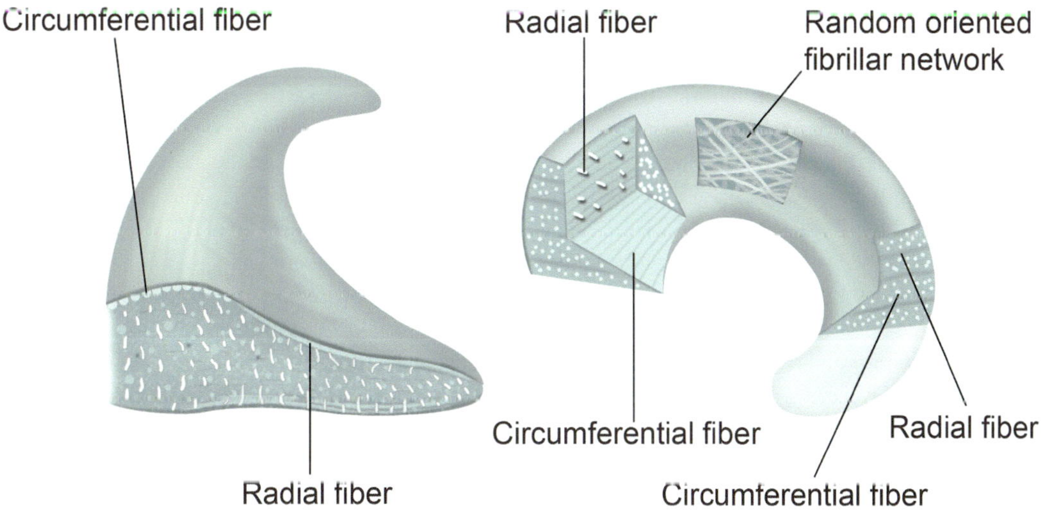

Fig. 2.9 Pattern of collagen fibers within meniscus. (**a**) The meniscus is composed of circumferential, radial fibers and random oriented fibrillar network. (**b**) The circumferential fibers are in the periphery, whereas the radial fibers extend from the circumferential fibers toward the central portion of the meniscus

circular or polygonal. Both of these have properties found in fibroblasts and chondrocytes. Both forms have rich endoplasmic retinacula and Golgi complex, with few mitochondria [43].

2.2.4 Blood Supply and Nerve Distribution

The blood supply of the entire meniscus at birth is abundant. Nine months after birth, central one-third of the meniscus loses almost all blood supply. This decrease in blood supply lasts until around the age of ten, which becomes very similar to adult meniscus [44]. This reduction in blood supply may be due to weight load and knee joint exercise. Only peripheral 10–25 percent of the lateral meniscus and 10–30 percent of the medial meniscus receive the blood supply in the human adult meniscus [45]. This blood supply is from the superior and inferior branches of the medial and lateral genicular arteries. The synovial membrane is briefly extended to the tibial and femoral articular surfaces of the meniscus but does rarely contribute to the blood supply of the meniscus. There is no blood supply of the meniscus in the popliteal hiatus, so the healing capacity at this area is low, and the possibility of re-tear of the lateral meniscus is high. Since the central zone of the meniscus is poorly supplied with blood, most of the nutrient supply is believed to be from the diffusion of joint fluids (Fig. 2.10).

The neural distribution of the meniscus has not yet been clarified, but it is thought that the distribution of nerve elements will usually be similar to the distribution of blood vessels. The joint capsule adjacent to the meniscus had many specialized receptors, such as axon, large bundle of nerves, free nerve endings, complex end bulbs and type 3 Golgi organ. However, this neural distribution did not extend to the meniscus itself [46]. Another study showed that the nerves ran with radial vessels in the peripheral zone of the meniscus, and the neural tissue passes through the peripheral one-third of the meniscus [47]. Accompanying to the blood supply, there are many nerve distributions in the anterior and posterior horn of the meniscus, and unlike other area, an axonal tissue was found even in the central one-third of this area. A study conducted a mapping of the neural sensory distribution of the internal structure of the knee, confirming that it was more painful when the probe was stressed at the peripheral zone rather than at the center [48]. The presence of mechanical receptors in the meniscus shows that they can play a role in the transmission of the efferent nerve of the knee joint. This kind of neural information can be important to the proprioception of the joint.

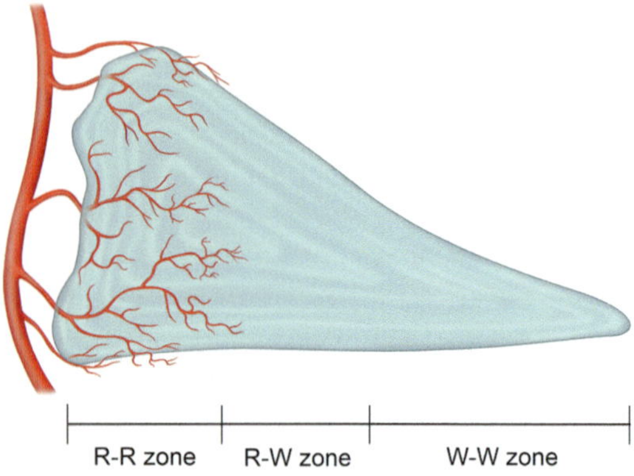

Fig. 2.10 Blood supply to the meniscus is from the superior and inferior branches of the medial and lateral genicular arteries. ***R-R*** red-red, fully within the vascular area; ***R-W*** red-white, at the border of the vascular area; and ***W-W*** white-white, within the avascular area

2.2.5 Biomechanics

Under load, the knee joint is subjected to axial compression. The compressive force is dispersed through the joint contact area, resulting in contact stress. The average contact stress is proportional to the load and inversely proportional to the joint contact area. In other words, the larger the contact area, the less stress the contact area receives. The concave medial tibial plateau is more congruent than the convex lateral tibial plateau. However, the bony structure of the knee joint does not provide the congruency of the joint contact surface. A sufficient joint contact area of the tibial plateau is not provided, and contact stress is not minimized without the meniscus. The meniscus is optimized for transmitting force through the knee joint by increasing the congruency of the articular surface. The average contact stress on the articular surface is reduced with the meniscus. The meniscus has a wedge-shaped cut surface for the femur and can be pushed out of the loading joint, which increases the circumferential tension of the meniscus. The anterior and posterior horn of the meniscus is attached to the tibia through ligamentous structures, which serve to hold the meniscus out to the increased circumferential tension. This is called a hoop stress. Thus, the ability to withstand a compressive load is due to circumferential stiffness resulting from the circumferentially oriented collagen fibers of the meniscus. The medial and lateral meniscus transmits loads from 50% to 70% in extension and increases to 85% in 90° flexion [49]. When the medial meniscus is removed, the contact area with the femur is reduced by 50–70%, and the contact stress is increased to 100%. The contact area will be reduced by 40–50% after the total meniscectomy of the lateral meniscus, increasing the contact stress in the lateral compartment by 200–300% [50]. The congruency of the articular surface with the meniscus plays an important role in the joint lubrication and supplying chondrocyte nutrition. The biomechanical changes that may occur after the meniscectomy affect the biochemical activity of the articular cartilage. Also, the meniscus plays an important role in shock absorption. It is also said that the degree of shock absorption after the meniscectomy is reduced by 20% compared to normal [51]. This shock absorption function is due to viscoelasticity caused by water contents in the meniscus. The meniscus also plays an important role in the stability of the joints. While the medial meniscectomy with intact anterior cruciate ligament does not affect the anterior-posterior translation of the joint, the anterior translation of the tibia increases to 58% in knee 90-degree flexion without the anterior cruciate ligament. The posterior horn of the medial meniscus was the most important structure to resist the anterior translation of the tibia in the knee joint without the anterior cruciate ligament. The medial meniscus at 134 N anterior load in the knee without the anterior cruciate ligament increases the resultant force by up to 52% at full extension and 197% in 60-degree flexions [52]. Similarly, the meniscus also acts as a secondary restraint in the internal and external rotation of the tibia, and the meniscectomy increases the rotation range of 5 degrees [53]. While the central two-thirds of the meniscus plays an important role in maximizing the area of joint contact and shock absorption, continuity of the peripheral zone is essential for the load transmission or joint stability. In a study conducted through MRI, the lateral meniscus at flexion moves posteriorly about 11.2 mm and the medial meniscus about 5.2 mm (Fig. 2.11) [54]. The arcuate ligament connects the lateral meniscus with the popliteus tendon, pulling back the meniscus at the time of internal tibial rotation occurring at the initial flexion of the knee joint. The mobility of the meniscus through the joint motion occurs more in the lateral meniscus.

2.2.6 Healing Response

The most important thing in the healing process of tissue is how easily cells and inflammatory mediators can access the damaged area. The formation of blood clots provides the backbone for substrate formation and becomes the chemical stimulus of the cell component for wound healing [55]. Adult meniscus is only supplied with blood at the peripheral 20–30%. If the meniscus is damaged at the central 70–80%, no blood clots are formed. Therefore, a healing process can take place in the peripheral zone where blood supply is made, but not in the central zone. According to the blood supply, the possibility of healing can be expected by dividing the meniscal tear into red-red, red white, and white white zones. In red-red zone where the blood is well supplied, healing process works well, but most of the meniscal tears occur in the red-white zone, causing the treatment to fall into a poor healing. Therefore, various attempts to obtain a good healing in this area are being made, such as a secure suture fixation, a careful rehabilitation and planned return to activity after surgery, and a biological stimulation using the blood clot. The extracellular matrix multiplication and

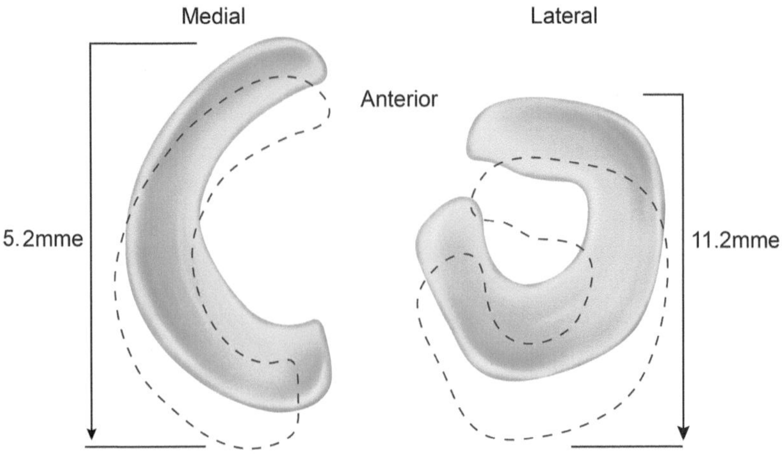

Fig. 2.11 The motion of the menisci during flexion. The lateral meniscus at flexion moves posteriorly about 11.2 mm and the medial meniscus about 5.2 m. ***mme*** mean meniscal excursion

synthesis occur when the meniscal cells are exposed to various healing factors observed in hematoma [43]. To promote healing, various methods are studied, such as fibrin clots, fibrin glue, cell growth factors, formation of vascular access channels, and inducing the synovial membrane bleeding through various methods. The method commonly used at present to provide hematoma to the tear site is stimulating the tear site and its surrounding the synovium by using a rasp or shaver [55]. However, the effect may not be efficient if the blood clots produced by natural bleeding are diluted by synovial fluids. Nevertheless, it is clinically understood that the healing potential is higher if the meniscal repair is performed simultaneously with the anterior cruciate ligament reconstruction than without the anterior cruciate ligament reconstruction. Therefore, sufficient blood clots can help heal. As well as the stability of the joint, the acute stage of the meniscal tear and the young age are considered positive factors for healing. The age-related degenerative changes of the meniscus have a negative effect on healing potential. From the point of view of rehabilitation and healing, the meniscal tear site reacts to normal physiological loading. The immobilization of the knee joint reduces the collagen formation in the meniscus, but the movement tends to prevent the reduction of the collagen formation [56].

References

1. Stockwell RA. The cell density of human articular and costal cartilage. J Anat. 1967;101(Pt 4):753–63.
2. Stockwell RA. Chondrocytes. J Clin Pathol Suppl (R Coll Pathol). 1978;12:7–13.
3. Buckwalter JA, Mankin HJ, Grodzinsky AJ. Articular cartilage and osteoarthritis. Instr Course Lect. 2005;54:465–80.
4. Aydelotte MB, Greenhill RR, Kuettner KE. Differences between sub-populations of cultured bovine articular chondrocytes. II. Proteoglycan metabolism. Connect Tissue Res. 1988;18(3):223–34.
5. Guerne PA, Blanco F, Kaelin A, Desgeorges A, Lotz M. Growth factor responsiveness of human articular chondrocytes in aging and development. Arthritis Rheum. 1995;38(7):960–8.
6. Martin JA, Buckwalter JA. Articular cartilage aging and degeneration. Sports Med Arthrosc Rev. 1996;4(3):263–75.
7. Martin JA, Ellerbroek SM, Buckwalter JA. Age-related decline in chondrocyte response to insulin-like growth factor-I: the role of growth factor binding proteins. J Orthop Res. 1997;15(4):491–8.
8. Meachim G. Effect of age on the thickness of adult articular cartilage at he shoulder joint. Ann Rheum Dis. 1971;30(1):43–6.
9. Gurr E, Mohr W, Pallasch G. Proteoglycans from human articular cartilage: the effect of joint location on the structure. J Clin Chem Clin Biochem. 1985;23(12):811–9.
10. Mow VC, Ratcliffe A, Poole AR. Cartilage and diarthrodial joints as paradigms for hierarchical materials and structures. Biomaterials. 1992;13(2):67–97.
11. Buckwalter JA, Rosenberg LA, Hunziker EB, et al. Articular cartilage: composition, structure, response to injury, and methods of facilitation repair. In: Ewing JW, editor. Articular cartilage and knee joint function:

basic science and arthroscopy. New York, NY: Raven Press; 1990. p. 19–56.
12. Sandell LJ. Molecular biology of collagens in normal and osteoarthritic cartilage. In: Kuettner KE, Goldberg VM, editors. Osteoarthritic disorders. Rosemont, IL: American Academy of Orthopaedic Surgeons; 1995. p. 131–46.
13. Marcelino J, McDevitt CA. Attachment of articular cartilage chondrocytes to the tissue form of type VI collagen. Biochem Biophys Acta. 1995;1249:180–8.
14. Schmid TM, Linsenmayer TF. Immunohistochemical localization of short chain cartilage collagen (type X) in avian tissues. J Cell Biol. 1985;100(2):598–605.
15. Roughley PJ, Lee ER. Cartilage proteoglycans: structure and potential functions. Microsc Res Tech. 1994;28:385–97.
16. Bayliss MT, Venn M, Maroudas A, Ali SY. Structure of proteoglycans from different layers of human articular cartilage. Biochem J. 1983;209(2):387–400.
17. Tang LH, Buckwalter JA, Rosenberg LC. The effect of link protein concentration on articular cartilage proteoglycan aggregation. J Orthop Res. 1996;14:334–9.
18. Guilak F, Ratcliffe A, Lane N, Rosenwasser MP, Mow VC. Mechanical and biochemical changes in the superficial zone of articular cartilage in canine experimental osteoarthritis. J Orthop Res. 1994;12(4):474–84.
19. Redler I, Mow VC, Zimny ML, Mansell J. The ultrastructure and biomechanical significance of the tidemark of articular cartilage. Clin Orthop Relat Res. 1975;112:357–62.
20. Oegema TR, Thompson RC. Histopathology and pathobiochemistry of the cartilage-bone interface in osteoarthritis. In: Kuettner KE, Goldberg VM, editors. Osteoarthritic disorders. Rosemont, IL: American Academy of Orthopaedic Surgeons; 1995. p. 205–17.
21. Buckwalter JA, Martin J, Mankin H. Synovial joint degeneration and the syndrome of osteoarthritis. Instr Course Lect. 2000;49:481–9.
22. Mow VC, Rosenwasser M. Articular cartilage: biomechanics. Injury and repair of the musculoskeletal soft tissues 1988:427–463
23. Rhee DK, Marcelino J, Baker M, Gong Y, Smits P, Lefebvre V, et al. The secreted glycoprotein lubricin protects cartilage surfaces and inhibits synovial cell overgrowth. J Clin Invest. 2005;115(3):622–31.
24. Hamerman D. The biology of osteoarthritis. N Engl J Med. 1989;320(20):1322–30.
25. Sokolove J, Lepus CM. Role of inflammation in the pathogenesis of osteoarthritis: latest findings and interpretations. Ther Adv Musculoskelet Dis. 2013;5(2):77–94.
26. Buckwalter JA. Mechanical injuries of articular cartilage. In: Finerman G, editor. Biology and biomechanics of the traumatized synovial joint. Ridge, IL: American Academy of Orthopaedic Surgeons; 1992. p. 83–96.
27. Buckwalter JA. Chondral and osteochondral injuries: mechanisms of injury and repair responses. Oper Tech Orthop. 1997;7(4):263–9.
28. Buckwalter JA, Einhorn TA, Bolander ME. Healing of musculoskeletal tissues. In: Rockwood CA, Green D, editors. Fractures. Philadelphia, PA: Lippincott; 1996. p. 261–304.
29. Berlet GC, Fowler PJ. The anterior horn of the medical meniscus. An anatomic study of its insertion. Am J Sports Med. 1998;26(4):540–3.
30. Johnson DL, Swenson TM, Livesay GA, Aizawa H, Fu FH, Harner CD. Insertion-site anatomy of the human menisci: gross, arthroscopic, and topographical anatomy as a basis for meniscal transplantation. Arthroscopy. 1995;11(4):386–94.
31. Simonian PT, Sussmann PS, van Trommel M, Wickiewicz TL, Warren RF. Popliteomeniscal fasciculi and lateral meniscal stability. Am J Sports Med. 1997;25(6):849–53.
32. Nathan PA, Cole SC. Discoid meniscus. A clinical and pathologic study. Clin Orthop Relat Res. 1969;64:107–13.
33. Sommerlath K, Gillquist J. The effect of a meniscal prosthesis on knee biomechanics and cartilage. An experimental study in rabbits. Am J Sports Med. 1992;20(1):73–81.
34. Nelson EW, LaPrade RF. The anterior intermeniscal ligament of the knee. An anatomic study. Am J Sports Med. 2000;28(1):74–6.
35. Kohn D, Moreno B. Meniscus insertion anatomy as a basis for meniscus replacement: a morphological cadaveric study. Arthroscopy. 1995;11(1):96–103.
36. Gupte CM, Bull AM, Thomas RD, Amis AA. The meniscofemoral ligaments: secondary restraints to the posterior drawer. Analysis of anteroposterior and rotary laxity in the intact and posterior-cruciate-deficient knee. J Bone Joint Surg Br. 2003;85(5):765–73.
37. Wan AC, Felle P. The menisco-femoral ligaments. Clin Anat. 1995;8(5):323–6.
38. Ingman AM, Ghosh P, Taylor TK. Variation of collagenous and non-collagenous proteins of human knee joint menisci with age and degeneration. Gerontologia. 1974;20(4):212–23.
39. Eyre DR, Wu JJ. Collagen of fibrocartilage: a distinctive molecular phenotype in bovine meniscus. FEBS Lett. 1983;158(2):265–70.
40. Cheung HS. Distribution of type I, II, III and V in the pepsin solubilized collagens in bovine menisci. Connect Tissue Res. 1987;16(4):343–56.
41. Bullough PG, Munuera L, Murphy J, Weinstein AM. The strength of the menisci of the knee as it relates to their fine structure. J Bone Joint Surg Br. 1970;52(3):564–7.
42. Beaupre A, Choukroun R, Guidouin R, Garneau R, Gerardin H, Cardou A. Knee menisci. Correlation between microstructure and biomechanics. Clin Orthop Relat Res. 1986;208:72–5.
43. Webber RJ, Harris MG, Hough AJ. Cell culture of rabbit meniscal fibrochondrocytes: proliferative and synthetic response to growth factors and ascorbate. J Orthop Res. 1985;3(1):36–42.

44. Petersen W, Tillmann B. Age-related blood and lymph supply of the knee menisci. A cadaver study. Acta Orthop Scand. 1995;66(4):308–12.
45. Arnoczky SP, Warren RF. Microvasculature of the human meniscus. Am J Sports Med. 1982;10(2):90–5.
46. Kennedy JC, Alexander IJ, Hayes KC. Nerve supply of the human knee and its functional importance. Am J Sports Med. 1982;10(6):329–35.
47. Day B, Mackenzie WG, Shim SS, Leung G. The vascular and nerve supply of the human meniscus. Arthroscopy. 1985;1(1):58–62.
48. Dye SF, Vaupel GL, Dye CC. Conscious neurosensory mapping of the internal structures of the human knee without intraarticular anesthesia. Am J Sports Med. 1998;26(6):773–7.
49. Radin EL, de Lamotte F, Maquet P. Role of the menisci in the distribution of stress in the knee. Clin Orthop Relat Res. 1984;185:290–4.
50. Watanabe Y, Scyoc AV, Tsuda E, Debski RE, Woo SL. Biomechanical function of the posterior horn of the medial meniscus: a human cadaveric study. J Orthop Sci. 2004;9(3):280–4.
51. Voloshin AS, Wosk J. Shock absorption of meniscectomized and painful knees: a comparative in vivo study. J Biomed Eng. 1983;5(2):157–61.
52. Allen CR, Wong EK, Livesay GA, Sakane M, Fu FH, Woo SL. Importance of the medial meniscus in the anterior cruciate ligament-deficient knee. J Orthop Res. 2000;18(1):109–15.
53. Wang CJ, Walker PS. Rotatory laxity of the human knee joint. J Bone Joint Surg Am. 1974;56(1):161–70.
54. Thompson WO, Thaete FL, Fu FH, Dye SF. Tibial meniscal dynamics using three-dimensional reconstruction of magnetic resonance images. Am J Sports Med 1991;19(3):210–215; discussion 5–6.
55. Ritchie JR, Miller MD, Bents RT, Smith DK. Meniscal repair in the goat model. The use of healing adjuncts on central tears and the role of magnetic resonance arthrography in repair evaluation. Am J Sports Med. 1998;26(2):278–84.
56. Dowdy PA, Miniaci A, Arnoczky SP, Fowler PJ, Boughner DR. The effect of cast immobilization on meniscal healing. An experimental study in the dog. Am J Sports Med. 1995;23(6):721–8.

Etiology and Risk Factors 3

Ok-Gul Kim and Seung-Suk Seo

Abstract

Knee osteoarthritis is one of the most common joint diseases in the world. It is known that there is no one cause of osteoarthritis in the knee but a combination of various risk factors. Risk factors of knee osteoarthritis can be divided into intrinsic factors and extrinsic factors (obesity, lifestyle, heavy physical work, exercise, and sports). Intrinsic factors can be further divided into systemic factors (age, gender, genetics, diet, bone density, and ethnic characteristics) and local factors (knee injury, ligament laxity, muscle weakness, malalignment). Among them, the main factors associated with knee osteoarthritis are previous knee trauma, obesity, female gender, hand osteoarthritis and older age. Besides abovementioned factors, various genetic and metabolic factors are extensively investigating to elucidate the association with knee osteoarthritis. Some systemic factors, such as age, gender, genetics, and ethnics are not modifiable, but other factors are modifiable. Patients with knee osteoarthritis develop physical disability, which increases all-cause mortality, especially cardiovascular disease. These modifiable factors, if properly corrected, could help a free from physical dysfunction and provides human well-being. In conclusion, the importance of preventing knee osteoarthritis by understanding the etiology and risk factors of osteoarthritis is important.

Keywords

Knee osteoarthritis · Risk factors · Previous knee trauma · Obesity · Female gender Genetics · Metabolism · Older age

O.-G. Kim (✉) · S.-S. Seo
Department of Orthopedics, Haeundae Bumin Hospital, Busan, South Korea
e-mail: geuley@bumin.co.kr

3.1 Etiology

Degenerative knee osteoarthritis (OA) can be divided into primary (or idiopathic) OA and secondary OA, depending on the causes. Primary OA occurs as a result of degeneration of the knee joint cartilage without specific causes. This is generally thought to be the result of wear, tear, and aging.

Among the many structures composing the knee joint, the hyaline joint cartilage is considered the major target for harmful effects that cause OA and the structure from which the disease originates. The structures that are making up the joint include its bony components covered with hyaline cartilage, its capsule, ligaments, and menisci, as well as the muscles that move it. These structures work organically for normal knee joint function. If it has a problem with one or more of these structures, knee OA may progress. Conversely, secondary knee arthritis occurs

S.-S. Seo (ed.), *A Strategic Approach to Knee Arthritis Treatment*,
https://doi.org/10.1007/978-981-16-4217-3_3

Table 3.1 Etiologies of secondary osteoarthritis of the knee

Post-traumatic	
Congenital/malformation of the limb	
Malposition	Varus Valgus
Postsurgical	
Metabolic disorders	Rickets Hemochromatosis Chondrocalcinosis Ochronosis Wilson disease Gout/Pseudogout
Endocrine disorders	Acromegaly Hyperparathyroidism Hyperuricemia
Inflammatory disorders	Rheumatoid arthritis Psoriatic arthritis
Aseptic osteonecrosis	
Others	Scoliosis Infectious arthritis Hemophilia Paget disease Sickle cell disease

as a result of degeneration of the knee joint cartilage for a known cause (Table 3.1).

However, it has been recently known that inflammation in bone and synovial tissues plays an important role in the development of OA. It is an important part of the development and progression of arthritis, and the degree of inflammation may vary depending on the specific congenital and local joint factors of the patient. Synovial macrophages are in charge of producing catabolism and pre-inflammatory mediators that cause inflammation, resulting in a negative balance of cartilage matrix breakdown and repair. Synovial inflammation is aggravated by cartilage debris and catabolic mediators entering the joint cavity, causing symptoms such as inflammatory pain and joint swelling and leads to the progression of arthritis. This can produce various clinical presentations for the same imaging picture and different timetables for the progression of the disease.

3.2 Risk Factors

Bone, cartilage, muscle, and other joint structures that make up the knee joint are biomechanical organs that maintain proper knee function and

Table 3.2 Risk factors of the knee osteoarthritis

Intrinsic factors		Extrinsic factors
Systemic factors	Local factors	
Age Gender (menopause) Genetics Diets Bone density Ethnic characteristics	Knee injury Ligament laxity Impairments in muscle function (muscle weakness) Malalignment (joint deformity)	Obesity Lifestyle (cultural and religious aspects) Heavy physical work Exercises and sports Smoking

prevent excessive weight loading. However, if the balances of the biomechanical function of the knee joint are broken due to various risk factors, joint degeneration and damage occur, and OA develops. Knee OA is a heterogeneous disease with various forms, each of which has its own risk factors working through its unique processes. These numerous risk factors can be largely categorized into intrinsic factors and extrinsic factors, and intrinsic factors can be further divided into systemic factors and local factors. Although each may occur individually, the progression of knee OA speeds up when systemic factors interact with local effects that affect the environment of the knee itself. Discussed below are some of the major risk factors, along with some supporting studies (Table 3.2).

3.2.1 Knee Injury

A 22-year prospective study of 98 Finnish participants conducted by doctors investigated the association of newly diagnosed OA cases using the information on disease history, symptoms, and standardized clinical physical examination [1]. According to the study, the risk factors for newly diagnosed OA showed a strong association with previous knee injuries and the heaviest category of physical stress at work (compared to the lightest category). A previous knee injury is the highest risk factor associated OA (OR (odds ratio) 3.86) [2]. A recent meta-analysis study of 24 observational studies with 20,997 participants concluded that previous knee injury is the most crucial risk factor for the development of knee

OA, regardless of study design and definition of knee injury [3]. The study also identified knee injuries as one of several modifiable risk factors for OA, emphasizing its prevention in future public health programs.

In an average 10-year follow-up study of 44 patients who underwent surgical treatment for knee dislocation, the incidence of OA was 23%, indicating a significant correlation between major knee injury and subsequent development of OA [4].

Anterior cruciate ligament (ACL) rupture and meniscal tear are also major risk factors for knee OA. ACL reconstruction improves joint stability, but in the long term, may not prevent knee OA and reinjuries. Eventually, it may not restore normal knee kinematics compared to conservative treatment [5]. ACL rupture is known to lead to early onset knee OA in 13% of patients 10–15 years after injury [6]. A study of 205 soccer players with ACL found that at 14-year follow-up, 41% of patients had advanced degenerative changes compared to 4% of noninjured knees [7]. In a similar study involving female soccer players, 51% of ACL ruptures were diagnosed with OA on radiographs 12 years later [8]. The risk of early onset of knee OA in patients with high physical activity was higher in patients with bone-patellar tendon bone technique than patients with semitendinosus and gracilis autogenous tendon technique during ACL reconstruction [9]. ACL rupture is associated with damage to cartilage, subchondral bone, collateral ligament, and meniscus in about 65–75%, in which case the prevalence of knee OA increases from 21% to 40% [6]. People who underwent partial meniscectomy during the reconstruction of the ACL had a significantly higher risk of developing signs of OA in the radiographs than those with normal meniscus [10].

In particular, the meniscal tear has a strong association with the incidence of knee OA. A multicenter study showed that untreated meniscus tears at 30-month follow-up had a 5.7 times higher OR than the incidence of knee OA [11]. In another study, a four-fold increase in the risk of knee OA after partial meniscectomy was observed at 16-year follow-up [12]. Total meniscectomy was found to be detrimental to the knee joint in that radiographic OA generally occurred 14 times more than people in the control group 20 years after the surgery [13].

Although it is generally believed that knee OA occurs due to abnormal biomechanical forces acting on an unstable knee after injury, some studies suggest additional or alternative mechanisms. Reports of ACL deficient knees [14] and meniscal injuries [15] confirmed that proteases and inflammatory cytokines that can directly damage cartilage are released into the joint after knee injury. In a rat modeled animal study, intra-articular inhibition of interleukin-1 reported considerably reduced synovitis and cartilage degradation after tibial plateau fracture [16].

3.2.2 Impairments in Muscle Function

Generally, muscle weakness, modified muscle activation patterns, and intrinsic sensory deficiencies are associated with knee OA. In particular, the weakness of the quadriceps muscle is mostly observed in symptomatic knee OA patients. The greater quadriceps muscle strength is associated with a lower risk for progression of tibiofemoral joint space narrowing and cartilage loss in women [17]. Strengthening of the quadriceps muscle is a key element in the conservative treatment and management of knee OA and is effective in improving pain, physical function, and quality of life [18]. This effect does not appear to be due to any structural changes found in knee MRI [19]. The basic mechanism is currently not fully understood, but one theory suggests that the knee extensor muscles absorb and stabilize the impact on the knee, whereas the lack of the muscles strength can cause excessive mechanical stress on the articular cartilage, thereby promoting OA progression, such as cartilage damage [18, 19].

3.2.3 Malalignment

It is well known that abnormal lower limb alignment causes asymmetrical increased compressive stress in the medial or lateral compartment, leading to arthritis with an increased structural breakdown of the knee joint. Knees from malalignment, varus and valgus deformity have a risk for progression of OA (RR 2.0 (1.3–2.8), 2.3 (1.4–3.1), and 1.7 (0.97–2.6), respectively) [20]. Medial compartment progression of knee OA was four times more common in patients with varus alignment, whereas lateral compartment progression of knee OA was five times more common in patients with external alignment [21].

3.2.4 Gender

Not only is OA in the knee joint more prevalent in women, but OA in the hip joint and hand are also more commonly seen in women compared to men [22], and the incidence of OA increases around women's menopause [23]. Although the opinion that hormone involvement causes different incidence rate of OA in men and women is dominant, the role of hormonal factors in the development of OA is not clear and still controversial [24]. The role of hormonal factors on knee OA will be described in detail below. In addition, the cause of women's high OA incidence may be explained by a decrease in the amount of cartilage, bone loss, and muscle strength loss [25]. Women in the severe OA group showed lower activity scores and more disabilities in their daily activities than men and were also reported to show more severe symptoms of OA [26]. In a 12-year prospective study of 315,495 Norwegians, knee arthroplasty cases doubled in women (0.55%) than men (0.28%) [27].

3.2.5 Menopause

Sex hormones play an important role in the causes of the rise in OA in postmenopausal women, and especially, estrogen deficiency contributes greatly to the development of osteoarthritis [28]. There is an estrogen receptor in subchondral osteoblasts, chondrocytes, and synoviocytes [29]. Estrogen mainly inhibits the expression of pro-inflammatory cytokines such as IL-1 and secretion into joints [30]. Several studies have reported that estrogen supplement reduces the incidence of OA, supporting the role of estrogen in OA [28]. Moreover, a decrease in ovarian function following menopause causes an increase in pre-inflammatory cytokines in the plasma [31]. However, due to the lack of clear conclusions on the effects of sex hormones on OA, further research is needed.

3.2.6 Age

Age may be one of the major risk factors for OA. The increased prevalence and incidence of OA with age increases not only in the knee but also in the hip and hand joints. The effect of age is greatest in the elderly (age 70–75 years) for knee OA [32]. The mechanisms suspected of causing joint damage have not been fully understood, but they are high due to thinning of cartilage, muscle atrophy, decreased proprioception and oxidative damage [33].

3.2.7 Heavy Physical Work

The relationship between heavy physical work and OA is a topic of great interest to many researchers. In particular, vibration, repetitive movements, a long period of kneeling, squatting, and standing have been shown to be associated with an increased risk for OA [34]. Frequent kneeling with a heavy object is another activity that is related to cartilage degeneration [35]. A German case-control study of 1310 patients with symptomatic knee OA and without OA suggested a dose-response relationship between knee flexion or squat and symptomatic knee OA [36]. However, occupational risks, such as climbing or running stairs or ladders, are not related to symptomatic knee OA [36]. A high body mass index(BMI) has a detrimental interaction with kneeling or squatting and lifting heavy objects [37].

3.2.8 Exercises and Sports

There is no clear conclusion as to whether exercise and sporting activities can be risk factors for

OA. Here, we will refer to related research. A cross-sectional study of 2439 participants with OA showed that non-professional running during life is not likely to increase the probability of occurrence in radiological OA, symptomatic OA or knee pain [38] Also, no relationship was found between short, medium distance running and OA, and long-distance running, barefoot running, and minimalistic shoes have not yet been clearly related to OA [39]. In reality, sports activities can have a protective effect on the knee joint if no traumatic injuries are involved [38]. This subject should be described in Chap. 4.

3.2.9 Obesity

In a recent meta-analysis including 22 studies, Obesity (body mass index (BMI) > 30 kg/m^2) is strongly associated with knee OA (pooled odds ratio [OR]: 2.66 [95% CI 2.15–3.28]), whereas the relationship between overweight (BMI > 25 kg/m^2) and knee OA is lower but still significantly associated with knee OA (pooled OR 1.98 [95% CI 1.57–2.20]) [22]. Several authors have shown a dose-response relationship between obesity and the risk of knee OA: with every 5 increase in BMI, the risk of OA increases by 35%. In the case of women, the association of OA occurrence with BMI increase was much greater than men. The risk increased further when BMI was combined with a high-intensity workforce, showing a 12-time increase for men and 16-time increase for women. 24.6% of patients with newly developed knee pain were associated with overweight or obesity [40]. There are also reports that excessive obesity not only causes knee OA, but may also lead to total knee arthroplasty. In a 12-year prospective study involving 315,495 Norwegians, an increase in BMI was reported to be directly related to the development of OA at the level requiring total knee arthroplasty [27]. Men with a BMI > 27 had a six-fold increase in the frequency of total knee arthroplasty compared to men with a BMI < 23. Women with a BMI > 26 have an 11-fold increase in the frequency of total knee arthroplasty compared to women with a BMI of 21 or less.

With an increased awareness of the relationship between obesity and inflammatory and metabolic activities, researchers reconsider the relationship between OA and obesity. The relationship between the incidence of knee OA and obesity is not necessarily determined by the severity of obesity. The development of OA in obesity appears to be closely related to the severity of obesity as well as the pathologic lipid and glucose metabolism abnormalities [41]. Cytokines closely related to adipose tissue, including leptin, adiponectin, and resistin, can affect knee OA development through direct joint breakdown or regulation of local inflammatory processes [41, 42]. Metabolic risk factors including obesity, hypertension, dyslipidemia, and glucose tolerance disorders (metabolic syndrome) increase the risk of OA as well as the progression of it [20]. This risk increases as the number of metabolic risk factors rise, showing a close relationship between these risk factors and OA [43]. Several studies have shown that weight loss improves knee function and reduces inflammation and knee pain. Obesity is a specific problem in Western nations, and it is one of the modifiable risk factors that can reduce the prevalence of OA in these nations. According to a study by Framingham, a weight loss of 5 kg reduced the risk of knee OA by 50% [44]. Efforts to lose weight are also essential in clinical practice (Fig. 3.1).

3.2.10 Genetics

A lot of research has been done recently to find specific genes related to knee OA development. A meta-analysis of 4 genome-wide association stud ies using a sample size of 6709 cases and 44,439 controls in the Caucasian population found an important susceptible locus for knee OA on chromosome 7q22 [45]. Other studies have discovered a possible role in OA for the genes encoding structural extracellular matrix components (such as DVWA) and molecules taking part in prostaglandin metabolism (DQB1 and BTNL2) [46]. A genetic polymorphism with a ~ 300 kilobase region in chromosome 7q22 is associated with

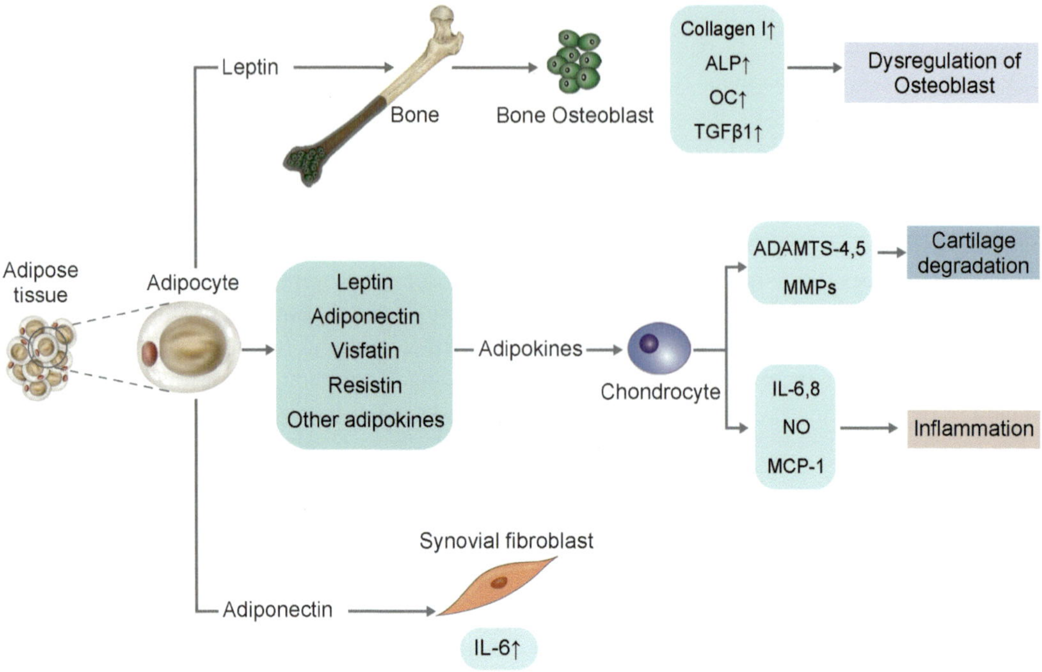

Fig. 3.1 The Influences of dysfunctional fat on synovial cells, chondrocytes, and bone. Dysfunctional adipose tissues produce pro-inflammatory adipokines excessively that interact with synovial cells, chondrocytes and bone by inducing several pro-inflammatory mediators (cytokines, reactive oxygen species, NO) and cartilage degradative factors (MMPs and ADAMTSs). *ADAMTS* a disintegrin and metalloproteinase with thrombospondin motifs, *ALP* alkaline phosphatase, *IL* interleukin, *MCP* monocyte chemoattractant protein, *MMPs* matrix metalloproteinases, *NO* nitric oxide, *OC* osteocalcin, *TGF* transforming growth factor

knee OA susceptibility [47]. Recently, genes encoding NCOA3, SULF2, and ALDH1A2 have all been revealed to be related to hip and hand OA, but not inevitably to knee OA [48].

3.2.11 Smoking

There are conflicting opinions on the relationship between smoking and OA development. In other words, it was not clear whether the fact that smoking increased or decreased the risk of knee OA. This can be attributed to the fact that smokers may have a different lifestyle than non-smokers. (e.g., less participation in intense physical activity). In a meta-analysis study analyzing the relationship between smoking and OA prevalence, several studies (n = 18) have shown conflicting results. However, the authors nonetheless reported smoking as having little or no protective effect against the prevalence of OA [2].

3.2.12 Diet

Some dietary factors suspected to increase the incidence of OA include a deficiency of vitamins D, C, and K and Certain food groups, such as fruits, milk/milk products, and meat/poultry are beneficial for knee OA [49]. However, more research is necessary to define a clearer relationship between OA and dietary factors.

3.3 Summary

Knee OA represents a large burden on healthcare with the aging of the population throughout the world. Treatment for knee OA is also important, but in recent years, a preventive approach is becoming more important. In other words, the best treatment for knee OA is prevention. This has led to renewed interest in the etiology and risk factors. In conclusion, healthcare personnel should try to prevent and treat knee OA by understanding the etiology and risk factors well.

References

1. Toivanen AT, Heliövaara M, Impivaara O, Arokoski JP, Knekt P, Lauren H, et al. Obesity, physically demanding work and traumatic knee injury are major risk factors for knee osteoarthritis—a population-based study with a follow-up of 22 years. Rheumatology. 2010;49(2):308–14.
2. Blagojevic M, Jinks C, Jeffery A, Jordan K. Risk factors for onset of osteoarthritis of the knee in older adults: a systematic review and meta-analysis. Osteoarthr Cartil. 2010;18(1):24–33.
3. Muthuri S, McWilliams D, Doherty M, Zhang W. History of knee injuries and knee osteoarthritis: a meta-analysis of observational studies. Osteoarthr Cartil. 2011;19(11):1286–93.
4. Fanelli GC, Sousa PL, Edson CJ. Long-term followup of surgically treated knee dislocations: stability restored, but arthritis is common. Clin Orthop Relat Res. 2014;472(9):2712–7.
5. Linko E, Harilainen A, Malmivaara A, Seitsalo S. Surgical versus conservative interventions for anterior cruciate ligament ruptures in adults. Cochrane Database Syst Rev. 2005;2
6. Slauterbeck JR, Kousa P, Clifton BC, Naud S, Tourville TW, Johnson RJ, et al. Geographic mapping of meniscus and cartilage lesions associated with anterior cruciate ligament injuries. JBJS. 2009;91(9):2094–103.
7. Von Porat A, Roos EM, Roos H. High prevalence of osteoarthritis 14 years after an anterior cruciate ligament tear in male soccer players: a study of radiographic and patient relevant outcomes. Ann Rheum Dis. 2004;63(3):269–73.
8. Lohmander L, Östenberg A, Englund M, Roos H. High prevalence of knee osteoarthritis, pain, and functional limitations in female soccer players twelve years after anterior cruciate ligament injury. Arthritis Rheum. 2004;50(10):3145–52.
9. Vairo GL, McBrier NM, Miller SJ, Buckley WE. Premature knee osteoarthritis after anterior cruciate ligament reconstruction dependent on autograft. J Sport Rehabil. 2010;19(1):86–97.
10. Magnussen RA, Mansour AA, Carey JL, Spindler KP. Meniscus status at ACL reconstruction is associated with the presence of radiographic signs of osteoarthritis at 5–10 year follow-up: a systematic review. J Knee Surg. 2009;22(1):347.
11. Englund M, Guermazi A, Roemer FW, Aliabadi P, Yang M, Lewis CE, et al. Meniscal tear in knees without surgery and the development of radiographic osteoarthritis among middle-aged and elderly persons: the Multicenter Osteoarthritis Study. Arthritis Rheum. 2009;60(3):831–9.
12. Englund M, Roos EM, Lohmander L. Impact of type of meniscal tear on radiographic and symptomatic knee osteoarthritis: a sixteen-year followup of meniscectomy with matched controls. Arthritis Rheum. 2003;48(8):2178–87.
13. Roos H, Laurén M, Adalberth T, Roos EM, Jonsson K, Lohmander LS. Knee osteoarthritis after meniscectomy: prevalence of radiographic changes after twenty-one years, compared with matched controls. Arthritis Rheum. 1998;41(4):687–93.
14. Irie K, Uchiyama E, Iwaso H. Intraarticular inflammatory cytokines in acute anterior cruciate ligament injured knee. Knee. 2003;10(1):93–6.
15. Scanzello CR, McKeon B, Swaim BH, DiCarlo E, Asomugha EU, Kanda V, et al. Synovial inflammation in patients undergoing arthroscopic meniscectomy: molecular characterization and relationship to symptoms. Arthritis Rheum. 2011;63(2):391–400.
16. Furman BD, Mangiapani DS, Zeitler E, Bailey KN, Horne PH, Huebner JL, et al. Targeting proinflammatory cytokines following joint injury: acute intra-articular inhibition of interleukin-1 following knee injury prevents post-traumatic arthritis. Arthritis Res Ther. 2014;16(3):R134.
17. Segal NA, Glass NA. Is quadriceps muscle weakness a risk factor for incident or progressive knee osteoarthritis? Phys Sportsmed. 2011;39(4):44–50.
18. Bennell KL, Wrigley TV, Hunt MA, Lim B-W, Hinman RS. Update on the role of muscle in the genesis and management of knee osteoarthritis. Rheum Dis Clin. 2013;39(1):145–76.
19. Jones G, Schultz MG, Dore D. Physical activity and osteoarthritis of the knee: can MRI scans shed more light on this issue? Phys Sportsmed. 2011;39(3):55–61.
20. Yusuf E, Bijsterbosch J, Slagboom PE, Rosendaal FR, Huizinga TW, Kloppenburg M. Body mass index and alignment and their interaction as risk factors for progression of knees with radiographic signs of osteoarthritis. Osteoarthr Cartil. 2011;19(9):1117–22.
21. Cerejo R, Dunlop DD, Cahue S, Channin D, Song J, Sharma L. The influence of alignment on risk of knee osteoarthritis progression according to baseline stage of disease. Arthritis Rheum. 2002;46(10):2632–6.
22. Silverwood V, Blagojevic-Bucknall M, Jinks C, Jordan J, Protheroe J, Jordan K. Current evidence on risk factors for knee osteoarthritis in older adults: a systematic review and meta-analysis. Osteoarthr Cartil. 2015;23(4):507–15.
23. Srikanth VK, Fryer JL, Zhai G, Winzenberg TM, Hosmer D, Jones G. A meta-analysis of sex differences prevalence, incidence and severity of osteoarthritis. Osteoarthr Cartil. 2005;13(9):769–81.
24. de Klerk BM, Schiphof D, Groeneveld FP, Koes BW, van Osch GJM, van Meurs JB, et al. No clear association between female hormonal aspects and osteoarthritis of the hand, hip and knee: a systematic review. Rheumatology. 2009;48(9):1160–5.
25. Hunter D. The epidemiology of osteoarthritis. Best Pract Res Clin Rheumatol. 2014;28:5–15.

26. Logerstedt DS, Zeni J Jr, Snyder-Mackler L. Sex differences in patients with different stages of knee osteoarthritis. Arch Phys Med Rehabil. 2014;95(12):2376–81.
27. Apold H, Meyer HE, Nordsletten L, Furnes O, Baste V, Flugsrud GB. Risk factors for knee replacement due to primary osteoarthritis, a population based, prospective cohort study of 315,495 individuals. BMC Musculoskelet Disord. 2014;15(1):217.
28. Arden N, Nevitt MC. Osteoarthritis: epidemiology. Best Pract Res Clin Rheumatol. 2006;20(1):3–25.
29. Tanko L, Søndergaard B-C, Oestergaard S, Karsdal M, Christiansen C. An update review of cellular mechanisms conferring the indirect and direct effects of estrogen on articular cartilage. Climacteric. 2008;11(1):4–16.
30. Richette P, Dumontier M-F, Tahiri K, Widerak M, Torre A, Benallaloua M, et al. Oestrogens inhibit interleukin 1β-mediated nitric oxide synthase expression in articular chondrocytes through nuclear factor-κB impairment. Ann Rheum Dis. 2007;66(3):345–50.
31. Pfeilschifter J, Köditz R, Pfohl M, Schatz H. Changes in proinflammatory cytokine activity after menopause. Endocr Rev. 2002;23(1):90–119.
32. Prieto-Alhambra D, Judge A, Javaid MK, Cooper C, Diez-Perez A, Arden NK. Incidence and risk factors for clinically diagnosed knee, hip and hand osteoarthritis: influences of age, gender and osteoarthritis affecting other joints. Ann Rheum Dis. 2014;73(9):1659–64.
33. Litwic A, Edwards MH, Dennison EM, Cooper C. Epidemiology and burden of osteoarthritis. Br Med Bull. 2013;105(1):185–99.
34. Yucesoy B, Charles LE, Baker B, Burchfiel CM. Occupational and genetic risk factors for osteoarthritis: a review. Work. 2015;50(2):261–73.
35. Hovis KK, Stehling C, Souza RB, Haughom BD, Baum T, Nevitt M, et al. Physical activity is associated with magnetic resonance imaging–based knee cartilage T2 measurements in asymptomatic subjects with and those without osteoarthritis risk factors. Arthritis Rheum. 2011;63(8):2248–56.
36. Klussmann A, Gebhardt H, Nübling M, Liebers F, Perea EQ, Cordier W, et al. Individual and occupational risk factors for knee osteoarthritis: results of a case-control study in Germany. Arthritis Res Ther. 2010;12(3):R88.
37. Palmer KT. Occupational activities and osteoarthritis of the knee. Br Med Bull. 2012;102(1):147–70.
38. Lo G, Driban J, Kriska A, Storti K, McAlindon T, Souza R et al. Habitual running any time in life is not detrimental and may be protective of symptomatic knee osteoarthritis: data from the osteoarthritis initiative: 2895. Arthritis Rheumatol. 2014;66.
39. Hansen P, English M, Willick SE. Does running cause osteoarthritis in the hip or knee? PM&R. 2012;4(5):S117–S21.
40. Andriacchi TP, Mündermann A, Smith RL, Alexander EJ, Dyrby CO, Koo S. A framework for the in vivo pathomechanics of osteoarthritis at the knee. Ann Biomed Eng. 2004;32(3):447–57.
41. Thijssen E, Van Caam A, Van Der Kraan PM. Obesity and osteoarthritis, more than just wear and tear: pivotal roles for inflamed adipose tissue and dyslipidaemia in obesity-induced osteoarthritis. Rheumatology. 2015;54(4):588–600.
42. Sowers MR, Karvonen-Gutierrez CA. The evolving role of obesity in knee osteoarthritis. Curr Opin Rheumatol. 2010;22(5):533.
43. Yoshimura N, Muraki S, Oka H, Tanaka S, Kawaguchi H, Nakamura K, et al. Accumulation of metabolic risk factors such as overweight, hypertension, dyslipidaemia, and impaired glucose tolerance raises the risk of occurrence and progression of knee osteoarthritis: a 3-year follow-up of the ROAD study. Osteoarthr Cartil. 2012;20(11):1217–26.
44. Christensen R, Bartels EM, Astrup A, Bliddal H. Effect of weight reduction in obese patients diagnosed with knee osteoarthritis: a systematic review and meta-analysis. Ann Rheum Dis. 2007;66(4):433–9.
45. Evangelou E, Valdes AM, Kerkhof HJ, Styrkarsdottir U, Zhu Y, Meulenbelt I, et al. Meta-analysis of genome-wide association studies confirms a susceptibility locus for knee osteoarthritis on chromosome 7q22. Ann Rheum Dis. 2011;70(2):349–55.
46. Valdes AM, Spector TD. Genetic epidemiology of hip and knee osteoarthritis. Nat Rev Rheumatol. 2011;7(1):23.
47. Consortium a, Collaborators a. Identification of new susceptibility loci for osteoarthritis (arcOGEN): a genome-wide association study. Lancet 2012;380(9844):815–823.
48. Loughlin J. Genetic contribution to osteoarthritis development: current state of evidence. Curr Opin Rheumatol. 2015;27(3):284.
49. Sanghi D, Mishra A, Sharma AC, Raj S, Mishra R, Kumari R, et al. Elucidation of dietary risk factors in osteoarthritis knee—a case-control study. J Am Coll Nutr. 2015;34(1):15–20.

4 Knee Osteoarthritis and Sports

Chang-Rack Lee

Abstract

There is much evidence to support the claim that regular exercise improves general health, and some activities are deemed to have beneficial effects for joints by increasing the circulation of synovial fluid and maintaining peri-articular muscle strength. However, in spite of such positive effects of exercise, there is some concern that increased participation in physical activity or sports can increase the incidence of osteoarthritis in the lower extremity joints. Although normal healthy joints can withstand repetitive loading during daily activities without the occurrence of osteoarthritis, long-term repetitive loading that exceeds the articular cartilage tolerance can play an important role in the occurrence or aggravation of osteoarthritis. Osteoarthritis is characterized by pain and impaired function and is a common chronic disease that has significant effects on one's quality of life. Although various factors such as age, gender, physical trauma, and genetics have been reported as risk factors for osteoarthritis, the correlation between physical activity and sports with osteoarthritis is not yet clear. In order to evaluate the correlation between physical activity or sports and osteoarthritis, various factors including age, types, and intensity of physical activity or sports participation, duration of the physical activity or sports participation, and joint injury history, etc. must be considered together. In this chapter, the effects of physical activity or sports participation on the onset of knee osteoarthritis will be described in the context of relevant published literature.

Keywords

Knee · Osteoarthritis · Physical activity
Sport activity · Knee injury

4.1 Experimental/Animal Studies

The key function of the articular cartilage is to protect the subchondral bones by resisting tensile, shear, and compressive forces. The amount and type of external mechanical loading on the joint are important factors that regulate the development and homeostasis of the articular cartilage. Generally, injury of the articular cartilage is not induced by contact stress generated by normal daily activities in normal and healthy joints [1]. According to a biomechanical study using a

C.-R. Lee (✉)
Department of Orthopedics, Inje University Busan Paik Hospital, Busan, South Korea
e-mail: leechangrack@inje.ac.kr

S.-S. Seo (ed.), *A Strategic Approach to Knee Arthritis Treatment*,
https://doi.org/10.1007/978-981-16-4217-3_4

cadaveric knee, the maximum contact stress exerted to the medial and lateral tibial plateau during walking was 5.6 ± 1.5 MPa and 7.3 ± 2.5 MPa, respectively, and 7.7 ± 2.9 MPa and 7.4 ± 2.3 MPa, respectively, for stair climbing [2]. The compressive stress exerted on a joint during physical activity can increase to the range of 10–20 MPa [3], and a study reported that contact stress of more than 25 MPa is necessary for the disruption of normal articular cartilage from a single impact [4–6]. However, some of the literature reports that articular cartilage damage or degeneration can occur even under contact stress of less than 25 MPa [3, 5, 7–10].

Moderate biomechanical loads on articular cartilage can stimulate the synthesis of chondrocyte sulfated-glycosaminoglycans and improve the quality of the articular cartilage [10, 11]. However, there is also some evidence to support the notion that joint loading generated by strenuous exercise is a risk factor for the damage to the articular cartilage or occurrence of osteoarthritis (OA). Numerous animal studies have assessed the effects of increased physical activity on the articular cartilage. Stress applied to the knee joint varies highly depending on the type of physical activity or sports involved. Moreover, since the intensity of such activities differs depending on the participants, it is difficult to execute a standardized animal experiment model that can cover all of the possible types and intensities of activities. The majority of animal studies have evaluated the effects of joint overuse on the articular cartilage in the format of applying repetitive loading or impacts to the knee joint or increasing the activity level of the animals. In addition, the majority of animal studies were conducted using dogs, rodents, rabbits, or sheep, and running was employed most commonly as the method of increasing the animals' activity level. One study reported that repeated movement of the knee from 80° flexion to full extension and impact loading at full extension induces formation of chondrocyte clusters, fibrillation of the matrix, thickening of subchondral bone, and articular cartilage damage such as penetration of subchondral capillaries into the calcified zone of articular cartilage in rabbits [12]. Newton et al. [13] evaluated the effects of life-long running on canine articular cartilage. Exercise was performed on a treadmill by dogs in the experimental group wearing a jacket weighing 130% of their body weight (11.5 kg) (3 km/hour for 75 minutes, 5 days a week for 527 weeks), while unrestricted activity in the cage was allowed for 550 weeks in the control group. In the evaluation of the articular cartilage of the knee joint on the 550th week of the study, there was no gross or microscopic difference between the two groups and also no difference in the mechanical properties of articular cartilage. Videman et al. [14] evaluated the effects of repetitive movements on the articular cartilage by dividing rabbits into two groups and having them run on treadmills with inclinations of 0° or 20°, respectively. According to their results, glycosaminoglycan metabolism of the articular cartilage decreased in the uphill running group and irregularities were observed in the articular cartilage under electron microscopy scanning. Vasan et al. [15] evaluated changes in the metabolism of articular cartilage in the femoral head after dogs underwent exercise on treadmills for 8 months. In this study, there was a reduction in the experimental group in hexosamine in the articulating area as well as the area surrounding the articulating area, along with a decrease in the size of the proteoglycan aggregates and monomers with incorporation of more radioactive sulfate. In addition, glycosaminoglycan chains from the articulating area were smaller than the control tissue with confirmation of an increase in chondroitin-4-sulfate synthesis. Kiviranata et al. [16, 17] evaluated the effects of running distance on the articular cartilage of canine knee joints and reported that moderate running exercise (4 km/day, 5 days a week) conducted by beagles for 40 weeks increased the proteoglycan content and thickness of the uncalcified cartilage in the lateral condyle and patella on the femur. However, it was also reported that the proteoglycan content and thickness of uncalcified cartilage in the medial femoral condyle were reduced by strenuous running exercise (20 km/day, 5 days a week) conducted for 15 weeks. Some researchers evaluated the effects of long-distance running on the metabolism of articular cartilage in the knees and hip joints of young beagles. Arokoski et al. [18] reported that there was no change in the thickness of knee joint articular cartilage after running exercise of 40 km/day for 15 weeks. However, running exercise induced a reduction in the glycosaminoglycan (GAG) content of the articular cartilage in the weight-bearing areas of the knee joint, and such change was observed mostly in the superficial zone of the articular cartilage. Evaluating the effects of long-distance running on the articular cartilage of the canine femoral head, it was reported that the femoral head articular cartilage displayed the greater capacity to adapt to increased mechanical loading with only minor biochemical changes in the structure and metabolism of the proteoglycans of the extracellular matrix [19]. The shape of the joint was proposed as the reason for the differences in the effects of running exercise on the metabolism of the articular cartilage between the hip and knee joints, with the assertion that the more congruent hip joint appears to protect the articular joint by minimizing local impacts. In addition, the results of this study differed from research by Vasan et al. [15] who reported that running exercise imparted negative effects such as a reduction in proteoglycan in the articulating area and the surrounding areas of the canine femoral head. The authors assumed that the running programs and the breeds and ages of the dogs, which were not the same, would have had some influence on such results.

Although there have been many other studies that evaluated the effects of exercise on the articular cartilage, the results are generally quite conflicting. In addition, since each of these studies used different types of animals, and the exercise type, intensities, durations, and frequencies of exercise, as well as evaluated outcomes were not the same, it is difficult to objectively assess the correlation between exercise and articular cartilage health. Nonetheless, since the majority of animal studies used running as the method of increasing physical activity, analysis of changes in the biochemical content or macroscopic and microscopic evaluation of articular cartilage according to the exercise dose could be meaningful. From such a perspective, a meta-analysis published recently evaluated the effects of daily exercise dose on the articular cartilage of the knee joint [20]. In this meta-analysis of 29 randomized controlled trials, there was no significant correlation between daily exercise dose and articular cartilage composition and thickness. However, the authors of this meta-analysis asserted that high amounts of daily exercise can have negative effects on articular cartilage matrix composition, while moderate amounts of daily exercise can have positive effects on articular cartilage matrix composition in healthy animals, although the effects of low daily amounts of exercise are inconclusive.

According to the animal studies that have been published thus far, repetitive loading or stress exerted on the knee joint appears to have some effect on the metabolism of the articular cartilage, although there is ongoing debate on this issue. However, since the exercise regimen used was not the same for all studies, and animals and humans have different knee joint biomechanics, it is difficult to conclude whether the results of such animal studies would be observed in human studies. Moreover, there remains inadequate evidence as to whether metabolic changes in the articular cartilage due to exercise accelerates the occurrence of OA. Accordingly, it is deemed that there is a need for a greater number of high-quality, randomized, and controlled studies in the future for this purpose.

4.2 The Role of Physical Activity or Sports Activity in the Development of Knee Osteoarthritis

Articular cartilage tolerance of chronic or repetitive stress in humans is yet to be clearly established. Although examination of the effects of physical activity or sports participation on the joints of human lower extremities including the knee has been carried out in numerous studies, there are extensive differences among study subjects (general population or elite athletes), activity levels (leisurely physical activity or sporting activity), activity types, and outcomes. The types and intensity of stress exerted on the knee joint vary for any given physical activity or sport. Even among participants of the same sport, the difference in the loading on the joint may be great depending on the activity levels involved. In addition, in order to evaluate the correlation between physical activity or sports participation and OA, it is necessary to consider not only the exercise pattern or intensity but also various other factors including the age, muscle strength, alignment, and joint stability of participants. Due to such numerous confounding factors, it is difficult to evaluate the effects of physical activity or sports on the development of knee OA. In spite of such limitations, there have been numerous cross-sectional, case-controlled, retrospective, and prospective cohort studies on this topic. Here, literature that is related predominantly to physical activity or sports and knee OA were reviewed.

4.2.1 General Population

4.2.1.1 Physical Activity (or Leisure/Recreational Physical Activity)

Physical activity is defined as any bodily movement produced by skeletal muscles that result in energy expenditure, and physical activity in daily life can be classified as occupational, sports, conditioning, household, or other activities [21]. Numerous studies have investigated the correlation between physical activity and occurrence of OA in the general population (Table 4.1), with many of these studies evaluating the level and quantity of physical activity by means of a questionnaire.

Cheng et al. [22] evaluated regular physical activity and self-reported physician-diagnosed OA of the knee and/or hip by following up 16,961 subjects aged 20 to 87 years for about 10 years (10.9 years for men and 9.9 years for women). This study reported that although there was a correlation between high levels of physical activity (running 20 miles or more per week) and OA in younger men under the age of 50 years, there was no correlation between such physical activity and knee or hip OA in women or older men, after having adjusted for differences among subjects in body mass index (BMI), smoking, and use of alcohol or caffeine. Hannan et al. [23] evaluated the habitual physical activity assessed during middle-age and radiographic knee OA experienced in later years for 1415 subjects from a Framingham study cohort with an average age of 73 years. The authors reported no correlation between the level of habitual physical activity and radiographic knee OA after having adjusted for subject differences in age, BMI, knee injury, smoking, and education. However, men with high levels of habitual physical activity had significantly elevated rates of asymptomatic osteophytes. As such, the authors reported that, although habitual physical activity may not cause severe or symptomatic knee OA, it could have some influence on the development of osteophytes. In addition, another study conducted with a Framingham study cohort reported that more than 4 hours of heavy physical activity per day is correlated with incidence of radiographic knee OA, and that heavy physical activity is an independent risk factor for the development of knee OA in the elderly people, especially among obese individuals [24]. Another study that evaluated the correlation between physical activity and radiological knee OA reported the mean amount of physical activity was associated with the prevalence of patellofemoral joint space narrowing in 257 middle-aged women who were followed up annually over a period of 11 years [25].

While the aforementioned studies reported that the increase in physical activity was somewhat associated with the occurrence of knee OA, some authors have reported that regular physical activity during leisure time may provide protection against knee OA. In a prospective study conducted on 8000 subjects representing the Finnish population over the age of 30 years, potential risk factors in the prediction of knee OA were analyzed. In the 22 years follow-up, knee OA was diagnosed in 95 of the 823 subjects (11.4%) who did not have knee OA at the baseline, and regular physical activity during leisure time including running, skiing, cycling, ball games, swimming, gymnastics, and weight lifting decreased the occurrence of knee OA [26]. However, it was

Table 4.1 The effect of physical activity on knee osteoarthritis in general population

Study	Follow-up	N (men/women)	Osteoarthritis	Association between PA and OA
Ageberg 2012 [31]	11 y	28,320 (60% women)	Severe knee or hip OA, defined as knee or hip replacement	No association between leisure time PA and risk for knee or hip replacement due to OA
Cheng 2000 [22]	Men: 10 y Women: 9.9 y	16,961 (12,888/4073)	Self-reported physician-diagnosed OA	High levels of PA Men under age 50: HR 2.4 (95% CI, 1.5–3.9) No relationship among older men and women
Felson 2007 [29]	9 y	1279	KL grade OARSIA	No relationship between recreational exercise and OA
Hannan 1993 [23]	NA	1404 (584/820)	KL grade 3 or 4 KL grade 2 with knee symptoms	No association between PA and knee OA Asymptomatic osteophyte: Men with high level PA-adjusted OR 2.14 (95% CI, 1.01–4.54)
Hart 1999 [30]	4 y	715 women	Osteophytes JSN	No association between PA and knee OA Walking (adjusted OR) Osteophytes: 0.60 (95% CI, 0.22–1.71) JSN: 0.38 (95% CI. 0.15–0.93) Sport (adjusted OR) Osteophytes: 1.23 (95% CI, 0.54–2.81) JSN: 0.98 (95% CI, 0.42–2.30)
Hootman 2003 [27]	12.8 y	5284 (4308/976)	Self-reported physician-diagnosed hip/knee OA	No association between PA and hip/knee OA
McAlindon 1999 [24]	10 y	470 (177/293)	Modified KL grade ≥ 2	Adjusted OR for ≥4 hours heavy PA/day compared with no heavy PA: 7.0 (95% CI, 2.4–20)
Mork 2012 [28]	17 y	15,191 women 14,766 men	Self-reported physician-diagnosed OA	Exercise intensity was not associated with risk of OA in any BMI category
Szoeke 2006 [25]	11 y	224 women	JSN, osteophytes	Adjusted OR Tibiofemoral joint Osteophytes: 6.99 (95% CI, 0.75–65.49) JSN: 0.96 (95% CI, 0.13–7.10) Patellofemoral joint Osteophytes: 1.19 (95% CI, 0.12–12.11) JSN: 17.17 (95% CI, 1.59–185.44) Total knee Osteophytes: 1.76(95% CI, 0.22–13.91) JSN 5.91 (95% CI, 0.87–40.10)
Toivanen 2010 [26]	22 y	823 (369/454)	Self-reported physician-diagnosed OA	Leisure time physical activity (adjusted OR) Little: 1 Irregular: 0.7 (95% CI, 0.4–1.3) Regular: 0.5 (95% CI, 0.3–1.0)
Wang 2011 [32]	4.8 y	39,023	Primary knee and hip replacement for OA	Increasing levels of total PA were associated with increased risk of primary knee replacement due to OA

BMI body mass index, *CI* confidence interval, *HR* hazard ratio, *JSN* joint space narrowing, *KL* Kellgren-Lawrence, *NA* not available, *OA* osteoarthritis, *OARSI* Osteoarthritis Research Society International Atlas, *OR* odds ratio, *PA* physical activity reported that physical stress at work is a risk factor for the occurrence of knee OA, and very heavy manual labor such as carrying furniture and engaging in forestry work are predictive of an extremely high risk of knee OA.

However, a correlation between physical activity and knee OA was not confirmed by other studies. In a longitudinal study of 5284 healthy adults without knee/hip OA, with an average follow-up period of 12.8 years, Hootman et al. [27] reported that participation in leisure time physical activity did not increase the risk of knee/hip knee OA. In a Norwegian HUNT study that included 15,191 women and 14,766 men with 11 years of follow-up, it was found that regular exercise did not increase the risks of knee and hip OA, irrespective of the intensity of that exercise [28]. In a longitudinal study of 1279 adults without OA, with an average of 9 year follow-up, it was reported that walking, jogging, or other self-reported physical activity neither increased nor reduced the risk of symptomatic or radiographic knee OA [29]. Another follow-up study over a period of 4 years conducted on 715 women from a Chingford cohort also reported that physical activity was not correlated with the presence of knee osteophytes or joint space narrowing [30].

Some authors have evaluated the correlation between physical activity and the risks of knee or hip replacement due to OA. Ageberg et al. [31] evaluated the correlation between leisure time physical activity and the risk of knee or hip replacement due to severe OA. In a prospective population-based cohort study of 28,320 participants with an average age of 58 years, with 11 years of follow-up, it was reported that higher leisure time physical activity could play a protective role for the hip against the necessity for hip replacements in women. In addition, it indicated that although there was a trend of higher risk of knee OA in accordance with higher leisure time activity levels, it was not significant. A prospective cohort study of 41,258 Australian adults reported that although there was a dose–response relationship between the total physical activity level and the risk of knee replacement, there was no relationship with hip replacement [32].

Mixed results have been reported on the correlation between physical activity and occurrence of OA in the general population. This is deemed to be the result of differences among studies in various aspects including the age of study subjects, diagnostic method and standards for OA, and follow-up periods. Moreover, these studies have limitations in assessing the correlation between knee OA and particular sports, since physical activity can include both occupational activity and sporting activity.

4.2.1.2 Sport Activity

Many studies have evaluated the correlation between participation in sports and knee OA (Table 4.2). Some of the authors of these studies reported that participation in sports increased the risks of knee OA. A population-based longitudinal study of 354 adults over the age of 55 years, with an average follow-up period of 5.1 years, evaluated risk factors for the incidence and progression of radiographic knee OA [33]. This study reported increased risk of incident radiographic knee OA in subjects with a history of regular sports participation. In addition, it reported that various risk factors for knee OA, including such a history of regular sports participation, appeared to have influence on the incidence rather than the radiographic progression. A case-controlled study conducted in Germany evaluated the dose–response relationships between sports participation and knee OA in male patients with knee OA [34]. In this study, a correlation was confirmed between participation in cycling and ball games (handball, volleyball, basketball), and symptomatic knee OA in the highest category of cumulative duration. Although there was a positive dose–response relationship in the second-highest category of duration (4000 to <7800 h) for soccer, the risk of knee OA did not increase significantly in the highest category (≥7800 h). Authors offered the "healthy athlete" effect, which signifies that athletes with knee problems might quit playing soccer at an earlier stage than those without knee problems, as the reason for the absence of a monotonic dose–response relationship in soccer. After adjustment for confounders, no correlation

Table 4.2 The effect of sport activity on knee osteoarthritis in general population

Study	Follow-up	N (men/women)	Osteoarthritis	Association between SA and OA
Chakravarty 2008 [40]	11.7 y	45 long-distance runners 53 controls	Modified KL grade total knee score (Osteophytes, JSN, sclerosis)	No association between long-distance running and accelerated radiographic OA
Cooper 2000 [33]	5.1 y	354 (99/255)	KL grade JSN, osteophytes	Regular sports participation (adjusted OR) Incident knee OA: 3.2 (95% CI, 1.1–9.1) Progressive knee OA: 0.7 (95% CI, 0.4–1.6)
Lane 1998 [39]	9 y	28 runners 27 controls (nonrunners)	total knee score (Osteophytes, JSN, sclerosis)	Progression of total knee scores: no difference between the runner and nonrunner groups
Lau 2000 [35]	NA	658 participants (control: 658)	KL grade 3 or 4	In women (adjusted OR) Regular sports activities Gymnastics: 7.4 (95% CI, 2.6–20.8) Kung fu: 22.5 (95% CI, 2.5–199)
Sandmark 1999 [36]	NA	325/300 (control: 264/284)	Prosthetic surgery due to primary femorotibial OA Knee OA	Relative risk Highly exposed to all kinds of sports (among men aged <65): 2.9 (95% CI, 1.3–6.5)
Thelin 2006 [37]	NA	825 (control: 825)	Ahlbäck level 1 and 2	Adjusted OR (previous knee injuries) Soccer: 0.94 (95% CI,0.61–1.44) Ice hockey: 1.64 (95% CI, 0.91–2.97) Tennis: 1.16 (95% CI, 0.55–2.46)
Vrezas 2010 [34]	NA	295 men (control: 327 men)	Radiographically confirmed knee OA	Adjusted OR Cycling (≥7000 h): 3.7 (95% CI, 1.7–7.8) Soccer (4000 to <7800 h): 2.2 (95% CI, 1.0–5.0) Ball games (≥2100 h): 4.0 (95% CI, 1.8–8.9) Apparatus gymnastics, shot put, javelin, hammer throwing, wrestling (≥2200 h): 0.9 (95% CI, 0.2–3.6) Weight lifting (≥1500 h): 0.6 (95% CI, 0.1–4.3) Body building, strength training (≥1700 h): 0.9 (95% CI, 0.3–3.0)

CI confidence interval, *h* hours, *JSN* joint space narrowing, *KL* Kellgren-Lawrence, *NA* not available, *OA* osteoarthritis, *OR* odds ratio, *SA* sport activity was reported between knee OA and high cumulative durations in sports including jogging/athletics, swimming, apparatus gymnastics, shot put, javelin, hammer throwing, wrestling, weight lifting, and bodybuilding/strength training. Another case-controlled study reported that the risks of knee OA increased in females regularly engaged in gymnastics or kung fu [35]. In addition, it reported that lifting heavy loads and walking upstairs frequently also increased the risks of knee OA. Sandmark et al. [36] evaluated the correlation between sports activities and knee OA by comparing 325 males and 300 females undergoing knee replacements due to primary knee OA with 264 males and 284 females without knee OA. This study reported an increase in the risk of severe knee OA in males over the age of 65 with high levels of participation in all kinds of sports. It also reported that although cross-country skiing, soccer, ice hockey/bandy, and track-and-field sports increased the risks of knee OA in men, jogging did not, while sports activities and moderated daily general physical activity did not increase the risks of knee OA in women. While many studies have reported that sporting activity is correlated with knee OA to a certain extent in the general population, some authors have provided evidence to cast doubt on such a correlation. Thelin et al. [37] evaluated the effects of sports participation and previous knee injuries on the occurrence of knee OA. 356 males and 469 females with an average age of 62.6 years were included in the case group of this case-controlled study which reported in a univariate analysis that although soccer, ice hockey, and tennis were found to increase the risks of knee OA in men, there was no correlation between any sports activities and knee OA after having adjusted for confounding factors including knee injuries.

Some studies have evaluated the risks of knee OA in non-elite long-distance runners. One of these studies evaluated the effects of repetitive external impact loading on bone and articular cartilage of knee joint using magnetic resonance imaging on 8 recreational or semi-professional marathon runners [38]. This study reported no pathological changes such as marrow edema, periosteal reactions, or joint effusions in pre-run and post-run scans of seven runners, with the exclusion of a subject who had undergone anterior cruciate ligament reconstruction. Lane et al. [39] evaluated the correlation over a 9-year follow-up period between running and radiographic knee OA progression in a prospective study of 28 runners and 27 non-runner controls who were matched in terms of their age, years of education, and occupation. In this study, both the runners and the non-runners had no progression of radiographic knee OA, and there was no significant difference between the 2 groups. Another prospective study evaluated the presence of differences in the progression of knee OA between 45 long-distance runners and 53 healthy non-runners with an average age of 58 through serial radiographic observation over an average period of 11.7 years [40]. This study reported no correlation between long-distance running and accelerated radiographic knee OA in healthy older individuals.

4.2.2 Elite Adult Athlete

There have been several studies evaluating the incidence of OA in lower extremity joints including the knee in former elite male athletes (Table 4.3). A case-controlled study conducted in Finland evaluated the cumulative 21-year incidence of hospital admissions for hip, knee, and ankle OA among 2049 male elite athletes and 1403 control subjects [41]. International-level athletes in endurance sports such as long-distance running and cross country skiing, power sports such as boxing, wrestling, weight lifting, and throwing, and team sports such as soccer, ice hockey, basketball, and track and field were included in this study. It reported that incidence of admission due to OA of lower extremity joints was higher than that of the controls in all types of sports, with participants in team sports and power sports being hospitalized at a relatively younger age in comparison to participants in endurance sports. Another study by the same authors that included 991 elite athletes and 577 control subjects evaluated the correlation between previous lower extremity loading and current self-reported

Table 4.3 Risk of knee osteoarthritis in elite adult athlete

Study	Follow-up	N	Osteoarthritis	Association between SA and OA
Drawer 2001 [48]	NA	185 soccer players	Questionnaire	The risk for soccer players of OA in at least one of the lower extremity joint is greater than for the general population
Elleuch 2008 [50]	>20 y	50 male former football players 50 male controls	KL grade	Radiologically confirmed OA: No difference between football players and controls KL grade ≥ 3 OA: more frequent in football players
Golightly 2009 [51]	NA	2538 NFL players	Self-reported physician-diagnosed OA	Arthritis prevalence ratio All ages group: 2.2 (95% CI, 2.1–2.3) Age < 60: 2.5 (95% CI, 3.3–3.7) Age < 50: 4.5 (95% CI, 4.1–4.9) Age < 40: 6.5 (95% CI, 5.7–7.5)
Iosifidis 2015 [44]	NA	218 former elite male athletes 181 male controls	Physician-diagnosed hip, knee, and ankle OA KL grade	Adjusted OR Clinical knee OA Athlete: 1.49 (95% CI, 0.81–2.73) Control: 2.42 ((95% CI, 1.39–4.21) Radiographic OA Athlete: 1.14 (95% CI, 0.67–1.92) Control: 2.11 (95% CI, 1.33–3.36)
Kettunen 2001 [42]	NA	991 former elite male athletes 577 male controls	Questionnaire (physician-diagnosed hip or knee OA) Hip and knee disability	Adjusted OR Endurance sports: 0.71 (95% CI, 0.32–1.60) Team sports: 1.76 (95% CI, 1.03–3.02) Track and field: 0.97 (95% CI, 0.51–1.84) Power sports: 1.25 (95% CI, 0.77–2.03) Shooters: 0.84 (95% CI, 0.27–2.55) All sports: 1.21 (95% CI, 0.82–1.79)
Klunder 1980 [47]	NA	57 male football players 57 male controls	JSN, sclerosis and/or subchondral cyst	No relationship between football players and controls
Konradsen 1990 [45]	NA	30 male runners 30 nonrunners	Ahlbäck grade	No differences between runner and controls with regard to grades of degenerative changes or osteophytosis

(continued)

Table 4.3 (continued)

Study	Follow-up	N	Osteoarthritis	Association between SA and OA
Kujala 1994 [41]	NA	2049 former male athletes 1403 male controls	Hospital admissions for hip, knee, and ankle OA	Adjusted OR Endurance sports: 1.73 (95% CI, 0.99–3.01) Mixed sports: 1.90 (95% CI, 1.24–2.92) Power sports: 2.17 (95% CI, 1.41–3.32) All sports: 1.97 (95% CI, 1.36–2.87)
Kujala 1995 [43]	NA	117 former top-level male athletes	KL grade	Adjusted OR Soccer: 5.21 (95% CI, 1.14–23.8)
Roos 1994 [49]	NA	286 former male soccer players (215 nonelite/ 71 elite) 572 controls	Ahlbäck grade	OR Soccer players: 4.4 (95% CI, 2.0–9.9) Elite players (compared with nonelite players): 3.7 (95% CI, 1.5–9.3) Nonelite players (compared with the controls): 2.7 (95% CI, 1.0–6.8)
Sandmark 2000 [52]	NA	290 male PE teachers and 281 PE female teachers (control: 255 male and 257 female)	Self-reported knee/hip OA	Prevalence ratio of symptomatic OA Men: 2.8 (95% CI, 1.6–4.8) Women: 3.2 (95% CI, 1.8–5.5)
Spector 1996 [46]	NA	81 female ex-elite athletes 977 age-matched female controls	KL grade Osteophytes, JSN,	Adjusted OR Tibiofemoral joint Osteophyte: 3.57 (95% CI, 1.89–6.71) JSN: 1.17 (95% CI, 0.71–1.94) Patellofemoral joint Osteophyte: 3.50 (95% CI, 1.80–6.81) JSN: 2.97 (95% CI, 1.15–7.67)
White 1993 [53]	NA	577 female PE teachers 305 female controls	X-rays (nil-to-minimal OA/ moderate-to-severe OA)	Lower prevalence of knee OA in PE teacher group

CI confidence interval, *JSN* joint space narrowing, *KL* Kellgren-Lawrence, *NA* not available, *NFL* National Football League, *PE* physical education, *OA* osteoarthritis, *OR* odds ratio hip and knee disability [42]. This study reported that, after adjusting for subject age, body mass index, and occupational group, although the team sport athletes had higher risks of knee disability in comparison to the control group, the risks in other sports athletes were similar to those of the control group. Kujala et al. [43] reported in an analysis of the correlation between different types of sports and knee OA in long-distance runners, soccer players, weight lifters, and shooters, that prevalence of tibio-femoral or patellafemoral OA was 3%, 29%, 31%, and 14% for the shooters, soccer players, weight lifters, and runners, respectively, while the prevalence of tibiofemoral OA was the highest for soccer players at 29% and the prevalence of patellofemoral OA was the highest for weight lifters at 28%. Iosifidis et al. [44] evaluated the prevalence of clinical and radiographic OA of the lower extremities in 281 former elite male athletes over the age of 40 and 181 male control subjects from the general population. This study included soccer, volleyball, martial arts, track and field, basketball players, and skiers. It was reported that although there was no significant difference in the prevalence of clinical OA between the two groups, the prevalence of radiographic OA was 36.6% for the former elite athletes, which was significantly higher than that of the control subjects at 23.9%. In particular, it reported that knee radiographic OA was more common for soccer and basketball players in comparison to the control subjects. The prevalence of clinical and radiographic OA was similar between the former athletes of different sports. Konradsen et al. [45] reported no significant difference in the grades of the degenerative changes and osteophytosis of hip and knee joints between 27 long-distance male runners and 27 nonrunners. Although the majority of studies that have evaluated the effects of sports participation on knee OA in elite athletes have focused on male athletes, some have used female elite athletes as subjects. In a retrospective cohort study that compared the risks of hip and knee OA between 81 ex-elite female athletes including 67 middle and long-distance runners and 14 tennis players, and 177 age-matched female control subjects, it was reported that the ex-athletes were 2-3 times at risk of radiologic OA in the hip and knee joints [46]. It also reported that the majority of radiologic features were in the early stages, with tennis players having more osteophytes in the tibio-femoral joints while runners were affected by patellofemoral joint disease.

Some authors have evaluated the risks of OA in the lower extremity joints of top-level soccer/football players. In a study that evaluated the prevalence of OA in the hip and knee joints of 57 retired football players with an average age of 56.4 and 57 control subjects, it was reported that although OA in the hip joint occurred more commonly for the football players in comparison to the control subjects, there was no difference in the knee OA between the two groups [47]. In a study of 185 retired professional soccer players conducted in the United Kingdom, it was reported that 32% of subjects were diagnosed with OA in at least one of the lower extremity joints, and knee OA was more common than OA of the ankle or hip joint [48]. Roos et al. [49] evaluated the prevalence of knee OA between former football players with an average age of 55 that included 215 non-elite and 71 elite players, and 572 age-matched control subjects. This study reported that a significant difference in the prevalence of knee OA between the two groups, with a rate of 1.6% for the control subjects and 7.0% for the football players. In addition, a significant difference between the elite players and non-elite players was confirmed, with a prevalence of 15.5% among elite players and 4.2% for non-elite players. The authors reported that although the risks of knee OA increased significantly for elite-level soccer players, there was no significant difference in the prevalence of knee OA between non-elite players and the control subjects when the study subjects with previous knee injuries were excluded. In a cross-sectional study of 50 male former top-level football players and 50 non-sporting volunteers, it was reported that the frequency of radiologically confirmed knee OA was higher for the football players group in comparison to the control group, although the difference was not statistically significant [50]. In addition, it was reported that although the proportion of the subjects having radiologically advanced OA was

80% in the football player group, significantly higher than 68% for the control group, the frequency and severity of pain were higher in the control group. In a cross-sectional study of 2356 retired National Football League (NFL) players in the United States, it was reported that the prevalence of arthritis was three times higher for retired NFL players in comparison to the general population, with the conclusion that such high prevalence can be contributed to the high incidence of injuries in the sport [51].

Some studies have evaluated the prevalence of knee OA among physical education teachers. In a study of 290 Swedish men and 281 Swedish women and 255 male and 257 female age-matched control subjects that compared the prevalence of OA in physical education teachers, it was reported that all of the male and female physical education teachers displayed a higher prevalence of symptomatic OA of the knee [52]. In another study, it was reported that although there was no significant difference in the prevalence of hip joint OA between female physical education teachers and age-matched women from the general population, female physical education teachers had a lower prevalence of knee OA [53].

4.2.3 Knee Injury

Many of the studies that have reported a correlation between physical activity or sports participation and knee OA did not make any considerations for joint injuries. However, joint injury is considered an important risk factor of OA [54–57]. In a 12-year follow-up study of female soccer players with anterior cruciate ligament injuries, it was reported that radiologic knee OA was confirmed in 82% of the players [58]. Moreover, a case-controlled study of 2432 retired NFL players reported that 7.7% of these players underwent knee replacement after retirement and that joint injury is a risk factor for knee replacement [59]. In one meta-analysis, the relative risk of the occurrence of OA of Kellgren and Lawrence grades II or higher on average 10 years after anterior cruciate ligament injury was 3.89 [60]. Therefore, in order to evaluate whether physical activity or sports participation itself increases the risks of knee OA, it is necessary to consider the effects of physical or sports-related joint injuries.

In some of the studies conducted on the general population, previous joint injuries were included as confounding variables in the analysis of the correlation between physical activity or sports participation and knee OA. However, a significant correlation between physical activity or sports participation and knee OA was not confirmed following adjustment for joint injuries in most of these studies [23, 26, 27, 37]. On the other hand, other studies reported that heavy physical activity or specific types of sports activities increase the risks of knee OA even after having made adjustment for joint injuries [24, 35]. Some of the literature evaluating the risks of knee OA in elite athletes with consideration of joint injury history has reported that radiographic knee OA was higher in comparison to the control group, after having excluded athletes with a history of joint injuries [43, 44].

4.2.4 Systematic Reviews and Meta-Analyses

In the middle of the 2000s, the OASIS group stated with a high degree of scientific evidence that sports and recreational activity are risk factors for knee OA, and that this risk correlates with the intensity and the duration of exposure [61]. However, it also stated with a high degree of scientific evidence that the risk of OA associated with sport is lower than the risks associated with trauma history and overweight. Several systematic reviews and meta-analysis of the correlation between physical activity or sports participation and knee OA were published thereafter. One systematic review evaluated the prevalence of chondral defects in athletes' knees among 732 men and 199 women from 11 case series [62]. The average age of the study subjects was 33, with 40% of the subjects consisting of professional athletes. In this study, the overall prevalence of full-thickness focal chondral defects in the knee was 36%, which is asserted to be higher than that of the general population. In addition, it reported meniscal tear as being the most common concomitant pathological finding. Although this systematic review did not make a direct comparison of prevalence between athletes and the general population, the fact that full-thickness focal chondral defects, deemed to be a potential risk factor for the development of OA, was confirmed in more than one-third of study subjects implies that the possibility of occurrence of early-onset knee OA in athletes in the future could be high. However, this study did not consider the effects of knee injuries and also had the limitation that research cited consisted of case series with level 4 evidence. Another systematic review concluded that although previous joint injuries and previous incidence of meniscectomy are related to increased risk of knee OA, there was an inconclusive correlation between physical activity or sports participation and knee OA [63]. In a systematic review and meta-analysis of the correlation between running and knee OA, it was asserted that a conclusion could not be reached as to whether running is associated with the diagnosis of knee OA. However, in a meta-analysis of three case-controlled studies, it was reported that runners had approximately 50% more reduced odds of undergoing surgery due to OA in comparison to control subjects. Such results differed from other prospective cohorts that reported that running increases the odds of OA diagnosis or that running was irrelevant to OA diagnosis [29, 64]. The authors described that the reason for the different outcomes was that the definitions of study designs, population, and outcomes were different. A systematic review of 17 studies that evaluated the correlation between participation in specific sports and knee OA reported that participants in soccer (elite and non-elite), elite-level long-distance running, competitive weight lifting, and wrestling had the increased prevalence of knee OA [65]. Some authors have systematically reviewed the literature evaluating the prevalence of knee OA in soccer players. One systematic review of 4 cross-sectional studies reported that the prevalence of knee OA in elite soccer players is in the range of 40–80%, which is higher than that of the general population [66]. In a systematic review that included 1576 former professional male soccer players and 2153 control subjects from 16 studies, it was reported that results of the prevalence of knee OA and knee replacement are contradictory [67].

4.3 Summary

The load exerted on the knee joint while walking is approximately three times one's body weight [68]. However, it is reported that the loads increase to approximately 4.3, 6, and 8 times body weight when climbing stairs, walking downstairs, and walking downhill, respectively. Furthermore, sports activities can increase the load exerted on the knee joint substantially more. The load exerted on the knee joint while jogging increases to nine times the body weight at each stride and to 14 times when an individual is running [68]. Although there is an extensive range of evidence stating that regular exercise is beneficial to general health, there is still no clear conclusion on the effects of long-term increase in physical activity or participation in recreational or competitive sporting activity on the joints of the lower extremity including the knees. Although abnormal biomechanical loading or stress exerted on the articular cartilage clearly appears to play a role in the development of OA, the pathophysiology of OA is yet to be understood clearly.

It was confirmed through some animal studies that repetitive loading or stress exerted on the knee joint affects the metabolism of articular cartilage. However, each of these studies used different animal types and exercise programs, and there are differences in the anatomical structure, biomechanics, and metabolism of the knee joints of animals and human beings. Although some studies have analyzed the correlation between physical activity or sports participation and knee OA in human subjects, they have produced conflicting results. This is deemed to be the result of differences between studies not only in the personal characteristics of study subjects including age, past family history of OA, alignment, body weight, and occupation, but also in various aspects such as types of physical activity or sports participation, duration of participation, exercise intensity, follow-up period, and methods of diagnosis of OA. In addition, many studies have evaluated the risk factors for knee OA based on self-reported data. However, one must keep in mind that such data has the possibility of recall bias. Another aspect that must be noted at the time of the evaluation of correlations between participation in physical or sporting activity and knee OA is joint injuries. Individuals who regularly participate in long-term physical or sporting activity may have a relatively higher risk of joint injuries in comparison to individuals who do not participate in physical or sporting activity. Although there is no clear standard on how severe knee trauma has to be defined as a joint injury, the joint injury itself is deemed to be an independent risk factor for OA.

It is difficult to reach conclusions on the correlation between physical activity or sports participation and knee OA due to various confounding factors such as joint injuries. However, based on the current literature, there is insufficient evidence for the assertion that physical or sports activity, which exerts low-to-moderate loading on the knee joint, increases the possibility of occurrence of knee OA. Nonetheless, it appears that participation in some types of sports such as football by elite athletes is associated with an increased risk of knee OA to a certain extent. However, more research is needed to reach a conclusion as to whether the risk of knee OA will also increase in elite athletes without joint injuries.

References

1. Buckwalter JA. Sports, joint injury, and posttraumatic osteoarthritis. J Orthop Sports Phys Ther. 2003;33(10):578–88.
2. Gilbert S, Chen T, Hutchinson ID, Choi D, Voigt C, Warren RF, Maher SA. Dynamic contact mechanics on the tibial plateau of the human knee during activities of daily living. J Biomech. 2014;47(9):2006–12.
3. Adams MA (2006) The mechanical environment of chondrocytes in articular cartilage. Biorheology 43(3,4):537–545.
4. Repo RU, Finlay JB. Survival of articular cartilage after controlled impact. J Bone Joint Surg Am. 1977;59(8):1068–76.
5. Brown TD, Shaw DT. In vitro contact stress distributions in the natural human hip. J Biomech. 1983;16(6):373–84.
6. Nelson BH, Anderson DD, Brand RA, Brown TD. Effect of osteochondral defects on articular cartilage. Contact pressures studied in dog knees. Acta Orthop Scand. 1988;59(5):574–9.
7. Brown TD, Anderson DD, Nepola JV, Singerman RJ, Pedersen DR, Brand RA. Contact stress aberrations following imprecise reduction of simple tibial plateau fractures. J Orthop Res. 1988;6(6):851–62.
8. Hadley NA, Brown TD, Weinstein SL. The effects of contact pressure elevations and aseptic necrosis on the long-term outcome of congenital hip dislocation. J Orthop Res. 1990;8(4):504–13.
9. Maxian TA, Brown TD, Weinstein SL. Chronic stress tolerance levels for human articular cartilage: two nonuniform contact models applied to long-term follow-up of CDH. J Biomech. 1995;28(2):159–66.
10. Siebelt M, Groen HC, Koelewijn SJ, de Blois E, Sandker M, Waarsing JH, Muller C, van Osch GJ, de Jong M, Weinans H. Increased physical activity severely induces osteoarthritic changes in knee joints with papain induced sulfate-glycosaminoglycan depleted cartilage. Arthritis Res Ther. 2014;16(1):R32.
11. Galois L, Etienne S, Grossin L, Cournil C, Pinzano A, Netter P, Mainard D, Gillet P (2003) Moderate-impact exercise is associated with decreased severity of experimental osteoarthritis in rats. Rheumatology (Oxford) 42 (5):692–693; author reply 693–694.
12. Dekel S, Weissman SL. Joint changes after overuse and peak overloading of rabbit knees in vivo. Acta Orthop Scand. 1978;49(6):519–28.
13. Newton PM, Mow VC, Gardner TR, Buckwalter JA, Albright JP. Winner of the 1996 Cabaud Award. The effect of lifelong exercise on canine articular cartilage. Am J Sports Med. 1997;25(3):282–7.
14. Videman T, Eronen I, Candolin T. Effects of motion load changes on tendon tissues and articular cartilage. A biochemical and scanning electron microscopic study on rabbits. Scand J Work Environ Health. 1979;5(suppl 3):56–67.
15. Vasan N. Effects of physical stress on the synthesis and degradation of cartilage matrix. Connect Tissue Res. 1983;12(1):49–58.
16. Kiviranta I, Tammi M, Jurvelin J, Arokoski J, Saamanen AM, Helminen HJ. Articular cartilage thickness and glycosaminoglycan distribution in the canine knee joint after strenuous running exercise. Clin Orthop Relat Res. 1992;283:302–8.
17. Kiviranta I, Tammi M, Jurvelin J, Saamanen AM, Helminen HJ. Moderate running exercise augments glycosaminoglycans and thickness of articular cartilage in the knee joint of young beagle dogs. J Orthop Res. 1988;6(2):188–95.
18. Arokoski J, Kiviranta I, Jurvelin J, Tammi M, Helminen HJ. Long-distance running causes site-dependent decrease of cartilage glycosaminoglycan content in the knee joints of beagle dogs. Arthritis Rheum. 1993;36(10):1451–9.

19. Lammi MJ, Hakkinen TP, Parkkinen JJ, Hyttinen MM, Jortikka M, Helminen HJ, Tammi MI. Adaptation of canine femoral head articular cartilage to long distance running exercise in young beagles. Ann Rheum Dis. 1993;52(5):369–77.
20. Bricca A, Juhl CB, Grodzinsky AJ, Roos EM. Impact of a daily exercise dose on knee joint cartilage – a systematic review and meta-analysis of randomized controlled trials in healthy animals. Osteoarthr Cartil. 2017;25(8):1223–37.
21. Caspersen CJ, Powell KE, Christenson GM. Physical activity, exercise, and physical fitness: definitions and distinctions for health-related research. Public Health Rep. 1985;100(2):126–31.
22. Cheng Y, Macera CA, Davis DR, Ainsworth BE, Troped PJ, Blair SN. Physical activity and self-reported, physician-diagnosed osteoarthritis: is physical activity a risk factor? J Clin Epidemiol. 2000;53(3):315–22.
23. Hannan MT, Felson DT, Anderson JJ, Naimark A. Habitual physical activity is not associated with knee osteoarthritis: the Framingham Study. J Rheumatol. 1993;20(4):704–9.
24. McAlindon TE, Wilson PW, Aliabadi P, Weissman B, Felson DT. Level of physical activity and the risk of radiographic and symptomatic knee osteoarthritis in the elderly: the Framingham study. Am J Med. 1999;106(2):151–7.
25. Szoeke C, Dennerstein L, Guthrie J, Clark M, Cicuttini F. The relationship between prospectively assessed body weight and physical activity and prevalence of radiological knee osteoarthritis in postmenopausal women. J Rheumatol. 2006;33(9):1835–40.
26. Toivanen AT, Heliovaara M, Impivaara O, Arokoski JP, Knekt P, Lauren H, Kroger H. Obesity, physically demanding work and traumatic knee injury are major risk factors for knee osteoarthritis—a population-based study with a follow-up of 22 years. Rheumatology (Oxford). 2010;49(2):308–14.
27. Hootman JM, Macera CA, Helmick CG, Blair SN. Influence of physical activity-related joint stress on the risk of self-reported hip/knee osteoarthritis: a new method to quantify physical activity. Prev Med. 2003;36(5):636–44.
28. Mork PJ, Holtermann A, Nilsen TI. Effect of body mass index and physical exercise on risk of knee and hip osteoarthritis: longitudinal data from the Norwegian HUNT Study. J Epidemiol Community Health. 2012;66(8):678–83.
29. Felson DT, Niu J, Clancy M, Sack B, Aliabadi P, Zhang Y. Effect of recreational physical activities on the development of knee osteoarthritis in older adults of different weights: the Framingham Study. Arthritis Rheum. 2007;57(1):6–12.
30. Hart DJ, Doyle DV, Spector TD. Incidence and risk factors for radiographic knee osteoarthritis in middle-aged women: the Chingford Study. Arthritis Rheum. 1999;42(1):17–24.
31. Ageberg E, Engstrom G, Gerhardsson de Verdier M, Rollof J, Roos EM, Lohmander LS. Effect of leisure time physical activity on severe knee or hip osteoarthritis leading to total joint replacement: a population-based prospective cohort study. BMC Musculoskelet Disord. 2012;13:73.
32. Wang Y, Simpson JA, Wluka AE, Teichtahl AJ, English DR, Giles GG, Graves S, Cicuttini FM. Is physical activity a risk factor for primary knee or hip replacement due to osteoarthritis? A prospective cohort study. J Rheumatol. 2011;38(2):350–7.
33. Cooper C, Snow S, McAlindon TE, Kellingray S, Stuart B, Coggon D, Dieppe PA. Risk factors for the incidence and progression of radiographic knee osteoarthritis. Arthritis Rheum. 2000;43(5):995–1000.
34. Vrezas I, Elsner G, Bolm-Audorff U, Abolmaali N, Seidler A. Case-control study of knee osteoarthritis and lifestyle factors considering their interaction with physical workload. Int Arch Occup Environ Health. 2010;83(3):291–300.
35. Lau EC, Cooper C, Lam D, Chan VN, Tsang KK, Sham A. Factors associated with osteoarthritis of the hip and knee in Hong Kong Chinese: obesity, joint injury, and occupational activities. Am J Epidemiol. 2000;152(9):855–62.
36. Sandmark H, Vingard E. Sports and risk for severe osteoarthrosis of the knee. Scand J Med Sci Sports. 1999;9(5):279–84.
37. Thelin N, Holmberg S, Thelin A. Knee injuries account for the sports-related increased risk of knee osteoarthritis. Scand J Med Sci Sports. 2006;16(5):329–33.
38. Hohmann E, Wortler K, Imhoff AB. MR imaging of the hip and knee before and after marathon running. Am J Sports Med. 2004;32(1):55–9.
39. Lane NE, Oehlert JW, Bloch DA, Fries JF. The relationship of running to osteoarthritis of the knee and hip and bone mineral density of the lumbar spine: a 9 year longitudinal study. J Rheumatol. 1998;25(2):334–41.
40. Chakravarty EF, Hubert HB, Lingala VB, Zatarain E, Fries JF. Long distance running and knee osteoarthritis. A prospective study. Am J Prev Med. 2008;35(2):133–8.
41. Kujala UM, Kaprio J, Sarna S. Osteoarthritis of weight bearing joints of lower limbs in former elite male athletes. BMJ. 1994;308(6923):231–4.
42. Kettunen JA, Kujala UM, Kaprio J, Koskenvuo M, Sarna S. Lower-limb function among former elite male athletes. Am J Sports Med. 2001;29(1):2–8.
43. Kujala UM, Kettunen J, Paananen H, Aalto T, Battie MC, Impivaara O, Videman T, Sarna S. Knee osteoarthritis in former runners, soccer players, weight lifters, and shooters. Arthritis Rheum. 1995;38(4):539–46.
44. Iosifidis MI, Tsarouhas A, Fylaktou A. Lower limb clinical and radiographic osteoarthritis in former elite male athletes. Knee Surg Sports Traumatol Arthrosc. 2015;23(9):2528–35.
45. Konradsen L, Hansen EM, Sondergaard L. Long distance running and osteoarthrosis. Am J Sports Med. 1990;18(4):379–81.
46. Spector TD, Harris PA, Hart DJ, Cicuttini FM, Nandra D, Etherington J, Wolman RL, Doyle DV. Risk of osteoarthritis associated with long-term weight-

bearing sports: a radiologic survey of the hips and knees in female ex-athletes and population controls. Arthritis Rheum. 1996;39(6):988–95.
47. Klunder KB, Rud B, Hansen J. Osteoarthritis of the hip and knee joint in retired football players. Acta Orthop Scand. 1980;51(6):925–7.
48. Drawer S, Fuller CW. Propensity for osteoarthritis and lower limb joint pain in retired professional soccer players. Br J Sports Med. 2001;35(6):402–8.
49. Roos H, Lindberg H, Gardsell P, Lohmander LS, Wingstrand H. The prevalence of gonarthrosis and its relation to meniscectomy in former soccer players. Am J Sports Med. 1994;22(2):219–22.
50. Elleuch MH, Guermazi M, Mezghanni M, Ghroubi S, Fki H, Mefteh S, Baklouti S, Sellami S. Knee osteoarthritis in 50 former top-level soccer players: a comparative study. Ann Readapt Med Phys. 2008;51(3):174–8.
51. Golightly YM, Marshall SW, Callahan LF, Guskiewicz K. Early-onset arthritis in retired National Football League players. J Phys Act Health. 2009;6(5):638–43.
52. Sandmark H. Musculoskeletal dysfunction in physical education teachers. Occup Environ Med. 2000;57(10):673–7. https://doi.org/10.1136/oem.57.10.673.
53. White JA, Wright V, Hudson AM. Relationships between habitual physical activity and osteoarthrosis in ageing women. Public Health. 1993;107(6):459–70.
54. Driban JB, Eaton CB, Lo GH, Ward RJ, Lu B, McAlindon TE. Association of knee injuries with accelerated knee osteoarthritis progression: data from the Osteoarthritis Initiative. Arthritis Care Res (Hoboken). 2014;66(11):1673–9.
55. Lotz MK, Kraus VB. New developments in osteoarthritis. Posttraumatic osteoarthritis: pathogenesis and pharmacological treatment options. Arthritis Res Ther. 2010;12(3):211.
56. Saxon L, Finch C, Bass S. Sports participation, sports injuries and osteoarthritis: implications for prevention. Sports Med. 1999;28(2):123–35.
57. Whittaker JL, Toomey CM, Woodhouse LJ, Jaremko JL, Nettel-Aguirre A, Emery CA. Association between MRI-defined osteoarthritis, pain, function and strength 3–10 years following knee joint injury in youth sport. Br J Sports Med. 2018;52(14):934–9.
58. Lohmander LS, Ostenberg A, Englund M, Roos H. High prevalence of knee osteoarthritis, pain, and functional limitations in female soccer players twelve years after anterior cruciate ligament injury. Arthritis Rheum. 2004;50(10):3145–52.
59. Davies MAM, Kerr ZY, DeFreese JD, Arden NK, Marshall SW, Guskiewicz KM, Padua DA, Pietrosimone B. Prevalence of and risk factors for total hip and knee replacement in retired national football league athletes. Am J Sports Med. 2019;47(12):2863–70.
60. Ajuied A, Wong F, Smith C, Norris M, Earnshaw P, Back D, Davies A. Anterior cruciate ligament injury and radiologic progression of knee osteoarthritis: a systematic review and meta-analysis. Am J Sports Med. 2014;42(9):2242–52.
61. Vignon E, Valat JP, Rossignol M, Avouac B, Rozenberg S, Thoumie P, Avouac J, Nordin M, Hilliquin P. Osteoarthritis of the knee and hip and activity: a systematic international review and synthesis (OASIS). Joint Bone Spine. 2006;73(4):442–55.
62. Flanigan DC, Harris JD, Trinh TQ, Siston RA, Brophy RH. Prevalence of chondral defects in athletes' knees: a systematic review. Med Sci Sports Exerc. 2010;42(10):1795–801.
63. Richmond SA, Fukuchi RK, Ezzat A, Schneider K, Schneider G, Emery CA. Are joint injury, sport activity, physical activity, obesity, or occupational activities predictors for osteoarthritis? A systematic review. J Orthop Sports Phys Ther. 2013;43(8):515–B519.
64. Kujala UM, Sarna S, Kaprio J, Koskenvuo M, Karjalainen J. Heart attacks and lower-limb function in master endurance athletes. Med Sci Sports Exerc. 1999;31(7):1041–6.
65. Driban JB, Hootman JM, Sitler MR, Harris KP, Cattano NM. Is participation in certain sports associated with knee osteoarthritis? A systematic review. J Athl Train. 2017;52(6):497–506.
66. Kuijt MT, Inklaar H, Gouttebarge V, Frings-Dresen MH. Knee and ankle osteoarthritis in former elite soccer players: a systematic review of the recent literature. J Sci Med Sport. 2012;15(6):480–7.
67. Lohkamp M, Kromer TO, Schmitt H. Osteoarthritis and joint replacements of the lower limb and spine in ex-professional soccer players: a systematic review. Scand J Med Sci Sports. 2017;27(10):1038–49.
68. Morrison JB. The mechanics of the knee joint in relation to normal walking. J Biomech. 1970;3(1):51–61.

5 Epidemiology and Pathogenesis

Young Choi

Abstract

It has been reported that radiologically, osteoarthritis is observed in 19.2% to 27.8% of patients over 45 years of age in the knee joint worldwide and in 37% of patients over 60 years of age. In Korea, it has been reported that radiologically, osteoarthritis occurred in 38.1% of population in a certain region over the age of 65, showing similar frequency compared to foreign countries. But, the incidence of osteoarthritis is affected by race, age, gender, genetics, obesity, and occupation. Direct health-care costs 1% and 2.5% of the gross domestic product but the national costs, together with the personal costs due to work loss and premature retirement are also substantial. The pathogenesis of osteoarthritis of the knee is explained by the damage of cartilage and the response of chondrocytes of cartilage (secreting various cytokines). It leads to reduction of anabolic and proliferative responses of cells. In the pathology of osteoarthritis of the knee, the key is hyaline cartilage, synovium, subchondral bone. The volume of hyaline cartilage damaged by osteoarthritis decreases. The loss of hyaline cartilage stimulates the formation of osteophytes at the joint margins. In the synovial membrane, synovial membrane cells are overproliferated leading to secrete excessive synovial fluid.

Keywords

Osteoarthritis · Knee · Incidence · Prevalence Pathogenesis · Pathology

Y. Choi (✉)
Department of Orthopedics, Kosin University Gospel Hospital, Busan, South Korea
e-mail: ks151635@kosinmed.or.kr

5.1 Epidemiology of Osteoarthritis of the Knee

5.1.1 Prevalence of Osteoarthritis of the Knee

To define radiographic osteoarthritis in epidemiologic studies, the World Health Organization (WHO) adopted the Kellgren and Lawrence score, which grades the severity of the disease from 0 to 4 by the appearance of osteophytes, joint space loss, sclerosis, and cyst [1–5]. It has been reported that radiologically, osteoarthritis is observed in 19.2% to 27.8% of patients over 45 years of age in the knee joint worldwide and in 37% of patients over 60 years of age [1, 5–7]. In Korea, it has been reported that radiologically, osteoarthritis occurred in 38.1% of population in a certain region over the age of 65, showing similar frequency compared to foreign countries [8–11].

S.-S. Seo (ed.), *A Strategic Approach to Knee Arthritis Treatment*,
https://doi.org/10.1007/978-981-16-4217-3_5

5.1.2 Incidence of Osteoarthritis of the Knee

The age-standardized incidence of patients with knee OA remained stable with 4.23% in 1996 and 3.75% in 2015 (AAPC = −0.5, 95%CI −1.4 to 0.5), but showed a positive trend between 2006 and 2015 from 3.05% to 3.75%, respectively (APC = 1.9, 95%CI 0.4 to 3.5). Between 2006 and 2015, this positive trend was higher for men (APC = 2.5, 95%CI 0.5 to 4.5) than for women (APC = 1.9, 95%CI 0.4 to 3.5) [7].

Other study used Spanish and UK general practice registry data to report on the incidence of osteoarthritis in the general population, and showed that the effects of age on individual risk of knee osteoarthritis in women follow similar patterns, with risk increasing rapidly (much more rapidly than in men) between the ages of 50 years and 75 years. This study reported peaks in incidence generally around the age of 75 years [4].

5.1.3 Socioeconomic Burden of Osteoarthritis of the Knee

Osteoarthritis is a common and disabling condition that represents a substantial and increasing health burden with notable implications for the individuals affected, health-care systems, and wider socioeconomic costs. Knee osteoarthritis accounts for approximately 85% of the burden of osteoarthritis worldwide. In terms of disability burden, osteoarthritis was responsible for the largest increases in years lived with disability at the global population level, relative to the other top 20 causes of disability, when comparing the period 1990–2005 with 2005–15 [4].

Sebbag et al. investigated the worldwide burden of musculoskeletal diseases between 2000 and 2015. They extracted Disease-Adjusted life years (DALYs) which combine the years of life lost (YLLs) and the years lived with disability (YLDs) of 183 countries from the WHO Global Health Estimates Database for 23 WHO categories of diseases. Based on these data the worldwide burden of musculoskeletal disorders as quantified using DALYs increased from 2000 to 2015, which was especially due to increase in YLDs. The median proportion of YLDs due to musculoskeletal disorders increased from 11.8% (8.3–15.1) in 2000 to 13.5% (9.6–16.6) in 2015 [5].

The medical cost of osteoarthritis in various high-income countries has been estimated to account for between 1% and 2.5% of the gross domestic product of these countries, with hip and knee joint replacements representing the major proportion of these health-care costs. These surgeries are clinically relevant and cost-effective treatment for end-stage osteoarthritis. However, they can only be considered cost-effective if the procedure is restricted to patients with more severely affected functional status. Although appropriate attention is given to direct health-care costs, the indirect costs due to work loss and premature retirement are also substantial and often ignored in considering disease burden. The national costs, together with the personal costs for patients with osteoarthritis, such as loss of income and the subsequent reductions in personal savings, greatly surpass the direct health-care costs [4].

5.2 Pathogenesis of Osteoarthritis of the Knee

As arthritis progresses, the continuity of cartilage matrix is lost along with changes in the surface of the joint, which leads to the change of biomechanical properties of the cartilage and destruction of joint (Fig. 5.1).

In the past, osteoarthritis was thought not to be inflammatory arthritis but recently, it has been recognized that substances involved in the inflammatory response are important for the development of osteoarthritis. When mechanical stimulation is transmitted to the cartilage, various factors and enzymes are secreted due to changes in the matrix production of cartilage cells [12–20]. Most of matrix that consists of cartilage are Type II collagen and proteoglycan, and these are destroyed by various factors and enzymes, leading to decrease of moisture content. Therefore, joint becomes vulnerable to loads. Matrix

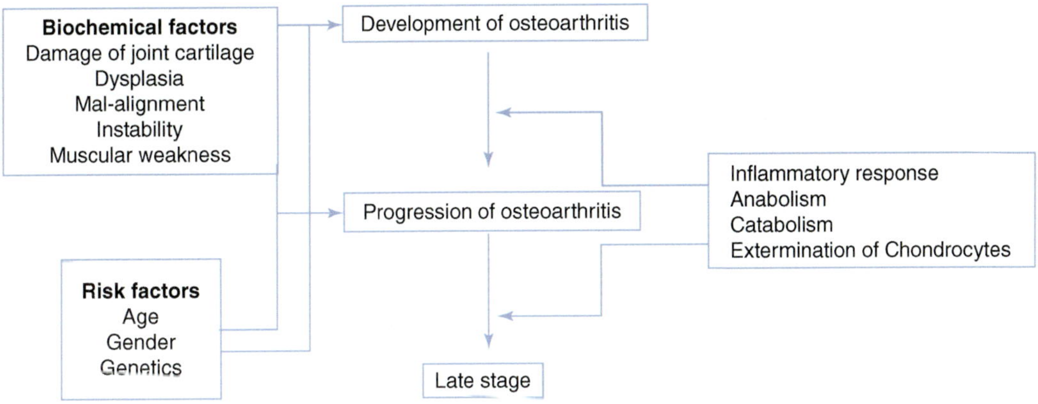

Fig. 5.1 The mechanisms of development and progression of osteoarthritis are a combination of biomechanical, biological, biochemical, and molecular biological factors and have mutual effects (Arthrology of the knee. second edition, p. 681)

metalloprotease (MMP) degrades cartilage matrix and causes irreversible fibrillation of joint cartilage [12–18, 21–23]. A large amount of nitric oxide (NO) is observed in osteoarthritis, which accelerates catabolism and is also involved in the killing of chondrocytes. Chondrocytes maintain a balance between degeneration and repair of cartilage matrix, but as the articular cartilage degrades, the catabolic ability of chondrocytes exceeds anabolic activity, leads to the loss of homeostasis. Osteoarthritis occurs when this balance is broken [12–18, 20, 24]. The two main pathological reactions that occur in chondrocytes of cartilage with osteoarthritis are premature senescence and apoptosis.

5.2.1 Damage and Change of Cartilage Matrix

Mechanical stimulation destroys the frame work of the matrix macromolecule at the molecular level and changes the level of moisture content [13, 25]. Although the concentration of type II collagen does not change, the relative concentration of the water content increases due to a decrease of proteoglycan aggrecan and a decrease in the length of the glycosaminoglycan chain. But the absolute amount of moisture and the ability to retain moisture content decreases, making it vulnerable to further damage. There is a rapid loss of proteoglycan content relative to collagen during the progression of osteoarthritis. However, while collagen content is initially maintained, collagen organization is severely perturbed. This results in a decrease in the tensile stiffness and strength provided by the normal 3D architecture of the collagen interfibrillar network. It causes a reduction in the compressive stiffness of the tissue, which can be identified clinically as the softening of early chondromalacia [12–18, 20].

5.2.2 Response of Chondrocytes to Tissue Damage

When tissue is damaged and chondrocytes detect the damage, both anabolic and catabolic processes increase. Factors involved in anabolic activity include IL-6, growth factor, insulin, insulin-like growth factor-l (IGF-l), and basic fibroblast growth factor, etc., and factors involved in catabolic activity include interleukin-1 (IL-1), tumor necrosis factor-α (TNF-α), etc. [12–18, 20, 24, 25].

5.2.2.1 IL-1, TNF α

The key inducers of catabolic processes in OA are Interleukin-1 (IL-1) and Tumor Necrosis Factor-α (TNF-α). IL-1 and TNF-α are synthesized by the same cell types, e.g., chondrocytes, osteoblasts, cells forming the synovial membrane, and mononuclear cells that were previously present in the joint or infiltrate its tissues during the inflammatory response [15]. These increase the secretion of degrading enzymes like matrix metalloproteinases (MMPs), aggrecanase, interleukin 8 (IL-8), interleukin 6 (IL-6), Prostaglandin E2 (PGE2), nitric oxide (NO). It increases the loss of glycoprotein from cartilage matrix, inhibits resynthesis, and prevents to replenish the loss of matrix components. It also promotes the production of Prostaglandin E2 (PGE2), which is closely related to the symptoms of osteoarthritis [12–18, 20, 25].

5.2.2.2 MMPs

MMPs are enzymes such as collagenase, stromelysin, gelatinase secreted from chondrocytes, synovial fluid, synovial membrane cells, etc., which destroy aggrecan and collagen in cartilage. It is also activated by IL-1, Tissue plasminogen activator, Matrix metalloproteinase activator, and inhibited by TGF-ß, Tissue inhibitor of metalloproteinase, and Plasminogen activator inhibitor [12–18, 20, 25]. Among MMPs, MMP-13 plays an important role in the process of degeneration in osteoarthritis. MMP-13 expression is more restricted to connective tissues. It has a much higher catalytic velocity rate compared with other MMPs over Col2 and gelatin, making it the most potent peptidolytic enzyme among collagenases. Clinical investigations revealed that patients with articular cartilage destruction had high MMP-13 expression, suggesting increased MMP-13 may be the cause of cartilage degradation [16, 20].

5.2.2.3 Nitric Oxide (NO)

Inhibits the synthesis of proteoglycan and collagen, activates MMP, and is upregulated by MMP to accelerate cartilage destruction. It also promotes the synthesis of PGE2 and Cyclooxygenase-2 (COX-2). It also plays an important role in the death of chondrocytes (apoptosis) [12–18, 20, 25].

5.2.2.4 Insulin, TGF

Insulin promotes the regeneration of joint cartilage. TGF-ß stimulates the synthesis of proteoglycan in joint cartilage and inhibits the destruction of cartilage by IL-1. Loss of TGF-ß signaling is associated with cartilage damage, which suggesting loss of the protective effect of TGF-ß during osteoarthritis progression. Additionally, TGF-ß is involved in early osteophyte formation [16]. TGF-1 stimulates cell differentiation and matrix generation in cartilage [14] (Table 5.1).

Table 5.1 Associated Cytolytic enzymes in cartilage metabolism

Cytokines of secretion response to cartilage and tissue damage		
Catabolic response	Inhibitory response	Anabolic response
IL-1, IL-6, TNF-α, IL-17, IL-18	IL-3, L-4, IL-10, IL-11, IL-13, IL-1 receptor antagonist, interferon-γ	IGF-1, TGF ß1, TGF ß2, TGF ß3, FGF-2, FGF-4, FGF-8, BMP-2, BMP-4, BMP-5, BMP-6, BMP-7, BMP-9, BMP-13

IL interleukin, *TNF* tumor necrosis factor, *IGF* insulin-like growth factor, *TGF* transforming growth factor, *FGF* fibroblast growth factor, *BMP* bone morphogenic protein

5.2.3 Reduction of Anabolic and Proliferative Responses of Cells

The anabolic and healing activity may last for several years opposed to catabolic, or even temporarily reverse the progression of arthritis. Anabolic activity occurs as the healing and remodeling process fails, resulting in gradual loss of articular cartilage and decreased anabolic and proliferative responses of chondrocytes. In addition, down regulation of the response to anabolic cytokine of cartilage cells is also a cause, which triggers the progression of arthritis. As the age increases, the composition ratio of cartilage matrix changes, and reactions to stimuli of anabolic enzymes of chondrocytes or cell activity decreases. These changes may be associated with the progression of arthritis [16] (Table 5.2).

Table 5.2 Differences between age-related and osteoarthritis in joint cartilage

	Joint surface	Cells/Cytokine mechanism	Changes in matrix
Aging course of joint state	– Localized stable fibrillation on the joint surface	– Chondrocytes decrease – Response to growth factors decrease – Decreased anabolic mechanism	– Decrease of moisture and huge proteoglycan decrease – Accumulation of matrix reductase – Thickened collagen fibers and heterogeneity – Relatively increase of the cross-linking of collagen – Decrease of tensile strength and stiffness
Pathogenesis of osteoarthritis	– Progressive fibrillation formation and extension to the subchondral bone – Cartilage defect or thin surface – Fibrous change of cartilage according to healing mechanism	– activated anabolic mechanism in early phase but gradually decreases – Loss of chondrocytes – Activated catabolic enzymes – Appearance of fibroblast-like cells in fibrocartilage tissue	– Increase of moisture and proteoglycan level in early phase – Lysis of collagen macromolecules – Progressive loss of proteoglycan – Permeability of water increases – Decrease of tensile strength, resistance, and stiffness

5.3 Pathology of Osteoarthritis of the Knee

Cartilage and surrounding tissues such as bones and synovial membranes are important in the development of osteoarthritis. Cartilage has an organized layered structure that can be functionally and structurally divided into four zones: the superficial zone, the middle (or transitional) zone, the deep zone, and the zone of calcified cartilage [21, 26]. The superficial zone is the articulating surface that provides a smooth gliding surface and resists shear. Also known as the tangential zone, this zone makes up approximately 10–20% of articular cartilage thickness. It has the highest collagen content of the zones; the collagen fibrils in this zone are densely packed and have a highly ordered alignment parallel to the articular surface. The chondrocytes in this layer, characterized by an elongated appearance histologically, preferentially express proteins that have lubricating and protective functions and secrete relatively little proteoglycan. Among the proteins involved in surface lubrication, superficial zone protein (SZP) has been identified as a functionally important molecule [21] (Figs. 5.2 and 5.3).

Macroscopically, cartilage changes in osteoarthritis can be seen as softening (chondromalacia), fibrillation, and erosions (ulceration). Histologic features of cartilage breakdown and failed repair include cartilage clefts, loss of the cartilage layers, cellular necrosis, chondrocyte cloning, and a duplication of the tidemark. It appears that the superficial zone is affected first in early osteoarthritis [21].

The most important factor is that as the transmission of load to the joint changes, it leads to a biochemical reaction within the joint. The biochemical changes caused by mechanical stimulation change the balance of destruction and synthesis of chondrocytes, cartilage matrix, and subchondral bones. The uncoupling of the normal balance of degradation and repair in the articular cartilage and subchondral bone leads to abrasion of articular cartilage with formation of new bone at and around joint surfaces. The end result is functional deterioration of the joint [17].

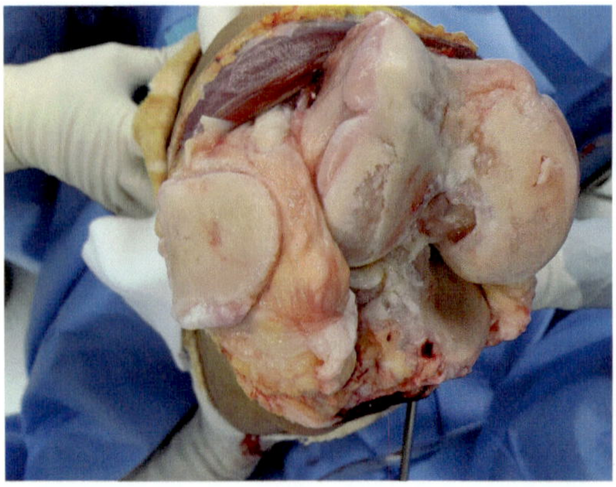

Fig. 5.2 In the later stages of osteoarthritis, the layers of the medial and lateral femoral condyle joint cartilage are lost. Thickening of the synovial membrane is observed

If the joints are young and healthy, the muscles around the joints, smooth lubrication of the joint surface, and sufficient ligament function can defend against damage whether the load to the joint changes [19]. If the movement physiologically occurred by joints is not controlled due to damaged and aged cartilage or ligaments, the transmission of loads on the joints changes and excessive loads are concentrated in one place, which leads to damage of joints, especially the hyaline cartilage [2]. These changes and loss of hyaline cartilage stimulate the formation of osteophytes at the joint margins. In the synovial membrane, synovial membrane cells are overproliferated leading to secrete excessive synovial fluid [26].

5.3.1 Hyaline Cartilage

Hyaline cartilage functions as a low-friction, wear-resistant tissue designed to bear and distribute loads. It is a highly specialized tissue with unique mechanical behavior and poor regenerative capacities [26]. The initial findings of osteoarthritis are fibrillation and disruption which looks like the cartilage surface is cracked where the hair sprouts roughly. As the disease progresses, irregularities of the surface form a cleft and most of the joint surface becomes rough and irregular. The fibrillation of cartilage progresses deeper and eventually forms a fissure, reaching the subchondral bone. As the fissure becomes deeper, the end of the fibrillated surface of cartilage falls off to make a float and the thickness of the cartilage becomes thin. In addition, as the matrix of cartilage is decomposed by enzymes, further reduction of the thickness of the cartilage layer occurs, leading to exposure of the bone under the cartilage (Figs. 5.4 and 5.5).

5.3.2 Synovium

Histologically, cells on the surface increase, and cells such as lymphocytes penetrate into the surface. Thickening of the synovial membrane and inflammatory changes promote formation of blood vessel and inflammatory responses. Inflammatory cells, such as macrophages, secrete angiogenic factors. Cells such as vascular endothelial cell or fibroblast, etc., induce secretion of substances that promote blood vessel formation like vascular endothelial growth factor (VEGF), basic fibroblast growth factor (bFGF), etc. [21].

5.3.3 Subchondral Bone

The subchondral bone represents the bony components located beneath the calcified cartilage and consists of the subchondral bone plate and the subchondral trabecular bone. The subchondral bone plate is a thin cortical lamella adjacent to the calcified cartilage [25]. Bone loss is enhanced by enzymes involved in cartilage

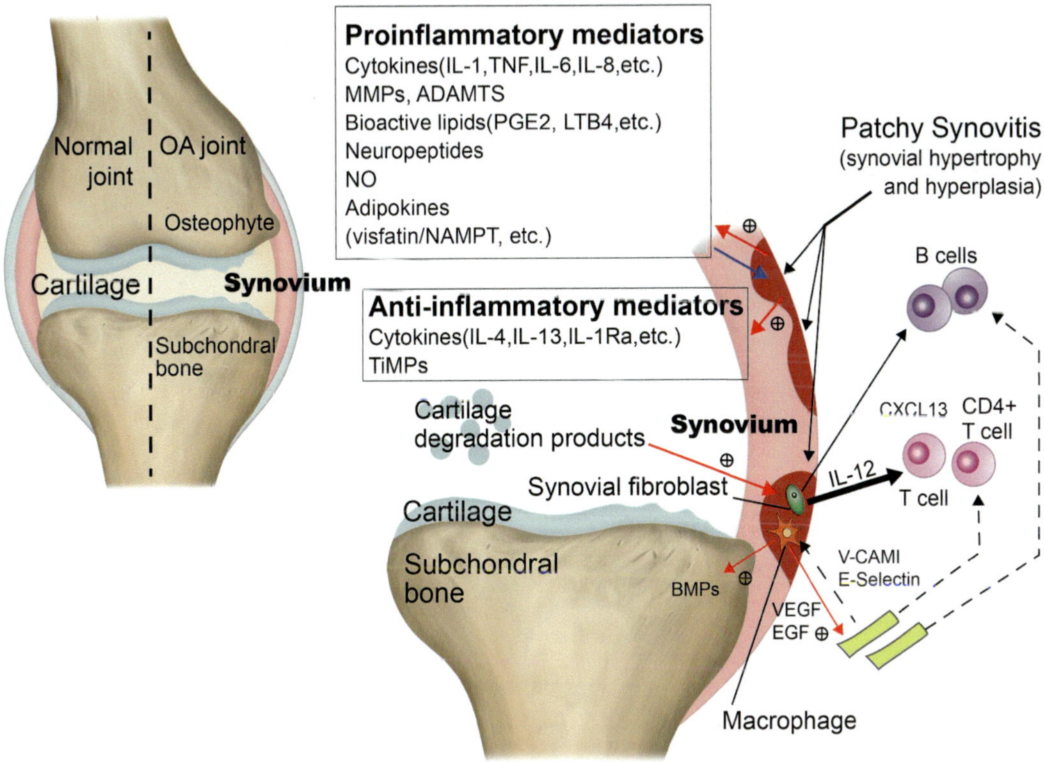

Fig. 5.3 Involvement of the synovium in OA pathophysiology. Products of cartilage breakdown that are released into the synovial fluid are phagocytosed by synovial cells, amplifying synovial inflammation. In turn, activated synovial cells in the inflamed synovium produce catabolic and proinflammatory mediators that lead to excess production of the proteolytic enzymes responsible for cartilage breakdown, creating a positive feedback loop. The inflammatory response is amplified by activated synovial T cells, B cells, and infiltrating macrophages. To counteract this inflammatory response, the synovium and cartilage may produce anti-inflammatory cytokines. In addition to these effects on cartilage inflammation and breakdown, the inflamed synovium contributes to the formation of osteophytes via BMPs. Abbreviations: *ADAMTS* a disintegrin and metalloproteinase with thrombospondin motifs, *BMP* bone morphogenetic protein, *CCL2* CC chemokine ligand 2, *CXCL13* CXC chemokine ligand 13, *EGF* endothelial growth factor, *GM CSF* granulocyte macrophage colony stimulating factor, *IL* interleukin, *IL 1Ra* IL 1 receptor antagonist, *LIF* leukemia inhibitory factor, *LTB4* leukotriene B4, *MMP* matrix metalloproteinase, *NAMPT* nicotinamide phosphoribosyl transferase (also called visfatin), *NO* nitric oxide, *NGF* nerve growth factor, *OA* osteoarthritis, *PGE2* prostaglandin E2, *TIMP* tissue inhibitor of metalloproteinase, *TNF* tumor necrosis factor, *vCAM 1* vascular cell adhesion molecule 1, *vEGF* vascular endothelial growth factor [20]

catabolism, and the formation of osteophytes and remodeling of subchondral bones by enzymes involved in anabolism occurs. As a result, sclerosis of subchondral bone appears relatively early in the progress of disease and osteophyte is formed by proliferation and thickening of bone around the joint. Occasionally, subchondral cysts are formed in the subchondral bone as well as sclerosis [26] (Figs. 5.6, 5.7, 5.8).

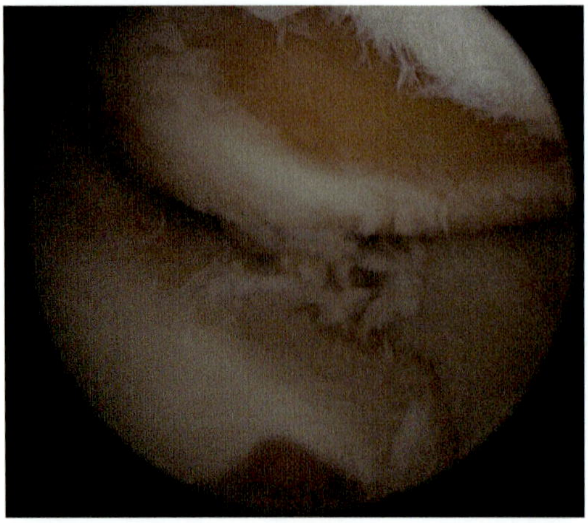

Fig. 5.4 Knee arthroscopic findings of female patient with synovitis. Showing chondral defects of medial femoral and tibial condyle

Fig. 5.5 Optical microscopic findings of cartilage matrix in osteoarthritis patients. Fibrillation and fissuring are formed on the surface of the articular cartilage. Apoptosis is observed along with proliferation of cartilage cells (H&E, ×100) (Orthopaedics seventh edition. Fig. III-17)

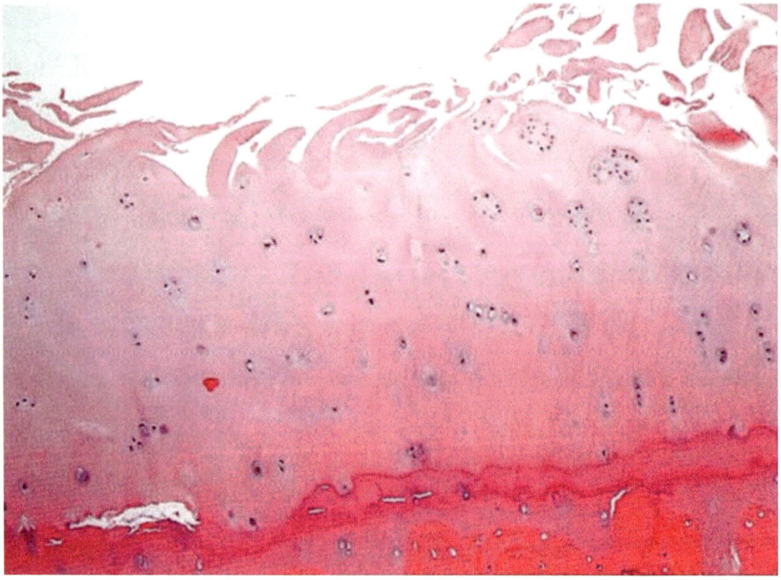

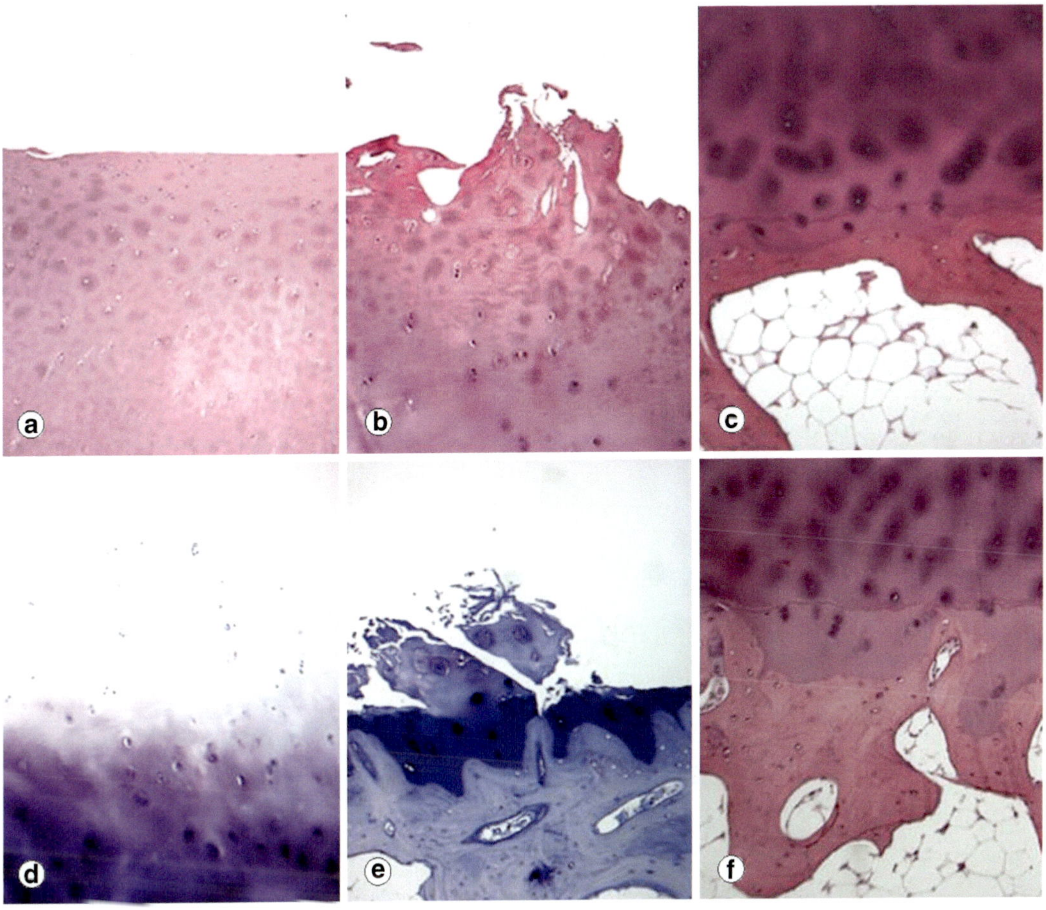

Fig. 5.6 Conventional histology shows fibrillation and matrix loss in OA cartilage (**b**) compared with normal cartilage (**a**). In severely damaged areas nearly all articular cartilage is destroyed (**e**). Also a moderate (**d**) to severe (**e**) loss of proteoglycans is found, as visualized by toluidine blue staining. Besides changes in articular cartilage, also changes in the subchondral bone are prominent, namely, thickening of the subchondral bone plate (**f**, OA; **c**, normal) (A Thomas et al. 175 – Pathogenesis and pathology of osteoarthritis; 2015. Fig173.4)

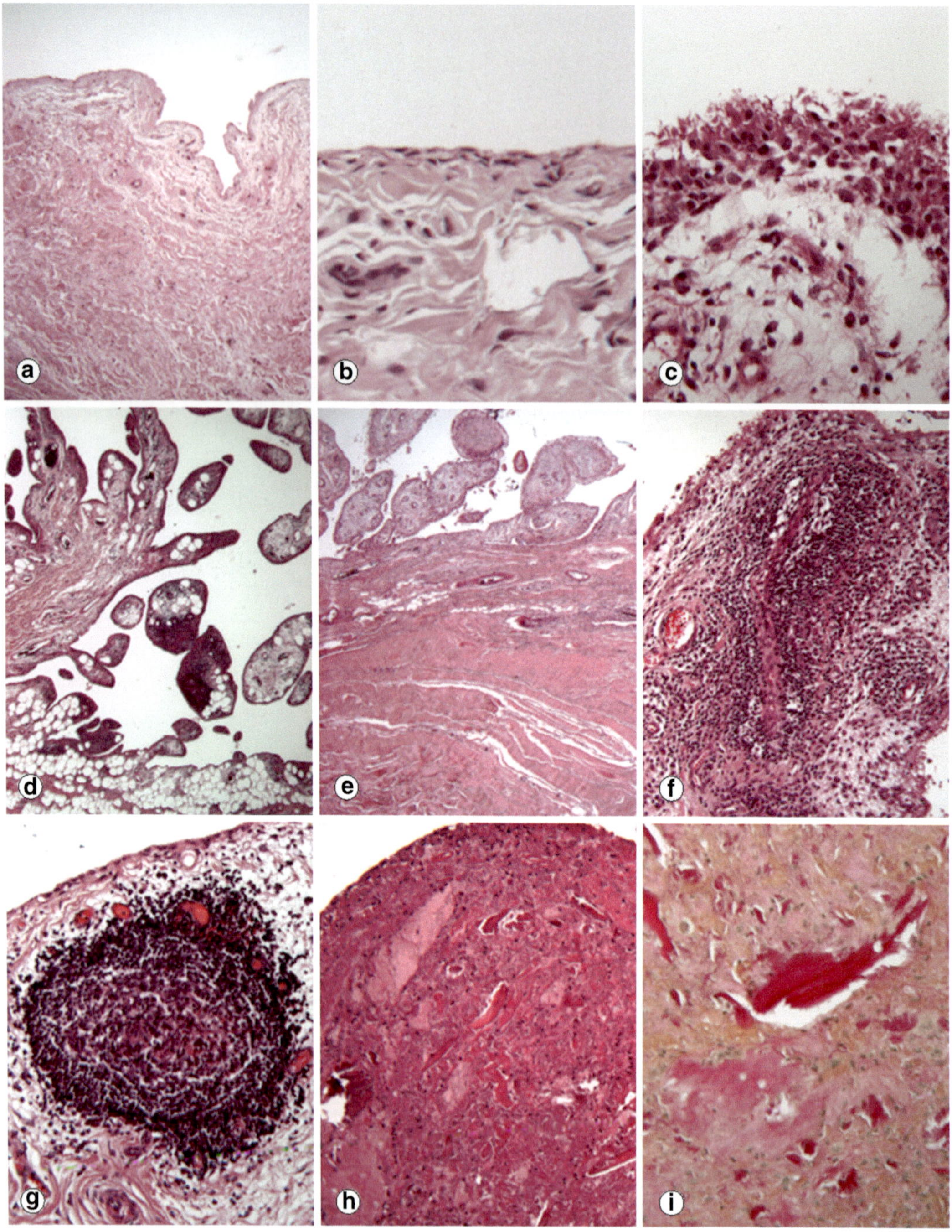

Fig. 5.7 (**a**, **b**) Normal synovial membrane shows a rather flat surface with a flat layer of inactive, non-proliferated layer of synoviocytes. In contrast, OA synoviocytes are at least in some cases severely activated and proliferated (**c**) similar to the situation found in rheumatoid arthritis. Most cases of late-stage OA synovial specimens show a moderate to abundant synovial hyperplasia (**d**, **e**) and often some sort of capsule thickening (**e**). A minority of cases of OA synovial membranes show mild to moderate (**f**, **g**) inflammatory infiltrates usually lying in aggregates around blood vessels (**f**). In part of the cases lymphoid follicles also are found (**g**). End-stage rapid progressive cartilage destruction leads to detritus-rich synovitis with cartilage and bone fragments incorporated in fibrinous exudate (**i**, van Gieson stain) or the synovial stroma (**h**) (Aigner T, Schmitz N, Salter D, editors. 175 Pathogenesis and pathology of osteoarthritis 2015)

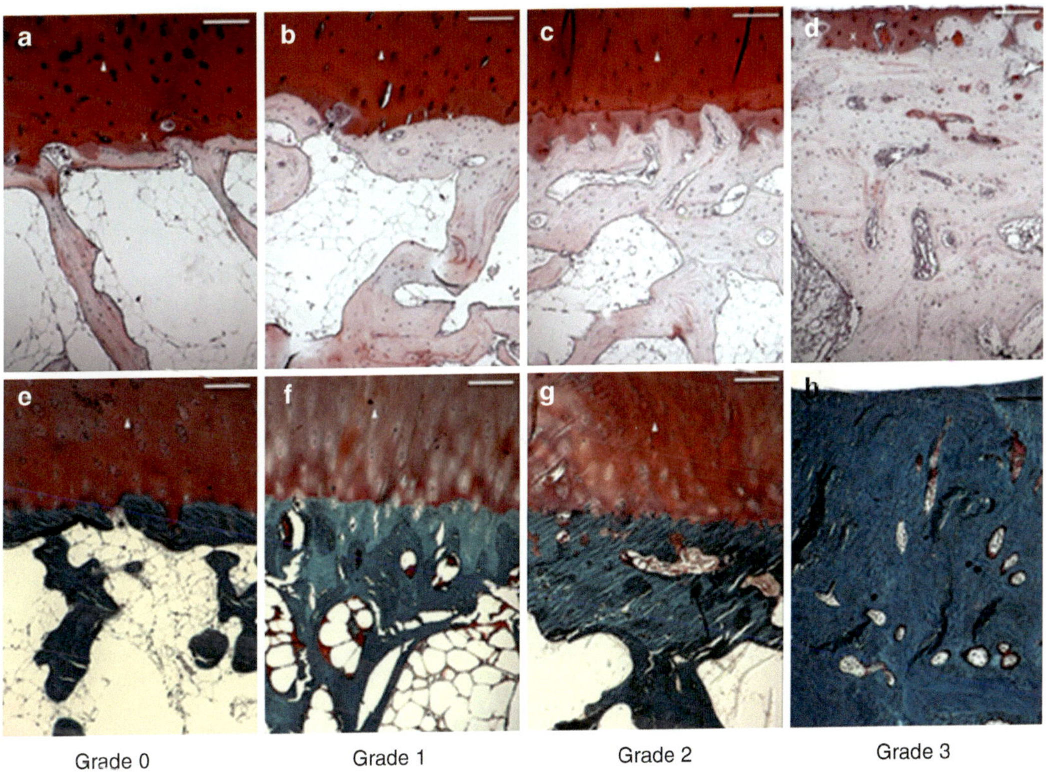

Fig. 5.8 Safranin O (**a**–**d**) and Masson's trichrome stained histological samples of subchondral bone grades. Images taken with a light microscope using digital camera. White triangle marks articular cartilage, white cross shows calcified cartilage. (**a** and **e**) Black asterisks marks fenestrae in subchondral bone plate connecting the articular cartilage to bone marrow in grade 0 and (**b** and **f**) grade 1. (**c** and **g**) Fibrillation on subchondral bone plate can be seen in grade 2. (**d** and **h**) Distinctive sclerosis and loss of articular cartilage mark late-stage OA in grade 3. Scale bar 200 μm (Aho OM, Finnilä M, Thevenot J, Saarakkala S, Lehenkari P. Subchondral bone histology and grading in osteoarthritis. PLoS One. 2017;12(3):e0173726)

5.4 Summary

The osteoarthritis, which is a common occurrence in the elderly population, is related to a variety of factors such as race, age, gender, genetics, obesity, and occupation. The pathogenesis of osteoarthritis of the knee is explained by the damage of cartilage and the response of chondrocytes of cartilage (secreting various cytokines). In the pathology of osteoarthritis of the knee, the key is hyaline cartilage, synovium, subchondral bone.

References

1. Palazzo C, Nguyen C, Lefevre-Colau MM, Rannou F, Poiraudeau S. Risk factors and burden of osteoarthritis. Ann Phys Rehabil Med. 2016;59(3):134–8.
2. Goldring MB, Goldring SR. Osteoarthritis. J Cell Physiol. 2007;213(3):626–34.
3. Zhang J, Song L, Liu G, Zhang A, Dong H, Liu Z, et al. Risk factors for and prevalence of knee osteoarthritis in the rural areas of Shanxi Province, North China: a COPCORD study. Rheumatol Int. 2013;33(11):2783–8.
4. Hunter DJ, Bierma-Zeinstra S. Osteoarthritis Lancet. 2019;393(10182):1745–59.

5. Kloppenburg M, Berenbaum F. Osteoarthritis year in review 2019: epidemiology and therapy. Osteoarthr Cartil. 2020;28(3):242–8.
6. Vina ER, Kwoh CK. Epidemiology of osteoarthritis: literature update. Curr Opin Rheumatol. 2018;30(2):160–7.
7. Spitaels D, Mamouris P, Vaes B, Smeets M, Luyten F, Hermens R, et al. Epidemiology of knee osteoarthritis in general practice: a registry-based study. BMJ Open. 2020;10(1):e031734.
8. Cho HJ, Morey V, Kang JY, Kim KW, Kim TK. Prevalence and risk factors of spine, shoulder, hand, hip, and knee osteoarthritis in community-dwelling Koreans older than age 65 years. Clin Orthop Relat Res. 2015;473(10):3307–14.
9. Kim I, Kim HA, Seo YI, Song YW, Jeong JY, Kim DH. The prevalence of knee osteoarthritis in elderly community residents in Korea. J Korean Med Sci. 2010;25(2):293–8.
10. Shin DW, Nam S, Bang YS, Lee JY. Estimation of the prevalence of Korean adults aged 50 years or more with knee osteoarthritis based on the data from fifth Korea National Health and Nutrition Examination Survey. J Korean Med Assoc. 2013;56(5):431–6.
11. Yoo JJ, Kim DH, Kim HA. Risk factors for progression of radiographic knee osteoarthritis in elderly community residents in Korea. BMC Musculoskelet Disord. 2018;19(1):80.
12. Adatia A, Rainsford KD, Kean WF. Osteoarthritis of the knee and hip. Part I: aetiology and pathogenesis as a basis for pharmacotherapy. J Pharm Pharmacol. 2012;64(5):617–25.
13. Brandt KD, Dieppe P, Radin EL. Etiopathogenesis of osteoarthritis. Rheum Dis Clin N Am. 2008;34(3):531–59.
14. Mora JC, Przkora R, Cruz-Almeida Y. Knee osteoarthritis: pathophysiology and current treatment modalities. J Pain Res. 2018;11:2189–96.
15. Lambova SN, Müller-Ladner U. Osteoarthritis – current insights in pathogenesis. Diagn Treatment Curr Rheumatol Rev. 2018;14(2):91–7.
16. Xia B, Di C, Zhang J, Hu S, Jin H, Tong P. Osteoarthritis pathogenesis: a review of molecular mechanisms. Calcif Tissue Int. 2014;95(6):495–505.
17. Kraus VB. Pathogenesis and treatment of osteoarthritis. Med Clin North Am. 1997;81(1):85–112.
18. Howell DS. Pathogenesis of osteoarthritis. Am J Med. 1986;80(4b):24–8.
19. Goldring SR. The role of bone in osteoarthritis pathogenesis. Rheum Dis Clin N Am. 2008;34(3):561–71.
20. Sellam J, Berenbaum F. The role of synovitis in pathophysiology and clinical symptoms of osteoarthritis. Nat Rev Rheumatol. 2010;6(11):625–35.
21. Pearle AD, Warren RF, Rodeo SA. Basic science of articular cartilage and osteoarthritis. Clin Sports Med. 2005;24(1):1–12.
22. Krasnokutsky S, Attur M, Palmer G, Samuels J, Abramson SB. Current concepts in the pathogenesis of osteoarthritis. Osteoarthr Cartil. 2008;16(Suppl 3):S1–3.
23. Sarzi-Puttini P, Cimmino MA, Scarpa R, Caporali R, Parazzini F, Zaninelli A, et al. Osteoarthritis: an overview of the disease and its treatment strategies. Semin Arthritis Rheum. 2005;35(1 Suppl 1):1–10.
24. Aigner T, Söder S, Gebhard PM, McAlinden A, Haag J. Mechanisms of disease: role of chondrocytes in the pathogenesis of osteoarthritis – structure, chaos and senescence. Nat Clin Pract Rheumatol. 2007;3(7):391–9.
25. Aigner T, Schmitz N, Salter D, editors. 175 Pathogenesis and pathology of osteoarthritis 2015.
26. Aho OM, Finnilä M, Thevenot J, Saarakkala S, Lehenkari P. Subchondral bone histology and grading in osteoarthritis. PLoS One. 2017;12(3):e0173726.

Radiographic Findings of the Knee Osteoarthritis

6

Sun Joo Lee

Abstract

Imaging is important for the diagnosis, prognosis, and follow-up of osteoarthritis (OA). The radiological evaluation of OA mainly consists of radiography, CT and MRI. Radiography and CT are useful tools for depicting bone shape, alignment, and osteophytes. On the other hand, MRI is a useful diagnostic tool for evaluating major anatomical structures, including articular cartilage, menisci, ligaments, synovium, capsular structures, and bone marrow in the knee. Typical findings of OA are joint space narrowing, subchondral sclerosis, and subchondral bone cyst in the area under pressure and osteophytes in the area without pressure. On the other hand, osteoporosis, bony erosion, and large amounts of joint effusion are not the typical findings of OA.

Keywords

OA · Radiography · CT · MRI

S. J. Lee (✉)
Department of Radiology, Inje University Busan Paik Hospital, Busan, South Korea
e-mail: tjswnlee@paik.ac.kr

6.1 Radiography

Image and pathologic changes are evaluated by dividing the knee into three sections, medial femorotibial compartment, lateral femorotibial compartment, and patellofemoral compartment. The ordinary radiographic imaging technique is limited in observing early changes of OA. The tunnel view technique, which obtains the image when the joint is bent, shows cartilage and bone changes that were not observed by ordinary techniques and visualized changes that occur in the posterior aspect of the femoral condyle. An image obtained during stress or weight loading may be additionally required. This image would be useful for evaluating cartilage loss and varus or valgus deformation. It also accurately shows the subluxation of the femur and tibia. While it would be ideal to obtain the weight-loaded image when standing only on the symptomatic leg, it is recommended to take standing tunnel projection or Rosenberg images of a joint in a standing position that is bent by 30–45° [1].

Image findings of the OA knees are clearly visible in the medial femorotibial compartment, and a single or two-compartment involvement is more typical than involvement in all three one. The normal joint cavity spacing is more than 3 mm on the standing image, but multiple joint space narrowing of less than 3 mm can be seen, and the spacing may sometimes become completely lost. Subchondral sclerosis is more com-

S.-S. Seo (ed.), *A Strategic Approach to Knee Arthritis Treatment*,
https://doi.org/10.1007/978-981-16-4217-3_6

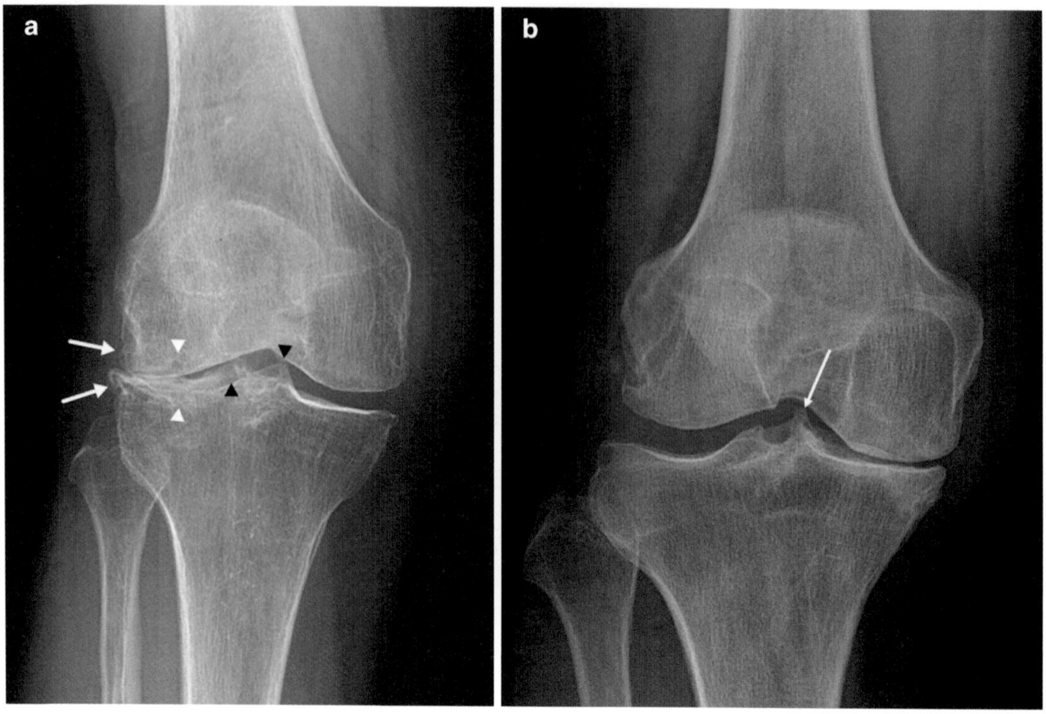

Fig. 6.1 (a) Standing AP radiograph of the right knee shows the irregular articular surface of the lateral femoral condyle and tibial plateau due to marginal (white arrowheads) and central osteophytes (black arrowheads) of the lateral tibiofemoral compartment. Note additional joint space narrowing and subchondral sclerosis (arrows) of the lateral compartment. (b) Standing AP radiograph of the right knee shows the tibial spine (arrow) sharp. Note joint space narrowing, subchondral sclerosis, and subchondral cysts in the medial tibiofemoral compartment

mon in the tibia than the femur. Osteophyte is observed at the edges of femur and tibia, while central osteophyte can occur at the femur that looks similar to the intraarticular loose body. Osteophyte makes the joint surface irregular and sharpens the tibial spine (Fig. 6.1). Other image findings of OA in the femorotibial compartment include condyle hypertrophy, medial compartment vacuum phenomenon, and meniscal calcification [2]. In the knee joint, the degree of OA is evaluated using the Kellgren-Lawrence class, which classified radiographic findings into four stages (Table 6.1) (Fig. 6.2) [3]. The Ahlbäck scoring system, which is used for defines OA with a global score. Rather than the presence of osteophytes, there is more emphasis on the narrowing of the joint space and wear of the bone (Table 6.2) (Fig. 6.3) [4]. Intraobserver reliability for KL was substantial for observer A (κ: 0.753) and moderate for observer B (κ: 0.573). Interobserver reliability for KL was moderate for both occasions (κ: 0.499 and 0.458, respectively). Intraobserver reliability for Ahlbäck was substantial for observer A (κ: 0.768) and moderate

Table 6.1 Kellgren-Lawrence grade

Grade 0	No radiographic features of OA
Grade 1	Doubtful joint space narrowing and possible osteophytic lipping
Grade 2	Definite osteophytes and possible joint space narrowing on weight-bearing radiograph
Grade 3	Multiple osteophytes, definite joint space narrowing, subchondral sclerosis, and possible bony deformity
Grade 4	Large osteophytes, marked joint space narrowing, severe sclerosis and definite bony deformity

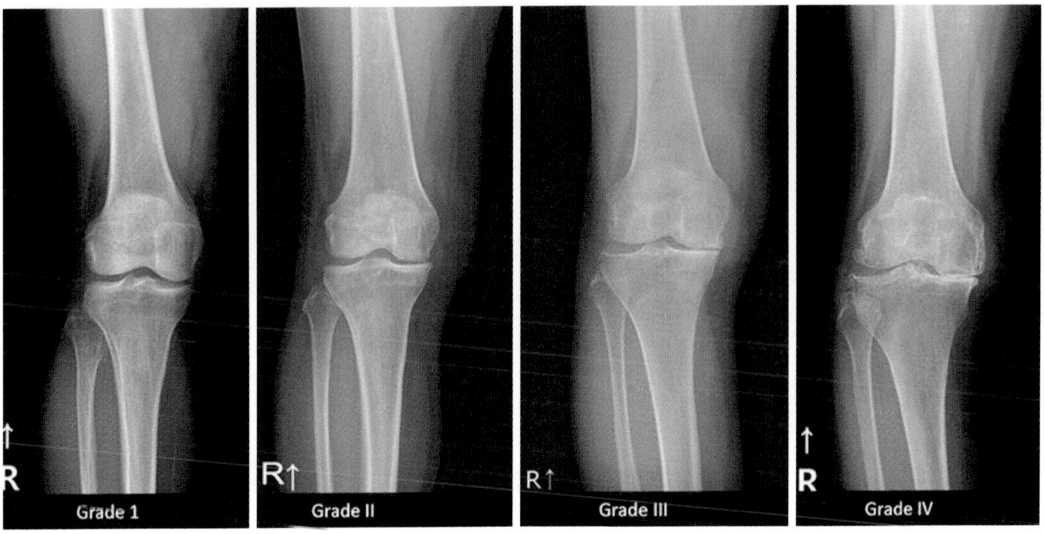

Fig. 6.2 Kellgren-Lawrence grading of the medial tibiofemoral compartment on standing AP radiograph

Table 6.2 Ahlbäck radiographic grading scale

Grade of osteoarthritis	Description
Grade 0	No radiographic findings of osteoarthritis
Grade I	Joint space narrowing <3 mm
Grade II	Joint space obliterated or almost obliterated
Grade III	Minor bone attrition (<5 mm)
Grade IV	Moderate bone attrition (5–15 mm)
Grade V	Severe bone attrition (>15 mm)

for observer B (κ: 0.561). Interobserver reliability for Ahlbäck was fair for both occasions (κ: 0.365 and 0.204, respectively). As the KL classification system is the most widely used, many studies have been performed on this system. The results of other studies of the inter- and intraobserver agreements in the KL grading scale were found to be almost perfect [4].

The patellofemoral compartment is also frequently involved by OA, and axial projection is an important examination technique. Cartilage erosion and subchondral sclerosis are predominant in the lateral patellar facet (Fig. 6.4), because of the wider articular surface and the force caused by the physiological varus. Changes in the patellofemoral joint are usually accompanied by femorotibial joints, especially the medial compartments. OA rarely develops only at patellofemoral joints alone, so if OA changes are seen only in patellofemoral joints, CPPD, Wilson disease, and hyperparathyroidism should be considered. Osteophyte may occur as an additional degeneration in the area where the quadriceps tendon attaches to the anterior aspect of the patella. When OA becomes severe, angulation, and subluxation accompany ligament changes. While varus alignment is more frequent than valgus alignment, the varus deformity is accompanied by lateral subluxation of the tibia (Fig. 6.5), and valgus deformity is typically accompanied by medial subluxation [5, 6].

6.1.1 Cartilage Abnormalities

The gradual loss of cartilage is depicted as joint space narrowing on the image and is the most basic finding of OA (Fig. 6.6). Joint space narrowing is localized in joints that receive severe pressure. Therefore, it is evident in the medial femorotibial joint in the knee [2].

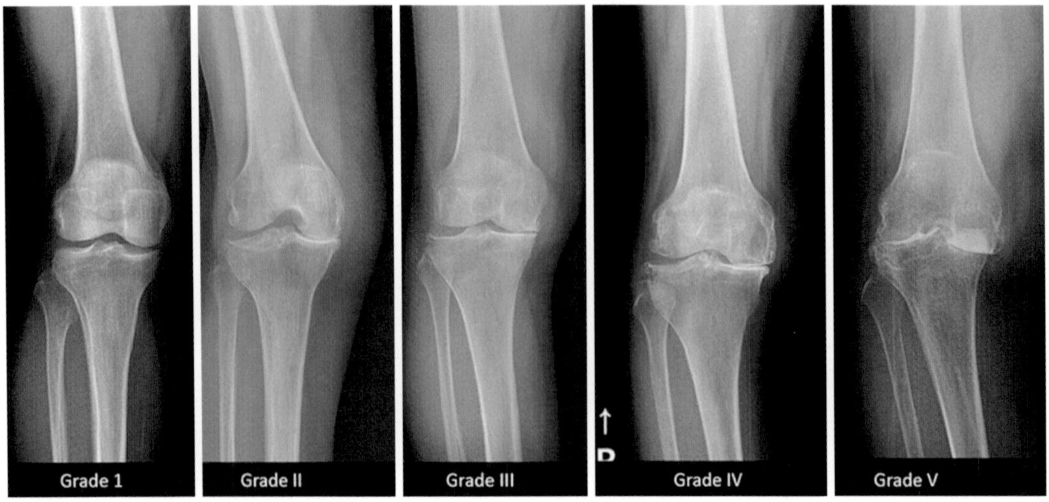

Fig. 6.3 Ahlbäck radiographic grading scale of the medial tibiofemoral compartment on standing AP radiograph

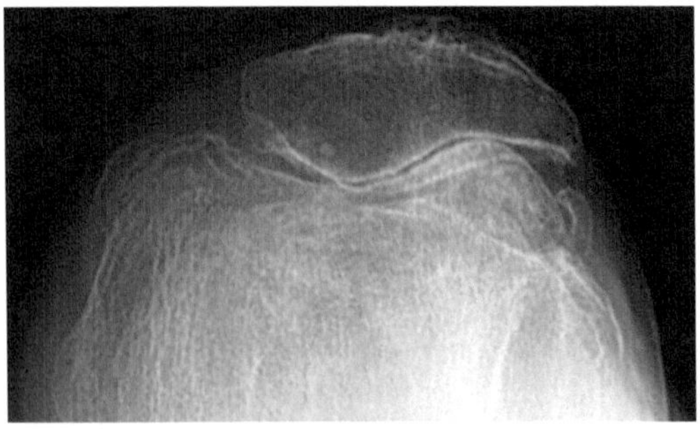

Fig. 6.4 Knee Merchant radiograph shows joint space narrowing, marginal osteophytes, and subchondral sclerosis in the lateral patellofemoral compartment

6.1.2 Subchondral Bone

Subchondral bone abnormalities can be divided into destructive phase (regressive remodeling) and productive phase (progressive remodeling), and both processes proceed simultaneously in different parts of the joint. The destructive phase occurs in areas under pressure due to bone eburnation, cyst formation, flattening, and deformation, and the productive phase such as osteophyte, occurs in areas that are not subject to joint pressure [7].

6.1.2.1 Subchondral Sclerosis

After cartilage loss, subchondral sclerosis can be seen on the image due to subchondral bone exposure according to bone eburnation (Fig. 6.6). Weak and congested subchondral bones are more vulnerable to deformation, and loss of cartilage and restriction of joint motion can cause fracture, flattening, and collapse of bone trabecula. Subchondral sclerosis and joint space narrowing are closely related. As the joint space becomes narrower, subchondral sclerosis tends to become more severe [8, 9].

6.1.2.2 Subchondral Cyst

Subchondral cysts take place in between thickened subchondral trabecula. They are histologically composed of internal mucus, adipose tissue, cartilage surrounded by fibrous elements and are accompanied by the sclerosis of the surrounding. There are two hypotheses about the mechanism of cyst formation. The first hypothesis is that the increased pressure in the joint pushes the synovial fluid through the cartilage, leading to cyst formation. Another hypothesis is the bone contusion, where cystic necrosis occurs due to an impact on the bone surface and

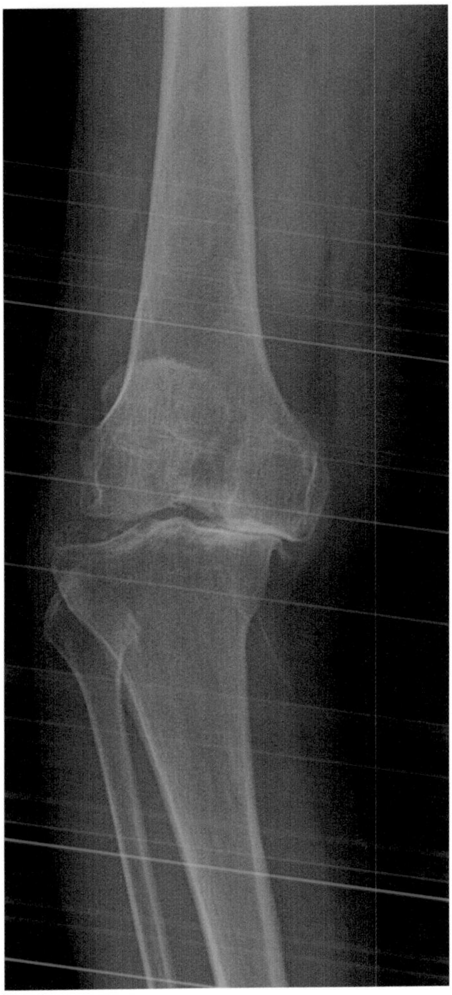

Fig. 6.5 Standing AP radiograph shows lateral subluxation of the tibia and varus deformity due to severe osteoarthritis of the knee

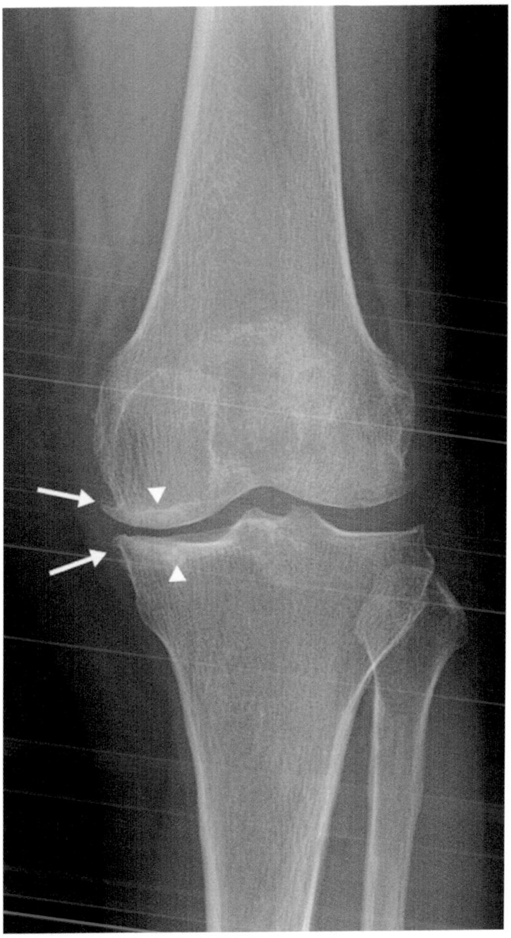

Fig. 6.6 Standing AP radiograph shows joint space narrowing, marginal osteophytes (arrows), and subchondral sclerosis (arrowheads) in the medial patellofemoral compartment

microfracture and blood flow failure in the subchondral bone [9]. Subchondral cysts are observed in various sizes and are accompanied by joint space narrowing and subchondral sclerosis (Fig. 6.7). There may or may not be communication with the joint cavity. If there is communication, gas in the joint may enter the cyst, forming a pneumatocyst [9].

6.1.3 Osteophyte

Osteophyte which increases the surface area of articular cartilage, cause reduction of the tension and increase of joint stability [8]. Osteophyte can be classified into marginal, central, periosteal, synovial, and capsular types. In radiographic images, the marginal osteophyte

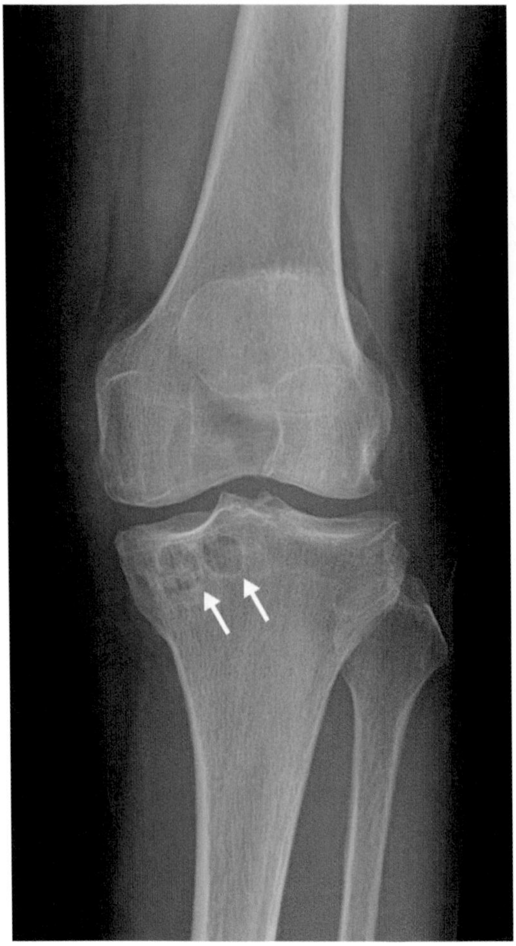

Fig. 6.7 Standing AP radiograph shows two small radiolucent lesions (arrows) with the thin sclerotic rim in the medial tibial subarticular area

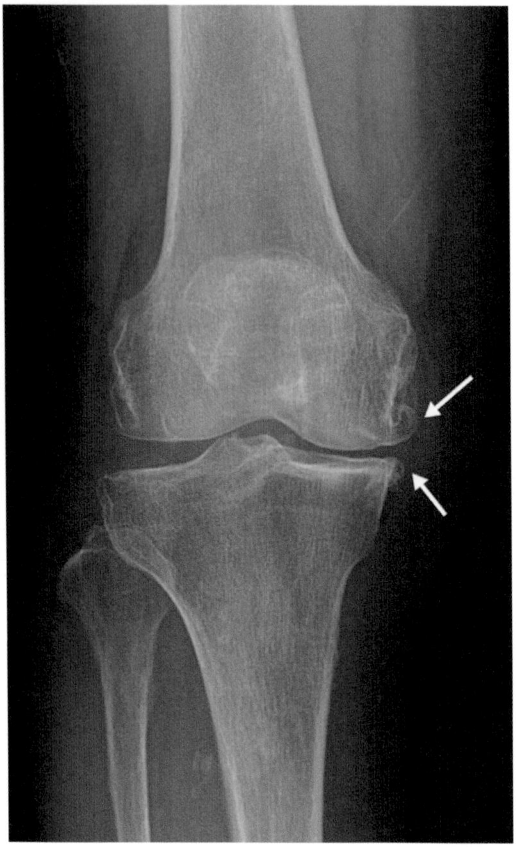

Fig. 6.8 Standing AP radiograph shows lip-shaped bone protrusions(arrows) at the edge of the femoral condyle and tibial plateau of the medial compartment

protrudes from the edge of the joint where there is no pressure (Fig. 6.8). They may be shown in various sizes, arising from one side of the joint, and can seem to have no relationship with subchondral sclerosis or cyst. Central osteophytes are rarely detected in OA, but they may arise from remaining cartilage in the center of the joint and are mainly observed in the knee or hip joint. Images of osteophyte show a rough outline of the joint surface, and small osteophytes can be mistaken for intraarticular loose body or cartilage calcification. The fact that osteophyte is connected to the original bone and is ossification rather than calcification, may help distinguish osteophyte [5, 7].

6.1.4 Synovitis

In OA, the synovial reaction consists of synovial hyperplasia, fibrosis, thickening of the synovial capsule, and activated synoviocyte. In some cases, there may be lymphocytic infiltrate such as plasma cells, B cells, and T cells. Synovium-induced pain is caused by irritation of the sensory nerve ending attached to the osteophyte in the synovium and synovial inflammation due to the secretion of prostaglandin, leukotrienes, proteinase, and neuropeptides. Synovitis and effusion are frequently observed in OA and are related to pain and clinical outcome. Synovitis facilitates the synthesis of cartilage matrix-degrading enzymes and secretes excessive synovial fluid, relaxing the joints and making them susceptible to damage. It also pushes the synovial fluid into the ulcer and erosion of the cartilage surface to further accelerate the degenerative change [10]. Synovitis can be seen as joint effusion on the image, but if it is not accompanied by trauma or rapid bony collapse, it is difficult to detect due to its small amount, and further findings can be observed with MRI [11].

6.1.5 Malalignment and Subluxation

In OA, malalignment and subluxation can be shown, especially in weight-bearing synovial joints. Angulation deformity is common, and varus deformity of the knee joint can be frequently observed in OA patients (Fig. 6.5). In addition, deformity and malignment of the joint may become severe due to rupture or distortion of the supporting structure of the joint capsule and ligaments [1, 5].

6.1.6 Intraarticular Loose Bodies

Intraarticular loose body is caused by transchondral fracture, cartilage surface disintegration, and synovial membrane metaplasia. Cartilage and bone debris remaining on the joint surface fall into the joint and accumulate on the synovial membrane, causing a local inflammatory reaction. This occurs mainly in the hip and knee joints, and on radiographic imaging, it appears as radiopaque density [2]. Lesions to be distinguished from loose bodies in OA include central osteophyte, meniscal calcification, ossification, and loose body can also take place in other diseases such as synovial osteochondromatosis and osteochondritis dissecans (Fig. 6.9) [1].

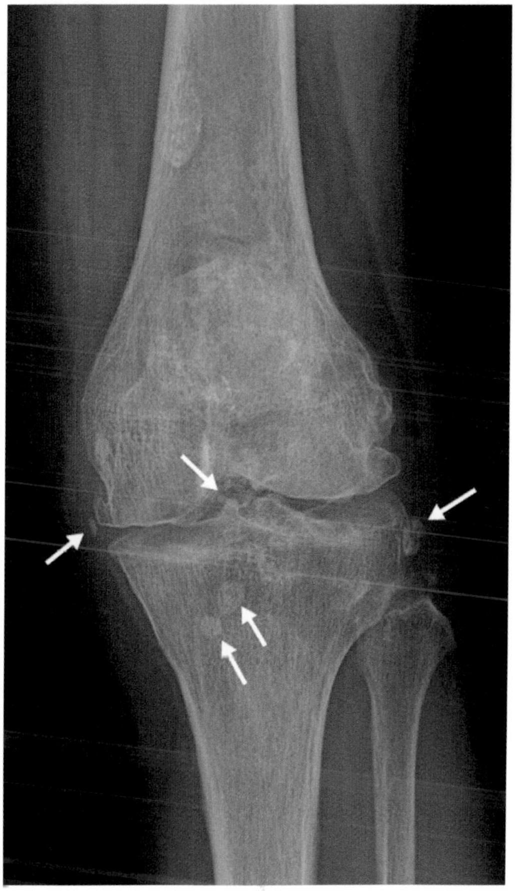

Fig. 6.9 Standing AP radiograph shows several ossified loose bodies (arrows) in the knee joint. Note mild joint space narrowing and marginal osteophytes

6.2 Computed Tomography (CT)

CT is useful for depicting cortical bone and soft tissue calcifications [12]. It also helps detailed evaluation of bone structures such as subchondral bone sclerosis, subchondral cysts, and osteophytes (Fig. 6.10). 3D CT is particularly helpful for orthopedic planning of arthroplasty

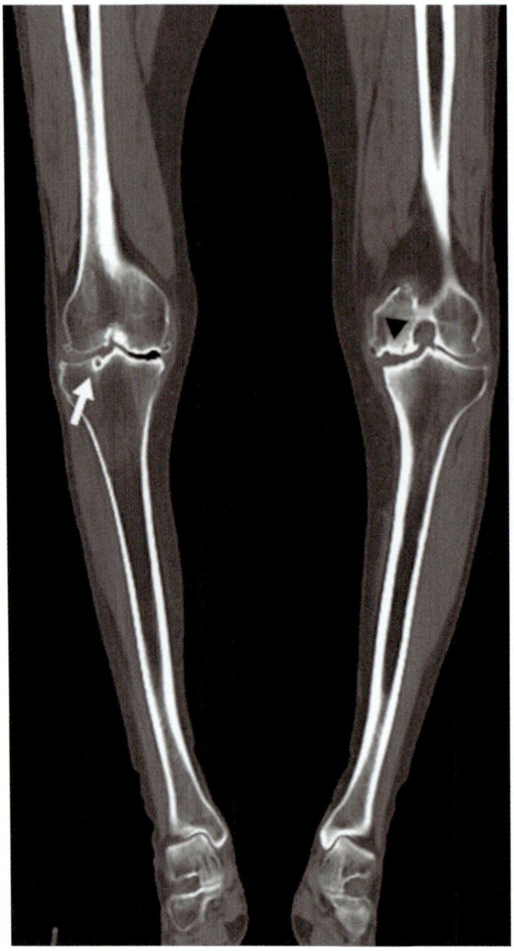

Fig. 6.10 Lower extremity CT image shows joint space narrowing, marginal osteophyte, and subchondral cyst (arrow) in the right knee. Note mild varus deformity, osteophyte, and irregular articular surface (arrowhead) of the left medial femoral condyle in the left knee

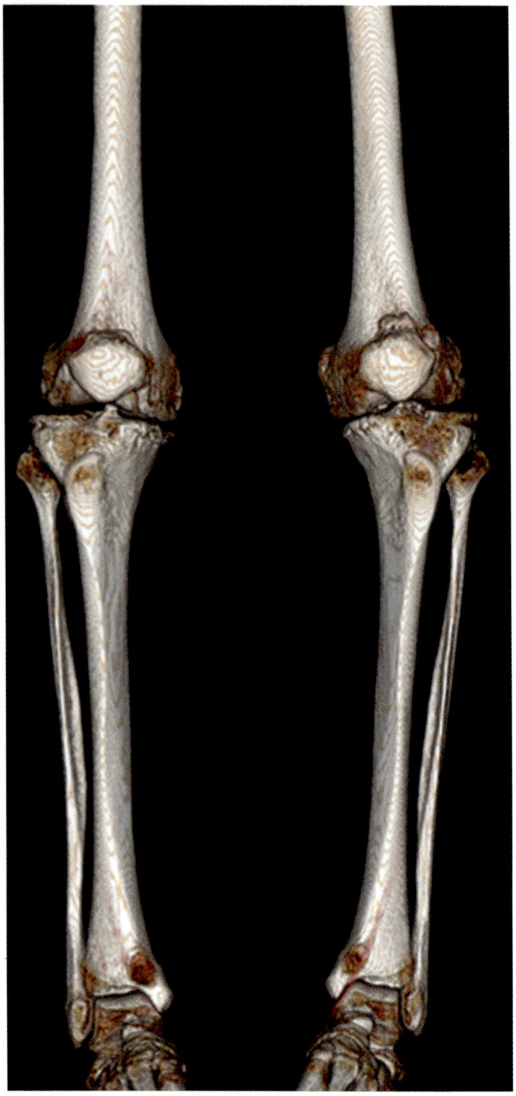

Fig. 6.11 Volume rendering 3D-CT image shows the overall outline and alignment of the bone well

(Fig. 6.11). However, due to limitations in the evaluation of soft tissue and ionizing radiation, CT is not routinely applied in clinical imaging of OA.

6.3 Magnetic Resonance Imaging (MRI)

Conventional radiography is the gold-standard for evaluating OA, but MRI-based OA studies have proven the limitations of radiography. Traditionally, cartilage has been considered a pivotal feature of OA and a major target of intervention. However, today OA is considered a whole joint disease that affects the bones, joints, and tissues around the joints [12–14]. Radiographic imaging is primarily used to diagnose OA, but MRI can simultaneously monitor various tissue changes, enable earlier detection of OA lesions, and can evaluate biochemical changes in joint tissues such as cartilage before morphological changes become apparent. Moreover, it can detect changes in the meniscus, ligaments, and soft tis-

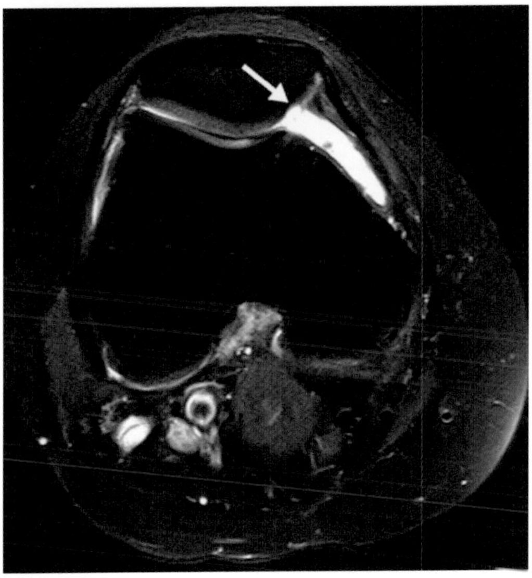

Fig. 6.12 Fat-suppressed proton density-weighted axial MR image shows focal articular cartilage defect in the medial patella (arrow)

sue related to OA. In MRI, appropriate pulse sequence protocols should be selected depending on the examination purpose. For example, focal cartilage defects, and bone marrow lesions are best evaluated using fluid-sensitive fast spin echo (FSE) sequences (T2-weighted, proton density (PD) weighted) with fat suppression. The fat suppression image darkens the signal intensity of bone marrow and surrounding tissue, making the cartilage signal intensity seem very high (Fig. 6.12). With this difference in signal intensity, diffuse, or focal lesions of cartilage can be accurately diagnosed, and cartilage lesions can be quantitatively measured before surgery. In MRI of patients with knee joint pain, cartilage lesion, bone marrow edema, osteophyte, subchondral sclerosis, meniscus lesion, joint effusion, and synovitis, findings were reported to have a strong correlation with the severity observed in radiographic imaging [15, 16].

6.3.1 MRI of Articular Cartilage

In evaluating the condition of articular cartilage, arthroscopy is highly accurate, but it is invasive and can only diagnose the case after the destruction of articular cartilage has already progressed, so MRI, a non-invasive diagnosis method, is most useful. MR microscopy (MRM) or microscopic MRI (mMRI) with increased resolution can distinguish the histological layers of articular cartilage and observe changes in the morphology or biochemistry of articular cartilage simultaneously, so it is widely used in research on the structure and early degeneration of articular cartilage. Particularly, quantitative MRM can detect the changes in early biochemical stages such as loss of glycosaminoglycan and enables early diagnosis before symptomatic or morphological changes appear on articular cartilage. Fat suppression T1-weighted gradient echo and proton density-weighted fast spin echo techniques are the most commonly used sequences for cartilage imaging [17]. Sensitivity to signals such as edema in the subchondral bone can be improved by adding fat suppression techniques to the FSE sequence using a fat selective presaturation pulse or a short tau inversion recovery sequence (STIR).

Advanced MRI techniques which offer a quantitative assessment of the biochemical composition of cartilage include delayed gadolinium-enhanced MRI of cartilage (dGEMRIC), T2 mapping, T1rho mapping, sodium MRI, and a few of the more novel methods [18, 19]. MRI parametric mapping techniques, such as cartilage transverse relaxation time (T2) mapping have the potential to identify the earliest stages of matrix degeneration that precede visible cartilage damage (Fig. 6.13). Cartilage T2 mapping uses intrinsic cartilage water as a probe to study the structural integrity of the extracellular matrix. Because it has a central role in the biomechanical properties of cartilage, water is an ideal biomarker of cartilage damage [20, 21]. Delayed gadolinium enhanced MR imaging of cartilage (dGEMRIC) is a technique used to measure the relative concentration of proteoglycan in articular cartilage in vivo using venous MR arthrography [22]. It is not only useful for tracking the progression or development of cartilage lesions, but also the progression of glycosaminoglycan synthesis and can help evaluate the success of cartilage regeneration noninvasively.

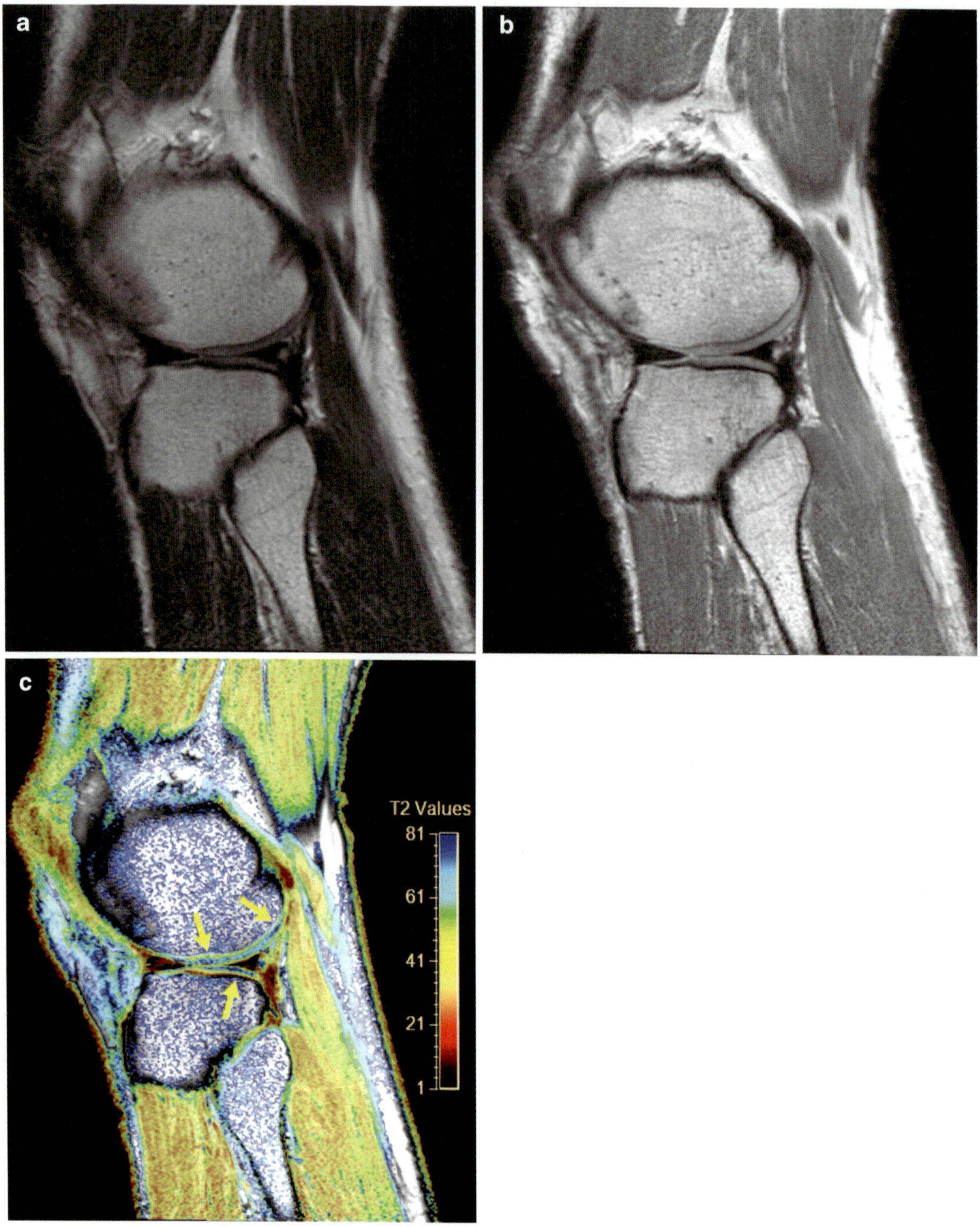

Fig. 6.13 Conventional T2-weighted (**a**) and PD-weighted (**b**) MR images may show no major morphological changes in the cartilage. Color T2 mapping (**c**) reveals high T2 relaxation value in the lateral femoral and tibial cartilage (arrows) that are also indicative of early OA

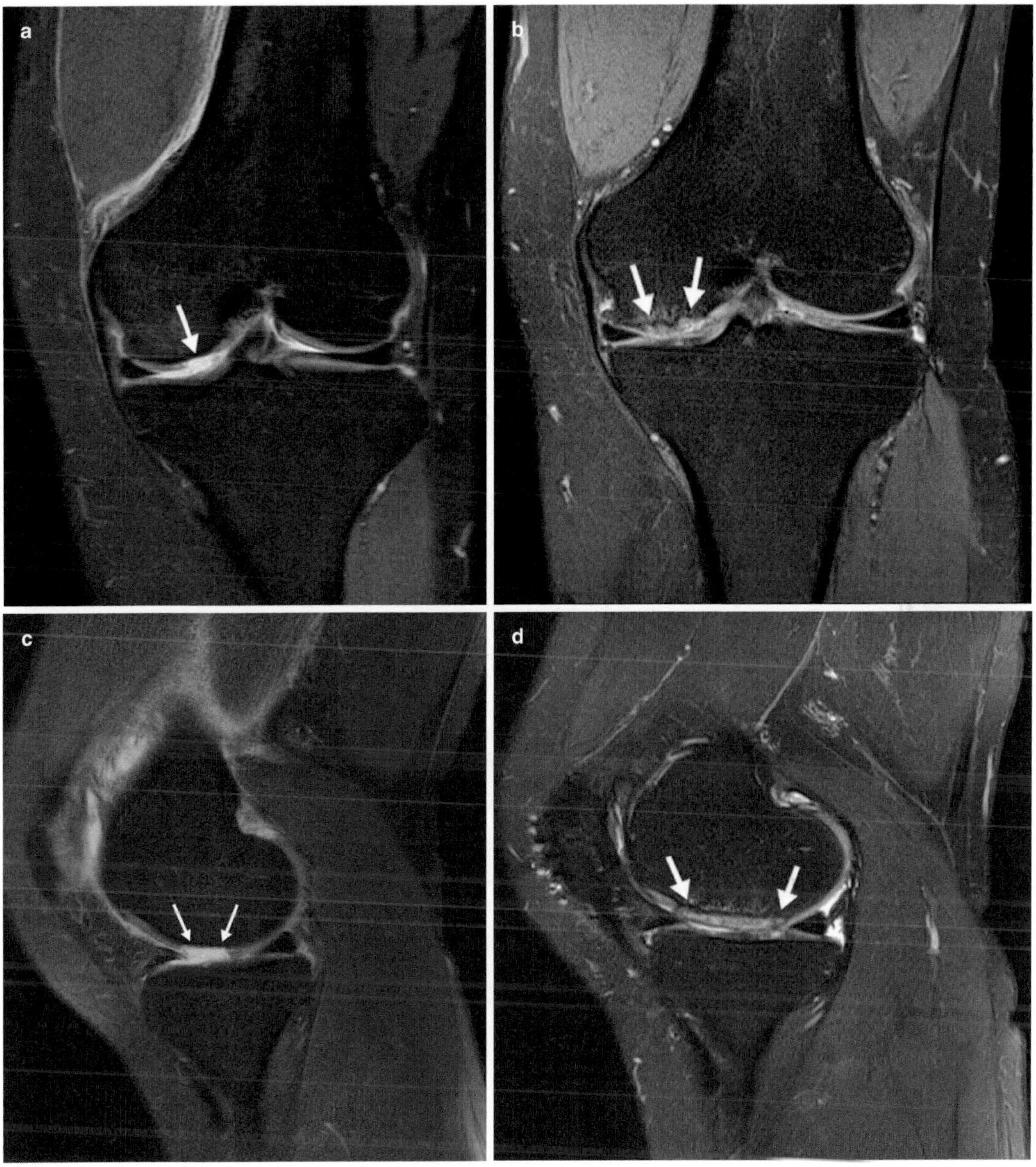

Fig. 6.14 Preoperative fat-suppressed PD weighted coronal (**a**), sagittal (**c**) MR images show focal articular cartilage defect (arrows) in the weight-bearing surface of the medial femoral condyle. At 14 months' follow-up after chondrocyte transplantation, postoperative fat-suppressed PD-weighted coronal (**b**), sagittal (**d**) MR images show isointense regenerated cartilage at the surgery site has smoothly covered the joint surface, but it is slightly hypertrophic (arrows). The regenerated cartilage and subchondral bone are well fused. Note mild subchondral bone marrow edema in the medial femoral condyle and tibial plateau

MRI is useful not only for the diagnosis of cartilage lesions, but also for treatment planning. Preoperative MRI is helpful in assessing the condition of articular cartilage in all compartments and detecting cartilage abnormalities to determine the feasibility of reconstruction. It is also valuable in evaluating the condition of regenerated articular cartilage after cartilage regeneration and identifying complications (Fig. 6.14) [23].

6.3.2 MRI-Based Diagnostic Criteria

MRI has become an important imaging tool in OA studies in recent years as it can evaluate articular cartilage, menisci, ligaments, synovium, capsular structures, fluid collections, and bone marrow lesions, which are not visible by radiography.

The MR-based diagnostic criteria of knee OA are as follows [14].

MR imaging-based diagnostic criteria: (proposed by the OARSI OA imaging working group)
(1) A definition of tibiofemoral OA on MRI = the presence of both group [A] features or one group [A] feature and two or more group [B] features.
Group [A] after exclusion of joint trauma within the last 6 months (by history) and exclusion of inflammatory arthritis (by radiographs, history, and laboratory parameters): (i) definite osteophyte formation, (ii) full-thickness cartilage loss.
Group [B]: (i) subchondral bone marrow lesion or cyst not associated with meniscal or ligamentous attachments, (ii) meniscal subluxation, maceration, or degenerative (horizontal) tear, (iii) partial-thickness cartilage loss (where full-thickness loss is not present), (iv) bone attrition.
(2) A definition of patellofemoral OA requires all of the following involving the patella and/or anterior femur: (i) definite osteophyte formation (ii) partial- or full-thickness cartilage loss

*OARSI (OA Research Society International)

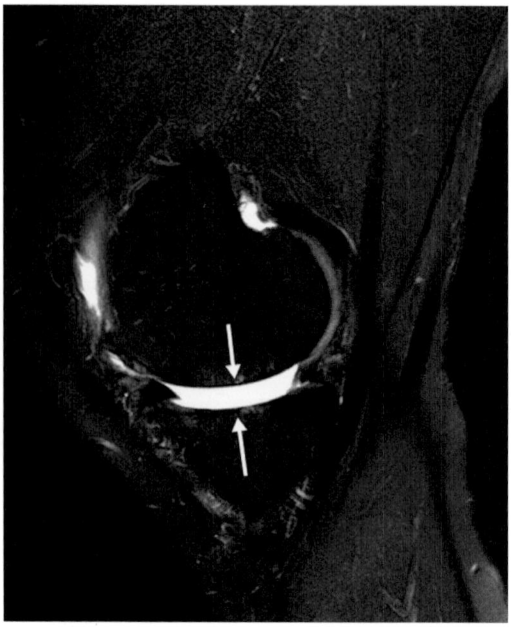

Fig. 6.15 Fat-suppressed T2-weighted sagittal MR image shows the fluid-filled area (arrows) in the medial tibiofemoral joint due to full-thickness cartilage loss

6.3.2.1 Cartilage Damage

Articular cartilage is one of the main tissues involved in the OA process. Since cartilage cannot be seen directly on radiographic imaging, MRI is optimal for morphological evaluation of cartilage. Choosing the appropriate pulse sequence is essential for the accurate evaluation of cartilage damage [13]. Although the clinical significance of the early stages of OA before the thinning of cartilage focal defect is unclear, high signal intensity can be observed inside the cartilage on the T2 weighted image. Once the morphological changes occur, the fluid signal fills the focal defects or thin regions of the cartilage (Fig. 6.15). In progressed OA, diffuse full-thickness cartilage loss may be seen, which appears as a bone-on-bone contact on radiographic imaging [13]. Numerous classification schemes exist for grading cartilage lesions, most of which take into account the size and/or depth of the lesion. The International Cartilage Repair Society (ICRS) has standardized the evaluation of articular cartilage injury based on the depth of the lesion, in which lesions are graded 0 to 4 based on the depth of the lesion (Table 6.3) (Fig. 6.16) [24]. Grade 1 and 2 lesions have an excellent prognosis. Grade 2 and 3 lesions may benefit from cartilage debridement or other more conservative surgical treatments. Grade 4 lesions extend into the subchondral bone and may require bone grafting if the bony defect is extensive. Subchondral marrow edema is more likely to be associated with higher-grade lesions [25].

6.3.2.2 Meniscal Lesions

MRI is the appropriate imaging test to evaluate the meniscus that carries out various functions including load-bearing, shock absorption, stability improvement, and lubrication. The normal meniscus demonstrates homogeneous low signal intensity on T1-, PD, T2-weighted images. Linear or complex high-intensity signals reaching the

Table 6.3 Articular Cartilage Lesion Classification according to the International Cartilage Repair Society (ICRS)

Grade	Description of the Condition of the Cartilage Tissue
0	Normal
1	Nearly normal. Superficial lesions. Soft indentation and/or superficial fissures and cracks.
2	Abnormal. Lesions extending down to <50% of cartilage depth.
3	Severely abnormal. Cartilage defects extending down >50% of cartilage depth as well as down to calcified layer and down to but not through the subchondral bone. Blisters are included in this grade.
4	Severely abnormal. Cartilage defects extending through the subchondral bone.

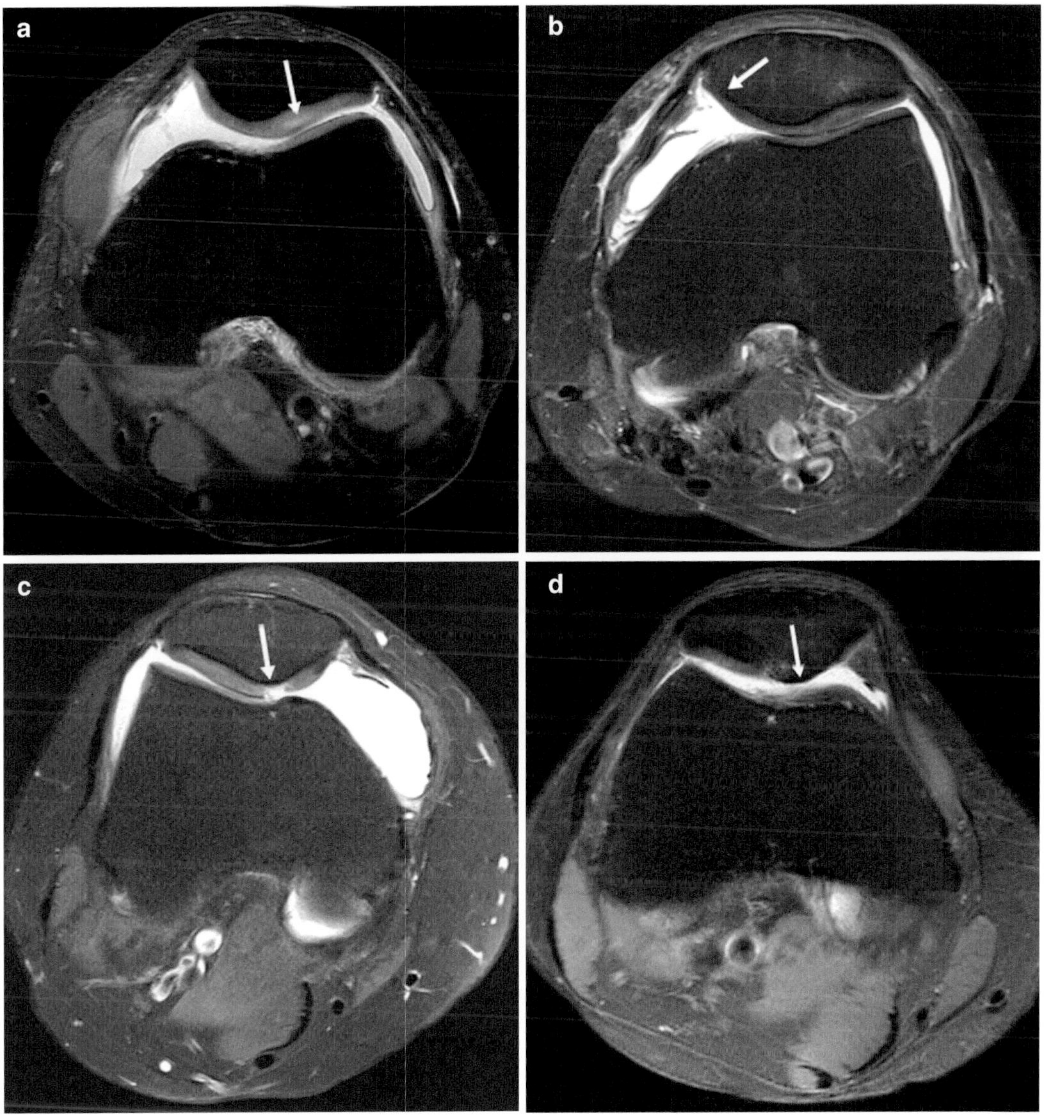

Fig. 6.16 Articular Cartilage Lesion Classification according to the International Cartilage Repair Society(ICRS). (**a**) Fat-suppressed PD-weighted axial MR image shows focal high signal intensity in the articular cartilage of the lateral facet of the patella (arrow) (grade 1). (**b**) Fat-suppressed PD-weighted axial MR image shows thinning of the articular cartilage (<50% of cartilage depth) in the medial facet of the patella(arrow) (grade 2). (**c**) Fat-suppressed PD-weighted axial MR image shows a focal defect of the articular cartilage (>50% of cartilage depth) in the central facet of the patella (arrow) (grade 3). (**d**) Fat-suppressed PD-weighted axial MR image shows the full-thickness cartilage defects extending through the subchondral bone in the medial and central facet of the patella (arrow) (grade 4)

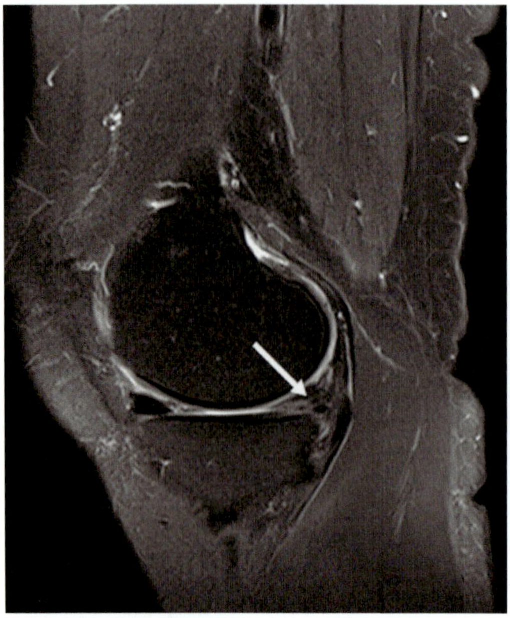

Fig. 6.17 Fat-suppressed proton density-weighted sagittal MR image shows complex tear (arrow) in the posterior horn of the medial meniscus. Note thinning of the articular cartilage in the medial compartment (grade 3)

articular surface on T2-weighted MRI are observed in horizontal cleavages, oblique, or complex tears, which are degenerative meniscal lesions (Fig. 6.17). Meniscal extrusion and meniscal root tear are also associated with OA [11, 12].

6.3.3 Intrameniscal Signal Intensity

The increased signal intensity inside the meniscus on the sagittal or coronal MRI is classified into three grades as follows (Fig. 6.18) [26].

- Grade 1: Globular signal intensity that is confined to the inside, not extending through the articular surface of the meniscus.
- Grade 2: Linear signal intensity that runs horizontally, also confined to the inside and not extending through the articular surface of the meniscus.
- Grade 3: Linear signal intensity extending through the articular surface of the meniscus.

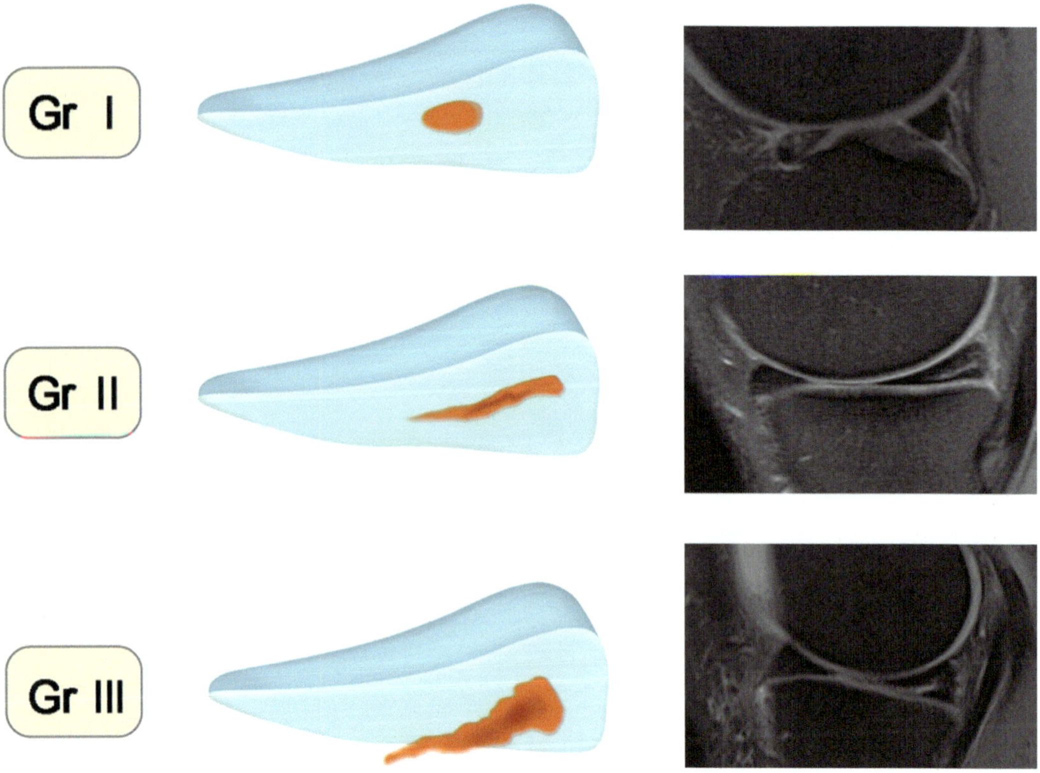

Fig. 6.18 Schema and correlated MRI findings of intrameniscal signal intensity classification

In the case of Grade 1 or 2, it is considered as an intrasubstance degeneration or myxoid degeneration rather than a tear [27]. Early degenerative changes progress in areas referred to as mucinous, myxoid, or hyaline degeneration, with an increase in intercellular mucoid ground substance. It is presumed to be a result of a simple aging process or wear and tear, but the obvious cause is still unknown. Generally, it does not cause any symptoms nor require any special treatment. Due to radially oriented collagen fiber or perimeniscal vessel, high signal intensity may arise at the junction between the meniscus and the joint capsule in normal conditions [28].

6.3.3.1 Bone Marrow Lesions

Bone marrow lesions show low signal intensity on T1 weighted image and unclear high signal intensity on subchondral bone on fluid-sensitive sequences. OA-related bone marrow lesions are accompanied by cartilage damage in the same area (Fig. 6.19). In OA, bone marrow lesions are associated with pain, while fluctuating over time. They are also accompanied by deterioration of joint space narrowing on radiographic imaging [29, 30].

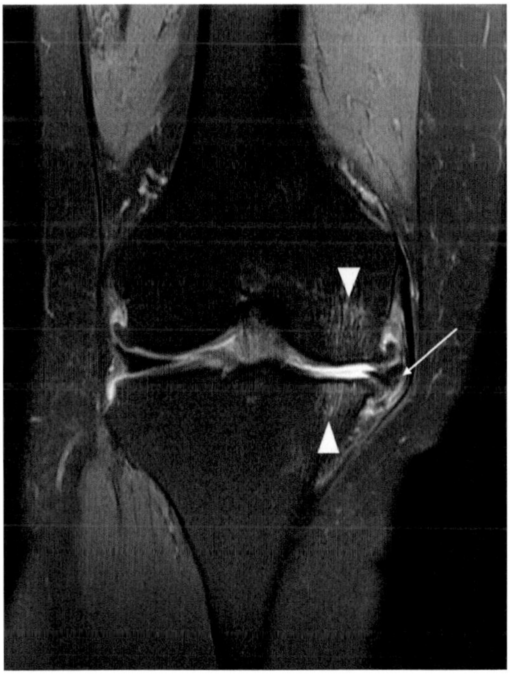

Fig. 6.19 Fat-suppressed proton density-weighted coronal MR image shows full-thickness cartilage loss with adjacent subchondral bone marrow edema (arrowheads) in the medial femoral condyle and tibial plateau. Note marginal osteophytes, meniscal degeneration (arrow), and medial extrusion of the medial meniscus

Differential diagnosis of bone marrow lesions is as follows [13].

• Traumatic bone marrow lesions
– Bone contusions, fractures, stress reactions
• Non-traumatic bone marrow lesions
– Avascular necrosis
– Spontaneous osteonecrosis of the knee (SONK)
– Bone marrow edema syndrome (including transient osteoporosis of the knee, regional migratory osteoporosis, complex regional pain syndrome, reflex sympathetic dystrophy)
– Inflammatory bone marrow lesions (such as chronic polyarthritis, reactive arthritis, rheumatoid arthritis, bacterial arthritis)
– Malignancy (lymphoma, myeloma, leukemia)
– Benign tumors (Langerhans cell histiocytosis, chondroblastoma, osteoid osteoma, osteoblastoma)

6.3.3.2 Subchondral Cyst

On MR imaging, this lesion appears as a well-defined circular boundary of water signal intensity on the pre-contrast imaging. Subchondral cysts usually exist along with bone marrow lesions and may occur within the bone marrow lesion area as well (Fig. 6.20) [9, 13].

6.3.3.3 Osteophytes

Osteophytes growing at the edge of the joint are characteristic features of OA [5]. It is well known that the presence of osteophytes on radiography defines an OA based on the KL grading system. Osteophytes can be detected by conventional radiography, but small ones are only seen on CT and MRI. The central part of the osteophyte shows the same signal intensity as the bone marrow, and the marginal area shows the same signal intensity as the cortical bone [31].

6.3.3.4 Joint Effusion and Synovitis

Joint effusion and synovitis are often accompanied by OA. Like synovitis in RA, synovitis in OA is best evaluated in contrast-enhanced MRI, which can discriminate contrast-enhanced synovium from non-enhanced synovial fluid (Fig. 6.21). Recent studies using contrast-

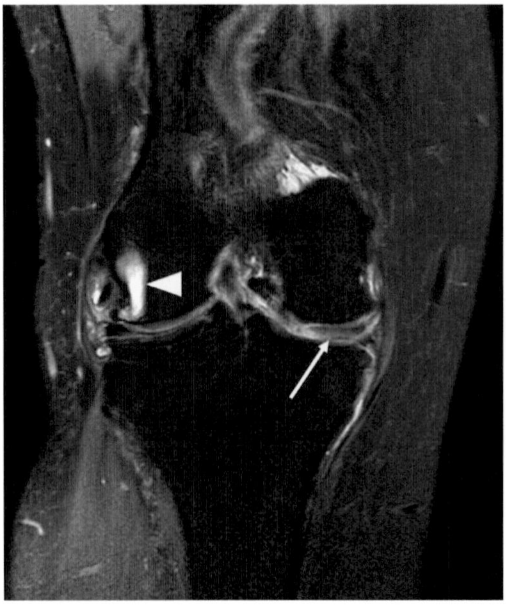

Fig. 6.20 Fat-suppressed proton density-weighted coronal MR image shows a hyperintense subchondral cyst (arrowhead) in lateral femoral condyle with thinning of adjacent articular cartilage. Note complex tear in the medial meniscus (arrow), thinning of the articular cartilage in the medial compartment

enhanced MRI showed that synovitis was increasingly associated with knee cartilage deterioration [32]. If contrast-enhanced MRI is not available, non-enhanced MRI can evaluate synovitis by using surrogate markers, such as a change in Hoffa fat pad signal. This can be called Hoffa synovitis and appears to be diffuse high signal intensity in the Hoffa fat pad on fluid-sensitive MRI [33]. A large amount of effusion is also associated with pain and stiffness in OA [11].

6.3.3.5 Ligaments

Rupture of the ligaments in and around the knee joint can lead to OA. The anterior, posterior cruciate ligament and collateral ligaments can be rupture. This ligament structure appears as a partial or complete discontinuity depending on the high signal intensity in the ligament on MRI [16]. Mucoid degeneration of the anterior cruciate ligament(ACL) is a disease that needs to be differentiated from partial rupture (Fig. 6.22). The exact pathogenesis of ACL mucoid degeneration is still unknown. Potential

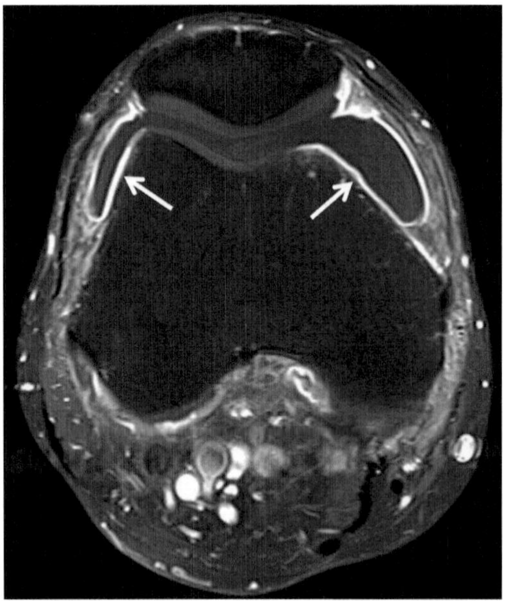

Fig. 6.21 Fat-suppressed Gd-enhanced T1-weighted axial MR image shows enhanced synovium (arrows)is distinguished from non-enhanced effusion

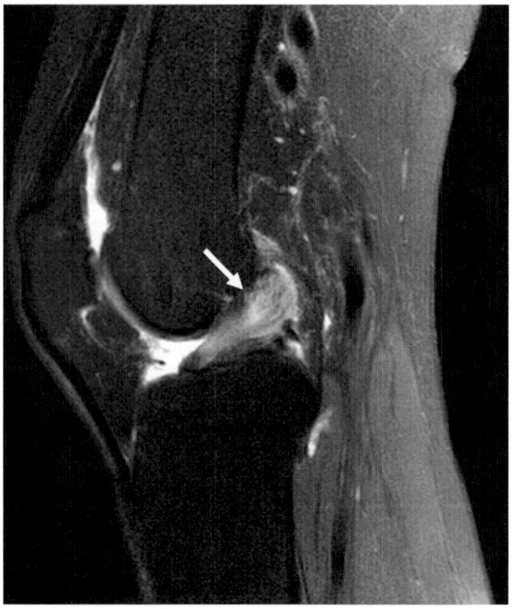

Fig. 6.22 Fat-suppressed proton density-weighted sagittal MR image shows swelling with high signal intensity in the anterior cruciate ligament without discontinuity of the fibers, which looks like a celery stalk (arrow)

causes include synovial lining defects causing exposure of the ACL to degradative synovial environment effects [34], the posttraumatic release of glycosaminoglycans by fibroblasts that become interspersed between ACL fibers [35], and congenital synovial tissue ectopia [36]. Mucus material is visible between the fiber bundles, but no disruption of the bundles is observed. Fat-suppressed PD MR image shows high signal intensity, but are not enhanced on contrast-enhanced images. The anterior cruciate ligament looks enlarged in the shape of a celery stalk. ACL mucoid degeneration at MR imaging in participants with or at risk for OA is associated with progression of medial tibiofemoral compartment joint space loss at radiography [37].

6.3.3.6 Bursitis and Loose Bodies

Bursitis can be shown in OA. Most cystic lesions appear to be encapsulated fluid collections showing low T1 and high T2 signals. Loose bodies are often seen, particularly in advanced OA (Fig. 6.23). In OA, loose bodies originate from chondral fragments, detached osteophytes, fragments of the meniscus. Differential diagnosis includes synovial osteochondromatosis, spontaneous osteonecrosis of the knee, RA, and calcium pyrophosphate dihydrate deposition disease, etc. [13].

6.3.3.7 Subchondral Attrition

Subchondral attrition is defined as flattening or depression of a subchondral osseous surface that is not associated with a fracture. This can be assessed by radiographic imaging, and while it may appear in knees of mild OA patients without joint space narrowing, subchondral attrition usually occurs in advanced knee osteoarthritis [13]. The exact mechanism of this OA finding is unknown, but subchondral microfracture and remodeling caused by changes in mechanical load might cause bone attrition. This has been demonstrated to be related to knee pain [38].

6.4 Summary

Radiography is the most commonly used imaging modality for OA evaluation in the knee due to lower cost and greater accessibility. It can be seen bony features, including osteophytes, subchondral sclerosis, and subchondral cysts. It can also

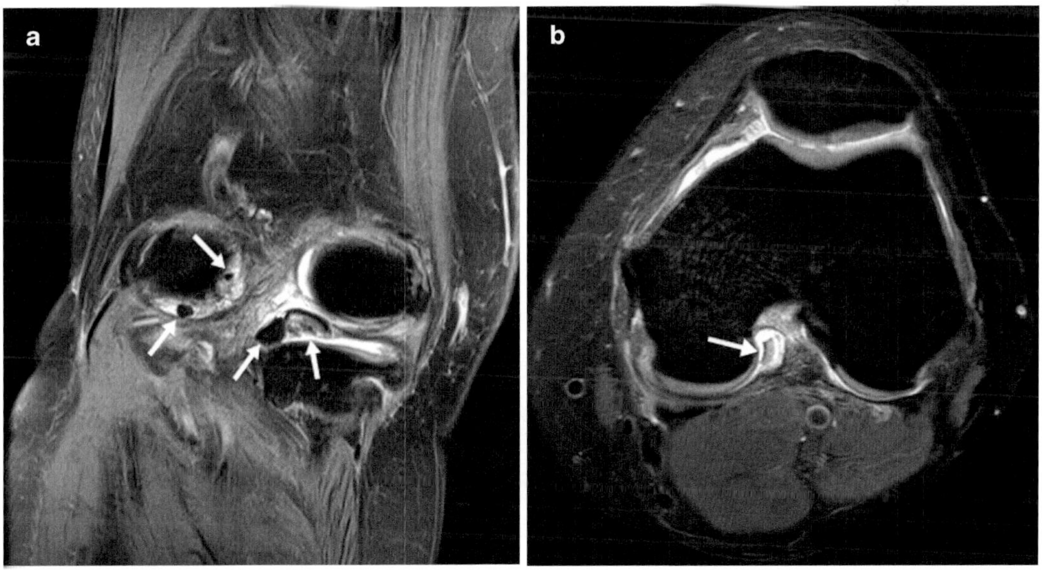

Fig. 6.23 (**a**) Fat-suppressed proton density-weighted coronal MRI image shows several small ovoid and globular loose bodies (arrows) in the knee. (**b**) Fat-suppressed proton density-weighted axial MRI image shows a small rectangular cartilage fragment (arrow) in the lateral aspect of the posterior medial femoral condyle

determine joint space width reflecting the status of not only cartilage but also menisci. However, the exact measurement of each of these articular structures is not possible with radiography. Progression of joint space narrowing is the most commonly used criterion for the evaluation of OA progression, and the complete loss manifested by bone-on-bone contact is one of the indicators for knee arthroplasty. MRI, which is becoming an increasingly more important imaging modality, can be seen non-osteochondral OA features that are not detected on radiography, including articular cartilage, menisci, ligaments, synovium, capsular structures, fluid collections, and bone marrow. Moreover, MRI has added to the understanding of the significance of these structures, such as explaining pain and structural progression, etc.

References

1. Resnick D. Degenerative disease of extraspinal locations. In: Diagnosis of bone and joint disorders, vol. 2. 4th ed. Philadelphia: Saunders; 2002. p. 1271–381.
2. Cooper C, Cushnaghan J, Kirwan JR, Dieppe PA, Rogers J, McAlindon T, et al. Radiographic assessment of the knee joint in osteoarthritis. Ann Rheum Dis. 1992;51(1):80–2.
3. Ball J, Jeffrey MR, Kellgren JH. The epidemiology of chronic rheumatism: Atlas of Standard Radiographs of Arthritis. Oxford: Blackwell Scientific Publications; 1963.
4. Özkan K, Baver A, Fatif Ç, Baris Y, Ferhat G, et al. Inter- and intraobserver reliabilities of four different radiographic grading scales of osteoarthritis of the knee joint. J Knee Surg. 2018;31(3):247–53.
5. Gupta KB, Duryea J, Weissman BN. Radiographic evaluation of osteoarthritis. Radiol Clin N Am. 2004;42(1):11–41.
6. McAlindon TE, Snow S, Cooper C, Dieppe PA. Radiographic patterns of osteoarthritis of the knee joint in the community: the importance of the patellofemoral joint. Ann Rheum Dis. 1992;51(7):844–9.
7. Nagaosa Y, Lanyon P, Doherty M. Characterisation of size and direction of osteophyte in knee osteoarthritis: a radiographic study. Ann Rheum Dis. 2002;61(4):319–24.
8. Milgram JW. Morphologic alterations of the subchondral bone in advanced degenerative arthritis. Clin Orthop Relat Res. 1983;173:293–312.
9. Radin EL, Rose RM. Role of subchondral bone in the initiation and progression of cartilage damage. Clin Orthop Relat Res. 1986;213:34–40.
10. Hunter DJ. Insights from imaging on the epidemiology and pathophysiology of osteoarthritis. Radiol Clin N Am. 2009;47(4):539–51.
11. de Lange-Brokaar BJ, Ioan-Facsinay A, Yusuf E, Kroon HM, Zuurmond AM, Stojanovic-Susulic V, et al. Evolution of synovitis in osteoarthritic knees and its association with clinical features. Osteoarthr Cartil. 2016;24(11):1867–74.
12. Guermazi A, Hayashi D, Eckstein F, Hunter DJ, Duryea J, Roemer FW. Imaging of osteoarthritis. Rheum Dis Clin N Am. 2013;39(1):67–105.
13. Hayashi D, Roemer FW, Jarraya M, Guermazi A. Imaging in osteoarthritis. Radiol Clin N Am. 2017;55(5):1085–102.
14. Hunter DJ, Arden N, Conaghan PG, Eckstein F, Gold G, Grainger A, et al. Definition of osteoarthritis on MRI: results of a Delphi exercise. Osteoarthr Cartil. 2011;19(8):963–9.
15. Alparslan L, Minas T, Winalski CS. Magnetic resonance imaging of autologous chondrocyte implantation. Semin Ultrasound CT MR. 2001;22(4):341–51.
16. Hayes CW, Jamadar DA, Welch GW, Jannausch ML, Lachance LL, Capul DC, et al. Osteoarthritis of the knee: comparison of MR imaging findings with radiographic severity measurements and pain in middle-aged women. Radiology. 2005;237(3):998–1007.
17. Disler DG, Peters TL, Muscoreil SJ, Ratner LM, Wagle WA, Cousins JP, et al. Fat-suppressed spoiled GRASS imaging of knee hyaline cartilage: technique optimization and comparison with conventional MR imaging. AJR Am J Roentgenol. 1994;163(4):887–92.
18. Burstein D, Gray M, Mosher T, Dardzinski B. Measures of molecular composition and structure in osteoarthritis. Radiol Clin N Am. 2009;47(4):675–86.
19. Matzat SJ, van Tiel J, Gold GE, Oei EH. Quantitative MRI techniques of cartilage composition. Quant Imaging Med Surg. 2013;3(3):162–74.
20. Gray ML, Burstein D, Xia Y. Biochemical (and functional) imaging of articular cartilage. Semin Musculoskelet Radiol. 2001;5(4):329–43.
21. Mosher TJ, Dardzinski BJ. Cartilage MRI T2 relaxation time mapping: overview and applications. Semin Musculoskelet Radiol. 2004;8(4):355–68.
22. Gillis A, Bashir A, McKeon B, Scheller A, Gray ML, Burstein D. Magnetic resonance imaging of relative glycosaminoglycan distribution in patients with autologous chondrocyte transplants. Investig Radiol. 2001;36(12):743–8.
23. Alparslan L, Winalski CS, Boutin RD, Minas T. Postoperative magnetic resonance imaging of articular cartilage repair. Semin Musculoskelet Radiol. 2001;5(4):345–63.
24. Brittberg M, Winalski CS. Evaluation of cartilage injuries and repair. J Bone Joint Surg Am. 2003;85-A(Suppl 2):58–69.
25. Kijowski R, Stanton P, Fine J, De Smet A. Subchondral bone marrow edema in patients with degeneration of the articular cartilage of the knee joint. Radiology. 2006;238(3):943–9.

26. Stoller DW, Martin C, Crues JV 3rd, Kaplan L, Mink JH. Meniscal tears: pathologic correlation with MR imaging. Radiology. 1987;163(3):731–5.
27. Kaplan PA, Nelson NL, Garvin KL, Brown DE. MR of the knee: the significance of high signal in the meniscus that does not clearly extend to the surface. AJR Am J Roentgenol. 1991;156(2):333–6.
28. Hauger O, Frank LR, Boutin RD, Lektrakul N, Chung CB, Haghighi P, et al. Characterization of the "red zone" of knee meniscus: MR imaging and histologic correlation. Radiology. 2000;217(1):193–200.
29. Zhang Y, Nevitt M, Niu J, Lewis C, Torner J, Guermazi A, et al. Fluctuation of knee pain and changes in bone marrow lesions, effusions, and synovitis on magnetic resonance imaging. Arthritis Rheum. 2011;63(3):691–9.
30. Edwards MH, Parsons C, Bruyere O, Petit Dop F, Chapurlat R, Roemer FW, et al. High Kellgren-Lawrence grade and bone marrow lesions predict worsening rates of radiographic joint space narrowing. SEKOIA Study J Rheumatol. 2016;43(3):657–65.
31. Hayashi D, Xu L, Roemer FW, Hunter DJ, Li L, Katur AM, et al. Detection of osteophytes and subchondral cysts in the knee with use of tomosynthesis. Radiology. 2012;263(1):206–15.
32. Hunter DJ, Guermazi A, Lo GH, Grainger AJ, Conaghan PG, Boudreau RM, et al. Evolution of semi-quantitative whole joint assessment of knee OA: MOAKS (MRI Osteoarthritis Knee Score). Osteoarthr Cartil. 2011;19(8):990–1002.
33. Hill CL, Gale DG, Chaisson CE, Skinner K, Kazis L, Gale ME, et al. Knee effusions, popliteal cysts, and synovial thickening: association with knee pain in osteoarthritis. J Rheumatol. 2001;28(6):1330–7.
34. Lancaster TF, Kirby AB, Beall DP, Wolff JD, Wu DH. Mucoid degeneration of the anterior cruciate ligament: a case report. J Okla State Med Assoc. 2004;97(8):326–8.
35. Roeser WM, Tsai E. Ganglion cysts of the anterior cruciate ligament. Arthroscopy. 1994;10(5):574–5.
36. Melloni P, Valls R, Yuguero M, Sáez A. Mucoid degeneration of the anterior cruciate ligament with erosion of the lateral femoral condyle. Skelet Radiol. 2004;33(6):359–62.
37. Robert MK, Nima HN, Frank WR, Bashir AZ, David JH, Ali G, et al. Association of mucoid degeneration of the anterior cruciate ligament at MR imaging with medial tibiofemoral osteoarthritis progression at radiography: data from the osteoarthritis initiative. Radiology. 2018;287(3):912–21.
38. Torres L, Dunlop DD, Peterfy C, Guermazi A, Prasad P, Hayes KW, et al. The relationship between specific tissue lesions and pain severity in persons with knee osteoarthritis. Osteoarthr Cartil. 2006;14(10):1033–40.

7 Diagnosis and Differential Diagnosis

Sang-Min Lee

Abstract

Knee osteoarthritis is a disease that causes structural and functional disorders of the joint due to damage to normal tissues; early diagnosis is difficult because it has various causes and vague symptoms. Even if it is detected early, the disease still needs further examination because of the lack of effective diagnostic tools for early diagnosis. To diagnose osteoarthritis, clinicians must systematically perform diagnostic procedures from detailed history taking to meticulous and thorough examination. Detailed history taking is important and should also include patient information such as ethnic information, age, sex, height, weight, and symptoms. Physical examination including inspection, palpation, and basic function examination is also performed. Plain radiographs are the basic imaging examination, and computed tomography and magnetic resonance imaging can be considered as necessary. Blood examination including white blood cell count, C-reactive protein level, erythrocyte sedimentation rate, rheumatoid factor level, uric acid level, and cartilage oligomeric matrix protein level; joint fluid analysis; and bone scan can be helpful for diagnosis and differential diagnosis. If other diseases causing arthritis are misdiagnosed as osteoarthritis, omitted or unnecessary treatment may adversely affect the patient, so the differential diagnosis should be considered. Therefore, prior to diagnosis of osteoarthritis, the possibility of rheumatoid arthritis, seronegative spondyloarthropathies, infectious arthritis, crystal-induced inflammatory arthropathy, spontaneous and secondary osteonecrosis, and other diseases should be considered.

Keywords

Knee osteoarthritis · Diagnosis · Physical examination · Alignment · Rheumatoid arthritis · Infectious arthritis · Arthropathy Osteonecrosis

7.1 Diagnosis

Knee osteoarthritis (OA) is known to be the clinical and pathological outcome of various disorders that induce structural and functional failure of the synovial joint [1]. The various causes of OA include disorders of the articular cartilage, ligaments, and joint capsule, synovial membrane inflammation, and subchondral bone calcification

S.-M. Lee (✉)
Department of Orthopedics, Pusan National University Yangsan Hospital, Yangsan, South Korea

Research Institute for Convergence of Biomedical Science and Technology, Pusan National University School of Medicine, Yangsan, South Korea
e-mail: dh62121@pusan.ac.kr

S.-S. Seo (ed.), *A Strategic Approach to Knee Arthritis Treatment*,
https://doi.org/10.1007/978-981-16-4217-3_7

Table 7.1 The American College of Rheumatology criteria for the diagnosis of knee OA

Using medical history and clinical examination
Pain in the knee and three of the following
1. Age > 50 years
2. Morning stiffness <30 min
3. Crepitus on active motions
4. Bony tenderness
5. Bony enlargement
6. No palpable warmth of synovium
Using medical history, clinical examination, and radiographic findings
Pain in the knee and one of the following
1. Age > 50 years
2. Morning stiffness <30 minutes
3. Crepitus on active motions and osteophyte
Using medical history, clinical examination, and laboratory findings
Pain in the knee and five of the following
1. Age > 50 years
2. Morning stiffness <30 min
3. Crepitus on active motions
4. Bony enlargement
5. No palpable warmth of synovium
6. ESR <40 mm/h
7. Rheumatoid factor < 1/40
8. Synovial fluid signs of osteoarthritis

ESR erythrocyte sedimentation rate

[2], and it occurs when the dynamic equilibrium between joint tissues break down and the self-repair system is overwhelmed [3]. Progression of OA may cause pain, physical disability, and psychological distress [4, 5].

Knee OA diagnosis is based on the history of the condition and clinical features (Table 7.1) [6]. Radiological testing such as X-ray and MRI is essential for the degree of involvement and diagnosis of the disease when evaluating patients with suspected osteoarthritis in the knee joint. Clinical findings and physical examination are important. Information about patient's ethnics, age, sex, body mass index (BMI), traumatic onset, difficulty in descending the stairs, and effusion should be also collected. Furthermore, radiologic findings and clinical features such as fixed flexion deformity, restricted flexion range of motion, and crepitus are known to be vital in predicting knee OA, with a sensitivity and specificity of 94% and 93%, respectively [7].

Knee OA can be diagnosed clinically and radiologically as well as based on diagnostic criteria such as the American College of Rheumatology (ACR) and European League Against Rheumatism (EULAR) diagnostic criteria [8]. The EULAR diagnostic criteria present three symptoms (persistent knee pain, limited morning stiffness, and reduced function) and three signs (crepitus, restricted movement, and bony enlargement), and patients showing all six symptoms and signs can be 99% accurately diagnosed with knee OA.

Knee OA can be classified as primary or secondary depending on the etiology. It may be induced by secondary factors such as obesity, fracture around the knee, ligament injury, and inflammatory or genetic factors; when these factors stimulate the progression of OA, such cases are considered secondary OA [9].

7.1.1 Evaluation and History Taking

The most basic aspect of diagnosing knee OA is detailed history taking. Because not all radiologic tests can be performed on all patients, knee OA cannot be diagnosed via radiologic assessment alone. It is also possible that clinical and radiological findings might be inconsistent; therefore, the cause of the symptoms should be determined, and differential diagnosis should be performed based on detailed history taking and clinical findings.

7.1.1.1 Patient Information

The first process involves obtaining patient information. Identifying the patient by confirming whether the patient's name, age, and ID number match the records is the most basic step in ensuring patient safety. Once the patient is identified, the patient's job, ethnics, and lifestyle should be additionally examined. Patients who engage in high-intensity manual labor for an extended period would be at an elevated risk for premature joint degenerative changes. Furthermore, kneeling and squatting with heavy lifting can accelerate the progression of OA.

7.1.1.2 Chief Complaint

It is important to obtain information on the specific site of pain: whether it is medial or lateral, the onset of the pain: gradual or sudden, the nature of the pain: focal or radiating, when the symptom exacerbates: whether the symptom improves with rest, whether it is exacerbated when walking, and the presence of swelling or instability. Chronic joint effusion may be observed in meniscus tear or knee OA, and inflammatory arthritis such as rheumatoid arthritis or goutic arthritis should be suspected when knee joints are repeatedly swollen.

7.1.1.3 History Taking

The main symptom of knee OA is pain. Pain on the knee occurs after a weight-bearing activity, and in the early stages, it improves with rest. This characteristic differentiates it from inflammatory arthritis, in which pain usually occurs early during an activity, and once arthritis progresses, pain does not easily improve with rest [10]. There may be persistent pain even at rest and at night with severe joint destruction or with acute inflammation.

The site of OA can be in the tibiofemoral or patellofemoral joint [11]. Patients with OA involving only the patellofemoral joint complain of pain around the patella, and the pain is typically exacerbated when climbing up and down the stairs. Arthritis affecting the tibiofemoral joint is more symptomatic and often causes walking dysfunction. Crepitus and swelling can be observed in the knee as arthritis progresses. When meniscus tear or loose body in the joint is also present, motor restriction or joint locking can also be observed. Disuse atrophy of the quadriceps femoris muscle can be developed with prolonged OA. Weakened quadriceps femoris, pain, and joint degeneration may cause the knee to give way. Substantial cartilage lost in one tibiofemoral compartment may also show progressive changes in the joint axis, such as genu valgum or genu varum (Fig. 7.1).

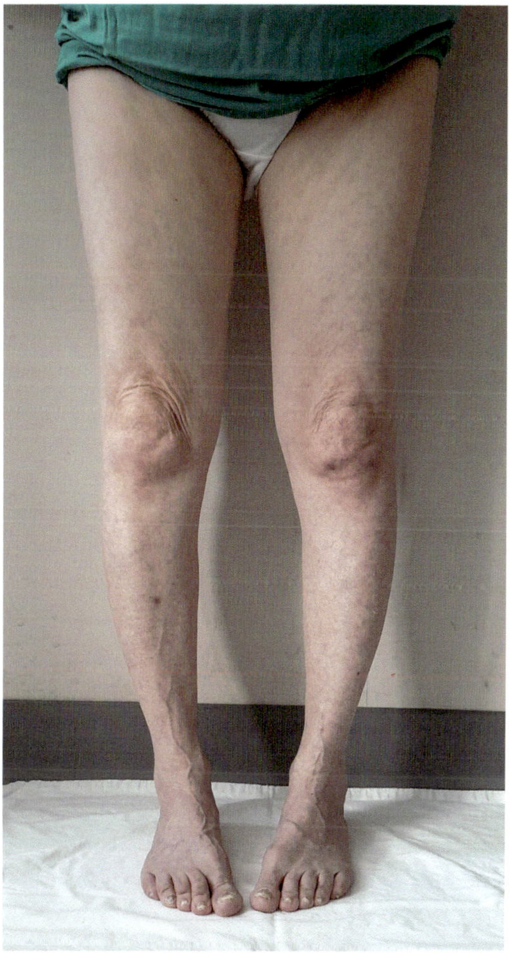

Fig. 7.1 Varus alignment shown in a patient with medial compartment osteoarthritis

7.1.2 Physical Examinations

7.1.2.1 Inspection

Clinicians should not solely rely on radiologic findings when examining a patient. Similar to history taking, physical examination is crucial in the diagnosis of knee OA [12, 13]. When performing physical examination, the entire knee should be exposed, and the anterior, medial, lateral, and posterior aspects of the knee should be visually inspected. The patient should be in an upright position with the patella facing forward and should be 2 feet apart with the toes pointing forward. While standing, the alignment of the patient's legs should be examined. The patient should be asked to walk to examine the presence of an antalgic or abnormal gait caused by neuropathy as well as lesions in any other parts, such as the spine, hip, and ankle. A gait cycle is broadly divided into the stance and swing phases, and most abnormal findings are observed in the stance phase, from the contact of the heel on the ground to the lifting of the tip of the toe off the ground.

Varus thrust refers to a lateral knee joint motion caused by increased varus in the stance phase, and OA with associated medial compartment erosion is known to be the most common cause [14]. Valgus thrust, the opposite of varus thrust, refers to a medial knee motion during weight-bearing; when valgus thrust occurs in both knee joints, individuals walk with their legs curved outward to prevent the knee joints from clashing into each other. Valgus thrust rarely occurs compared to varus thrust, and it contributes to the onset or progression of lateral OA by increasing the load transmitted onto the lateral tibiofemoral compartment of the knee [15].

To measure the range of motion of the knee joint, the patient should be asked to lie down on an examination bed, and the lateral angle between the thigh and lower leg is measured using a goniometer. An approximately 5-degree hyperextension is normal, but restrictions in extension or flexion compared to the healthy knee may indicate internal joint abnormalities such as meniscus tear or OA.

7.1.2.2 Palpation

Because the knee joint has thin soft tissue except on its posterior aspect, abnormalities can be palpated unless in cases of severe obesity. During palpation, a clinician should screen for bony tenderness around the joint line, examine whether a crackling or grinding sound (crepitus) is heard when the knee is flexed or extended or during weight-bearing, and screen for any bony enlargement in the joint line [5]. Particularly, tenderness and osteophyte in the joint line are serious indications of OA diagnosis. Patellofemoral joint line tenderness is usually observed in patients with patellofemoral pain. Joint effusion refers to increased joint fluid within the joint, and it indicates a problem within the joint such as synovitis. Though a joint effusion is commonly observed in meniscal tear or OA, it may be also caused by inflammatory arthritis, hemarthrosis, or abscess due to infection.

7.1.2.3 Basic Function Examination

Muscle power or joint balance and stability should be performed to assess muscle strength and proprioception. In particular, quadriceps weakness is a characteristic feature of knee OA. Reduced quadriceps strength is one of the initial clinical findings observed before the patient experiences symptoms or disability from knee OA, and it plays an important role in disease development [5].

7.1.2.4 Image Finding

Radiological findings are used to confirm OA and examine the involved compartments and degree of progression. However, the severity of the pain and joint injury on radiological findings are not always consistent. Plain radiographs for evaluating the knee OA include a supine knee anterior-posterior, lateral view, and merchant view which visualize patellofemoral joint. Rosenberg view which is posterior-anterior radiograph with weight-bearing and 45 degrees of knee flexion is helpful for detecting an early chondral loss in the medial and lateral femoral condyle. Standing whole leg radiographs should be taken to assess alignment abnormalities of the lower limbs. For OA, plain radiographs in the weight-bearing position may be more beneficial, and the findings show typical joint space narrowing in the medial, lateral, and patellofemoral compartments, subchondral bone sclerosis, subchondral bone cyst, osteophyte in the joint edges, and irregular joint surface [9, 16]. The Kellgren–Lawrence classification system, which classifies the severity of arthritis based on radiographic findings, is widely used. MRI can detect early arthritic changes as well as abnormalities of the articular cartilage, subchondral bone, meniscus, and other soft tissues. Detailed radiologic assessment and radiologic staging were described in the previous chapter.

7.1.2.5 Alignment of the Knee Joint

The alignment of the knee joint can be evaluated in the coronal and sagittal planes, and whole leg weight-bearing radiographs are generally used for this purpose. In the standing position, a neutral alignment of the knee joint in the coronal plane places the weight-bearing axis on the center of the knee joint, but deviation of the center of the knee joint from the weight-bearing axis leads to a malalignment on the coronal plane. Varus alignment shows a lateral displacement of the center of the knee joint from the weight-bearing axis, while valgus alignment shows a medial displacement of the center of the knee joint from the weight-bearing axis. In varus, there is increased weight placed on the medial compartment; therefore, the risk for medial compartment arthritis is increased, while in valgus, there is increased weight placed on the lateral compartment and thus the risk of lateral compartment arthritis is elevated [17, 18]. Many patients with OA who complain of pain show varus alignment. The alignment angle can be deviated from the normal without symptoms in young adults, but increasing degree of misalignment facilitates joint sub luxation and may accelerate arthritis due to abnormal increase of loading.

In a normal alignment of the knee joint in the sagittal plane, the center of the knee joint is immediately behind the weight-bearing axis. Flexion contracture occurs when the center of the knee joint is anterior to the weight-bearing axis, while recurvatum occurs when the center of the knee joint is posterior to the weight-bearing axis. In such misalignment, the posterior joint capsule and ligament cannot act to support the body weight, which would cause difficulty in maintaining posture and cause a dysfunction of normal kinematics.

7.1.2.6 Laboratory Findings

Blood test results are generally normal in knee OA and they are mostly used to exclude other conditions, such as infection, gout, and rheumatoid arthritis, as opposed to diagnosing knee OA itself. Parameters such as white blood cell (WBC) count, C-reactive protein (CRP), erythrocyte sedimentation rate (ESR), and rheumatoid factor (RF) may be conducive to differential diagnosis. Joint fluid analysis examines the joint fluid in the knee joint via aspiration. In knee OA, results generally indicate no inflammation, with a WBC (mostly monocytes) count of below 200 mm^3. A recent study has reported the potential utility of cartilage oligomeric matrix protein (COMP) as a diagnostic and prognostic biomarker of knee OA. The median serum COMP levels were significantly higher in the knee OA group than in the control group, and had positive correlations with age, BMI, and pain scores, suggesting their usefulness in the diagnosis of knee OA. However, COMP levels were not significantly correlated with the radiological grade and were high during the first 3 years of the disease, suggesting a limitation [19, 20]. Matrix metalloproteinases suppress chondrocyte synthesis of type II collagen and aggrecan, which is required to restore the extracellular matrix. It is also found during the turnover of osteoarthritic joints, fragments of extracellular matrix molecules, and other degradation products of cartilage metabolism and the cartilage matrix that are released into the synovial fluid and thereafter into the blood serum. However, it seems that further research on this topic is needed [21–23].

7.1.2.7 Bone Scintigraphy

Bone scintigraphy generates functional images that reflect metabolic activities of the bones. It is easily accessible in the clinical settings and is useful in differentiating the type of bone trauma including bone metastases, stress fracture, plantar fasciitis, Paget's disease, and osteomyelitis [24]. Bone scintigraphy uses ^{99m}Technetium labeled methylene diphosphonate (99mTc-MDP), a compound that relatively binds less to the organic phase, and is absorbed by and quickly accumulated in the mineral phase of the bone [24]. OA also includes bone reactivity such as osteophyte formation around the joint and subchondral sclerosis. Progressive OA is characterized by high bone turnover and release of bone minerals, which increases the likelihood of bonding with 99mTc-MDP; therefore, the technique can be useful for diagnosis [25].

7.2 Differential Diagnosis

The key aspects of differential diagnosis for degenerative knee OA are medical history and physical examination. First, clinicians should determine whether it is monoarthritis or polyarthritis and whether the onset is acute or chronic. Acute onset within several hours to 1 week typically indicates inflammatory arthritis, particularly bacterial infection, while slow onset suggests degenerative arthritis. Septic arthritis can be suspected in the presence of fever, chills, and infection in other parts of the body. Rheumatoid arthritis can initially be suspected if there are symmetrical polyarthritis symptoms that persist for more than 1 month. Ankylosing spondylitis or Reiter's syndrome can be suspected in the presence of repeated low back pain and lumbar stiffness in addition to knee pain. Psoriatic arthritis, which is related to psoriasis, is characterized by scaly skin rashes and a small number of involved joints. In gouty arthritis, the characteristic monosodium urate monohydrate crystals can be observed in the joint fluid using a polarizing microscope. Tuberculous arthritis and pigmented villonodular synovitis can be differentiated from other oncologic disorders using tissue biopsy. Additionally, knee joint fluid analysis can be helpful for differential diagnosis of inflammatory, septic arthritis, among others (Table 7.2).

Clinicians should note that knee pain may also be caused by a lumbar or an ipsilateral hip joint disorder and should rule out pain originating from periarticular soft tissues, such as tendons or bursa.

7.2.1 Rheumatoid Arthritis

Severity and onset of symptoms and family history are helpful in diagnosing rheumatoid arthritis. In general, rheumatoid arthritis involves multiple joints, and patients complain of pain in several joints. However, rheumatoid arthritis, which only complains of knee symptoms for weeks to months before symptoms begin in other joints, is also not uncommon. Rheumatoid arthritis is characterized by synovial deposition of mononuclear phagocytes, lymphocytes, plasma cells, and polynuclear leukocytes, and as the disease progresses, the synovial tissue swells and enlarges, and the villi protrude into the joint. Rheumatoid arthritis does not show consistent clinical manifestations; some cases end up with synovitis, while other cases may progress aggressively and cause structural injuries of the joint within 2 years of onset [26]. The 2010 ACR and EULAR diagnostic criteria for rheumatoid arthritis are helpful in the diagnosis [27]; According to these criteria, rheumatoid arthritis can be diagnosed with a score of 6 or higher out of 10 for joint involvement (A), RF and anti-citrullinated protein antibody (B), ESR, CRP (C), and symptom duration (D) (Table 7.3). Blood examination includes RF and anti-cyclic citrullinated peptide antibodies.

Table 7.2 Characteristics of joint fluid analysis

	Normal	Non-inflammatory	Inflammatory	Septic arthritis	Hemorrhagic
Viscosity	High	High	Low	Low	Low
Color	Colorless	Straw or yellow	Yellow or white	Various	Blood
Transparency	Transparent	Transparent	Light transmittable	Opaque	Various
White blood cells per mm^3	~200	200–3000	2000–75,000	>100,000, mostly	Various
Polymorphonuclear leukocytes	≤25%	≤25%	>50%	>75%	Various
Glucose	90% of blood	90% of blood	75% of blood	50% of blood	Various
Culture result	Negative	Negative	Bacteria negative	Bacteria positive	Negative

Table 7.3 The 2010 American College of Rheumatology/European League Against Rheumatism classification criteria for rheumatoid arthritis (Aletaha et al. [27])

	Score
Target population (who should be tested?): Patients who 1. have at least one joint with definite clinical synovitis (swelling)[a] 2. with the synovitis not better explained by another disease[b] Classification criteria for RA (score-based algorithm: add score of categories A–D; a score of ≥6/10 is needed for classification of a patient as having definite RA)[c]	
A. Joint involvement[d]	
1 large joint[e]	0
2–10 large joints	1
1–3 small joints (with or without involvement of large joints)[f]	2
4–10 small joints (with or without involvement of large joints)	3
>10 joints (at least 1 small joint)[g]	5
B. Serology (at least one test result is needed for classification)[h]	
Negative RF and negative ACPA	0
Low-positive RF or low-positive ACPA	2
High-positive RF or high-positive ACPA	3
C. Acute-phase reactants (at least one test result is needed for classification)[i]	
Normal CRP and normal ESR	0
Abnormal CRP or abnormal ESR	1
D. Duration of symptoms[j]	
<6 weeks	0
≥6 weeks	1

RA rheumatoid arthritis, *RF* rheumatoid factor, *ACPA* anti-citrullinated protein antibody, *CRP* C-reactive protein, *ESR* erythrocyte sedimentation rate

aThe criteria aim at classification of newly presenting patients. In addition, patients with erosive disease typical of RA with a history compatible with prior fulfillment of the 2010 criteria should be classified as having RA. Patients with longstanding disease, including those whose disease is inactive (with or without treatment), and who, based on retrospective available data, have previously fulfilled the 2010 criteria should be classified as having RA

[b]Differential diagnoses vary among patients with different presentations, but may include conditions such as systemic lupus erythematosus, psoriatic arthritis, and gout. If the relevant differential diagnoses that need to be considered are unclear, an expert rheumatologist should be consulted

[c]Although patients with a score of 6/10 cannot be classified as having RA, their status can be reassessed and the criteria might be fulfilled cumulatively over time

(continued)

Table 7.3 (continued)

[d]Joint involvement refers to any swollen or tender joint on examination, which may be confirmed by imaging evidence of synovitis. Distal interphalangeal joints, first carpometacarpal joints, and first metatarsophalangeal joints are excluded from the assessment. Categories of joint distribution are classified according to the location and number of involved joints, with placement into the highest category possible based on the pattern of joint involvement

[e]"Large joints" refer to shoulders, elbows, hips, knees, and ankles

[f]"Small joints" refer to the metacarpophalangeal joints, proximal interphalangeal joints, second through fifth metatarsophalangeal joints, thumb interphalangeal joints, and wrists

[g]In this category, at least one of the involved joints must be a small joint; the other joints can include any combination of large and additional small joints, as well as other joints not specifically listed elsewhere (e.g., temporomandibular, acromioclavicular, and sternoclavicular)

[h]Negative refers to international unit (IU) values that are less than or equal to the upper limit of normal (ULN) for the laboratory and assay; low-positive refers to IU values that are higher than the ULN but ≤3 times the ULN for the laboratory and assay; high-positive refers to IU values that are >3 times the ULN for the laboratory and assay. Where RF information is only available as positive or negative, a positive result should be scored as low-positive for RF

[i]Normal/abnormal is determined by local laboratory standards

[j]Duration of symptoms refers to patient self-report of the duration of signs or symptoms of synovitis (e.g., pain, swelling, tenderness) of joints that are clinically involved at the time of assessment, regardless of treatment status

7.2.2 Seronegative Spondyloarthropathies

Seronegative spondyloarthropathies are a group of disorders related to rheumatoid arthritis that involve joints of the spine and extremities, particularly the knee [28]. The prevalence of the disease is increased among individuals with the human lymphocyte antigen (HLA)-B27 gene. Ankylosing spondylitis, Reiter's syndrome, and psoriatic arthritis fall under this category, and they are characterized by chronic synovitis in the involved joint. The pathology of synovitis is consistent with that of rheumatoid arthritis; therefore, the disease cannot be differentiated based on synovial biopsy; clinical diagnosis is required.

Ankylosing spondylitis involves the sacroiliac joint, joints of the extremities, and knee joint. It generally affects men in their 20s and 30s. It involves the sacroiliac joint at the time of onset; therefore, low back pain and lumbosacral stiffness are characteristic symptoms. If inflammatory arthritis of a single knee joint is accompanied by low back pain, the diagnosis for ankylosing spondylitis may be frequently missed because the symptoms are masked. The disease triggers pain at the tendon and ligament insertion on the bone, and particularly, patients complain of multiple pain sites such as the Achilles tendon insertion. Patients exhibit spastic gait, where they compensate for spinal stiffness with knee flexion to maintain a standing posture and walk. HLA-B27 can be tested for diagnostic purposes, and most patients are diagnosed based on history, physical examination, and radiologic findings.

Reiter's syndrome is a disease that asymmetrical arthritis occurs in a small number of joints following an infection of the urogenital or gastrointestinal tract, and inflammation of the eyes, mucosa, and skin may occur. Asymmetrical arthritis occurs in a small number of joints 1–3 weeks after urethritis or gastrointestinal tract infection, and the knee joint is commonly involved. Inflammation at tendon or ligament insertion of a bone, such as the Achilles tendon, is also common. Radiographs show sacroiliac joint involvement in 70% of the patients, and 80% of the patients are positive for HLA-B27.

The concept of psoriatic arthritis emerged as it had been reported that psoriasis was associated with inflammatory arthritis. Various types of arthritis occur in the extremities or spinal joints, but unlike other spinal arthritis, sacroiliac arthritis is rare. The diagnosis can be made based on psoriasis in the skin or fingernails and toenails with polyarthritis. Synovial findings are similar to those of rheumatoid arthritis.

7.2.3 Infectious Arthritis

Infection of the knee joint can affect individuals of any age; however, it most commonly affects immunocompromised patients with cancer, diabetes mellitus, alcoholism, acquired immunodeficiency syndrome, or corticosteroid therapy. In septic arthritis, sudden pain or swelling often occurs in the knee joint without trauma [29]. During physical examination, the knee is warm and swollen, and the patient experiences intense pain even with slight motion of the knee joint. Septic arthritis that occurs after an invasive procedure is believed to be a common cause. This is because the use of intraarticular injection and acupuncture for degenerative arthritis is increasing in the aged population and the knee joint is vulnerable to microbial infiltration and trauma [30].

When patients present to the hospital, systemic symptoms are not uncommon, with fever, sweat, and chills presented in 34%, 15%, and 6% of cases, respectively; however, fever is not an essential criterion for the diagnosis of septic arthritis [31]. Arthrocentesis is required for the diagnosis, and the joint fluid is turbid. In septic arthritis, the WBC count in the fluid exceeds 50,000 per mm^3 (50×10^9 per L); however, the WBC count may be below 28,000 per mm^3 in immunocompromised individuals. Particularly, more than 90% (0.90) polymorphonuclear cells strongly indicate acute septic arthritis. Although the likelihood is low, it cannot be completely ruled out even in normal patients with a WBC count of below 50,000 per mm^3 [32]. Common pathogens include *Staphylococcus aureus*, Streptococcus species, *Haemophilus influenzae*, and *Neisseria gonorrhoeae*.

7.2.4 Crystal-Induced Inflammatory Arthropathy

Acute inflammation, pain, or sudden swelling that is nontraumatic may indicate septic arthritis as well as crystal-induced inflammatory arthropathy such as gout or pseudogout. The latter commonly affects the knee joint and is characterized by heat sensation and increased WBC count, showing similar symptoms with those of septic arthritis. Crystal arthritis and septic arthritis are differentiated based on synovial analysis, by confirming crystals and positivity on culture test. Acute gout, an inflammatory crystal arthropathy, is spontaneously resolved within an average of 1–2 weeks [33, 34]. However, if gouty attack occurs more frequently, persists longer, and is not completely resolved, these lead to chronic gouty arthropathy. Gouty arthropathy is characterized by joint space narrowing but not periarticular osteopenia, which contrasts with rheumatoid arthritis. In gout, monosodium urate crystal precipitates can be observed in the knee joint fluid using a polarized microscope, and in pseudogout, calcium pyrophosphate crystals are observed.

7.2.5 Spontaneous and Secondary Osteonecrosis

Osteonecrosis of the knee is a disease that causes knee pain, similar to that generated by OA; it can be classified into spontaneous and secondary osteonecrosis. Although the exact etiology of osteonecrosis is still unknown, medical conditions such as blood diseases, steroid use, systemic lupus erythematosus, organ transplantation, Casson's disease, Gaucher's disease, and alcohol overuse are some known causes.

Spontaneous osteonecrosis is three times more common among women, and most patients are 60 years or older. In general, sudden knee joint pain is caused by mild trauma or abnormal behavior, and pain is mostly severe. The disease exacerbates proportionately with activity, and the symptoms tend to be worse at night. While the medial femoral condyle is the typical site affected, it is also relatively common in the tibial condyle and lateral femoral condyle, as well as in the patella. Recently, it has been reported that spontaneous osteonecrosis of the knee (SONK) is a subchondral insufficiency fracture (SIF) that has progressed into collapse with secondary necrosis. Because proven microtraumatic origin of SONK and the histopathologic and MRI features unite it with SIF, this notion is currently accepted [35].

Secondary osteonecrosis mostly affects young patients under 55 years, and most patients have risk factors including trauma, use of corticoste roids, sickle cell anemia, collagen vascular disease, and alcoholism. Multiple joints are affected in many cases, and more than 80% of secondary osteonecrosis cases in the knee joint are bilateral, with a 60–90% probability of involving an additional joint [36]. Radiologic evaluation is important in the diagnosis of knee osteonecrosis. Bone scan is essential for the diagnosis of osteonecrosis, and MRI is crucial for staging and differential diagnosis of osteonecrosis, as it enables a detailed observation of the changes in the subchondral bone related to osteonecrosis.

7.2.6 Other Diseases to Be Diagnosed Differentially

In many cases, it is difficult to differentiate symptoms of meniscal tear in older adults with OA from progressive OA and spontaneous osteonecrosis. Even if a patient complains of severe pain in the knee without trauma, there are many difficulties in determining the cause if the cause of the symptoms such as an additional meniscal tear, exacerbation of an existing disease, and loose body in the joint have not been identified. If the symptoms are not severe, observing clinical progress for an appropriate period of time will help with clinical treatment and prognosis.

One or more bursae are present around the knee joint, and some are connected to the knee joint. Depending on their location, they are called the suprapatellar bursa, prepatellar bursa, infrapatellar bursa, popliteal cyst, pes anserine bursa, medial collateral ligament bursa, and iliotibial bursa. As the medial collateral ligament bursa is commonly shown on an MRI of a normal joint, it must be differentiated from meniscal tear and medial collateral ligament tear. Iliotibial band syndrome causes lateral knee pain that is related to repeated motion. Its etiology is chronic infection of the iliotibial bursa due to friction between the iliotibial band and lateral femoral epicondyle. Patients complain of local pain in the distal iliotibial band between the epicondyle and Gerdy tubercle. Anserine bursitis shows swelling and tenderness on the medial aspect of the knee joint.

Connective tissue diseases, such as lupus, may show inflammatory arthritis of the knee joint. Fortunately, arthritis is rare, and this disease can be suspected in the presence of systemic joint symptoms.

Lyme disease is a complex multiorgan infection caused by *Borrelia burgdorferi*, a spirochete found in ticks. The pathogen circulates in the blood and causes rash and pain at the infection site, and following a migrating joint pain, unilateral or bilateral knee chronic synovitis ultimately develops.

7.3 Summary

Diagnosis of OA is made by combining patient's detailed medical history and physical examination, radiological examination, and blood test results. Knee OA should not be diagnosed by radiological changes alone, as they are detected after the disease has progressed. Moreover, since most elderly people are accompanied by degenerative changes in their knee joints, differential diagnosis with other diseases that cause degenerative changes in the knee is of great importance, especially in the elderly. Misdiagnosis can be harmful to patients if it does not provide proper treatment. Therefore, differential diagnosis of rheumatoid arthritis, seronegative spondyloarthropathies, infectious arthritis, crystalline inflammatory arthropathy, spontaneous and secondary osteonecrosis, and other diseases should be considered.

References

1. Nuki G. Osteoarthritis: a problem of joint failure. Z Rheumatol. 1999;58:142–7.
2. Bijlsma JW, Berenbaum F, Lafeber FP. Osteoarthritis: an update with relevance for clinical practice. Lancet. 2011;377:2115–26.
3. Eyre DR. Collagens and cartilage matrix homeostasis. Clin Orthop Relat Res. 2004;427:S118–22.
4. Guccione AA, Felson DT, Anderson JJ, Anthony JM, Zhang Y, Wilson PW, et al. The effects of specific medical conditions on the functional limitations of elders in the Framingham Study. Am J Public Health. 1994;84:351–8.
5. Altman R, Asch E, Bloch D, Bole G, Borenstein D, Brandt K, et al. Development of criteria for the classification and reporting of osteoarthritis. Classification of osteoarthritis of the knee. Diagnostic and Therapeutic Criteria Committee of the American Rheumatism Association. Arthritis Rheum. 1986;29:1039–49.
6. Heidari B. Knee osteoarthritis diagnosis, treatment and associated factors of progression: Part II. Caspian J Inter Med. 2011;2:249–55.
7. Peat G, Thomas E, Duncan R, Wood L. Is a false-positive clinical diagnosis of knee osteoarthritis just the early diagnosis of preradiographic disease? Arthritis Care Res (Hoboken). 2010;62:1502–6.
8. Zhang W, Doherty M, Peat G, Bierma-Zeinstra MA, Arden NK, Bresnihan B, et al. EULAR evidence-based recommendations for the diagnosis of knee osteoarthritis. Ann Rheum Dis. 2010;69:483–9.
9. Arya RK, Jain V. Osteoarthritis of the knee joint: an overview. J Ind Acad Clin Med. 2013;14:154–62.
10. Michael JW-P, Schlüter-Brust KU, Eysel P. The epidemiology, etiology, diagnosis, and treatment of osteoarthritis of the knee. Dtsch Ärtzebl Int. 2010;107:152–62.
11. Kuttner JH, Goldberg VM. Osteoarthritic disorders. Am Acad Ortho Surg. 1995; Rosemont xxi–v.
12. Kornaat PR, Bloem JL, Ceulemans RY, Riyazi N, Rosendaal FR, Nelissen RG, et al. Osteoarthritis of the knee: association between clinical features and MR imaging findings. Radiology. 2006;239:811–7.
13. Bedson J, Croft PR. The discordance between clinical and radiographic knee osteoarthritis: a systematic search and summary of the literature. BMC Musculoskelet Disord. 2008;9:116.
14. Kuroyanagi Y, Nagura T, Kiriyama Y, Matsumoto H, Otani T, Toyama Y, et al. A quantitative assessment of varus thrust in patients with medial knee osteoarthritis. Knee. 2012;19:130–4.
15. Chang A, Hochberg M, Song J, Dunlop D, Chmiel JS, Nevitt M, et al. Frequency of varus and valgus thrust, and factors associated with thrust presence in persons with or at higher risk of developing knee osteoarthritis. Arthritis Rheum. 2010;62:1403–11.
16. Parmet MS, Lynm C, Glass RM. Osteoarthritis of the knee. JAMA. 2003;289:1068.
17. Cooke TD, Scudamore RA, Bryant JT, Sorbie C, Siu D, Fisher B. A quantitative approach to radiography of the lower limb. Principles and applications. J Bone Joint Surg Br. 1991;73:715–20.
18. Hsu RW, Himeno S, Coventry MB, Chao EY. Normal axial alignment of the lower extremity and load-bearing distribution at the knee. Clin Orthop Relat Res. 1990;255:215–27.
19. Verma P, Dalal K. Serum cartilage oligomeric matrix protein (COMP) in knee osteoarthritis: a novel diagnostic and prognostic biomarker. J Orthop Res. 2013;31:999–1006.
20. Andersson ML, Thorstensson CA, Roos EM, Petersson IF, Heinegard D, Saxne T. Serum levels of cartilage oligomeric matrix protein (COMP) increase temporarily after physical exercise in patients with knee osteoarthritis. BMC Musculoskelet Disord. 2006;7:98.

21. Aigner T, Soeder S, Haag J. IL-1beta and BMPs--interactive players of cartilage matrix degradation and regeneration. Eur Cell Mater. 2006;12:49–56; discussion 56
22. Song SY, Han YD, Hong SY, Kim K, Yang SS, Min BH, et al. Chip-based cartilage oligomeric matrix protein detection in serum and synovial fluid for osteoarthritis diagnosis. Anal Biochem. 2012;420:139–46.
23. Goldring SR, Goldring MB. The role of cytokines in cartilage matrix degeneration in osteoarthritis. Clin Orthop Relat Res. 2004;427:S27–36.
24. Love C, Din AS, Tomas MB, Kalapparambath TP, Palestro CJ. Radionuclide bone imaging: an illustrative review. Radiographics. 2003;23:341–58.
25. Bettica P, Cline G, Hart DJ, Meyer J, Spector TD. Evidence for increased bone resorption in patients with progressive knee osteoarthritis: longitudinal results from the Chingford study. Arthritis Rheum. 2002;46:3178–84.
26. Harris ED Jr. Rheumatoid arthritis: pathophysiology and implications for therapy. N Engl J Med. 1990;322:1277–89.
27. Aletaha D, Neogi T, Silman AJ, Funovits J, Felson DT, Bingham CO III, et al. 2010 rheumatoid arthritis classification criteria: an American College of Rheumatology/European League Against Rheumatism collaborative initiative. Arthritis Rheum. 2010;62:2569–81.
28. Taurog JD. Immunology, genetics, and animal models of the spondyloarthropathies. Curr Opin Rheumatol. 1990;2:586–91.
29. McCune WJ, Golbus J. Monoarticular arthritis. In: Kelley WN, editor. Textbook of rheumatology. 5th ed. Philadelphia: Saunders; 1997. p. 371–80.
30. Seo SS, Ha DJ, Kim CW, Kim KW, Seo JH. Etiologic transition of septic arthritis of the knee. J Korean Knee Soc. 2008;20:44–9.
31. Mathews CJ, Weston VC, Jones A, Field M, Coakley G. Bacterial septic arthritis in adults. Lancet. 2010;375:846–55.
32. Coutlakis PJ, Roberts WN, Wise CM. Another look at synovial fluid leukocytosis and infection. J Clin Rheumatol. 2002;8:67–71.
33. Choi HK, Mount DB, Reginato AM, American College of Physicians; American Physiological Society. Pathogenesis of gout. Ann Intern Med. 2005;143:499–516.
34. Martinon F, Glimcher LH. Gout: new insights into an old disease. J Clin Invest. 2006;116:2073–5.
35. Gorbachova T, Melenevsky Y, Cohen M, Cerniglia BW. Osteochondral lesions of the knee: Differentiating the most common entities at MRI. Radiographics. 2018;38:1478–95.
36. Jones JP Jr. Concepts of etiology and early pathogenesis of osteonecrosis. Instr Course Lect. 1994;43:499–512.

Non-Pharmacologic Management 8

Soung-Kyun Hong and Seung-Suk Seo

Abstract

Knee OA has been known as a degenerative change in which various causes, such as aging, obesity, and inflammatory changes, are compounded, resulting in repeated wear and tear of articular cartilage. In addition to pain, physical symptoms of knee OA include reduced muscle strength and range of motion, reduced lower limb balance due to decreased proprioception, and walking disability. Non-pharmacologic treatment is necessary to treat physical symptoms caused by knee OA. Non-pharmacologic treatment includes patient education, weight loss, exercise therapy, and physical therapy. Knee OA is a chronic disease, so it is important for patients to understand their condition and change their lifestyle. Therefore, patient education is necessary. Losing weight is an essential factor in improving pain caused by knee OA. Losing weight requires exercise therapy as well as diet therapy. Exercise therapy also helps strengthen muscles around the knee, improve the range of exercise and improve the sense of balance in the lower extremities. Physical therapy is useful for improving the pain and function of OA. Many kinds of the instrument are needed for physical therapy. Various methods are used for such non-pharmacologic treatments, but not only one method is used for treatment, but a combination of different treatment methods depending on the patient's condition can lead to better treatment.

Keywords

Knee OA · Non-pharmacologic management Exercise · Weight loss · Physical therapy

8.1 Introduction

Osteoarthritis (OA) of the knee is a progressive and debilitating condition characterized by marked pain and stiffness, which frequently causes physical disability [1]. Especially, joint pain and functional problem are the main symptoms of knee OA [2]. More than 50 modalities of non-pharmacological, pharmacological, and surgical therapy for OA are described in the medical literature [3]. The non-pharmacological treatment is usually useful for patients with low-grade knee OA [4]. Strategies for relieving pain, minimizing disability and slowing disease progression are key elements of conservative, non-surgical

S.-K. Hong (✉)
Department of Physical Therapy, Woosuk University, Jeonju, South Korea
e-mail: popory77@woosuk.ac.kr

S.-S. Seo
Department of Orthopedics, Haeundae Bumin Hospital, Busan, South Korea

S.-S. Seo (ed.), *A Strategic Approach to Knee Arthritis Treatment*,
https://doi.org/10.1007/978-981-16-4217-3_8

management of knee OA. Osteoarthritis Research Society International (OARSI)'s guidelines recommend land-based exercise (walking, strengthening exercise, yoga, cycling, etc.), hydrotherapy, massage, manual therapy, heat therapy, assistive aids (brace, cane, wedge, insole, taping) and especially strong bodyweight management for the patient with knee OA as a non-pharmacological methods [5]. In addition, National institute for Health and Care Excellence (NICE) also recommended weight loss, exercise, electrotherapy, using aids and devices [6]. Although there are no curative methods for knee OA, non-pharmacologic treatment for knee OA is supposed to reduce pain and improve joint mobility functional impairment [7].

8.2 Weight Loose and OA

OA is characterized by gradual degenerative changes in the articular surface and is often involved in the weight-bearing joint [8]. Therefore, the weight gain stress on the knees, which further accelerates knee OA. Obesity is associated with a three to four-fold increased risk of knee pain with a disability that has an attributable fraction estimate for raised body mass index (BMI) of 36% (27%–44%) [9]. Three to five times the body weight passes through the knee joint during ambulation [10]. In various studies about weight loss effect in overweight and obese patients with knee OA showed similar results; compared with no weight loss or under 10% weight loss, 10% weight loss resulted in less pain and inflammation, better function, improved health-related quality of life, and reduced knee joint loads [11, 12]. The standard of care for elderly, overweight, and obese adults with knee OA should include, at minimum, a 10% weight loss. Furthermore,, losing 20% compared with 10% of baseline body weight in overweight and obese adults with knee OA has the added benefit of significantly improved physical health-related quality of life and a 25% reduction in pain and improvement in function [13]. In the Framingham Study, a 12-lb weight loss reduced knee OA risk by 50% [14]. Christensen et al. [15] found that rapid diet-induced weight reductions of 10% improved function by 28% with 2.2% body fat reduction and 9.4% improvement in WOMAC (The Western Ontario and McMaster Universities Osteoarthritis Index) scores.

Although, significant weight loss in older adults could exacerbate bone loss and increase the risk of hip fracture [16]; however, obesity can make it worse because it increases the load on the lower limb bones. Despite controversies about weight reduction's effect on the risk of hip fractures, weight loss interventions may have small to moderate improvements on pain and disability for OA compared to minimal care [17].

When considering exercise to lose weight in knee OA patients, the following should always be considered:

1. Selection of appropriate program (composition of exercise)
2. Frequency according to the composition of the exercise (time and duration)
3. Intensity according to the composition of exercise (weight and amount of exercise, appropriate rest time)
4. Continuous feedback with experts (whether it is appropriate for the patient's characteristics or exercise) (Fig. 8.1)

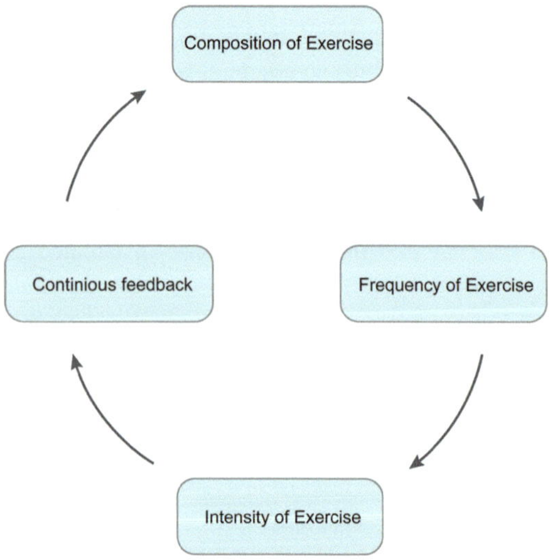

Fig. 8.1 Consideration for weight control exercise

8.3 Exercise for OA

8.3.1 Selection of Appropriate Program (Composition of Exercise)

One of the most important treatments in the symptomatic knee OA is weight loss. Weight loss is a helpful treatment in terms of functional recovery and pain control in patients. Additionally, obesity increases circulating levels of tumor necrosis factor-α, interleukin-6, C-reactive protein, and other proinflammatory cytokines that may promote cartilage matrix degeneration [18]. So, the first goal for weight loss is to select an appropriate exercise program for symptom improvement in patients with knee OA and to identify the patient's goal accurately. American College of Rheumatology (ACR) has published 2019 ACR/AF guidelines for the management of knee OA (Table 8.1). This new guideline suggests for the first time that patients will be directly involved in disease treatment. Additionally, a remarkable new guideline is that exercise therapy, which can be used by most patients with knee OA, is a very important treatment for patients with knee OA, as its effectiveness is demonstrated through evidence presented through various reviewed literature.

The appropriate exercise for the patient with knee OA, regardless of the level of activity, should be individualized and patient centered, taking into account the patient's age, mobility, functional level, comorbidity, and preferences.

In conclusion, appropriately designed exercise is a powerful intervention method for weight control, and if attention is paid to appropriate exercise according to the patient's personal condition, lifestyle, and background, it can bring a higher effect.

Table 8.1 Summary of 2019 American College of Rheumatology/Arthritis Foundation Guideline for the Management (non-pharmacological) of osteoarthritis of knee

Interventions	Recommendation
Exercise (aerobic exercise, strengthening)	Strongly recommended
Balance training	Recommended
Self-management program	Strongly recommended
Yoga	Recommended
Cognitive behavioral therapy	Recommended
Cane	Strongly recommended
Tibiofemoral knee braces	Strongly recommended
Patellofemoral braces	Recommended
Kinesiotaping	Recommended
Modified shoes	Recommended against
Lateral and medial wedged insoles	Recommended against
Acupuncture	Recommended
Thermal intervention	Recommended
Radio frequency ablation	Recommended
Massage therapy	Recommended against
Manual therapy with/without exercise	Recommended against
Pulsed vibration therapy	Recommended against
Transcutaneous electrical nerve stimulation	Strongly recommended against

8.3.2 Basic Composition of Exercise for Weight Reduction

The basic composition of the exercise program consists of a warm-up period (around 10 min), an endurance period (20–60 min), and a cool-down (5–10 min).

The purpose of warm-up may reduce the susceptibility to musculoskeletal injuries by increasing connective tissue extensibility, improving joint range of motion and function, and enhancing muscular performance [19]. Warm-up should start with a low-intensity exercise of 5–10 min, stretching exercise, or a light bare-handed exercise, and it is recommended to start with an exercise that can increase heart rate enough for main exercise [20].

The main exercise is the process of starting exercise in earnest, raising cardiopulmonary capacity and creating muscle strength, and it is a process of continuously exercising 20–60 min or more or collecting at least 10 min of exercise several times during a day. Additionally, for the effect of exercise, medium-intensity exercise (walking speed of 5–6 km/h per hour) should be continued for at least 30 min, and in the case of high-intensity exercise (intensity of 70–90% of the maximum heart rate), it is effective only to continue exercise for at least 20 min [19]. The most effective way to maximize the effectiveness of exercise that can help to recovering your body's function is naturally to use large muscles group through the exercise that moves the body as active as possible [20].

Cool down is an exercise that reduces the intensity of the muscles that have become excited in stages and the intensity of the heart and lungs and includes exercises such as slow walking and yoga.

8.3.2.1 Aerobic Exercise

For weight loss that affects degenerative knee OA, aerobic exercise is recommended as an effective type of exercise suitable for individuals along with dietary therapy [20]. Aerobic exercise is a form of exercise that obtains energy required during exercise through aerobic energy metabolism and refers to exercise that lasts for about 5 min or more. This is one of the methods for synthesizing ATP (adenosine triphosphate), energy for muscle contraction activity, and it is made in the mitochondria by the complex interaction of the Krebs cycle and the electron transport chain. Pyruvate is converted to high-energy molecules like NADH, GTP, and FADH2 through catalyzation by TCA/Krebs cycle enzymes. NADH generated is shuttled to complex I and is converted to NAD+ driving oxidative phosphorylation. Transfer of electrons through the chain maintains the membrane potential via proton pumping into the intermembrane space (IMS). In this final step, ADP is phosphorylated to form ATP via complex V (ATP synthase) (Fig. 8.2).

General aerobic exercise is known as effective management of patients with knee OA by nearly all international guidelines [21]. Effective aerobic exercises commonly used for weight loss include lightly outdoor exercises such as walking, running, swimming, and jumping rope, and indoor aerobic exercises such as treadmills, stationary bicycles, and stair steppers. Randomized clinical trials of walking exercise have shown significant short-term improvements in pain, functional status, and quality of life in the patient with knee OA [22, 23]. Among these various exercises, it is first necessary to consider various conditions such as the patient's physical condition, temporary, or permanent dysfunction, the patient's surrounding environment, and the patient's goals. Most of all, what produces the most effective results is to do an exercise consistently.

However, as an absolute contraindication of aerobic exercise, it should not be performed if the resting heart rate is 100 bpm or higher, the systolic blood pressure is 200 mmHg or higher, and the diastolic blood pressure is 120 mmHg or higher. Especially, patients with underlying diseases related to heart conditions or with signs of risk of heart disease should always monitor blood pressure and heart rate. Physicians should also educate patients on how to measure their heart rate and blood pressure. Considering the age of most patients, an aquatic exercise can also be helpful, which can reduce the force on the joints due to weight and the force required for movement. Subjective pain decreases through water exercise, and the sensory feeling increases due to the turbulence flow, pressure, and temperature of the water. Additionally, the buoyancy of water decreases weight load and reduces joint compression. As a result, it helps patients complaining of knee pain due to knee OA [24]. The use of aquatic exercise can provide positive physical activity and basic strength to start ground exercise for patients who are unable to exercise due to pain or knee OA. However, it should not be forgotten that this improvement of function in the water is the beginning of allowing the patient to carry out an exercise that can be done on the ground as soon as possible. The positive effect of aerobic exercise for weight loose include increased vital capacity, endurance, muscle strength, weight loss and less exertion at a given workload.

8.3.2.2 Range of Motion (ROM) and Anaerobic Exercise

Aerobic exercise can increase cardiorespiratory and aerobic exercise capacity. However, it is difficult to create an effective increase in muscle strength or functional capacity with aerobic exercise alone. Resistance exercise (anaerobic exer-

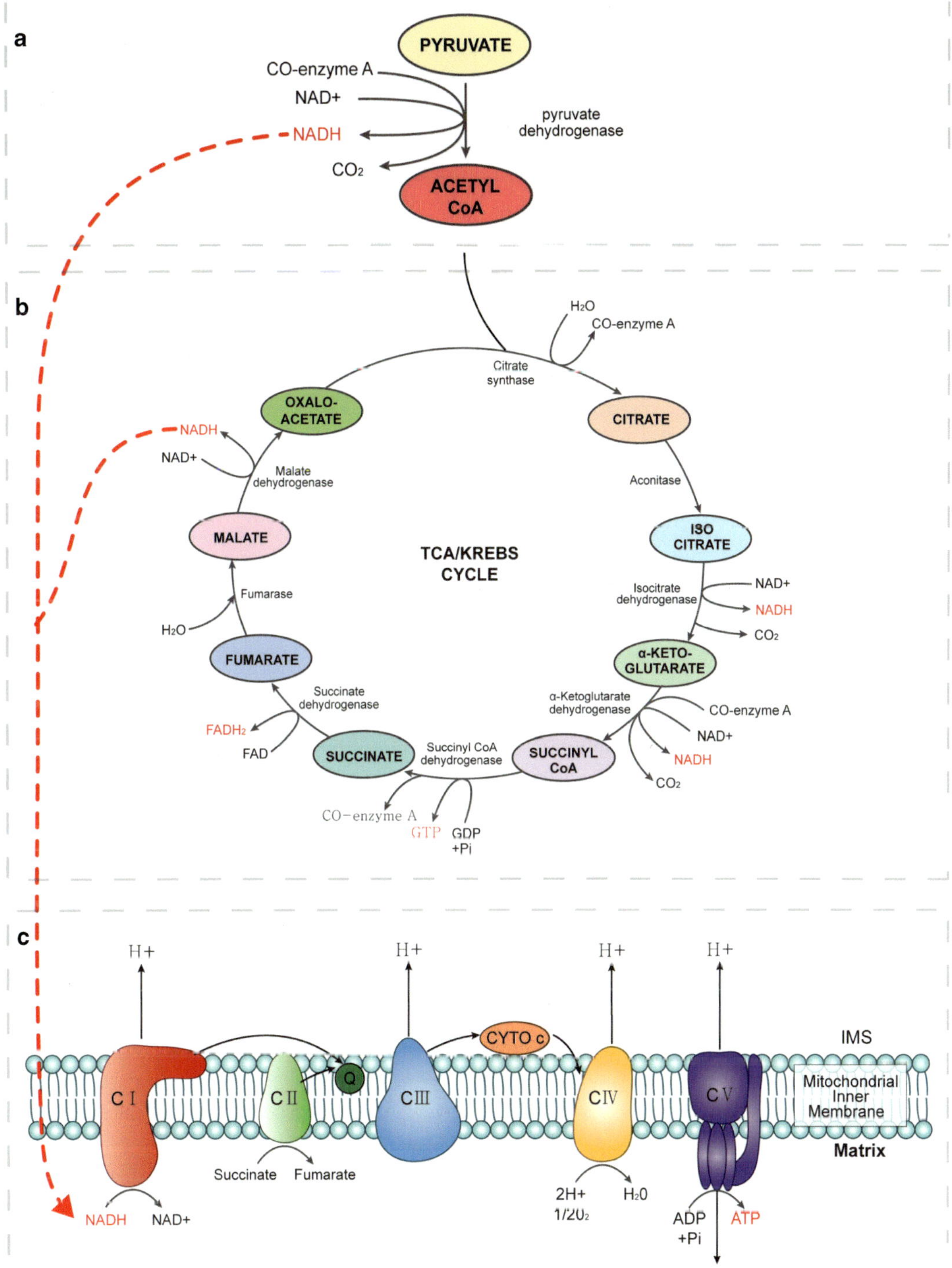

Fig. 8.2 Bioenergetics of the electron transport chain and the TCA/Krebs cycle. (**a**) Stage 1: The generation of a key two-carbon molecule, acetyl-CoA, (**b**) Stage 2: The oxidation of acetyl-CoA in the Krebs cycle, (**c**) Stage 3: The process of oxidative phosphorylation (i.e., ATP formation) in the electron transport chain (i.e., respiratory chain)

cise) can help increase not only strength but also reduce weight [25].

According to OARSI recommendations, strength training refers to an exercise aimed to increase muscle strength, and it is known to reduce pain in the knee and improve the function of the knee joint. In particular, it is important to increase muscle strength by targeting various lower limb muscle groups, including quadriceps, and it is possible to increase the muscle strength through various types of exercise equipment or movements [3]. The limited mobility and adhesion of soft tissues caused by inflammation of the joints and surrounding tissues can affect a variety of symptoms in knee OA patients [26]. The result of adhesions can lead to changes in the biomechanical forces on articular surfaces, restricting joint movement leading to another symptom like a limited range of motion [27, 28]. The loss in ROM of the knee OA is a primary factor that leads to muscular weakness during isokinetic exercise [29]. The first aim of management is to improve joint mobility and ROM by reducing soft tissue contracture and improving function. In athletics with knee OA, the extensibility of the joint capsule, hip flexor, quadriceps, hamstrings, gastrocnemius, and soleus muscle length is very important because they affect the function of the knee. Anaerobic exercise(resistance/strength exercise) also has positive effects on pain scores and functional outcomes in knee OA [30–32]. The resistance/strength exercise program should include resistance load, number of repetitions, movement speed, and session frequency. Because the weakness of the quadriceps muscle is highly correlated with knee OA and disability of the knee [33, 34], many of the resistance-training protocols have focused on quadriceps strengthening and stabilization and have shown good clinical benefit. However, there are precautions before exercise prescription. In individuals with malaligned or overly loosened knees, increased quadriceps strength is associated with the progression of knee OA [35].

Stretching

When subjected to immobilization or inactivity, the periarticular connective tissue becomes fibrotic, resulting in capsular adherence, adaptive shortening of muscles and consequent limitation of ROM [36]. For this, stretching exercises are recommended initially. Stretching exercises restore limited ROM after damage to bones or ligaments due to OA, correct posture, and prevent injury to reduce associated pain. In addition, it can protect joint wear and increase flexibility, and maintain the strength of major joints at an appropriate level, not only for the elderly with OA but also for the elderly without joint pain [37]. Additionally, low-intensity stretching exercises performed while sitting or lying on a mat without having to prepare a separate exercise place have no weight bearing, no risk of falling, and are simple and easy to learn. Therefore, it can be applied not only to the elderly but also to people who are overweight. And it is a highly recommended exercise method because you can keep exercising continuously because you are interested [38]. In addition, for those who have difficulty continuing exercise due to the burden of knee pain caused by standing motions for a long time, sitting stretching exercises will be suitable [39]. Therefore, for patients with knee OA who have to practice continuous symptom management behavior for life as a chronic disease, stretching exercise can be helpful to reinforce changes in symptom management behavior to improve health and quality of life. The major muscles involved in the movement of the knee joint such as paraspinal muscle, gluteus, iliopsoas, hamstrings, quadriceps, hip adductors and gastrocnemius should be stretched during exercise.

Stretching exercise consists of five methods, repeated three times and sustained for 30 s of each time. Unilateral exercises are performed alternately, allowing the contralateral limb to rest during execution. Participants must be correctly positioned, and the responsible physiotherapist has to guide body awareness, breathing, and alignment throughout the therapy. After completing each exercise, relax the muscle (Fig. 8.3).

Selective Muscle Training

Several lower extremity muscle groups support the knee joint from own weight and gravity. The two main muscle groups that control the knee joint movement and stability are the quadriceps and the hamstrings. The quadriceps and hamstring muscles have the potential to provide dynamic frontal plane knee stability because of their abduction and/or adduction moment arms [40]. Using a neuromuscular biomechanical model, the quadriceps and hamstring muscles not only have the potential to support frontal plane moments but also provide support to abduction-adduction moments [41].

Muscle weakness or dysfunction is involved in the pathogenesis of knee OA [42, 43]. Knee extensor and knee flexor strengths are both lost with the progress of symptomatic knee OA [44–46]. Because the lower limb musculature is the natural brace of the knee joint, important muscle dysfunction may arise from either quadriceps weakness or weakness of the hamstrings relative to the quadriceps [42, 47]. Additionally, the ratio of the quadriceps to hamstring muscle strength is important for the stability of the knee and for protection from excessive stress [48, 49]. The strength of both quadriceps and hamstring muscles is associated with incident symptomatic knee OA but not radiographic OA [47].

For selective muscle strength training, isometric exercises are recommended initially, because they employ less joint motion and are less likely to aggravate symptoms [50]. In addition, isometric exercise may be helpful to improve muscle tone, strength, and static endurance and to prepare joints for more vigorous exercise or activity. Isometric contractions performed at 70% of the maximal voluntary contraction, held for 6 seconds and 5–10 times/day, can increase strength and endurance significantly. Additionally,

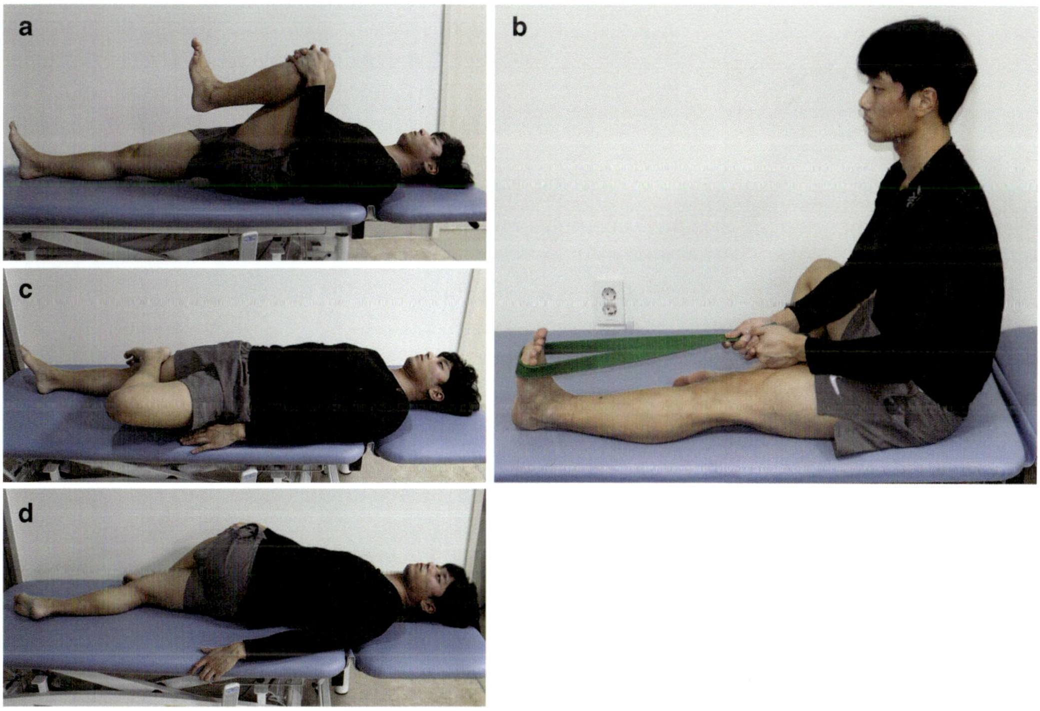

Fig. 8.3 Stretching Exercise. (**a**) Paraspinal and gluteus maximus stretched by alternate limbs, (**b**) Paraspinal, hamstring, and gastrocnemius stretched by alternate limbs, (**c**) Hip adductors stretched by alternate limbs, (**d**) Glutes stretched by alternate limbs, (**e**) Quadriceps stretched by alternate limb

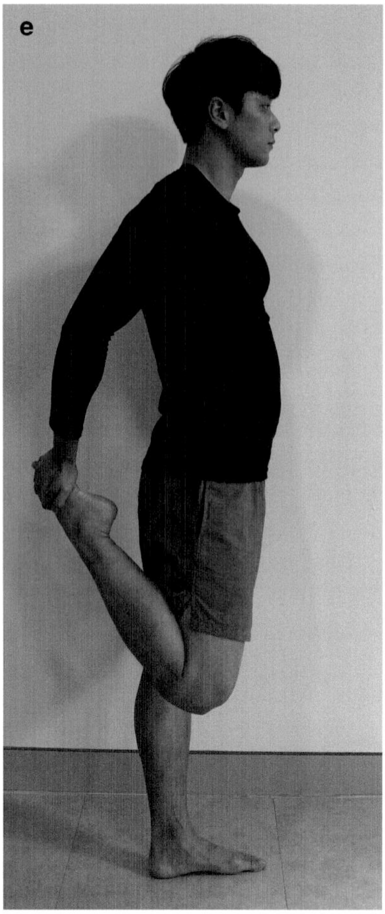

Fig. 8.3 (continued)

Isometric contraction at more than 40% maximal voluntary contraction constricts blood flow through the contracted muscle. Figure 8.4 Contain instructions for isometric quadriceps and hamstring exercise for the patient with knee OA.

For quadriceps isometric exercise, with your knees straight and ankle dorsiflexion, press the floor. And for hamstring isometric exercise, bring up your knee and place your heel on the ground. Push your heel directly down to fire those hamstrings. So pushing down and hold and relax.

Proprioceptive Exercise (Balance Training)

Proprioception can be defined as the ability to recognize and to locate the body in relation to its position and orientation in space [51, 52]. Proprioception ability is essential to motor control and joint stability during daily activities and sports practice [53]. However, OA patients have decreased joint position sense [54]. Joint position sense plays a very important role in improving the induction and promotion of voluntary or involuntary movements by sending basic information to the motor control areas such as balance and vestibular sense [55].

Therefore, it is very important to increase the positional sense of patients with knee OA through exercise to enhance the proprioceptive sense. These exercises improve an individual proprioception feedback circle. The brain sends signals to either contract or relaxes the muscles. The joints movement response is detected by the sensory nervous system and reported back to the brain for fine-tuning and improvement with repetition of the process (Fig. 8.5).

Figure 8.6 contain instructions for a progressive proprioceptive exercise for the patient with knee OA.

The exercise consists of three stages. Stage 1 is static phage for progress the base of support. Patients maintain balance on the progressively unstable surface of the balance board. If the patient adapts to it, progress to a unilateral stance. Stage 2 is dynamic progress of center of gravity. Add arm and leg movements while balancing on the progressively unstable surface of the balance board. For an additional challenge, incorporate a flex bar or dumbbell(soft weight). Stage 3 is functional movement to perform functional movements(lunge, step, push, squat, pull, etc.) on the progressively unstable surface on balance board.

8.3.3 Exercise Dosing (Intensity/Frequency of Aerobic/Anaerobic Exercise)

8.3.3.1 Aerobic Exercise

If you have organized the type of exercise and the appropriate exercise program, the next step is to determine the intensity or frequency of the exercise. The frequency and intensity of exercise refer to the number of exercises per week, and the amount of exercise required to achieve the best effect.

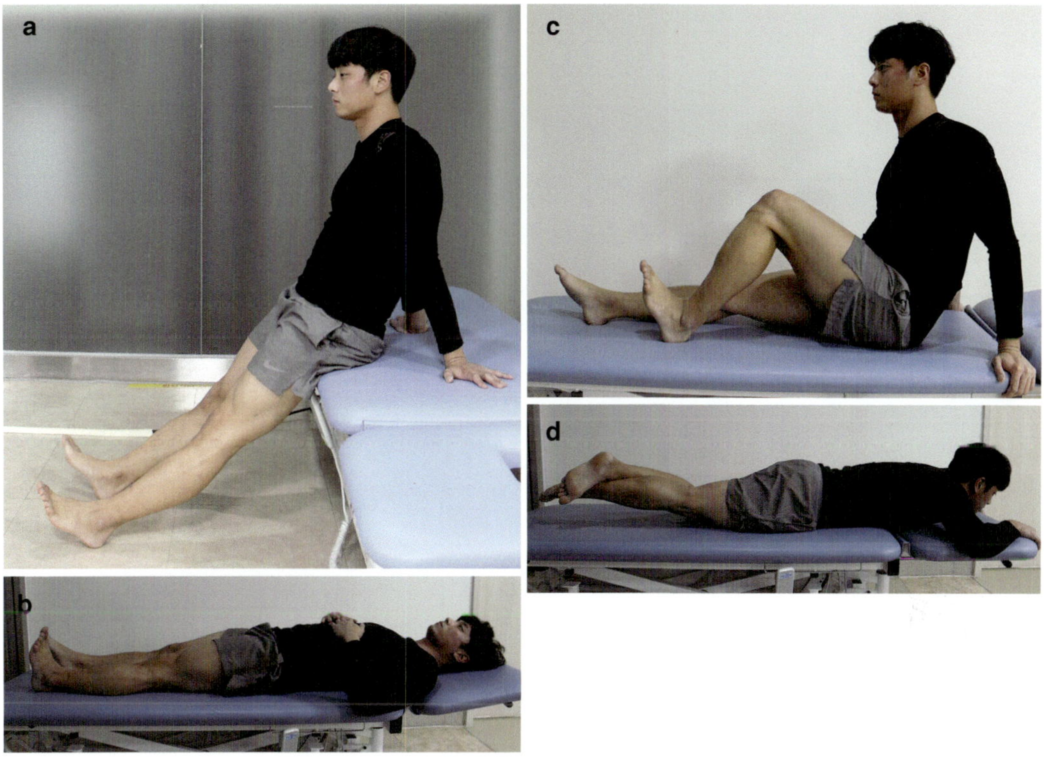

Fig. 8.4 Isometric exercise on quadriceps and hamstring with knee OA. (**a**) Sit position for isometric exercise on quadriceps, (**b**) Lie position for isometric exercise on quadriceps, (**c**) Sit position for isometric exercise on the hamstring, (**d**) Lie position for isometric exercise on hamstring

Fig. 8.5 Proprioception feedback circle

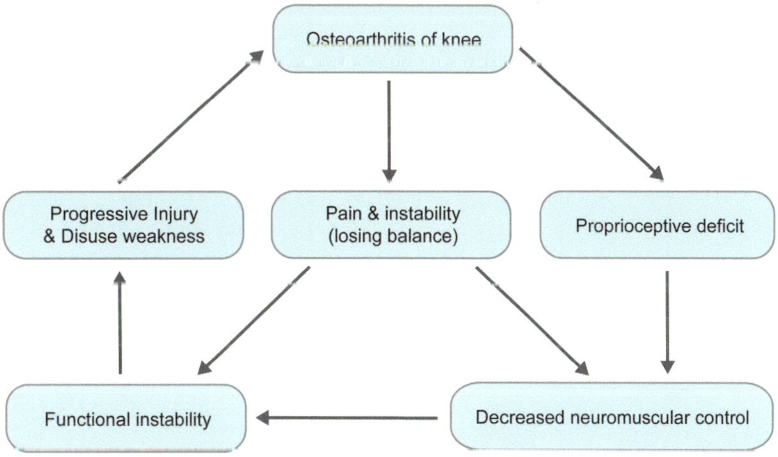

What dose of appropriate exercise is required for patients with OA? There are many ways to determine the intensity of exercise. The first method is the recommended method according to the weight loss program guideline of the American College of Sports Medicine (ACSM). That guideline recommends an exercise 3 to 5 times a week with a target heart rate of 70–85% of the patient's maximum heart rate. This is known as the intensity and frequency to achieve

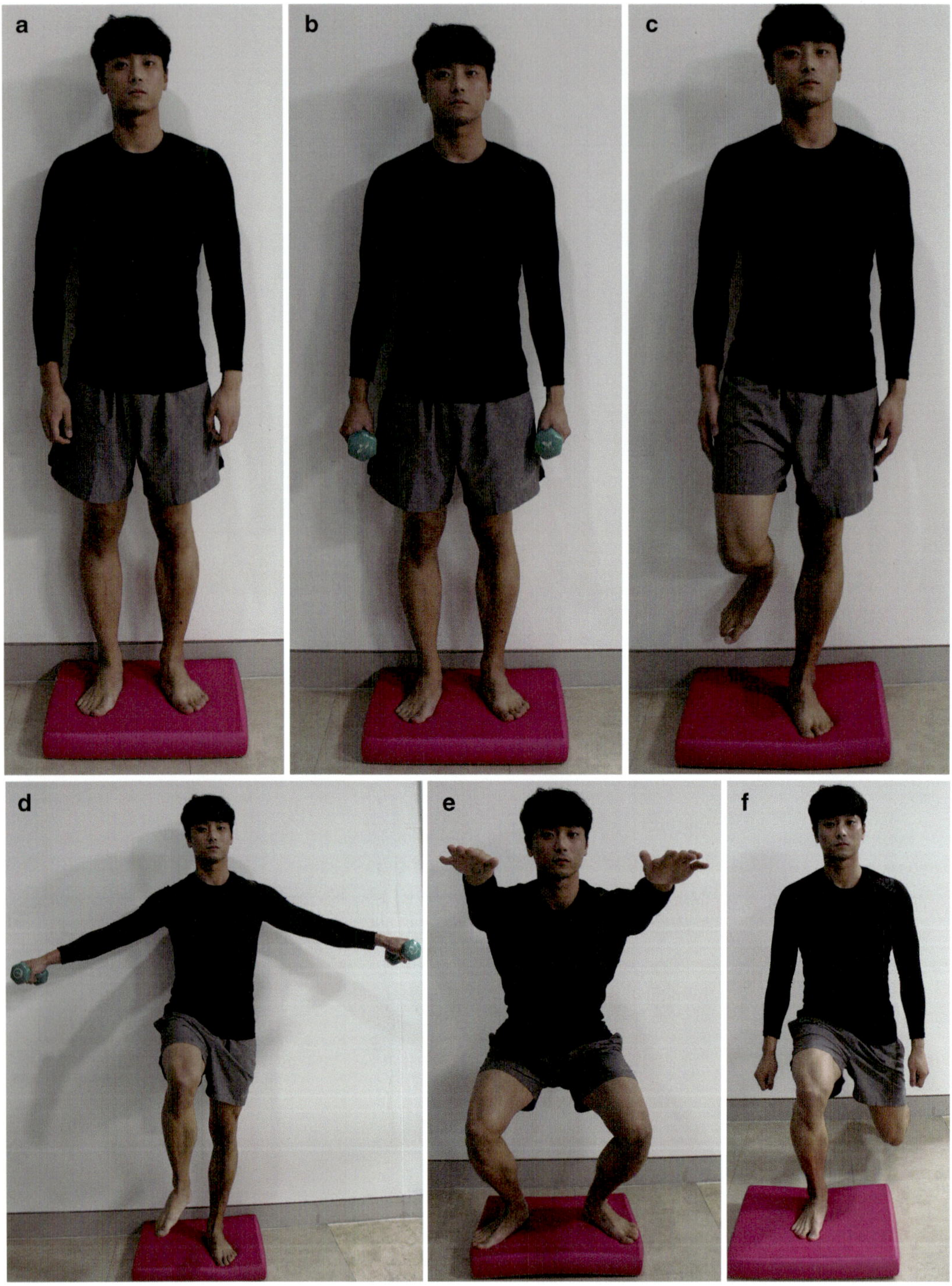

Fig. 8.6 Progressive proprioceptive exercise. (**a**) Static: Progress the base of support, (**b**) Static: Progress the base of support with weight, (**c**) Dynamic: Progress of Center of Gravity, (**d**) Dynamic: Progress of Center of Gravity with weight, (**e, f**) Functional: Add functional movement

the ideal exercise effect in weight loss and fitness of OA patients for symptom relief. Patient with OA of lower extremity joints which are able to perform the moderate-to-vigorous exercise, i.e., 70 ~ 85% of maximal heart rate for 20–60 min at least 3 days per week, can improve their fitness and health without exacerbating their joint pain or increasing their need for analgesic drugs [56]. In a study of aerobic exercise in a patient with knee or hip OA, patients were randomized into three treatment groups for a 12-week program of aerobic walking, aerobic pool exercise and nonaerobic ROM exercise. Exercise heart rate ranges of 60–80% of the maximum heart rate achieved on the baseline graded exercise test were assigned individually to those who participated in the aerobic exercises (walking and pool exercise). The aquatics and walking exercise groups showed significant improvement over the control group in aerobic capacity, 50-foot walking time, depression, anxiety, and physical activity after the 12-week exercise program [57].

A simple and traditional method for determining a patient's desired target heart rate is:

$$\max \mathbf{heart\ rate}(\mathbf{220}-\mathbf{age})\times \mathbf{The\ target\ intensity}(\mathbf{70}-\mathbf{85\%})$$

Another method is Karvonen's method [58]. Karvonen's method determines the heart rate of exercise training (target heart rate) as follows:

$$\mathbf{Target\ heart\ rate}=\mathbf{Rest\ heart\ rate}+(\max \mathbf{heart\ rate}-\mathbf{Rest\ heart\ rate})\times \mathbf{K}$$

Where K is the coefficient determined by a value ranging from 0.6 to 0.8, which is decided according to the experience of the physician [59]. Karvonen's method is convenient, however it fails to take into account individuals with scattered heart rate responses [60] (Table 8.2).

8.3.3.2 Anaerobic Exercise

When developing a resistance exercise program, you should include resistance load, number of repetitions, the velocity of movement and frequency of sessions. Individual strength and overall knee evaluation must be preceded. The application of resistance can be applied by weight, free weight, machine, or band. When considering muscle strength, it is important to consider the muscles that are important for weight-bearing function activities, such as the quadriceps muscle, hip abductor muscle, hip extensor muscle, hamstring, and calf muscle. Initiation of a resistance-training program requires assessment of strength, full knee ROM, knee pain throughout ROM, and the patient's knee function like WOMAC score. Studies of resistance generally report exercise intensity as a percentage of 1RM in which the exercises are performed. The term "repetition maximum" (RM) refers to the maximal number of times a load can be lifted before fatigue using appropriate form and technique (1RM = the maximum load that can be lifted once with proper form) [61]. The RPE (relative perceived exertion) scale, another method used as the intensity of resistance exercise, can also be used effectively [62] (Table 8.3).

However, the RPE scale is the patient's sub jective awareness; thus it may show a difference from the intensity felt by the patient's physical condition. For example, even if the patient's physical condition shows a moderate heart rate, there is a disadvantage in that the RPE scale can be high depending on the patient's individual awareness. In another way, the general recommendations of exercise intensity for the general people are known as performing exercises 3 days a week, 2–3 sets per exercise, and 8–15 repetitions per set [26]. Farr

Table 8.2 Calculation of target heart rate during 75% intensity exercise for 60 years old (Ex. 80 bmp resting heart rate)

	Age	Max heartrate	Rest heartrate	Target intensity(%)	Target heartrate
Traditional method	60	220–60 = 160		×0.75	(220–60) × 0.75 = 120
Karvonen method	60	220–60 = 160	80	×0.75	0.75 × [(220 – 60) – 80] + 80 = 140

Table 8.3 Borg's RPE (relative perceived exertion) scale. 1982

Rating	Perceived exertion
6	No exertion
7	Extremely light
8	
9	Very light
10	
11	Light
12	
13	Somewhat hard
14	
15	Hard
16	
17	Very hard
18	
19	Extremely hard
20	Maximal exertion

et al. studied at a randomized control trial of progressive resistance training improves overall physical activity levels in 171 patients with early OA of the knee [63]. A resistance-training session including a leg press, leg curl, hip abduction, adduction, straight leg lift, incline dumbbell press, seated row, and calf raise were performed three times a week for 1 h per day for 3 months. After the training (at both 3 and 9 months), the resistance-training group compared to a control group (self-management group) had improvement in functional status and symptoms on the knee OA.

High-resistance training also has been shown similar effects of low-resistance training. Jan et al. conducted the investigation of clinical effects of high- and low-resistance training for patients with knee OA [31]. The two groups performed isokinetic knee flexion and extension training at high resistance (60% of 1RM) and low resistance (10% of 1RM) over three times per week. After the training, both groups improved compared to a control group that did not perform any resistance exercise. Cycling also has shown similar benefits. Both high- and low-intensity cycling show benefits, are well tolerated, and do not appear to increase daily acute pain [64].

8.3.4 Continuous Feedback from Experts

Feedback through experts is one of the most important variables affecting exercise performance and learning ability. It plays a role in returning information on the results and evaluation of exercise performance to the learner and is evaluated as one of the important strategies among various intervention strategies for continuing and maintaining exercise [65].

Martin et al. found that the reinforcement method of providing praise and feedback on exercise intensity to participants has a positive effect on exercise continuation, and it has been shown that when given individually than in a group, results are more effective [66]. Furthermore, previous studies have demonstrated that motor learning improves function with feedback compared to without feedback [67]. Therefore, providing feedback for lower extremity exercise to patients with knee OA is effective in correcting improper movements, improving performance, and maintaining or developing confidence and persistence in exercise for patients who cannot continue exercise due to the burden and fear of exercise. The timing and method of providing this feedback should be given immediately after the subject has made an effort to achieve the learning objectives and when teaching a new content or next level task for the first time. After the subject has completed the task, it should be checked immediately and given back feedback. In addition, even if the subject is experiencing difficulties with a given amount of exercise or exercise time, it should be encouraged to seek feedback from health care providers [68].

In conclusion, it is difficult for an unskilled subject to recognize errors in his or her performance results, and it is difficult to plan a specific next reaction. When specific information about the response result is provided by an external stimulus such as feedback, it can be changed into a technical action, so this feedback information corrects the learner's incorrect behavior and improves performance, and continuous feedback corrects performance errors.

8.4 Pain Control (Factor Management)

8.4.1 Thermal therapy

Application of heat therapy has been used in the management of knee OA symptoms for a long time. Heat therapy is commonly used in physical rehabilitation for patients with OA to relieve pain [69]. Heat can be administered by a variety of methods, including the application of superficial heat (infrared), hot packs, immersion in warm water and paraffin bath [3]. Heat increases the extensibility of collagen tissue by enhancing the viscous flow of collagen fibers and subsequently relaxing the tension. Heat increases blood circulation through vessel dilation, reduces nociception and ischemia caused by muscle spasms. Additionally, heat stimulates the free nerve endings and peripheral nerves by a gating mechanism or increased secretion of endorphin. As such, heat is effective in controlling pain, and the superficial heat can elevate the temperature of the soft tissue 3° at a depth of 1 cm beneath the surface. Especially, moist heat elevates the superficial temperature more than dry heat and is often preferable for reducing joint pain. However, care must be taken to avoid burn injury during heat therapy, particularly over bony prominences [70].

Despite the effectiveness of heat treatments, there is still much debate about the effectiveness of superficial heating therapy [71]. Superficial heating modality for symptomatic knee OA did not induce clinically relevant changes. These results are due to the inherent nature of this method, where heat transfer is not delivered in depth [72]. However, superficial heating therapy may still be beneficial in combination with other rehabilitative treatments. Cetin et al. found that hot packs combined with isokinetic exercise improved physical performance and alleviated joint pain in patients with knee OA compared with only receiving isokinetic exercise [73] (Table 8.4).

Deep heating therapy is also effectiveness. Deep heating therapy, such as short-or micro-wave diathermy or ultrasound, can affect the viscoelastic properties of deep joint. Especially, ultrasound penetrates more deeply than either short- or micro-wave diathermy [74]. Pain in patients with knee OA can be significantly reduced by either ultrasound and diathermy, especially if these are combined with an analgesic or an NSAID [75]. Recently study also reported that the application of 4-week localized microwave diathermy has been shown to improve pain and physical function in patients with symptomatic knee OA, with benefits, retained over a 12-week follow-up [76]. Deep heating therapy has contraindication in a patient with a local malignancy or bleeding diathesis [77]. Additionally, care must be taken if the patient has poor circulation or sedated, sensation impaired. Mechanisms of action of heat therapy are still under investigation. However, it is believed that the increases in local blood flow secondary to tissue heating may convey most benefits [78].

8.4.2 Cold Therapy

Cryotherapy is used in rehabilitation to reduce inflammation, pain, and edema, which in turn facilitates improvement in mobility. Techniques for cryotherapy include the application of cold or ice packs, ice massage, or local sprays such as rapid cooling nitrogen gas or carbon dioxide gas. Superficial cooling can decrease muscle spasm and increase the pain threshold [79]. Vasoconstriction and metabolic activity, as a result of the cold application, produce decreased local blood flow and help control swelling and reduce pain [80], thus leading to possible improvement in range of motion and function. The application of cold, however, should not be used in patients with Raynaud's phenomenon, cold hypersensitivity and cryoglobulinemia, or paroxysmal cold hemoglobinuria [81].

Table 8.4 Physiological change of thermotherapy

Change factor	Muscle spasm	Nociceptor	Blood flow	Metabolic rate	Collagen elasticity	Joint stiffness	Edema
Result	Decrease	Decrease	Increase	Increase	Increase	Decrease	Increase

8.4.3 Electrical Stimulated Therapy (TENS)

One of the important objectives of OA management is to relieve pain and to maintain or improve function. Various modalities in physiotherapy have been suggested to improve the clinical course of knee OA, with potentially fewer adverse effects than medical treatment [82]. Transcutaneous electrostimulation, the application of any electrical current through the skin with the aim of pain modulation, is a frequently used modality in knee OA [83]. It is based on the "Gate-Control Theory" of pain perception as described by Melzack and Wall [84]. However, the value of TENS as reported in the literature is controversial [85].

8.5 Assistive Aids

8.5.1 Walking Assistive Devices (Canes, Walker)

Almost half of knee OA patients with pain and impaired body function use walking aids to improve their ability to walk. Walking aids include such devices as cane, crutch, walker, brace, and orthopedic orthosis. These aids can be used to substitute for impairments in range of motion, muscle strength, joint stability, coordination, and endurance [86]. If the patients with OA have a problem own low extremities, a cane or walker may be used for their balance. If a cane is used to relieve weight-bearing in a patient with unilateral OA, it should be placed in the contralateral hand. Because the base of support on the uninvolved side is increased, the patient's weight to be shifted toward that side. Held in the contralateral hand, walking canes can decrease medial compartmental knee load during walking by up to 17% [87]. The cane should be fitted properly. Cane recommended length is defined by the distance from the greater trochanter or the ulnar styloid process [88]. However, the use of longer canes is very common in the general population [89]. The adoption of longer canes may limit the individual to bear the bodyweight on this device due to increased elbow flexion from the ideal angle of 20°–30° and raised shoulder [90]. According to a study of the relationship between pain and cane, use of a cane for 8 weeks by 21 obese or overweight patients with painful knee OA was found to produce an immediate lateral shift in the vertical forces through the knee which, was then maintained when walking without cane. Peak vertical force across the knee decreased 12%, and the center of pressure in the painful extremity was shifted laterally in 22% if frequent cane users. Half of those who used the cane>4 days per week reported a decrease in pain by 20% or more [91]. Based on these data, cane is a non-pharmacological treatment option that can improve symptoms and function for the patient with knee OA.

8.5.2 Knee Brace

Knee braces are commonly used for knee OA, and the AAOS recommends bracing for biomechanical stability in knee OA [92]. Knee OA with malalignment can cause significant pain and dysfunction, and knee braces have been shown to help with stability and function in such cases [93, 94]. In the case of knee OA with severe varus deformity, the use of a specially designed valgus brace can reduce joint pain and improve knee function and quality of life [95]. Because the brace creates valgus thrust, it reduces the load on the medial tibiofemoral compartment. Kirkley et al. performed a randomized controlled trial comparing unloader braces and neoprene sleeves to a control group [96].

There were significant differences in pain after the 6-min walk test and 30-s stair-climbing test with the unloader brace when compared to neoprene sleeves at 6 months. When comparing braced to unbraced patients, there were significant differences in WOMAC function scores. Chughtai et al. randomized 36 patients with Kellgren-Lawrence grades 3–4 knee OA to receive either a pneumatic unloader brace with conventional treatment or just conventional treatment. At a follow-up of one year, there were significantly fewer patients who received injections and less subsequent TKAs in the brace group [97]. Consequently, braces help knee OA patients achieve marked improvements in pain, function, and may prolong their time to a TKA.

8.5.3 Wedged Insoles

About the importance of biomechanical factors in the pathogenesis of OA, many experts have shown interest in biomechanical approaches to the treatment of knee OA, which reduce joint loading and correct malalignment. The load on the knee in patients with varus OA is almost ten times higher in the medial compartment than in the lateral compartment. This increased load is a result of the high load on the inner compartment in static and dynamic gait activities, and approximately 60–80% of the load across the knee is transferred to the medial compartment [98]. As a result, when the medial compartment of the knee joint is narrowed, the articular cartilage degenerates, the outer soft tissues become loose, and the mechanical body alignment moves in the inward direction. Because the length of the moment arm at the knee joint for ground repulsion was increased, the affected side of patients with varus knee OA produced higher endogenous torque than the non-affected side, so the treatment approach also focused on reducing the moment arm which can ultimately reduce the load on the joints [99]. One of the ways to reduce the moment arm that can reduce the load on the joint is high tibial osteotomy (HTO). HTO, which plays a role in the realignment of the knee joint, has been successfully applied to patients with medial compartment knee OA [100]. The other way is wedged insole. In various studies, they have found that lateral wedge insoles improve pain and walking ability. Toda et al. reported a decrease in pain among patients who used a lateral wedge insole in a controlled [101], and in Sasaki's study, the insole group showed significantly greater improvement of pain and walking ability [102]. When walking with the lateral wedge footrest, the weight of the foot is transmitted from the outside of the foot in the initial stance phase, and the pronation occurring in the subtalar joint produces the valgus of the calcaneus and the medial rotational force of the tibia. At this time, valgus torque occurs in the ankle joint, and large valgus torque is generated mainly in the stance phase [103]. In other words, when wedged insole is used, it has the effect of erecting the talus vertically in the direction of the tibia by transforming the spatial position of the lower extremities during the initial stance phase [104]. Therefore, by reducing the force applied to the medial compartment and lateral collateral ligaments of the knee joint and the iliotibial band, it reduces not only the force acting on the medial compartment about 16% of body weight, but also pain [105].

8.5.4 Taping

The abnormal position of the patella is one of the most dangerous causes of structural deterioration of the knee joint, and it causes structural and functional loss of the joint [106]. It is estimated that abnormal alignment on the lateral joint surface of the patella is the main cause of pain [107], and changes in the contact surface of the patella or changes in muscle strength of the quadriceps muscle increase the compression force on the lateral joint surface of the patella, thus affecting degenerative knee OA [108]. If patellofemoral joint malalignment occurs, the contact surface between the patella and femoral trochlea is reduced, and the pressure of the patella-femoral joint is increased. Therefore, in patients with knee OA, it is very important to correct the position of the patella in the knee joint of patients with knee OA. Warden et al. conducted that a systematic review and meta-analysis of patellar taping and bracing for treatment of chronic knee pain [109]. In this study, the medial-directed taping group significantly reduced pain compared to the non-tapping group. A common problem among patients with patella-femoral pain is a weakness of the quadriceps muscle. Therefore taping can change the length of the VMO (Vastus Medialis Oblique) to activate the VMO and induce alignment of the patella, thereby increasing the strength of the quadriceps muscle [110].

The method of applying taping has the advantages of easy treatment and non-expensive. Additionally, patients can learn to apply their own tape after minimal instruction.

8.6 Summary

Knee OA represents a collection of structural changes that lead to pain and knee dysfunction due to various causes. Therefore, it is most important to devise various intervention strategies to improve the patient's symptoms, such as reduced muscle strength and range of motion, balance, pain, etc., which can reduce the quality of life, and physical ability and functional status. In conclusion, for the treatment of knee OA, healthcare providers should help patients recover symptoms and functions by selecting various knowledge and appropriate management methods such as education, weight loss, exercise therapy, physical therapy, etc.

References

1. Cherian JJ, Jauregui JJ, Leichliter AK, et al. The effects of various physical non-operative modalities on the pain in osteoarthritis of the knee. Bone Joint J. 2016;98(1):89–94.
2. Altman RD, Hochberg M, Murphy WAJR, et al. Atlas of individual radiographic features in osteoarthritis. Osteoarthr Cartil. 1995;3(Suppl. A):3–70.
3. Zhang W, Moskowitz RW, Nuki G, et al. OARSI recommendations for the management of hip and knee osteoarthritis, Part I: critical appraisal of existing treatment guidelines and systematic review of current research evidence. Osteoarthr Cartil. 2007;15:981–1000.
4. Vaishya R, Pariyo GB, Agarwal AK, Vijay V. Non-operative management of osteoarthritis of the knee joint. J Clin Orthop Trauma. 2016;7(3):170–6.
5. Royal Australian College of General Practitioners. Guideline for the management of knee and hip osteoarthritis. 2018.
6. National institute for Health and Care Excellence. Osteoarthritis: care and management. Clinical guideline [CG177]. 2014.
7. Solomon L, Warwick D, Nayagam S. Apley's system of orthopaedics and fractures. 9th ed. pp. 85–86. 2010.
8. McAlindon TE, Wilson PW, Aliabadi P, et al. Level of physical activity and the risk of radiographic and symptomatic knee osteoarthritis in the elderly: the Framingham study. Am J Med. 1999;106:151–7.
9. Webb R, Brammah T, Lunt M, et al. Opportunities for prevention of 'clinically significant' knee pain: results from a population-based cross sectional study. J Pub Health. 2004;26(3):277–84.
10. Morrison JB. The mechanics of the knee joint in relation to normal walking. J Biomech. 1970;3:51–61.
11. Messier SP, Mihalko SL, Legault C, et al. Effects of intensive diet and exercise on knee, joint loads, inflammation, and clinical outcomes among overweight and obese adults with knee osteoarthritis: the IDEA randomized clinical trial. JAMA. 2013;310:1263–73.
12. Atukorala I, Makovey J, Lawler L, et al. Is there a dose-response relationship between weight loss and symptom improvement in persons with knee osteoarthritis? Arthritis Care Res. 2016;68:1106–14.
13. Messier SP, Resnik AE, Beavers DP, et al. Intentional weight loss in overweight and obese patients with knee osteoarthritis: is more better? Arthritis Care Res. 2018;70(11):1569–75.
14. Felson D, Zhang Y. Weight loss reduces the risk for symptomatic knee osteoarthritis in women the Framingham study. Ann Int Med. 1992;116(7):535–9.
15. Christensen R, Astrup A, Bliddal H. Weight loss: the treatment of choice for knee osteoarthritis? A randomized trial. Osteoarthr Cartil. 2005;13(1):20–7.
16. Langlois JA, Mussolino ME, Visser M, et al. Weight loss from maximum body weight among middle-aged and older white women and the risk of hip fracture: the NHANES I epidemiologic follow-up study. Osteoporos Int. 2001;12:763–8.
17. Robson EK, Hodder RK, Kamper SJ, et al. Effectiveness of weight loss interventions for reducing pain and disability in people with common musculoskeletal disorders: a systematic review with meta-analysis. J Orthop Sports Phys Ther. 2020;50(6):319–33.
18. Park H, Park J, Yu R. Relationship of obesity and visceral adiposity with serum concentrations of CRP, TNF-α and IL-6. Diab Res Clin Pract. 2005;69(1):29–35.
19. Pollock ML, Gaesser GA, Butcher JD, et al. The recommended quantity and quality of exercise for developing and maintaining cardiorespiratory and muscular fitness, and flexibility in healthy adults. Med Sci Sports Exerc. 1998;30(6):975–91.
20. American College of Sports Medicine. ACSM's guidelines for exercise testing and prescription. 9th ed. Philadelphia: Wolters Kluwer Health/Lippincott Williams & Wilkins; 2014. p. 162–93.
21. O'Connor SR, Tully MA, Ryan B, et al. Walking exercise for chronic musculoskeletal pain: systematic review and meta-analysis. Arch Phys Med Rehabil. 2015;96:724–34.
22. Ettinger WH Jr, Burns R, Messier SP, et al. A randomized trial comparing aerobic exercise and resistance exercise with a health education program in older adults with knee osteoarthritis. The Fitness Arthritis and Seniors Trial(FAST). JAMA. 1997;277:25–31.

23. Hiyama Y, Yamada M, Kitagawa A, et al. A four-week walking exercise programme in patients with knee osteoarthritis improves the ability of dual task performance: a randomized controlled trial. Clin Rehabil. 2012;26:403–12.
24. McNeal RL. Aquatic therapy for patients with rheumatic disease. Rheum Dis Clin N Am. 1990;16(4):915–29.
25. Villareal DT, Aguirre L, Gurney AB, et al. Aerobic or resistance exercise, or both, in dieting obese older adults. N Engl J Med. 2017;376(20):1943–55.
26. Jayabalan P, Ihm J. Rehabilitation strategies for the athletic individual with early knee osteoarthritis. Curr Sports Med Rep. 2016;15(3):177–83.
27. Deyle GD, Allison SC, Matekel RL, et al. Physical therapy treatment effectiveness for osteoarthritis of the knee: a randomized comparison of supervised clinical exercise and manual therapy procedures versus a home exercise program. Phys Ther. 2005;85:1301–17.
28. Deyle GD, Henderson NE, Matekel RL, et al. Effectiveness of manual physical therapy and exercise in osteoarthritis of the knee: a randomized, controlled trial. Ann Intern Med. 2000;132:173–81.
29. Mangione KK, Axen K, Haas F. Mechanical unweighting effects on treadmill exercise and pain in elderly people with osteoarthritis of the knee. Phys Ther. 1996;76:387–94.
30. Topp R, Woolley S, Hornyak J, et al. The effect of dynamic versus isometric resistance training on pain and functioning among adults with osteoarthritis of the knee. Arch Phys Med Rehabil. 2002;83:1187–95.
31. Jan MH, Lin JJ, Liau JJ, et al. Investigation of clinical effects of high and low-resistance training for patients with knee osteoarthritis: a randomized controlled trial. Phys Ther. 2008;88(4):427–36.
32. Baker KR, Nelson ME, Felson DT, et al. The efficacy of home based progressive strength training in older adults with knee osteoarthritis: a randomized controlled trial. J Rheumatol. 2001;28(7):1655–65.
33. Slemenda C, Brandt K, Heilman DK, et al. Quadriceps weakness and osteoarthritis of the knee. Ann Int Med. 1997;127(2):97–104.
34. McAlindon TE, Cooper C, Kirwan JR, Dieppe PA. Determinants of disability in osteoarthritis of the knee. Ann Rheum Dis. 1993;52:258–62.
35. Sharma L, Dunlop DD, Cahue S, et al. Quadriceps strength and osteoarthritis progression in malaligned and lax knees. Ann Int Med. 2003;138(8):613–9.
36. Weng MC, Lee CL, Chen CH, et al. Effects of different stretching techniques on the outcomes of isokinetic exercise in patients with knee osteoarthritis. Kaohsiung J Med Sci. 2009;25(6):306–15.
37. McDonald CM. Limb contractures in progressive neuromuscular disease and the role of stretching, orthotics, and surgery. Phys Med Rehabil Clin N Am. 1998;9(1):187–211.
38. Roddy E, Zhang W, Doherty M. Aerobic walking or stretching exercise for osteoarthritis of the knee? A systematic review. Ann Rheum Dis. 2005;64(5):544–8.
39. Bennell K, Hinman R. Exercise as a treatment for osteoarthritis. Curr Opin Rheumatol. 2005;17(5):634–40.
40. Lloyd DG, Buchanan TS. Strategies of muscular support of varus and valgus loads at the human knee. J Biomech. 2001;34:1257–67.
41. Lloyd DG, Buchanan TS, Besier TF. Neuromuscular biomechanical modeling to understand knee ligament loading. Med Sci Sports Exerc. 2005;37:1939–47.
42. Sharma L, Pai YC, Holtkamp K, et al. Is knee joint proprioception worse in the arthritic knee versus the unaffected knee in unilateral knee osteoarthritis? Arthritis Rheum. 1997;40:1518–25.
43. Slemenda C, Brandt KD, Heilman DK, et al. Quadriceps weakness and osteoarthritis of the knee. Ann Intern Med. 1997;127:97–104.
44. Tan J, Balci N, Sepici V, et al. Isokinetic and isometric strength in osteoarthrosis of the knee. A comparative study with healthy women. Am J Phys Med Rehabil. 1995;74:364–9.
45. Hall KD, Hayes KW, Falconer J. Differential strength decline in patients with osteoarthritis of the knee: revision of a hypothesis. Arthritis Care Res. 1993;6:89–96.
46. Costa RA, de Oliveira LM, Watanabe SH, et al. Isokinetic assessment of the hip muscles in patients with osteoarthritis of the knee. Clinics. 2010;65:1253–9.
47. Segal NA, Torner J, Felson D, et al. The effect of thigh strength on incident radiographic and symptomatic knee osteoarthritis in the Multicenter Osteoarthritis (MOST) study. Arthritis Rheum. 2009;61:1210–7.
48. Hayes KW, Falconer J. Differential muscle strength decline in osteoarthritis of the knee. A developing hypothesis. Arthritis Care Res. 1992;5:24–8.
49. Adegoke BO, Mordi EL, Akinpelu OA, et al. Isotonic quadriceps-hamstring strength ratios of patients with knee osteoarthritis and apparently healthy controls. Afr J Biomed Res. 2007;10:211–6.
50. Minor MA, Hewett JE, Webel RR, et al. Exercise tolerance and disease related measures in patient with rheumatoid arthritis and osteoarthritis. J Rheumatol. 1988;15:905–11.
51. Dover G, Powers ME. Reliability of joint position sense and force-reproduction measures during internal and external rotation of the shoulder. J Athl Train. 2003;38(4):304–10.
52. Simon AM, Ferris DP. Lower limb force production and bilateral force asymmetries are based on sense of effort. Exp Brain Res. 2008;187(1):129–38.
53. Riemann B, Lephart S. The sensorimotor system, Part II. the role of proprioception in motor control and functional joint stability. J Athl Train. 2002;37:80–4.
54. Skinner HB, Barrack RL, Cook SD. Age-related decline in proprioception. Clin Orthop. 1984;184:208–11.

55. Torres R, Durate JA, Cabri JM. An acute bout of quadriceps muscle stretching has no influence on knee joint proprioception. J Hum Kinet. 2012;34(1):123–30.
56. Fox KR. The effects of exercise on self-perceptions and self-esteem. In: Biddle SJ, Fox KR, Boutcher SH, editors. Physical activity and psychological well-being, vol. 13. London: Routledge; 2000. p. 81–118.
57. Minor MA, Webel RR, Kay DR, et al. Efficacy of physical conditioning exercise in patients with rheumatoid arthritis and osteoarthritis. Arthritis Rheum. 1989;32(11):1396–405.
58. Karvonen MJ, Kentala E, Mustala O. The effects of training on heart rate. Ann Med Exp Fenn. 1957;35:307–15.
59. Miller WC, Wallace JP, Eggert KE. Predicting max HR and the HR-Vo_2 relationship for exercise prescription in obesity. Med Sci Sports Exerc. 1993;25:1077–81.
60. Whipp BJ, Davis JA, Torres F, Wasserman K. A test to determine parameters of aerobic function during exercise. J Appl Physiol. 1981;50:217–21.
61. Vincent KR, Vincent HK. Resistance exercise for knee osteoarthritis. PM&R. 2012;4(5):45–52.
62. Borg GA. Psychophysical bases of perceived exertion. Med Sci Sports Exerc. 1982;14(5):377–81.
63. Farr JN, Going SB, McKnight PE, et al. Progressive resistance training improves overall physical activity levels in patients with early osteoarthritis of the knee: a randomized controlled trial. Phys Ther. 2010;90:356–66.
64. Mangione KK, McCully K, Gloviak A, et al. The effects of high intensity and low-intensity cycle ergometry in older adults with knee osteoarthritis. J Gerontol A Biol Sci Med Sci. 1999;54(4):184–90.
65. Sidentop PJ. Academic learning time: reflection and prospests. J Teach Phys Educ. 1983;2(4):3–7.
66. Martin J, Dubbert PM, Katell AD, et al. The behavioral control of exercise in sedentary adults: studies 1 through 6. J Consult Clin Psychol. 1984;52:795–811.
67. Reeve TG, Dornier LA, Week DJ. Precision of knowledge of results: consideration of requirements imposed by the task. Res Q Exerc Sport. 1990;61:285–90.
68. American College of Sports Medicine. ACSM's guidelines for exercise testing and prescription. 9th ed. Philadelphia: Wolters Kluwer Health/Lippincott Williams & Wilkins; 2014. p. 355–82.
69. APTA. 2001 American Physical Therapy Association. Guide to physical therapist practice: part one: a description of patient/client management. American Physical Therapy Association: Alexandria, VA; 2001.
70. Hollander JL, Horvath SM. Changes in joint temperature produced by diseases and by physical therapy. Arch Phys Med Rehabil. 1949;30:437–40.
71. Bannuru RR, Osani MC, Vaysbrot EE, et al. OARSI guidelines for the non-surgical management of knee, hip, and polyarticular osteoarthritis. Osteoarthr Cartil. 2019;27(11):1578–89.
72. Rabini A, Piazzini DB, Tancredi G, et al. Deep heating therapy via microwave diathermy relieves pain and improves physical function in patients with knee osteoarthritis: a double-blind randomized clinical trial. Eur J Phys Rehabil Med. 2012;48(4):549–59.
73. Cetin N, Aytar A, Atalay A, Akman MN. Comparing hot pack, short-wave diathermy, ultrasound, and TENS on isokinetic strength, pain, and functional status of women with osteoarthritic knees: a single-blind, randomized, controlled trial. Am J Phys Med Rehabil. 2008;87:443–51.
74. Lehmann JF, Masock AJ, Warren CG, Koblanski JN. Effect of therapeutic temperatures on tendon extensibility. Arch Phys Med Rehab. 1970;51(8):481–7.
75. Svarcova J, Trnavsky K, Zvarova J. The influence of ultrasound, galvanic currents and shortwave diathermy on bain intensity in patients with osteoarthritis. Scand J Rheumatol Suppl. 1987;67:83–5.
76. Giombini A, Di Cesare A, Di Cesare M, et al. Localized hyperthermia induced by microwave diathermy in osteoarthritis of the knee: a randomized placebo-controlled double-blind clinical trial. Knee Surg Sports Traumatol Arthrosc. 2011;19:980–7.
77. Lehmann JF, Krusen FH. Biophysical effects of ultrasonic energy on carcinoma and their possible significance. Arch Phys Med Rehab. 1955;36(7):452–9.
78. Giombini A, Giovannini V, Di Cesare A, et al. Hyperthermia induced by microwave diathermy in the management of muscle and tendon injuries. Br Med Bull. 2007;83:379–96.
79. Miglietta O. Action of cold on spasticity. Am J Phys Med Rehab. 1973;52(4):198–205.
80. Benson TB, Copp EP. The effects of therapeutic forms of heat and ice on the pain threshold of the normal shoulder. Rheumatology. 1974;13(2):101–4.
81. Olson JE, Stravino VD. A review of cryotherapy. Phys Ther. 1972;52(8):840–53.
82. Jamtvedt G, Dahm KT, Christie A, et al. Physical therapy interventions for patients with osteoarthritis of the knee: an overview of systematic reviews. Phys Ther. 2008;88(1):123–36.
83. Vance CG, Baebara AR, Nicole PB, et al. Effects of transcutaneous electrical nerve stimulation on pain, pain sensitivity, and function in people with knee osteoarthritis: a randomized controlled trial. Phys Ther. 2012;92(7):898–910.
84. Melzack R, Wall P. Pain mechanisms: a new theory. Science. 1965;150:971–7.
85. Griffin JW, McClure M. Adverse responses to transcutaneous electrical nerve stimulation in a patient with rheumatoid arthritis. Phys Ther. 1981;61(3):354–5.
86. Van der Esch M, Heijmans M, Dekker J. Factors contributing to possession and use of walking aids among persons with rheumatoid arthritis and osteoarthritis. Arthritis Rheum. 2003;49(6):838–42.

87. Simic M, Bennell KL, Hunt MA, et al. Contralateral cane use and knee joint load in people with medial knee osteoarthritis: the effect of varying body weight support. Osteoarthr Cartil. 2011;19(11):1330–7.
88. Camara CT, de Freitas SM, de Lima WP, et al. Comparison of two methods for estimating adjustable one-point cane length in community-dwelling older adults. Physiother Res Int. 2015;22(1):9. https://doi.org/10.1002/pri.1641.
89. Lam R. Practice tips: choosing the correct walking aid for patients. Can Fam Physician. 2007;53(12):2115–6.
90. Li ZY, Chou C. The effect of cane length and step height on muscle strength and body balance of elderly people in a stairway environment. J Physiol Anthropol. 2014;33:6.
91. Lee SM, Heiney C, Perell KL, et al. Effect of cane use on lower limb biomechanics and pain in knee osteoararthritis. Arthritis Rheum. 2009;60(suppl):s309.
92. Jevsevar DS. Treatment of osteoarthritis of the knee: evidence-based guideline. J Am Acad Orthop Surg. 2013;21(9):571–6.
93. Yu SP, Williams M, Eyles JP, et al. Effectiveness of knee bracing in osteoarthritis: pragmatic trial in a multidisciplinary clinic. Int J Rheum Dis. 2016;19:279–86.
94. Larsen BL, Jacofsky MC, Brown JA, et al. Valgus bracing affords short-term treatment solution across walking and sit-to-stand activities. J Arthroplast. 2013;28:792–7.
95. Matsuno H, Kadowaki KM, Tsuji H. Generation II knee bracing for server median compartment osteoarthritis of ths knee. Arch Phys Med Rehabil. 1997;78:745–9.
96. Kirkley A, Webster-Bogaert S, Litchfield R, et al. The effect of bracing on varus gonarthrosis. J Bone Joint Surg Am. 1999;81:539–48.
97. Chughtai M, Bhave A, Khan SZ, et al. Clinical outcomes of a pneumatic unloader brace for Kellgren-Lawrence grades 3 to 4 osteoarthritis: a minimum 1-year follow-up study. J Knee Surg. 2016;29:634–8.
98. Prodromos CC, Andriacchi TP, Galante JO. A relationship between gait and clinical changes following high tibial osteotomy. J Bone Joint Surg. 1985;67(A):1188–94.
99. Wang JW, Kuo KN, Andriacchi TP, Galante JO. The influence of walking mechanics and time of proximal tibial osteotomy. J Bone Joint Surg. 1990;72(A):905–9.
100. Steppacher SD, Tannast M, Ganz R, Siebebrock KA. Mean 20-year follow-up of Bernese periacetabular osteotomy. Clin Orthop Relat Res. 2008;466:1633–44.
101. Toda Y, Segal N. Usefulness of an insole with subtalar strapping for analgesia in patients with medial compartment osteoarthritis of the knee. Arthritis Rheum. 2002;4:468–73.
102. Sasaki T, Yasuda K. Clinical evaluation of the treatment of osteoarthritic knees using a newly designed wedged insole. Clin Orthop Relat Res. 1987;221:181–7.
103. Kerrigan CK, Lelas JL, Goggins J. Effectiveness of a lateral-wedge insole on knee varus torque in patients with knee osteoarthritis. Arch Phys Med Rehabil. 2002;83:889–93.
104. Yasuda K, Sasaki T. The mechanics of treatment of the osteoarthritic knee with a wedged insole. Clin Orthop. 1987;215:162–72.
105. Sasaki T, Yasuda K. Clinical evaluation of the treatment of osteoarthritic knees using a newly designed wedged insole. Clin Orthop Rel Res. 1987;221:181–7.
106. Pelletier JP, Martel-Pelletier J, Abramson SB. Osteoarthritis, an inflammatory disease: potential implication for the selection of new therapeutic targets. Arthritis Rheum. 2001;44(6):1237–47.
107. McConnell J. The management of chondromalacia patellae: a long term solution. Aust J Physiother. 1986;32(4):215–23.
108. Elahi S, Cahue S, Felson DT, et al. The association between varus–valgus alignment and patellofemoral osteoarthritis. Arthritis Rheum. 2000;43(8):1874–80.
109. Warden SJ, Hinman RS, Watson MA Jr, et al. Patellar taping and bracing for the treatment of chronic knee pain: a systematic review and meta-analysis. Arthritis Rheum. 2008;59:73–83.
110. Ernst GP, Kawaguchi J, Saliba E. Effect of patellar taping on knee kinetics of patients with patellofemoral pain syndrome. J Orthop Sports Phys Ther. 1999;29:661–7.

9 Pharmacologic Treatment

Ki-Bong Park

Abstract

Osteoarthritis (OA) of the knee is one of the common diseases found in the outpatient clinic, and patients with OA of the knee mainly complain of pain and dysfunction. Non-operative treatment options include lifestyle correction and physical therapy, as well as pharmacologic treatment consisting of topical, oral, and injection treatments. In order to select the appropriate pharmacologic treatment modality for patients with OA of the knee, a comprehensive understanding of the classification, mechanism of action, effects, and side effects of each drug is required. In addition, it is necessary to check the underlying disease, age, and weight of each patient. In this chapter, we will look at the contents of the pharmacologic treatment for OA of the knee. In particular, the characteristics of drug according to classification, recent international guidelines for pharmacologic treatment, and patient characteristics to be considered when selecting a drug are addressed. The recent international guidelines for the pharmacologic treatment of OA can help us identify expert opinions on the various treatment options. An individual approach to the patients is most beneficial in patients with knee OA and the treatment plan should be based on this principle. Selection of pharmacologic treatment according to the individual characteristics of patients was introduced according to the items of obesity, post-traumatic OA, and status with just waiting for arthroplasty in young patients. In addition, the individual characteristics of elderly patients were also introduced according to the items of hypertension, gastrointestinal ulcer, anticoagulation therapy, impaired renal function, and advanced age over 75 years of age.

Keywords

Knee · Osteoarthritis · Pharmacologic management · Drug characteristics International guideline · Patient characteristics

Knee osteoarthritis (OA) is one of the most common musculoskeletal diseases. It frequently induces intense pain and functional impairment. To date, there is no definitive treatment able to slow down the structural progression. Only the symptomatic part of knee OA is accessible to treatment [1]. Non-operative treatments are usually the first choice for the management of knee OA, especially in the early phase when no clear lesions or combined abnormalities need to be

K.-B. Park (✉)
Department of Orthopedics, Ulsan University Hospital, University of Ulsan College of Medicine, Ulsan, South Korea
e-mail: kbpark@uuh.ulsan.kr

S.-S. Seo (ed.), *A Strategic Approach to Knee Arthritis Treatment*,
https://doi.org/10.1007/978-981-16-4217-3_9

addressed surgically [2]. Non-operative treatment options were categorized as three groups: non-pharmacological treatment, pharmacologic treatment including dietary supplements, and injection treatment. Pharmacologic treatment modalities may be categorized as either symptom- or structure-modifying. Symptom-modifying drugs alleviate pain, reduce stiffness, improve mobility, and enhance patient's well-being. Analgesics (including opioids and acetaminophen), non-steroidal anti-inflammatory drugs (NSAIDs), cyclooxygenase-2 (COX-2) inhibitors, and corticosteroids comprise this category. Structure-modifying drugs, which are still under development, may arrest or slow the progression of OA and/or enhance the reparative processes of the disease.

9.1 Type of Drugs for OA Treatment

The categories of pharmacologic treatment modalities for OA can be summarized as Table 9.1.

Symptomatic drugs are usually divided into drugs with a rapid onset of action (Symptomatic Rapid Acting Drugs for OA, SYRADOA) and with a slow onset of action (Symptomatic Slow Acting Drugs for OA, SYSADOA). SYRADOA included NSAIDs, paracetamol or other analgesics, opioids, and corticosteroids. SYSADOA included glucosamine and chondroitin sulfate. And, drugs with potential beneficial effect on the joint structure (Disease-Modifying OA Drugs, DMOADs) may be developed in the future.

Table 9.1 Classification of pharmacological treatment of osteoarthritis

Categories	Effects
Symptom-modifying agents	On symptoms (pain, functional disability)
	• Rapid onset of action
	• Slow onset of action
Structure-modifying agents	On the progression of the pathological changes in osteoarthritis

9.1.1 Topical Agents

9.1.1.1 Topical Capsaicin

Capsaicin, the active component of chili peppers, is used as an analgesic in topical ointments to relieve pain. It caused an initial excitation of the neurons and a period of enhanced sensitivity. After repeated applications, a refractory period with reduced sensitivity is followed by persistent desensitization, possibly due to depletion of substance P [3].

In a systematic review, Mason L et al. concluded that for every 8 patients with musculoskeletal pain using capsaicin 0.025% for 4 weeks, one additional patient would benefit. However, around one third of patients experienced local adverse events with capsaicin, which would not have been the patient with placebo [3].

Kosuwon W et al. evaluated the efficacy of 0.0125% capsaicin gel compared to a placebo in patients with mild to moderate knee OA. They reported that the respective mean difference of visual analog scale (VAS) and total Western Ontario and McMaster Universities Osteoarthritis Index (WOMAC) score in the capsaicin group vs. the placebo group was statistically significant, and the burning sensation—the only adverse event—reported by patients in the capsaicin group, was less disturbing than in previous studies. Therefore, they concluded that 0.0125% capsaicin gel was an effective treatment in mild to moderate knee OA [4].

9.1.1.2 Topical NSAIDS

NSAIDs can be divided into topical NSAIDs applied to the skin and oral NSAIDs taken orally, and oral NSAIDs will be discussed in detail in Sect. 9.1.2.2.

Topical NSAIDs have been shown to provide analgesia through the same mechanism of action as oral NSAIDs, but because the activity of topical NSAIDs is effectively confined to the application site, systemic exposure—and consequently, the risk for gastrointestinal (GI), cardiovascular (CV), and renal toxicity—has been shown to be much lower than that observed with oral NSAIDs [5]. Therefore, topical NSAIDs are recommended in international and national guidelines as an early treatment option for the symptomatic management of knee OA and may be used ahead of oral NSAIDs due to their superior safety profile about CV and GI adverse events and renal toxicity.

Tugwell PS et al. compared the safety and efficacy of a topical diclofenac solution and oral diclofenac in relieving the symptoms of knee OA, in a randomized, double-blind trial. They reported that topical diclofenac solution produced relief of symptoms equivalent to oral diclofenac, with minor local skin irritation, but significantly reduced incidence of diclofenac-related GI adverse events and abnormal laboratory values [6]. Simon LS et al. conducted double-blind, randomized controlled trial of topical diclofenac in a vehicle solution containing dimethyl sulfoxide in patients with knee OA [7]. They reported that topical diclofenac was superior to placebo for pain, physical function, overall health, and Patient Global Assessment (PGA) and fewer digestive system and laboratory abnormalities were observed with topical diclofenac than with oral diclofenac. They concluded that topical diclofenac in a vehicle solution containing dimethyl sulfoxide is an effective treatment option for knee OA with efficacy similar to, but tolerability better than oral diclofenac. Rother M et al. compared topical ketoprofen and oral celecoxib and placebo for relief of signs and symptoms in knee OA and reported that topical ketoprofen is superior to placebo and comparable with celecoxib in relieving pain associated with an acute flare of OA [8].

9.1.1.3 Relative Efficacy of Topical Capsaicin and NSAIDs

In a recent network meta-analysis, Persson MSM et al. included 17 randomized controlled trials and compared the efficacy of topical capsaicin with topical NSAIDs for pain relief in OA. They concluded that topical capsaicin and NSAIDs in licensed doses may be equally effective for pain relief in OA. However, there were no significant differences in pain relief between topical capsaicin and NSAIDs (overall: effect size (ES) 0.04, 95% confidence interval (CI) −0.26 to 0.33; as licensed: ES −0.09, 95% CI −0.34 to 0.16) [9].

9.1.2 Symptomatic Rapid Acting Drugs of Osteoarthritis

Analgesics such as acetaminophen, NSAIDs, and opioids are the main pharmacologic treatment options for OA.

9.1.2.1 Acetaminophen

Acetaminophen (paracetamol) is widely used as the first-line analgesic for OA, is available over the counter, and is safe for most people to take. Acetaminophen is usually preferred to NSAIDs because of its better harms profile, especially in people at risk of GI bleeding.

Case JP et al. had a randomized, double-blind, placebo-controlled trial of diclofenac sodium and acetaminophen in patients with knee OA [10]. They reported that at 2 and 12 weeks, clinically and statistically significant improvements were seen in the diclofenac-treated group; however, no significant improvements were seen in the acetaminophen-treated group. This study concluded that diclofenac is effective in the symptomatic treatment of OA of the knee, but acetaminophen is not.

In a recent Cochrane review, Leopoldino AO et al. compared the effectiveness of paracetamol and placebo in the patients with knee OA [11]. They searched seven scientific databases for relevant studies, including randomized controlled trials of participants with knee OA irrespective of the intensity or duration of symptoms. The main outcomes were pain intensity, physical function, quality of life, adverse events, serious adverse events, withdrawal because of adverse events and liver toxicity. They reported that paracetamol provides only minimal improvements in pain and function for people with knee OA, with no increased risk of adverse events overall. Current clinical guidelines consistently recommend paracetamol as the first-line analgesic medication for hip or knee OA, given its low absolute frequency of substantive harm. However, they are less certain if paracetamol use increases the risk of serious adverse events, withdrawals due to adverse events, and rate of abnormal liver function tests.

9.1.2.2 Oral NSAIDs

Oral NSAIDs are drugs commonly used for pain relief, anti-inflammatory, and antipyretic. NSAIDs work by inhibiting the COX isoforms COX-1 and COX-2, thereby reducing levels of prostaglandins and other products, such as thromboxane. COX-1 is constitutively expressed in a variety of tissues. Its products have many functions, including platelet aggregation and gastric mucosal protection. COX-2 is endogenous only in the brain, and thus other tissues have to induce it through inflammation. COX-2 overexpression is likely induced by pro-inflammatory cytokines such as IL-1β and tumor necrosis factor (TNF)-α, and thus COX-2 may be more representative of an inflammatory response.

NSAIDs reduce the synthesis of prostaglandin (PG) from arachidonic acid by inhibiting COX. PG is changed back to thromboxane, prostacyclin, etc. to promote vasodilation and platelet aggregation, and NSAIDs inhibit it, thereby showing various clinical usefulness such as antipyretic, analgesic, anti-inflammatory effects, blood vessel control, and platelet function control (Fig. 9.1).

The main types of NSAIDs include: high-dose aspirin, ibuprofen, naproxen, diclofenac, celecoxib, etoricoxib, and indomethacin.

Since aspirin was first sold in 1899, NSAIDs are the most commonly prescribed drugs in the world. Some NSAIDs can be purchased at pharmacies without a separate prescription from a doctor and are widely used in daily life in various dosage forms such as oral drugs, injections, and external preparations.

Side effects of GI bleeding and gastric ulcer were first reported, and then various side effects have been reported in the CV system, renal urinary system, and hematology system. And, concerns about the safety of NSAIDs have increased since rofecoxib withdrew the product license in 2004. Merck & Co. announced a voluntary withdrawal of rofecoxib (Vioxx®) from the market because Adenomatous Polyp Prevention on VIOXX trial (APPROVe) study showed an unexpected high incidence of CV event. The trial found an incidence of adverse thromboembolic events in patients taking rofecoxib 25 mg/day that was 3.9 times greater than the incidence in those taking a placebo. After that, the relationship between COX-2 inhibitors and their CV adverse effects is an area of growing concern [12]. Currently, there are two COX-2 inhibitors (celecoxib and valdecoxib) approved for use by US FDA and another (etoricoxib) approved by the European Regulatory Authority.

A review of the use of NSAIDs for knee OA selected 16 double-blind randomized controlled trials [13]. Significant design flaws in individual studies made it impossible to distinguish a difference between equivalent recommended doses of NSAIDs. Instead, the authors recommended that NSAID selection should be based on physician preference, patient acceptability, safety, and efficacy.

9.1.2.3 Opioids

Opioids are considered as powerful pain relief substances that are used for cancer pain or OA pain. Opioids include codeine, hydromorphone, oxycodone, morphine, and others. They can be taken in oral, injectable, or patch form [14].

Among OA patients who fail to respond adequately to pharmacologic modalities, including oral NSAIDs, the European Society for Clinical and Economic Aspects of Osteoporosis, Osteoarthritis and Musculoskeletal Diseases (ESCEO) algorithm recommends the short-term use of weak opioids, such as tramadol, as one of the last pharmacological treatments [15]. Opioids should be reserved only for situations where non-opioid treatments are contraindicated, such as advanced kidney disease or prior GI bleed or CV history.

The prevalence of opioid use was 40% in the US patients with knee OA and nearly a third of Canadian pre-surgical patients with end-stage knee OA [16, 17]. In southern Sweden, every fourth patient with knee or hip OA has opioids dispensed over a 1-year period, and 12% of incident opioid dispensations are attributable to OA and/or its related comorbidities [18]. In Korea, 12.2% of knee OA patients were treated with opioids as an early treatment, and tramadol was used more commonly than stronger opioids [19].

Tramadol is a centrally acting analgesic with opioid agonist properties that acts on the neuro-

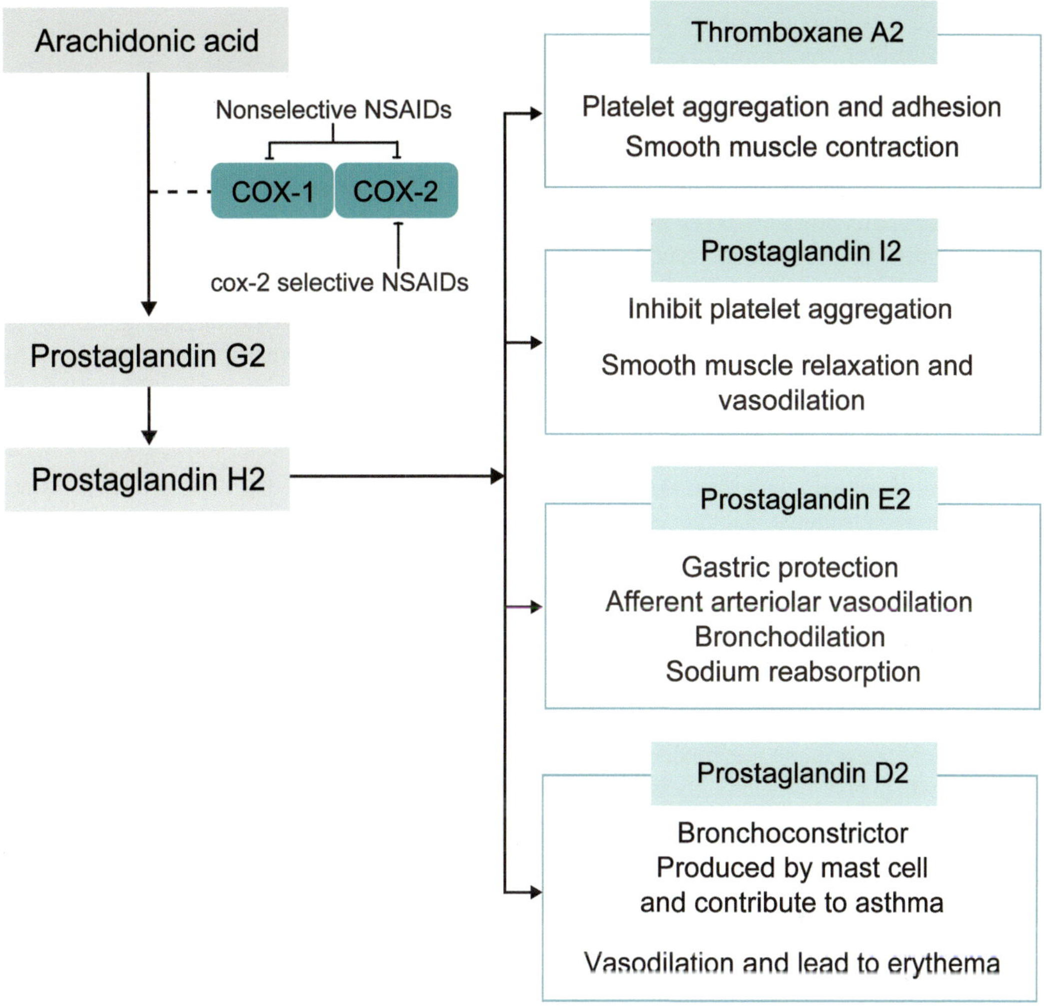

Fig. 9.1 Pathway of prostanoid formation and illustration of functions. *NSAIDs* non-steroidal anti-inflammatory drugs, *COX* cyclooxygenase

transmission of serotonin and norepinephrine. In addition, tramadol modifies the transmission of pain impulses by inhibition of monoamine reuptake. Tramadol rarely causes the adverse events of respiratory depression and physical dependence commonly associated with conventional opioid drugs, since its analgesic effects are through both weak opioid and non-opioid mechanisms [20]. Tramadol is not attributed with the GI and CV adverse events associated with NSAIDs [21]. Sustained release (SR) formulations of tramadol may improve tramadol tolerability and reduce the incidence of adverse events [22]. SR formulations are associated with prolonged effective plasma levels of tramadol, while preventing the high plasma peaks associated with adverse events seen with the immediate-release formulations [22, 23]. Zeng C et al. compared mortality within 1 year after initial tramadol prescription with 5 other pain relief medications (naproxen, diclofenac, celecoxib, etoricoxib, or codeine) among patients aged 50 years and older with OA [24]. They revealed that initial prescription of tramadol was associated with a significantly higher rate of mortality over 1 year of follow-up compared with commonly prescribed NSAIDs, but not compared with codeine.

Opioids can help relieve severe pain of knee OA, but the use of opioids may be impeded by non-serious adverse events, predominantly drowsiness, nausea, and constipation. In addition, they carry a well-established risk of respiratory depression, dependence, and have the potential for abuse. Not only is the potential for adverse effects and abuse concerning, but also recent evidence suggests that preoperative use of opioids is associated with worse postoperative outcomes [25].

A recent Cochrane systematic review showed that opioids yielded a small clinical benefit, but with a high risk of side effects, including opioid dependence in patients with knee OA [14, 26]. Smith SR et al. summarized the comparative effectiveness of oral NSAIDs and opioids in reducing knee OA pain and reported that NSAIDs and opioids offer similar pain relief in OA patients [27]. In the study about initial analgesic prescriptions for OA conducted in the United Kingdom, Zeng C et al. reported that oral/transdermal opioid prescription was higher among the elderly (≥65 years), women, obesity, current smoker, and patients with GI, CV, or chronic kidney disease [28].

9.1.2.4 Corticosteroids

Corticosteroids, also called steroids, are used for symptom improvement in knee OA, with several studies confirming the efficacy of intra-articular injection [29]. Glucocorticoids have a role in managing inflammatory arthritis, because of their anti-inflammatory and immunosuppressive functions. Additionally, oral corticosteroids may have analgesic efficacy.

Abou-Raya A et al. investigated the efficacy of daily low-dose oral prednisolone in patients with moderate to severe knee OA [30]. Patients were randomized as intervention group received 7.5 mg/day of prednisolone and control group received placebo for 6 weeks. Prednisolone group showed clinical relevant reduction for knee pain, physical function, patient global assessment, and 6-min walk distance at 6 weeks. Steroids do not tend to cause significant adverse events if they are taken for a short term at a low dose. However, Apostu D et al. represented corticosteroids are one of the currently available systemic drugs that impair cartilage healing [31].

9.1.3 Symptomatic Slow Acting Drugs for Osteoarthritis

Compounds in symptomatic slow acting drugs for OA (SYSADOA) class include glucosamine, chondroitin sulfate, avocado/soybean unsaponifiables (ASU), and diacerein [32]. Use of SYSADOA is characterized by both a delay in improvement of symptoms and a carryover effect of that improvement. The current evidence suggests that chondroitin falls into the symptom-modifying category, and glucosamine and diacerein into the structure-modifying category. One of the main proposed advantages of these medications over traditional medical therapies is their safety profile [33].

9.1.3.1 Glucosamine

Glucosamine hydrochloride (GHCl) is a simple molecule obtained by extraction processes and used as a nutraceutical or over-the-counter product. Conversely, glucosamine sulfate is a more complex molecule, which can be obtained only by a proprietary semi-synthetic route and stabilization process and that is found only in the prescription drug product, i.e. prescription crystalline glucosamine sulfate (pCGS) [34, 35]. Only pCGS is shown to deliver consistently high glucosamine bioavailability and plasma concentration in humans, which corresponds to demonstrated clinical efficacy.

Glucosamine sulfate can supplement the cartilage matrix, delay the cartilage degradation, and promote the synthesis of proteoglycan in chondrocytes, which is a nutritional drug for cartilage [36]. Glucosamine sulfate is able to alleviate the symptoms of pain, delay and alter the pathological process of OA, specifically supply the cartilage matrix in articular cartilage, and restore the normal metabolism. Thus, it is an effective drug that can block the vicious circle of OA and promote the cartilage repair. As a specific inhibitor of COX-2 and an NSAID, etoricoxib has analgesic, anti-inflammatory, and antipyretic effects [37], which has been widely used to relieve pain, reduce morning stiffness, and improve the joint function of OA patients.

9.1.3.2 Chondroitin Sulfate

Chondroitin sulfate belongs to the group of glycosaminoglycans and is a major component of articular cartilage. The effect of chondroitin sulfate is possibly the result of the stimulation of the synthesis of proteoglycans and the decrease in catabolic activity of chondrocytes by inhibiting the synthesis of proteolytic enzymes and other factors that contribute to cartilage matrix damage and cause the death of these cells. Chondroitin sulfate was also shown to exert anti-inflammatory activity. In addition, it acts on osteoarthritic subchondral bone osteoblasts by modulating the osteoprotegerin/receptor activator of NF-kappaB ligand ratio in favor of reduced bone resorption. It is noteworthy to mention that a head-to-head comparison of the effects of chondroitin sulfate of different origins and levels of purity on human osteoarthritic cartilage revealed the existence of a disparity in effects [38].

In a recent Cochrane review, Singh JA et al. revealed that chondroitin (alone or in combination with glucosamine) was better than placebo in improving pain in participants with OA in short-term studies and chondroitin had a lower risk of serious adverse events compared with control [33].

9.1.3.3 Avocado Soybean Unsaponifiables

Essentially, 'avocado soybean unsaponifiables (ASU)' are the fraction of avocado and soybean oil which, after hydrolysis, is not producing soap [39]. ASU has been shown in vitro to inhibit the pro-inflammatory cytokines interleukin-1 (IL-1), IL 6, IL-8, and MMPs. It has likewise demonstrated anabolic ability by stimulating chondrocyte collagen synthesis in vitro. A recent investigation showed that ASU stimulated aggrecan production and restored aggrecan production after IL-1β treatment. In addition, ASU decreased MMP-3 production and stimulated TIMP production [40, 41].

A systematic review, which included 4 randomized, placebo-controlled, double-blind trials of ASU, reported that 3 trials suggested efficacy of ASU for improving the symptoms of OA [39]. Another systematic review and meta-analysis from RCT examined the efficacy and safety of ASU in patients with hip or knee OA. This meta-analysis suggests a beneficial effect of ASU treatment in symptomatic knee OA but not in hip OA. Additionally, adverse events were similar in patients receiving ASU or placebo [42].

9.1.3.4 Diacerein

Diacerein is a drug with IL-1 inhibitory activity and is known as SYSADOA with anti-inflammatory, anti-catabolic, and pro-anabolic properties on cartilage and synovial membrane. It has also recently been shown to have protective effects against subchondral bone remodeling [43].

Pelletier JP et al. conducted a randomized, double-blind, placebo-controlled trial to evaluate the efficacy and safety of diacerein in patients with knee OA [44]. This study reported that 100 mg/day diacerein was significantly superior to placebo using VAS assessment of pain on movement as the primary criterion and the WOMAC score, the WOMAC sub-scores, and the VAS assessment of handicap as the second criteria. They concluded that diacerein was shown to be an effective treatment for symptoms in patients with knee OA.

European Society for Clinical and Economic Aspects of Osteoporosis and Osteoarthritis (ESCEO) constituted a panel of 11 experts to better define the real place of diacerein in the armamentarium for treating OA. Based on a literature review of clinical trials and meta-analyses, the ESCEO confirms that the efficacy of diacerein is similar to that of NSAIDs after the first month of treatment and superior to that of paracetamol. Additionally, diacerein has shown a prolonged effect on symptoms of several months once treatment was stopped [43].

An international, multicenter, double-blind, randomized study investigated whether diacerein has comparable efficacy with celecoxib in pain reduction for treatment in symptomatic knee OA patients. In this study, patients were randomized to 6 months of treatment with diacerein 50 mg once daily for 1 month and twice daily thereafter, or celecoxib 200 mg once daily. This study showed that in the per protocol population, the adjusted mean change from baseline in the WOMAC pain score was −11.1 with diacerein and −11.8 with celecoxib and the intergroup difference was 0.7 (95% CI: −1.8, 3.2; $P = 0.597$), meeting the non-inferiority margin. Therefore, this study concluded that diacerein was non-inferior to celecoxib in reducing knee OA pain and improving physical function [45].

9.1.3.5 Safety of SYSADOAs

A comprehensive meta-analysis of randomized placebo-controlled trials was performed to assess the safety of SYSADOAs [46]. This meta-analysis did not identify any safety issue associated with glucosamine sulfate, chondroitin sulfate, and avocado soybean unsaponifiables. Diacerein is associated with significantly more adverse events than placebo, particularly regarding the GI and renal and urinary systems. Therefore, the usefulness of diacerein should be considered, taking into account its benefit:risk profile according to individual patient characteristics.

9.1.4 Disease-Modifying Osteoarthritis Drugs

OA therapy has evolved in the past few decades from symptomatic treatment to possible disease-modifying solutions. Ideal disease-modifying osteoarthritis drugs (DMOADs) have chondroprotective, anti-inflammatory, and analgesic effects. Although a number of potential DMOADs have been investigated for OA, no pharmacological agent has yet been approved by regulatory agencies as a DMOAD [47, 48]. However, DMOADs are one of the emerging therapeutic agents that address patients with difficult-to-treat OA as well as the possibility of altering progression of disease. Although there may not yet be DMOADs, there have been several trials reported over the past year [49]. There certainly is a medical need for academia and the pharmaceutical industry to develop drugs that have cartilage-regenerating properties and that translate into changes of structure of joints and improvement of symptoms for patients affected by OA [50]. Regulatory agencies require that the drug has to show changes in joint space width on X-ray and improvement in symptoms in large phase 3 trials before a DMOAD can obtain marketing authorization [51].

9.1.4.1 REG-O3 Chimeric Peptide Combining Growth Hormone and Somatostatin Sequences

REG-O3 is a 24-amino acid chimeric peptide combining a sequence derived from growth hormone and an analog of somatostatin, molecules displaying cartilage repair and anti-inflammatory properties, respectively. This study showed REG-O3 was able to significantly improve weight bearing as efficiently as dexamethasone and hyaluronic acid. REG-O3 (25 μg) was also able to significantly decrease OARSI histological global score as well as degeneration of both cartilage and matrix while the other treatments did not. The authors provided evidence of a remarkable protecting effect of REG-O3 on pain/knee joint function and cartilage/matrix degradation in ACLT/pMMx model of rat OA. REG-O3 thus displays an interesting profile as a DMOAD [52].

9.1.4.2 Neural EGFL Like 1 (NELL-1)

Li C et al. demonstrated that neural EGFL-like 1 (NELL-1) has an anti-inflammatory role to protect articular cartilage from aggravated OA progression and pro-chondrogenic effects by using a loss- of-function Nell-$1^{+/6R}$ mouse model [53]. They concluded that NELL-1 is a promising pro-chondrogenic, anti-inflammatory dual-functional DMOADs candidate for preventing and suppressing arthritis-related cartilage damage.

9.1.4.3 Duloxetine

Duloxetine is the most studied of this class of DMOADs with regard to treatment of pain associated with OA. Duloxetine is a balanced and potent reuptake inhibitor of serotonin (5-HT) and norepinephrine (NE). Aside from its indications in major depressive disorders and generalized anxiety disorders, it has been approved for treatment of diabetic peripheral neuropathic pain, fibromyalgia, and chronic low back pain.

Although OA pain has traditionally been considered as peripheral/nociceptive pain that results from inflammation or mechanical damage in peripheral tissues, emerging evidence suggests that central sensitization is also an important mechanism underlying OA pain. Central sensitization involves the impaired activity of descending inhibitory pathway. 5-HT and NE are key neurotransmitters in the descending inhibitory pathway and thus involved in pain modulation [54]. The chronic pain experienced by individuals with OA has been partially attributed to a biological process called central sensitization, which may be driven by painful stimuli that originate from damaged bone and joint tissue [55]. Central sensitization has been observed both in animal and human models of OA [56–58].

The initial placebo-controlled trial study by Chappel et al. and the second study by Chappel et al. revealed that the duloxetine group showing a significant improvement compared with the placebo group in average pain score, WOMAC scores, and Patient Global Impression of Severity index [59, 60]. These two 13-week studies led to the approval by the FDA of duloxetine for the treatment of chronic knee pain due to OA.

Given its utility in managing central and neuropathic pain syndromes, there have been three large placebo-controlled, randomized clinical trials assessing duloxetine as treatment for symptomatic knee OA. Enteshari-Moghaddam A et al. reported that both gabapentin and duloxetine have similar and acceptable effects in pain reduction and improvement of functional status in patients with knee OA [61]. Cehn L et al. reported that duloxetine is effective in the management of chronic pain and loss of physical function in knee OA with acceptable adverse events despite having no advantage in treating joint stiffness [62]. Randomized, placebo-controlled trial assessed the efficacy of duloxetine in patients with pain due to knee OA and showed pain reduction was significantly greater with duloxetine compared with placebo at 14 weeks. In patients with ≥3 painful sites, pain reduction was significantly greater with duloxetine. These results suggest that duloxetine may be an effective choice of analgesic for patients with knee OA [63].

In randomized, double-blind, placebo-controlled trial, Chappell AS et al. evaluated the efficacy and safety of duloxetine in the treatment of chronic pain due to OA of the knee [60]. Patients treated with duloxetine had significantly greater improvement at all-time points on Brief Pain Inventory (BPI) average pain and had significantly greater improvement on BPI pain severity ratings, WOMAC total and physical functioning scores, and Clinical Global Impressions of Severity (CGI-S) at the study endpoint. They concluded that treatment with duloxetine 60–120 mg QD was associated with significant pain reduction and improved function in patients with pain due to OA of the knee. Nevertheless, frequency of treatment-emergent nausea, constipation, and hyperhidrosis was significantly higher in the duloxetine group.

9.1.5 Medications Utilization in Patients with Knee OA

Zeng C et al. examined trends in the initial prescription of commonly prescribed analgesics and patient- as well as practice-level factors related to their selection in incident OA [28]. Initial analgesic prescription included oral non-selective NSAID, oral selective cyclooxygenase-2 inhibitor, topical NSAID, paracetamol, topical salicylate or oral/transdermal opioid within 1 month after OA diagnosis. They reported that the incidence of oral NSAID prescriptions decreased whereas other analgesic prescriptions, including oral opioid prescriptions, increased.

9.2 International Clinical Guidelines for Knee OA

9.2.1 International Clinical Guidelines

International guidelines for the management of patients with knee OA recommended to start with

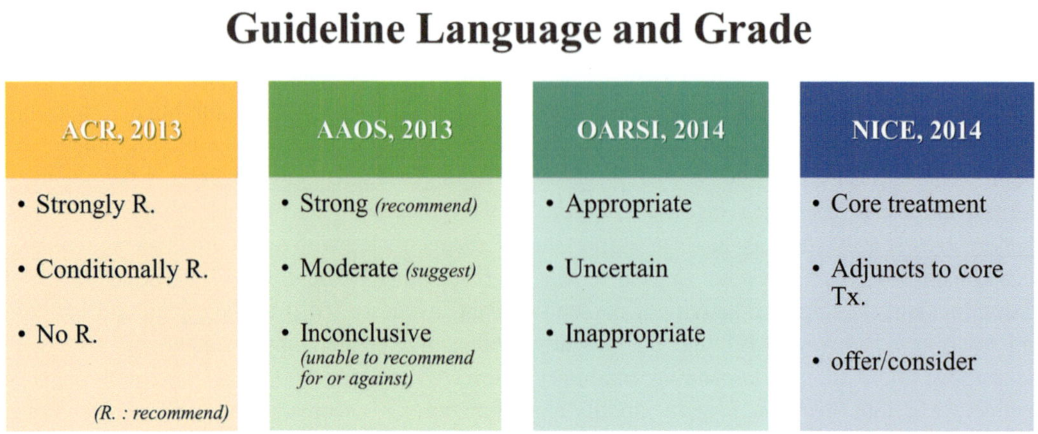

Fig. 9.2 Language used in each international guidelines. *ACR* American College of Rheumatology, *AAOS* American Academy of Orthopaedic Surgeons, *OARSI* Osteoarthritis Research Society International, *NICE* United Kingdom's National Institute for Health and Care Excellence

non-operative treatments, and using surgical intervention only if a patient does not respond sufficiently to non-operative treatment options. In the last 10 years, currently available guidelines for OA management include those developed by the American College of Rheumatology (ACR, 2013), the American Academy of Orthopaedic Surgeons (AAOS, 2013), the Osteoarthritis Research Society International (OARSI, 2014), the United Kingdom's National Institute for Health and Care Excellence (NICE, 2014) and the European Society for Clinical and Economic Aspects of Osteoporosis, Osteoarthritis and Musculoskeletal Diseases (ESCEO, 2014) [15, 64–67]. Collectively, these guidelines reflect the experience of physicians across a variety of medical disciplines. However, they differ in their scope and are reliant on the therapeutic options that were available at the time they were developed. Before interpreting the contents of the guidelines, it is necessary to understand the guideline language and grade of each guideline (Fig. 9.2).

The ACR guideline used guideline languages as "strongly recommend," "conditionally recommend" and "no recommend" for each item. The AAOS guideline used "strong" means recommend, "moderate" means suggest, and "inconclusive" means unable to recommend for or against. The OARSI guideline used "appropriate," "uncertain," and "inappropriate." The NICE guideline used "core treatment," "adjuncts to core treatment," and "off/consider."

9.2.1.1 Acetaminophen

ACR guideline conditionally recommended acetaminophen as treatment modality of knee OA. They permitted the use of acetaminophen with full dosage up to 4000 mg/day. AAOS guideline summarized acetaminophen as "inconclusive" along with opioids and pain patch as the treatment modality of knee OA. NICE guideline offered paracetamol in addition to core treatment (Fig. 9.3).

9.2.1.2 Topical Capsaicin

ACR guideline conditionally recommended that health care provider do not use topical capsaicin. OARSI guideline recommended that the use of topical capsaicin is "appropriate" in knee-only OA patients without relevant comorbidities and "uncertain" in multi-joint OA patients and patients with relevant comorbidities. NICE guideline considered topical capsaicin as an adjunct to core treatments for knee or hand OA.

9.2.1.3 Non-selective NSAIDs

ACR guideline "strongly recommended" the concomitant use of non-selective NSAIDs with proton pump inhibitors (PPI) for knee OA

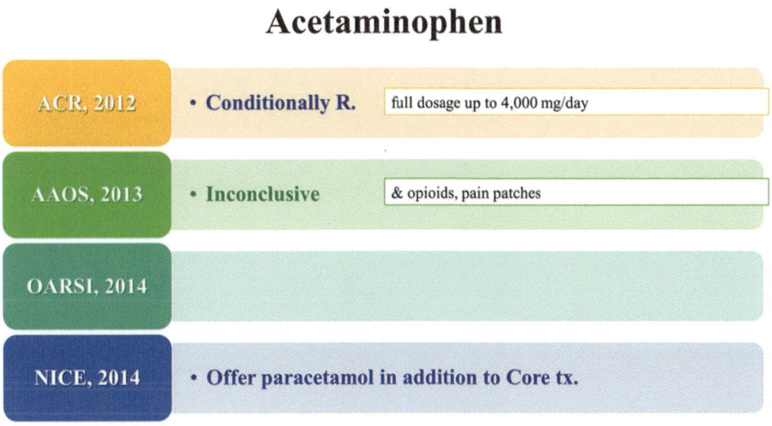

Fig. 9.3 Recommendations of each international guideline for acetaminophen

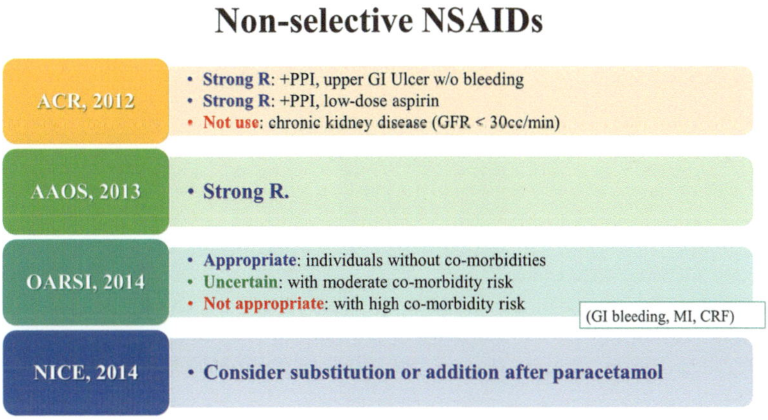

Fig. 9.4 Recommendations of each international guideline for non-selective non-steroidal anti-inflammatory drugs. *PPI* proton pump inhibitor, *GI* gastrointestinal, *GFR* glomerular filtration rate

patients with upper GI ulcer without bleeding or patients taking low-dose aspirin. But, ACR guideline not recommended non selective NSAIDs to chronic renal failure (CRF) patients with a glomerular filtration rate (GFR) of 30 or less. AAOS guideline strong recommended non-selective NSAIDs without any further comment. OARSI guideline divided the recommended degree of non-selective NSAIDs use according to the degree of risk of comorbidities. They recommended that the use of the non-selective NSAIDs is "appropriate" in patients without comorbidities and "uncertain" in patients with moderate comorbidity risk. But, they recommended that the use of non-selective NSAIDs is "not appropriate" in patients with high comorbidity risk, for examples, GI bleeding or myocardial infarction, and CRF. NICE guideline considered non-selective NSAIDs as substitution or addition after paracetamol (Fig. 9.4).

9.2.1.4 COX-2 Inhibitors

ACR guideline strongly recommended the use of COX-2 inhibitors for knee OA patients with upper GI ulcer without bleeding and the concomitant use with PPI for patients with upper GI bleeding. But, they strongly recommended to not use COX-2 inhibitors for knee OA patients taking low-dose aspirin. OARSI guideline recommended that the use of COX-2 inhibitors is "appropriate" in patients without comorbidities and "uncertain" in patients with moderate comorbidity risk. However, they recommended that the use of COX-2 inhibitors is "not appropriate" in patients with high comorbidity risk. NICE guideline considered COX-2

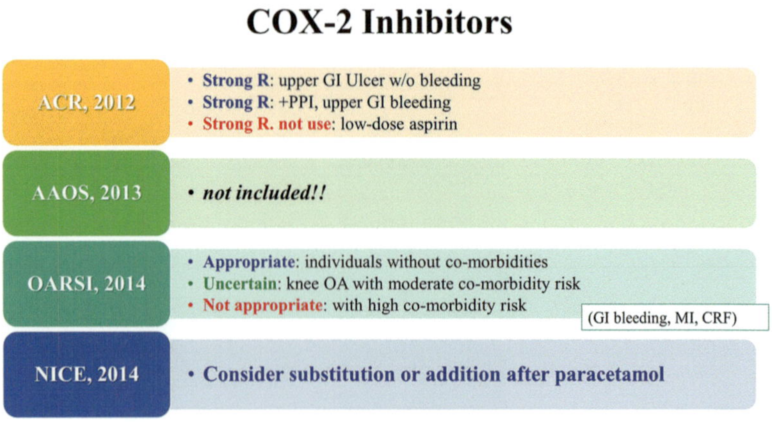

Fig. 9.5 Recommendations of each international guideline for cyclooxygenase-2 inhibitors. *GI* gastrointestinal, *PPI* proton pump inhibitor, *OA* osteoarthritis, *MI* myocardial infarction, *CRF* chronic renal failure

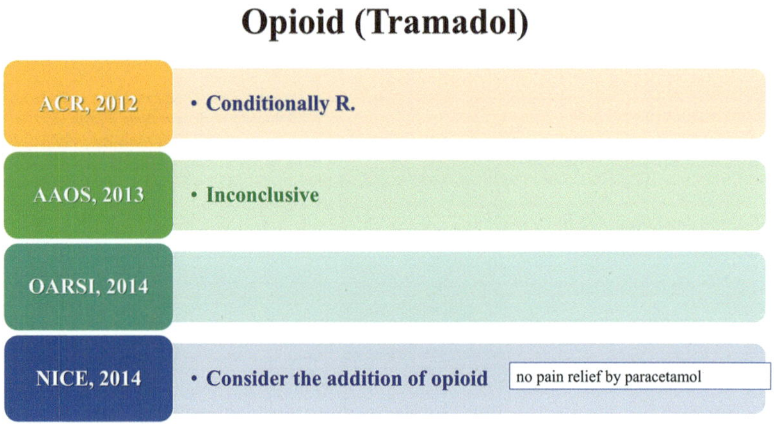

Fig. 9.6 Recommendations of each international guideline for opioid (tramadol)

inhibitors as substitution or addition after paracetamol (Fig. 9.5).

9.2.1.5 Opioid (Tramadol)

ACR guideline conditionally recommended the use of opioid for knee OA patients. AAOS guideline indicated that the use of opioid was "inconclusive" in knee OA patients. NICE guideline considered the addition of opioid to patients who had no pain relief by paracetamol (Fig. 9.6).

9.2.1.6 Dietary Supplements

Dietary supplements are products intended to supplement the diet. They are not drugs and, therefore, are not intended to treat, diagnose, mitigate, prevent, or cure diseases. Unlike drugs, which must be approved by the US FDA before they can be marketed, dietary supplements do not require premarket review or approval by the FDA.

The four international clinical guidelines have summarized the position on glucosamine and chondroitin in patients with knee OA as follows. ACR guideline conditionally not recommended the use of the glucosamine and chondroitin for knee OA patients. AAOS guideline strongly not recommended and NICE guideline not offered the use of dietary supplements for knee OA patients. OARSI guideline divided the benefits achievable from dietary supplement use into symptom relief and disease modification. They said that the use of glucosamine and chondroitin was "uncertain" in terms of symptom relief and "not appropriate" in terms of disease modification (Fig. 9.7).

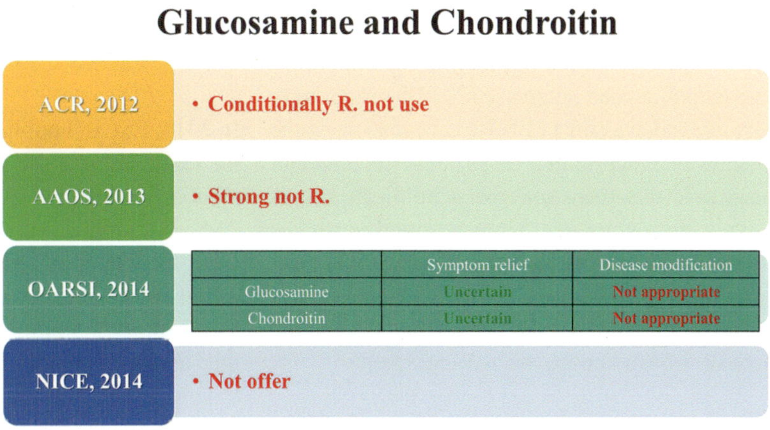

Fig. 9.7 Recommendations of each international guideline for glucosamine and chondroitin

9.2.2 Update Guidelines (I): ACR 2012 and ACR 2019

In January 2020, the ACR updated official guideline—which was last released in 2012—after reviewing the scientific literature on OA treatment that has come out in the past few years. The current version is "2019 American College of Rheumatology/Arthritis Foundation Guideline for the Management of OA of the Hand, Hip, and Knee" and appears in the journal Arthritis Care & Research [68]. Therefore, we would like to summarize the updates in pharmacologic management compared to the existing guidelines [64].

Category changed slightly from "non-pharmacologic modalities" and "pharmacologic modalities" in 2012 to "physical, psycho-social, and mind-body approaches" and "pharmacologic management" in 2019. The words used in the ACR guideline are as follows. "Strongly recommended," "conditionally recommended," "conditionally recommended against," "strongly recommended against."

9.2.2.1 Topical NSAIDs

Currently, only the NICE and AAOS recommend topical NSAIDs as the first-line treatment for OA of the knee. Additionally, EULAR guidelines recommend these agents as a first-line option for OA of the hand. Other guidelines, such as ACR, recommend topical NSAIDs as first-line treatment only for select, high-risk patient populations. Topical NSAIDs have been changed from "conditionally recommended (2012)" to "strongly recommended (2019)." Under the principle of "medications with the least systemic exposure are preferable," it is strongly recommended to use oral NSAIDs before using them.

9.2.2.2 Acetaminophen

Acetaminophen was not changed to "conditionally recommended" in both the 2012 and 2019 guideline. However, in the 2019 guideline, references were added to very small effect size in clinical trials, ineffective as monotherapy (meta-analysis), patient panel (ineffective), intolerance of contraindications to the use of NSAIDs, regular monitoring for hepatotoxicity, etc.

9.2.2.3 Oral NSAIDs

Oral NSAIDs have been changed from "conditionally recommended (2012)" to "strongly recommended (2019)." In the 2019 guideline, oral NSAIDs remain the mainstay of the pharmacologic management. However, only the efficacy of the short-term use was recognized, and the relative merits of different NSAIDS were not addressed.

9.2.2.4 Duloxetine

Duloxetine has been changed from "no recommended (2012)" to "conditionally recommended (2019)."

9.2.2.5 Glucosamine

Glucosamine has been changed from "conditionally recommended not to use (2012)" to "strongly recommended against (2019)." The reason for the change of glucosamine to strongly recommend against is that there may be a publication bias with discrepancies in efficacy reported in studies that were industry sponsored as opposed to publicly funded, and lack of a clear biologic understanding of how efficacy would vary with the type of salt studied has been mentioned.

9.2.2.6 Chondroitin Sulfate

Chondroitin sulfate has been changed from "conditionally recommended not to use (2012)" to "strongly recommended against (2019)."

9.2.3 Update Guidelines (II): OARSI 2019

Whereas the earlier versions of OARSI guideline allowed recommendations to be predicated on the distribution of OA and various comorbidity profiles, these updated OARSI guidelines have taken a more patient-centered approach [66, 69]. Updated OARSI guidelines provide guidance for 4 comorbidities that are common in patients with OA and confound its treatment—(1) gastrointestinal comorbidities, (2) cardiovascular comorbidities, (3) frailty, and (4) widespread pain and/or depression.

The list of "Recommended Treatments for knee OA" is shown in Table 9.2.

9.2.4 Update Guidelines (III): ESCEO 2019

In 2014, ESCEO published recommendations for the treatment of knee OA in the form of a treatment algorithm (Fig. 9.8).

Since publication of the 2014 recommendation, considerable new evidence has been published, particularly regarding the safety of many medications commonly used to treat OA [70]. In this update, ESCEO has revisited the ESCEO treatment recommendations and has developed an updated stepwise algorithm of recommendations based upon application of the Grading of Recommendations Assessment, Development and Evaluation (GRADE) process [71]. The strength of recommendation was determined as "strong" rather than "weak", if at least 75% of the working group members rated a recommendation as "strong".

9.2.4.1 Paracetamol (Acetaminophen)

The ES of paracetamol on pain is 0.14 (95% CI 0.05–0.22), which translates to no detectable clinical effect (<0.2), and no significant effect on stiffness and physical function in knee OA patients. The ESCEO gives a weak recommendation that paracetamol should not be used on a regular basis as STEP 1 background treatment of knee OA.

9.2.4.2 SYSADOA

Prescription crystalline glucosamine sulfate (pCGS) has a small ES on pain of 0.27 (95% CI

Table 9.2 The Osteoarthritis Research Society International (OARSI)'s recommended treatments, by treatment type, for knee osteoarthritis

Treatment type	No comorbidities	Gastrointestinal	Cardiovascular	Frailty	Widespread pain/ depression
Topical NSAIDs	Strong	Strong	Strong	Strong	Conditional
Oral NSAIDs	Conditional	Conditionally R. (Non-selective NSAIDs + PPI or selective COX-2 inhibitors)	Not (due to evidence associating NSAID use with heightened cardiovascular risk)	Not	Conditional
Duloxetine					Conditional

NSAIDs non-steroidal anti-inflammatory drugs, *PPI* proton pump inhibitor, *COX* cyclooxygenase

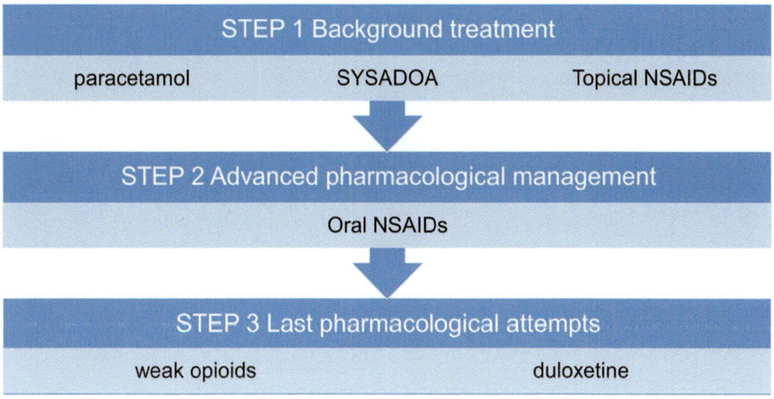

Fig. 9.8 European Society for Clinical and Economic Aspects of Osteoporosis, Osteoarthritis and Musculoskeletal Diseases (ESCEO)'s recommendations for the treatment of osteoarthritis of the knee in the form of a treatment algorithm. *SYSADOA* symptomatic slow acting drugs for osteoarthritis, *NSAIDs* non-steroidal anti-inflammatory drugs

0.12–0.43), which is greater than paracetamol (ES 0.14) and similar to NSAIDs (ES 0.32). The ES of chondroitin 4&6 sulfate on pain is reportedly variable [33, 66]. The ESCEO affords a strong recommendation to the use of pCGS and prescription chondroitin sulfate as STEP 1 background therapy for the treatment of knee OA and discourages the use of other glucosamine formulations. However, the ESCEO gives a weak recommendation that a combination of glucosamine and chondroitin sulfate should not be used in STEP 1 background therapy. And, the ESCEO gives a weak recommendation to the use of ASU and diacerein as alterative STEP 1 therapy.

9.2.4.3 Topical NSAIDs

Topical NSAIDs are as effective as oral NSAIDs, with a pooled ER for pain relief of 0.44 (95% CI, 0.27–0.62) and the ESCEO affords a strong recommendation to the use of topical NSAIDs as cyclic add-on analgesia in STEP 1.

9.2.4.4 Oral NSAIDs

Oral NSAIDs have a small to moderate effect on pain relief in OA, with ES ranging between 0.35 (95% CI, 0.31–0.40) for OA approved daily doses of celecoxib 200 mg/day, and 0.57 (95% CI 0.45–0.69) or 0.58 (95% CI 0.43–0.74) for maximally approved daily doses of diclofenac 150 mg/day or etoricoxib 60 mg/day [72]. Therefore, the ESCEO affords a strong recommendation to the use of oral NSAIDs (selective or non-selective) as STEP 2 therapy.

9.2.4.5 Short-Term Weak Opioids

Opioids significantly decrease pain intensity (ES −0.79; 95% CI, −0.98 ~ −0.59) and have small benefit on function (ES −0.31, 95% CI, −0.39 ~ −0.24). Therefore, the ESCEO gives a weak recommendation to the use of short-term weak opioids in STEP 3 therapy.

9.2.4.6 Others

The ESCEO gives a weak recommendation that 'the use of duloxetine as an alternative to weak opioids in STEP 3 therapy' and 'the use of classical oral or transdermal opioids in end-stage knee OA patients for whom surgery is contraindicated'.

9.3 How to Prescribe Medications to Knee OA Patients with Specific Situations

The choice of medications to use in clinical practice depends on individual patient characteristics and medical history. Several patient factors have been identified to increase the risk of CV, GI, and renal complications. Currently available guidelines for OA management recommend that patients are assessed for risk factors and the risk:benefit ratio of treatment is determined before making treatment decisions.

9.3.1 Young Patients

The treatment of OA of the knee in the young, active patient remains a challenge to the orthopedic surgeon. Initial nonsurgical management with exercise, activity modification, NSAIDs, and viscosupplementation may improve symptoms but will not dramatically alter the natural history of the disease process [73]. The number of young patients affected by knee OA is increasing exponentially, due to the increasing number of individuals involved in physically demanding careers and sporting lifestyles [73, 74]. National Health Interview Survey data from 2007 to 2008 in the USA show an estimated incidence of diagnosed symptomatic knee OA [75]. The largest increase is seen between the ages of 55–64, followed by the next largest increase between the ages of 45–54. This symptomatic knee OA can be seen from a young age. Khanna V et al. excluded trauma, fracture, infection, rheumatoid arthritis, and gout and defined Kellgren-Lawrence grade of 2 or higher as primary knee OA [76]. They reported that the incidence of primary knee OA under the age of 40 as 6.5%. Losina E et al. reported that about 5% of cases in the US population are diagnosed with knee OA at 50 years old, and about 9% at 60 years old, indicating that knee OA is diagnosed in a relatively young age group [75].

9.3.1.1 Obesity

Obesity is increasing worldwide, and the purpose of obesity treatment is not just to lose weight, but also to prevent the occurrence of obesity-related diseases (Fig. 9.9).

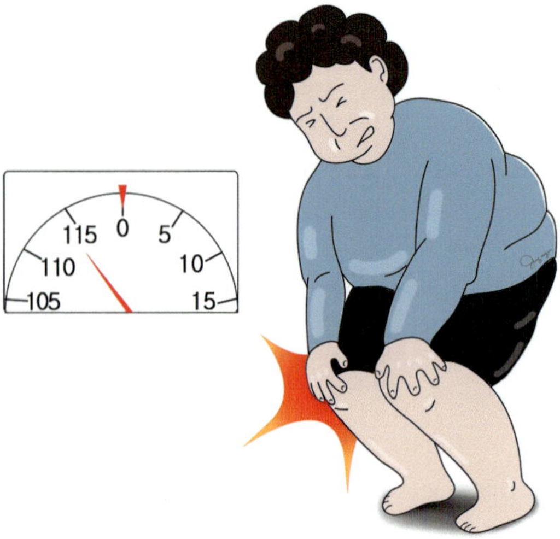

Fig. 9.9 Obese patient suffers from pain due to osteoarthritis in the knee joint

The close association between OA and obesity is well established. Mechanisms linking obesity and OA involve multifactorial phenomena such as systemic factors (i.e., adipokines and pro-inflammatory cytokines), hormonal disturbances (hyperinsulinemia) and muscle changes (i.e., sarcopenia and lower muscular tone). The concomitant increasing prevalence of the two diseases has major health, social and economic consequences [77]. The odds ratio for knee OA of overweight compared to normal weight is 2.18, odds ratio of obesity is 2.63. You can see that the odds ratio of overweight or obesity is larger than the odds ratio of 1.84 of female gender, which is well known as a risk factor of knee OA [78].

It is well known that weight loss is important in patients with knee OA. Although patients who received advice were more likely to make an attempt to do so, only 42% of obese patients were advised by their physician to lose weight [79]. Referring to the previously reviewed update guideline, weight loss should be recommended when all patients with symptomatic knee OA [64], body mass index (BMI) > 25 [65], obese >30 or overweight > 25 [67]. A standard of about 5% weight loss should be presented over a period of about 5 months [66].

The basic treatment for obesity is lifestyle correction such as diet and exercise therapy, but it is difficult to achieve sufficient weight loss effect with existing lifestyle therapy, so appropriate obesity medication is required. The ideal obesity treatment drug has few side effects, has good weight loss effect, and can maintain weight loss for a long time, but there are currently not many safe and effective obesity treatment drugs, so there is a great demand for the development of a new treatment for obesity.

To date no specific recommendation for the pharmacologic management of obese patients with OA has been published. Conrozier T recommended that NSAIDs and corticosteroids must be avoided, especially in obese patients with metabolic syndrome [77]. And, the author recommended that in such patients SYSADOA and some anti-oxidant drugs (i.e., curcumin, ginger extracts, copper) may be helpful, thanks to their excellent benefit/risk ratio and their mode of action which may have a positive impact on both OA and obesity-related metabolic disorders.

In recent years, the US FDA has withdrawn several therapeutic options for obesity due to their side effects, but has approved four novel anti-obesity agents. Until recently, Orlistat was the only drug approved for the management of long-term obesity, but the US FDA approved the novel anti-obesity drugs lorcaserin and phentermine/topiramate in 2012, and naltrexone/bupropion and liraglutide in 2014.

Orlistat is the only drug approved by the FDA for long-term treatment of obesity. Orlistat is a potent and selective inhibitor of pancreatic lipase that reduces intestinal digestion of fat [80]. A 4-year double-blind, randomized, placebo-controlled trial with orlistat in overweight patients achieved a weight loss during the 4 years of 6.9% below baseline in the orlistat-treated group compared with 4.1% below baseline in the placebo-treated group [81]. Fecal fat loss and related GI symptoms are common initially, but they subside as patients learn to use the drug.

The selective serotonin receptor agonist lorcaserin, in conjunction with lifestyle modification, was approved by the FDA in 2012 for weight management. Lorcaserin was in clinical use for 8 years and was withdrawn because of concerns regarding an excess in cancer risk after long-term use [82].

Topiramate is an anticonvulsant drug that is approved for use in certain types of epilepsy and it was shown to reduce food intake, but was not developed clinically because of the side effects at the doses selected for trial. In a randomized, double-blind, placebo-controlled, dose-ranging trial, Bray GA et al. evaluated the efficacy and safety of topiramate for weight loss in healthy obese subjects [83]. Patients were randomly assigned 5 groups: topiramate at 64 ~ 384 mg/d or placebo and mean percent weight loss from baseline to week 24 was −2.6% in placebo group vs. −5.0%, −4.8%, −6.3%, and −6.3% in the 64, 96, 192, and 384 mg/d topiramate groups, respectively. And, the most frequent adverse events were paresthesia, somnolence, and difficulty with concentration, memory, and attention.

Phentermine/topiramate (PHEN/TPM) is a new, once-daily, controlled-release, combination weight-loss product approved as an adjunct to diet and exercise for chronic weight management of obese or overweight patients with weight-related comorbidities. Smith SM et al. reviewed the pharmacology, efficacy, and safety of PHEN/TPM in the management of obese patients [84]. In Phase III trials, treatment with PHEN/TPM consistently demonstrated statistically significant weight loss compared with placebo. After 56 weeks of treatment, percent weight loss achieved with PHEN/TPM was 10.6%, 8.4%, and 5.1% with 15/92 mg, 7.5/46 mg, and 3.75/23 mg, respectively. The 52-week extension study showed maintained weight loss over 2 years with 9.3% and 10.5% weight loss from baseline for 7.5/46 mg and 15/92 mg PHEN/TPM. Adverse reactions occurring in 5% or more of study subjects included paresthesia, dizziness, dysgeusia, insomnia, constipation, and dry mouth.

The fixed combination of extended-release naltrexone and bupropion has been developed for the treatment of adults who are obese or overweight with at least weight-related comorbidity, such as type 2 diabetes mellitus, hypertension, or dyslipidemia, as an adjunct to diet and lifestyle modifications and was approved for use in the USA in 2014. In 56-week phase III trials in these patient populations, oral naltrexone extended-release/bupropion extended-release 32/360 mg/day was significantly more effective than placebo with regard to percentage body weight reductions from baseline and the proportion of patients who achieved body weight reductions of ≥5 and ≥ 10%.

Liraglutide is glucagon-like peptide-1 (GLP-1) agonist that has a 97% homology to GLP-1. In a double-blind, placebo-controlled 20-week trial, Astrup A et al. reported that daily injections of liraglutide at 1.2 ~ 3.0 mg produced weight losses of −4.8 ~ −7.2 kg in comparison with −2.8 kg in the placebo group and −4.1 kg in the orlistat group [85].

9.3.1.2 Post-Traumatic Osteoarthritis

Post-traumatic OA (PT-OA) is believed to be an end-stage organ failure of injured joint (Fig. 9.10).

In particular, it occurs frequently after intra-articular fracture (IAF), and about 77% of IAF is known to occur in patients under the age of 45, and PT-OA is known to occur in about 23–44% of IAF of the knee. PT-OA occurs in younger age groups, around 9–14 years of age, compared to primary OA [86]. However, there is a therapeutic dilemma as an approach to young PT-OA, which requires clinically meaningful pain relief and functional improvement, while ensuring long-term treatment safety.

The traditional first approach is nonsurgical treatments, but it is impossible to correct the underlying pathology, which leads to persistent abnormal joint loading, with the limitation that continued disease progression cannot be prevented.

Schmal H et al. conducted a systematic review—9 clinical studies in humans—to summarize the current status of anti-inflammatory therapy for PT-OA [87]. The majority of the analyses (n = 6) focused on the intra-articular (IA) application of hyaluronic acid and 1 study stated positive results of IA administration of interleukin 1 receptor antagonist and 1 study revealed that platelet-rich plasma relieved symptoms. But, there were no studies which evaluated the effects of oral medications to prevent or treat PT-OA.

9.3.1.3 Just Waiting for Arthroplasty

Certain countries use "age" as one of the criteria for determining whether total knee arthroplasty (TKA) can be operated in addition to the Kellgren-Lawrence grade of X-rays. As a result, even with advanced OA findings on X-rays, younger patients may not receive surgical treatment and endure symptomatic treatment (Fig. 9.11).

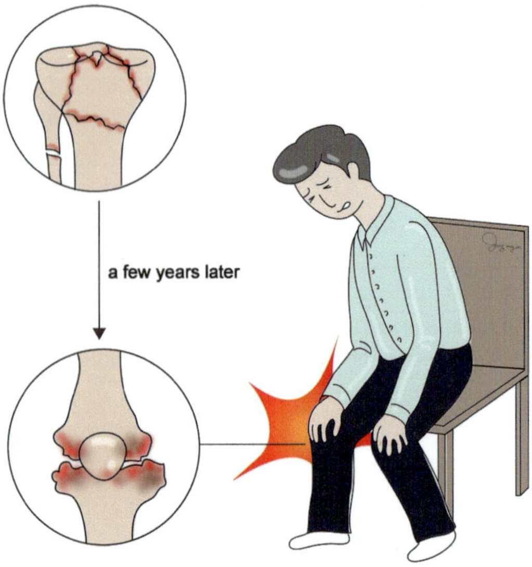

Fig. 9.10 Patient with an intra-articular fracture of the knee suffers from post-traumatic osteoarthritis after several years

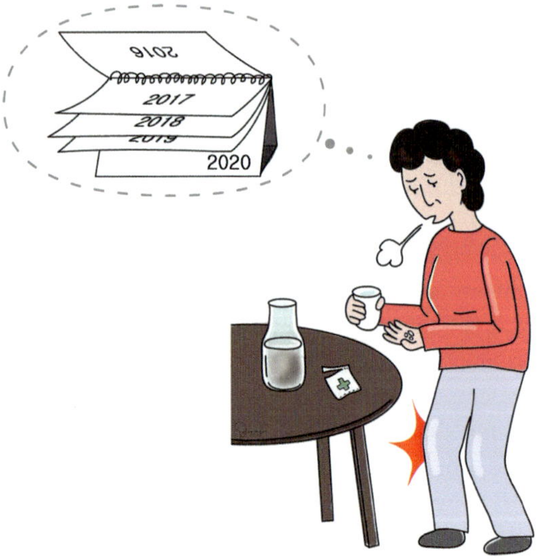

Fig. 9.11 Patient of a relatively young age to undergo total knee arthroplasty is waiting for the passing of time with only medication

Scott CEH et al. presented the results of a survey using the "EuroQol five-dimension (EQ-5D) questionnaire" for patients waiting for arthroplasty surgery [88]. In questionnaire's interpretation of the score, "1" means full health, and "0" means death. If the score comes out as "negative scores," it can be interpreted as "worse than death (WTD)," which means that it means a so-called sick condition rather than dying. They surveyed 2168 patients awaiting total knee arthroplasty surgery, of whom 57% were female and the average age was 69 years. Of these, about 12% were found to be waiting for total knee arthroplasty in the health state of "WTD."

Symptoms such as pain and restriction of joint motion and the degree of radiological OA are severe, but there are cases where TKA is not available due to problems such as age and insurance, and patients in this situation are called "treatment gap" for knee OA. Li CS et al. conducted a survey of orthopedic surgeons and published the following results [89]. When asked "Perceive a need for better treatments for younger (<60 years old) OA patients not suitable for unicompartmental knee arthroplasty (UKA) or TKA", about 84% of all respondents answered yes. "Do you perceive a treatment gap?" About 68% of all respondents answered yes. When asked, "What is the most important thing for successful intervention for patients within the gap?" 45% of all respondents answered 'pain relief'. Thirty percent of respondents answered 'an alternative such as UKA or high tibial osteotomy (HTO) for younger patients' and 24% of respondents answered 'reduce use of conservative treatments'. Therefore, for younger knee OA patients who are in the "treatment gap" while waiting for arthroplasty in "WTD" status, appropriate medication to provide pain relief or other surgical options should be considered. There were studies which explored the relative efficacy of oral pharmacologic interventions in the treatment of knee OA.

da Costa BR et al. conducted a network meta-analysis to assess the effectiveness of different preparations and doses of NSAIDs on OA pain [72]. They included 76 randomized trials with a total of 58,451 patients and compared six interventions (diclofenac 150 mg/day, etoricoxib 30 mg/day, 60 mg/day, and 90 mg/day, and rofecoxib 25 mg/day and 50 mg/day). Among maximally approved daily doses, diclofenac 150 mg/day and etoricoxib 60 mg/day had the highest probability to be the best intervention, both with 100% probability to reach the minimum clinically important difference. Jung et al. conducted a systematic literature review and revealed that etoricoxib had the highest ranking for improving WOMAC pain followed by naproxen, acetaminophen, and celecoxib [90]. In the subgroup analysis, the top three ranked interventions were etoricoxib, celecoxib, and aceclofenac in the higher pain group, and tramadol, celecoxib, and diclofenac in the lower pain group.

9.3.2 Elderly Patients and Comorbid Disease

When medical professionals prescribe OA medications, they need to know the types of medications that can be used for various comorbid diseases that elderly patients have, and also know the interactions with medications currently being used for those comorbid diseases (Fig. 9.12).

Higuera CA et al. surveyed the comorbidity prevalence of 502 elderly patients 65 years of age or older who received TKA or total hip arthroplasty, and published as shown in Fig. 9.13 [91].

Therefore, we would like to introduce the knee OA pain management of elderly patients with comorbidity of hypertension (Rank 1st),

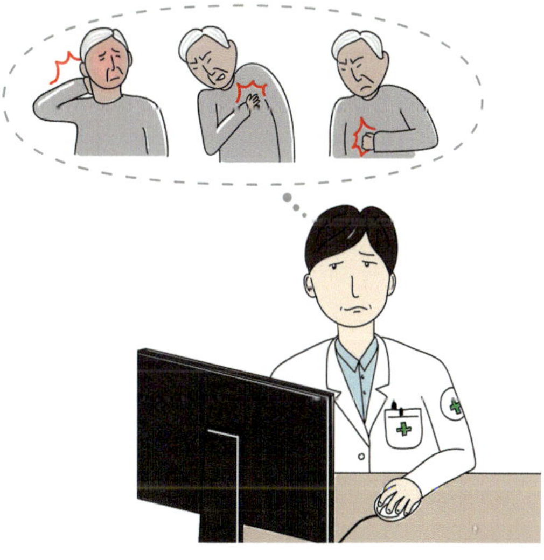

Fig. 9.12 Doctor who is contemplating what drugs to prescribe for elderly patient with osteoarthritis of the knee and various underlying disease

Fig. 9.13 Comorbidity prevalence of elderly patients who received arthroplasty. *DVT* deep vein thrombosis

Rank / 25	Comorbidity	Rate
1st	**hypertension**	82%
3rd	coronary artery disease	25%
5th	diabetes mellitus	22%
6th	**esophagogastroduodenal ulcer disease**	23%
13th	**history of DVT/ pulmonary embolism**	9%
18th	**renal disease**	5%
19th	**liver disease**	3%

ulcer disease (6th), oral anticoagulant (13th), and renal disease (18th).

9.3.2.1 Hypertension (HTN)

The authors who studied the interaction between non-selective NSAIDs and antihypertensive drugs reported that systolic blood pressure increased by 10 mmHg on average when non-selective NSAIDs were used in patients taking antihypertensive drugs such as angiotensin-converting-enzyme inhibitor (ACEi), angiotensin receptor blockers (ARB), beta blockers, calcium antagonists, diuretics. These results can be interpreted that non-selective NSAIDs interfere with the effects of antihypertension drugs [92].

White WB et al. evaluated the effects of specific CO-2 inhibitors compared with placebo on 24-h blood pressure (BP) levels in ACEi-treated patients with HTN. They involved 178 men and women with essential HTN who were treated and controlled with lisinopril monotherapy (10–40 mg daily). Patients received either 400 mg celecoxib or placebo for 4 weeks. Mean changes from baseline in the 24-h systolic and diastolic BP were 2.6/1.5 ± 0.9/0.6 mmHg on celecoxib versus 1.0/0.3 ± 1/0.6 mmHg on placebo ($p = 0.34$ for systolic BP; $p = 0.45$ for diastolic BP). They concluded that high doses of celecoxib have no significant effect on the antihypertensive effect of the ACEi [93].

Bingham CO III et al. compared etoricoxib and celecoxib in patients excluding congestive heart failure, unstable angina, and uncontrolled hypertension and reported similar mean changes in BP from baseline between etoricoxib and celecoxib [94].

9.3.2.2 Ulcer Disease

Gastrointestinal (GI) tolerability is an important treatment consideration when choosing non-selective NSAIDs for elderly arthritis patients [95]. Several patient factors have been identified to increase the risk of upper GI complications, including advanced age, a history of GI ulcer, and concomitant treatment with corticosteroids, aspirin, or anticoagulant [96]. Visser LE et al. reported the results of a survey of 100 patients over the age of 55 with serious GI complications [97]. Serious GI complications were GI hemorrhage, symptomatic ulcer, and intestinal perforation, and the average age of the patients was 75 years. Among them, prescriptions of contraindicated drugs were most common with aspirin at 51%, followed by NSAIDs at 49%. Specifically, the proportion of patients taking anti-ulcer drugs while taking NSAIDs was only 35%. Zeng C et al. reported that only 38% of patients with history of GI disease and 21% of patients without it had co-prescription of gastro-protective agent with oral NSAIDs [28]. Mallen SR et al. conducted a systematic review—21 trials—to compare the GI tolerability of the COX-2 inhibitor (celecoxib) and non-selective NSAIDs in patients with arthritis aged 65 years or older [95]. And, they revealed that the combined incidence of GI intolerability adverse events was reported by significantly fewer patients treated with celecoxib (16.7%) than naproxen (29.4%), ibuprofen (26.5%), or diclofenac (21.0%). The discontinuation rate due to GI intolerability adverse events was significantly lower for celecoxib versus naproxen and ibuprofen.

9.3.2.3 Oral Anti-Coagulant (OAC)

NSAIDs are known to increase the risk of bleeding due to the nature of the drug's mechanism, and the risk of bleeding is further increased, especially when used with anticoagulants (Fig. 9.14).

In a post-hoc analysis of NSAIDs in the RE-LY (Randomized Evaluation of Long Term Anticoagulant Therapy) trial, Kent AP et al. compared dabigatran etexilate (DE) 150 and 110 mg twice daily with warfarin in patients with atrial fibrillation [98]. The results of this study revealed that major bleeding was significantly elevated with NSAID use (hazard ratio [HR]: 1.68; 95% CI: 1.40 to 2.02; $p < 0.0001$). GI major bleeding was significantly elevated with NSAID use (HR: 1.81; 95% CI: 1.35 to 2.43; $p < 0.0001$). The rate of stroke or systemic embolism (stroke/SE) with NSAID use was significantly elevated (HR: 1.50; 95% CI: 1.12 to 2.01; $p = 0.007$). They concluded that the concomitant OAC (DE 110 or 150 mg twice daily, or warfarin) and NSAIDs therapy in patients with atrial fibrillation increased risk of major bleeding, and stroke/systemic embolism.

9.3.2.4 Impaired Renal Function

The management of knee OA pain in patients with chronic kidney disease (CKD) is challenging and safe analgesic choices are limited. These patients have increased susceptibility to adverse drug effects due to altered drug metabolism and excretion, and there are limited safety data for use in this population despite a high pain burden. NSAIDs have long been regarded as dangerous for use in this population because of risk for nephrotoxicity and thus alternative analgesics, including opioids, have become more commonly used for pain control. NSAID use has been associated with acute kidney injury, progressive loss of glomerular filtration rate in CKD, electrolyte derangements, and hypervolemia with worsening of heart failure and hypertension [99].

In a systemic review to estimate the strength of association between chronic NSAIDs use and CKD progression, regular-dose NSAID use did not significantly affect the risk of accelerated CKD progression; pooled odds ratio (OR) = 0.96 (95%CI: 0.86–1.07), but high-dose NSAID use

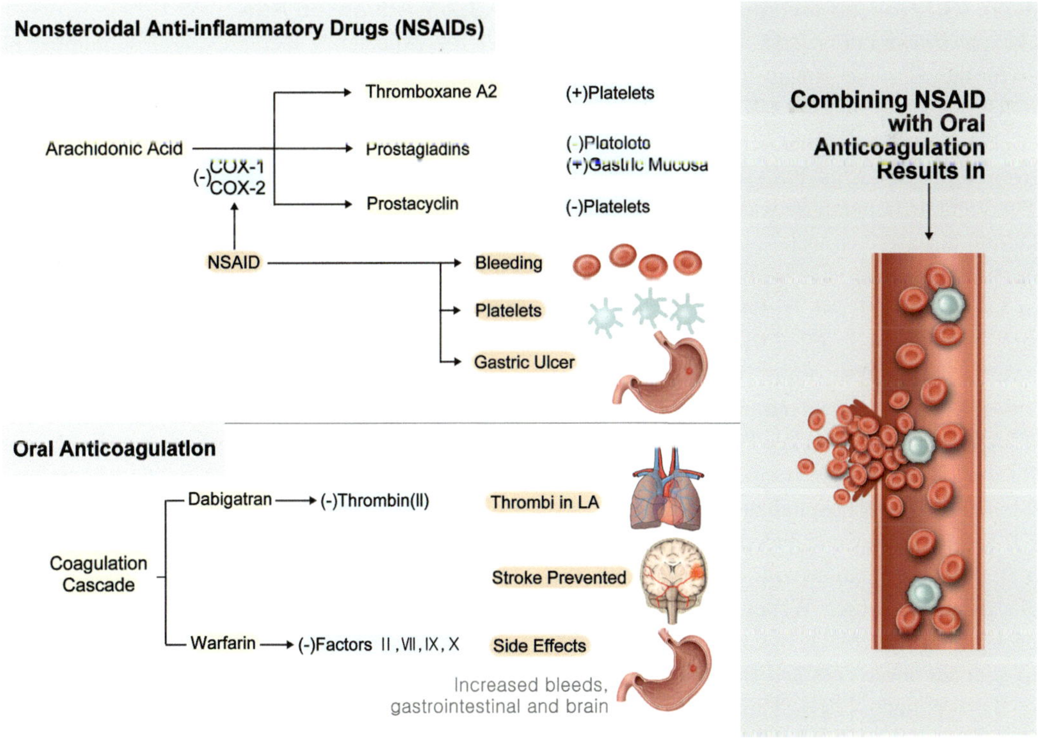

Fig. 9.14 Mechanism of action for non-selective non-steroidal anti-inflammatory drugs and oral anticoagulation therapy

Fig. 9.15 Non-steroidal anti-inflammatory drugs use in chronic kidney disease patients according to the five stages. *CKD* chronic kidney disease, *eGFR* estimated glomerular filtration rate, *NSAIDs* non-steroidal anti-inflammatory drugs

CKD stage	eGFR (ml/min)	Recommendations
1	> 90	favor NSAIDs - greater pain control - fewer side effects
2	60~89	favor NSAIDs - greater pain control - fewer side effects
3a	45~59	favor NSAIDs - greater pain control - fewer side effects
3b	30~44	avoid NSAIDs
4	15~29	avoid NSAIDs
5	< 15	avoid NSAIDs
All CKD with chronic use of NSAIDs		close monitoring of eGFR (every 3 months)

significantly increased the risk of accelerated CKD progression; pooled OR = 1.26 (95%CI: 1.06–1.50). The authors concluded that the avoidance of NSAIDs in the medium term is unnecessary in patients with moderate to severe CKD, if not otherwise contraindicated. As the definition of high-dose of NSAID use remains unclear, the lowest effective dose of NSAIDs should be prescribed where indicated [100].

We showed recommendations about NSAIDs use in CKD patients according to the five stages [101] as shown in Fig. 9.15.

In the Chronic Renal Insufficiency Cohort (CRIC) study with 3939 CKD patients, Zhan M et al. conducted a comparative analysis of harm from opioids versus NSAIDs in CKD [102]. Time-updated opioid use was associated with the kidney disease composite outcome, kidney failure with kidney replacement therapy, death (HRs of 1.4 [95% CI, 1.2–1.7], 1.4 [95% CI, 1.1–1.7], and 1.5 [95% CI, 1.2–2.0], respectively), and hospitalization (rate ratio [RR], 1.7; 95% CI, 1.6–1.9) versus opioid nonusers. Time-updated NSAID use was associated with increased risk for the kidney disease composite (HR, 1.2; 95% CI, 1.0–1.5) and hospitalization (RR, 1.1; 95% CI, 1.0–1.3). They concluded that opioid use had a stronger association with adverse events than NSAIDs. Meuwesen WP et al. investigated the prescribing of NSAIDs in CKD patients in order to generate awareness and improve the outcome of these patients [103]. This study showed that most NSAID prescriptions (52 ~ 63%) were for patients aged 35 ~ 64 years. Diclofenac (34.3%) was the single most frequently prescribed NSAID, but the COX-2-inhibitors were the preferred NSAID class to be prescribed. They concluded that even though NSAIDs are regarded as nephrotoxic drugs, every three to four patients with CKD in South Africa are being prescribed NSAIDs in dosages similar to, and exceeding, the recommended daily dosages for patients with a normal kidney function.

9.3.2.5 Advanced Age

As life expectancy increases, a large number of populations experience pain from OA in various joints, including the knee. Although TKA is the final treatment modality for advanced knee OA, it is well known that surgical treatments cannot be selected for all patients. Higuera CA et al. reported old age and complications of TKA [93]. They studied the relative risk according to age in 304 patients over 65 years old and reported that the results shown in Table 9.3 were obtained.

Patients were approximately 40% more likely to have any complication per every 10 years of life. Therefore, in the case of advanced age, you will need to be aware of the risks of complications of TKA and try appropriate pharmacologic management. Huang WN et al. evaluated the effectiveness and tolerability of etoricoxib in extremely elderly patients aged 79 years or older (mean age 85.9, range 79 ~ 96 years) [104]. Patients who responded inadequately to NSAIDs or other analgesics were switched to etoricoxib, 60 mg once daily for 4 weeks. They reported that pain and disability scores measured by WOMAC

Table 9.3 Relative risk for complications after total knee arthroplasty with increasing age

All complications	Relative risk (95% confidence interval)	*p*-value
Age (per 10 years)	1.39 (1.17 ~ 1.66)	0.0003
65 ~ 74 years (reference)	1.00	
75 ~ 84 years	1.43 (1.14 ~ 1.80)	0.002
≥85 years	1.25 (0.79 ~ 1.98)	0.35

index were lower after treatment (pain, $p \leq 0.001$; disability, $p = 0.020$) and no adverse events were reported. They concluded that pain relief, joint function, quality of life, and treatment satisfaction improved significantly in elderly patients with OA after etoricoxib administration.

9.4 Summary

The goal of the pharmacologic management of knee OA is to minimize pain and optimize function. The guidelines for the pharmacologic management of OA can help you identify expert opinions on the various treatment options. However, it is important to recognize that there are differences between the guidelines and the individual treatment experiences, and select treatment modalities by referring to the guidelines. In the real world, the treatment of OA of the knee in the young, active patient remains a challenge to the orthopedic surgeon, and the presence of comorbidities in elderly patients often impacts treatment choices, particularly with respect to pharmacologic therapy. Although various pharmacologic treatment options are available for knee OA patients, an individualized approach to the patients is most beneficial in patients with knee OA and the treatment plan should be based on this principle. The choice of the pharmacologic treatment of OA should always be based on the professional judgment of the physician and the patient's condition and preference.

References

1. Eymard F, Chevalier X. Pharmacological treatments of knee osteoarthritis. Rev Prat. 2019;69(5):515–9.
2. Kon E, Filardo G, Drobnic M, Madry H, Jelic M, van Dijk N, Della VS. Non-surgical management of early knee osteoarthritis. Knee Surg Sports Traumatol Arthrosc. 2012;20(3):436–49.
3. Mason L, Moore RA, Derry S, Edwards JE, McQuay HJ. Systematic review of topical capsaicin for the treatment of chronic pain. BMJ. 2004;328(7446):991.
4. Kosuwon W, Sirichatiwapee W, Wisanuyotin T, Jeeravipoolvarn P, Laupattarakasem W. Efficacy of symptomatic control of knee osteoarthritis with 0.0125% of capsaicin versus placebo. J Med Assoc Thail. 2010;93(10):1188–95.
5. Balmaceda CM. Evolving guidelines in the use of topical nonsteroidal anti-inflammatory drugs in the treatment of osteoarthritis. BMC Musculoskelet Disord. 2014;15:27.
6. Tugwell PS, Wells GA, Shainhouse JZ. Equivalence study of a topical diclofenac solution (pennsaid) compared with oral diclofenac in symptomatic treatment of osteoarthritis of the knee: a randomized controlled trial. J Rheumatol. 2004;31(10):2002–12.
7. Simon LS, Grierson LM, Naseer Z, Bookman AA, Zev SJ. Efficacy and safety of topical diclofenac containing dimethyl sulfoxide (DMSO) compared with those of topical placebo, DMSO vehicle and oral diclofenac for knee osteoarthritis. Pain. 2009;143(3):238–45.
8. Rother M, Lavins BJ, Kneer W, Lehnhardt K, Seidel EJ, Mazgareanu S. Efficacy and safety of epicutaneous ketoprofen in Transfersome (IDEA-033) versus oral celecoxib and placebo in osteoarthritis of the knee: multicentre randomised controlled trial. Ann Rheum Dis. 2007;66(9):1178–83.
9. Persson MSM, Stocks J, Walsh DA, Doherty M, Zhang W. The relative efficacy of topical non-steroidal anti- inflammatory drugs and capsaicin in osteoarthritis: a network meta-analysis of randomised controlled trials. Osteoarthr Cartil. 2018;26(12):1575–82.
10. Case JP, Baliunas AJ, Block JA. Lack of efficacy of acetaminophen in treating symptomatic knee osteoarthritis: a randomized, double-blind, placebo-controlled comparison trial with diclofenac sodium. Arch Intern Med. 2003;163(2):169–78.
11. Leopoldino AO, Machado GC, Ferreira PH, et al. Paracetamol versus placebo for knee and hip osteoarthritis. Cochrane Database Syst Rev. 2019;2(2):CD013273.
12. Fitzgerald GA. Coxibs and cardiovascular disease. N Engl J Med. 2004;351(17):1709–11.
13. Watson M, Brookes ST, Faulkner A, Kirwan J. Non-aspirin, non-steroidal anti-inflammatory drugs for treating osteoarthritis of the knee. Cochrane Database Syst Rev. 2007;1:CD000142.

14. da Costa BR, Nüesch E, Kasteler R, et al. Oral or transdermal opioids for osteoarthritis of the knee or hip. Cochrane Database Syst Rev. 2014;9:CD003115.
15. Bruyère O, Cooper C, Pelletier JP, et al. An algorithm recommendation for the management of knee osteoarthritis in Europe and internationally: a report from a task force of the European Society for Clinical and Economic Aspects of Osteoporosis and Osteoarthritis (ESCEO). Semin Arthritis Rheum. 2014;44(3):253–63.
16. Wright EA, Katz JN, Abrams S, Solomon DH, Losina E. Trends in prescription of opioids from 2003-2009 in persons with knee osteoarthritis. Arthritis Care Res (Hoboken). 2014;66(10):1489–95.
17. Power JD, Perruccio AV, Gandhi R, et al. Factors associated with opioid use in presurgical knee, kip, and spine osteoarthritis patients. Arthritis Care Res (Hoboken). 2019;71(9):1178–85.
18. Thorlund JB, Turkiewicz A, Prieto-Alhambra D, Englund M. Opioid use in knee or hip osteoarthritis: a region-wide population-based cohort study. Osteoarthr Cartil. 2019;27(6):871–7.
19. Cho SK, Jung SY, Choi S, et al. Factors related to the use of opioids as early treatment in patients with knee osteoarthritis. Arthritis Res Ther. 2019;21(1):222.
20. Grond S, Sablotzki A. Clinical pharmacology of tramadol. Clin Pharmacokinet. 2004;43(13):879–923.
21. Cepeda MS, Camargo F, Zea C, Valencia L. Tramadol for osteoarthritis. Cochrane Database Syst Rev. 2006;3:CD005522.
22. Raber M, Schulz HU, Schürer M, Krupp S, Momberger H. Pharmacokinetic properties of tramadol sustained release capsules. 3rd communication: investigation of relative bioavailability under steady state conditions. Arzneimittelforschung. 1999;49(7):594–8.
23. Cnota PJ, Nowak H, Tagarro I, et al. Tramadol SR formulations: pharmacokinetic comparison of a multiple-units dose (capsule) versus a single-unit dose (tablet). Clin Drug Investig. 2005;25(7):435–43.
24. Zeng C, Dubreuil M, LaRochelle MR, et al. Association of tramadol with all-cause mortality among patients with osteoarthritis. JAMA. 2019;321(10):969–82.
25. DeMik DE, Bedard NA, Dowdle SB, Burnett RA, McHugh MA, Callaghan JJ. Are we still prescribing opioids for osteoarthritis? J Arthroplast. 2017;32(12):3578–82.
26. Nüesch E, Rutjes AW, Husni E, Welch V, Jüni P. Oral or transdermal opioids for osteoarthritis of the knee or hip. Cochrane Database Syst Rev. 2009;4:CD003115.
27. Smith SR, Deshpande BR, Collins JE, Katz JN, Losina E. Comparative pain reduction of oral nonsteroidal anti-inflammatory drugs and opioids for knee osteoarthritis: systematic analytic review. Osteoarthr Cartil. 2016;24(6):962–72.
28. Zeng C, Zhang W, Doherty M, et al. Initial analgesic prescriptions for osteoarthritis in the United Kingdom, 2000-2016. Rheumatology (Oxford). 2020.
29. Bellamy N, Campbell J, Robinson V, Gee T, Bourne R, Wells G. Intraarticular corticosteroid for treatment of osteoarthritis of the knee. Cochrane Database Syst Rev. 2006;2:CD005328.
30. Abou-Raya A, Abou-Raya S, Khadrawi T, Helmii M. Effect of low-dose oral prednisolone on symptoms and systemic inflammation in older adults with moderate to severe knee osteoarthritis: a randomized placebo-controlled trial. J Rheumatol. 2018;45(12):1713.
31. Apostu D, Lucaciu O, Mester A, et al. Systemic drugs with impact on osteoarthritis. Drug Metab Rev. 2019;51(4):498–523.
32. Henrotin Y, Marty M, Mobasheri A. What is the current status of chondroitin sulfate and glucosamine for the treatment of knee osteoarthritis? Maturitas. 2014;78(3):184–7.
33. Singh JA, Noorbaloochi S, MacDonald R, Maxwell LJ. Chondroitin for osteoarthritis. Cochrane Database Syst Rev. 2015;1:CD005614.
34. Sun Y, Wang C, Gong C. Repairing effects of glucosamine sulfate in combination with etoricoxib on articular cartilages of patients with knee osteoarthritis. J Orthop Surg Res. 2020;15(1):150.
35. De Wan M, Volpi G, Inventors; Rottapharm, assignee. A method of preparing mixed glucosamine salts.: US patent 5,847,107. https://patents.google.com/patent/US5847107A/en. Accessed 8 January 2019. USA patent 5,847,107.1998.
36. Bruyère O, Altman RD, Reginster JY. Efficacy and safety of glucosamine sulfate in the management of osteoarthritis: evidence from real-life setting trials and surveys. Semin Arthritis Rheum. 2016;45(4 Suppl):S12–S7.
37. Zhang S, Zhang Y, Liu P, Zhang W, Ma JL, Wang J. Efficacy and safety of etoricoxib compared with NSAIDs in acute gout: a systematic review and a meta-analysis. Clin Rheumatol. 2016;35(1):151–8.
38. Martel-Pelletier J, Kwan Tat S, Pelletier JP. Effects of chondroitin sulfate in the pathophysiology of the osteoarthritic joint: a narrative review. Osteoarthr Cartil. 2010;18(Suppl 1):S7–S11.
39. Ernst E. Avocado-soybean unsaponifiables (ASU) for osteoarthritis - a systematic review. Clin Rheumatol. 2003;22(4–5):285–8.
40. Henrotin YE, Sanchez C, Deberg MA, et al. Avocado/soybean unsaponifiables increase aggrecan synthesis and reduce catabolic and proinflammatory mediator production by human osteoarthritic chondrocytes. J Rheumatol. 2003;30(8):1825–34.
41. Mauviel A, Daireaux M, Hartmann DJ, Galera P, Loyau G, Pujol JP. Effects of unsaponifiable extracts of avocado/soy beans (PIAS) on the production of collagen by cultures of synoviocytes, articular chondrocytes and skin fibroblasts. Rev Rhum Mal Osteoartic. 1989;56(2):207–11.
42. Simental-Mendía M, Sánchez-García A, Acosta-Olivo CA, et al. Efficacy and safety of avocado-

soybean unsaponifiables for the treatment of hip and knee osteoarthritis: a systematic review and meta-analysis of randomized placebo-controlled trials. Int J Rheum Dis. 2019;22(9):1607–15.
43. Pavelka K, Bruyère O, Cooper C, et al. Diacerein: benefits, risks and place in the management of osteoarthritis. an opinion-based report from the ESCEO. Drugs Aging. 2016;33(2):75–85.
44. Pelletier JP, Yaron M, Haraoui B, et al. Efficacy and safety of diacerein in osteoarthritis of the knee: a double-blind, placebo-controlled trial. The Diacerein Study Group. Arthritis Rheum. 2000;43(10):2339–48.
45. Pelletier JP, Raynauld JP, Dorais M, et al. An international, multicentre, double-blind, randomized study (DISSCO): effect of diacerein vs celecoxib on symptoms in knee osteoarthritis. Rheumatology (Oxford). 2020.
46. Honvo G, Reginster JY, Rabenda V, et al. Safety of symptomatic slow-acting drugs for osteoarthritis: outcomes of a systematic review and meta-analysis. Drugs Aging. 2019;36(Suppl 1):65–99.
47. van Helvoort EM, Popov-Celeketic J, Eijkelkamp N, et al. Canine IL4-10 fusion protein provides disease modifying activity in a canine model of OA; an exploratory study. PLoS One. 2019;14(7):e0219587.
48. Roemer FW, Kwoh CK, Hayashi D, Felson DT, Guermazi A. The role of radiography and MRI for eligibility assessment in DMOAD trials of knee OA. Nat Rev Rheumatol. 2018;14(6):372–80.
49. Smelter E, Hochberg MC. New treatments for osteoarthritis. Curr Opin Rheumatol. 2013; 25(3):310–6.
50. Flechsenhar K, Ried JS, Driban JB, Price LL, McAlindon T. Sample size calculations for detecting disease-modifying osteoarthritis drug effects on the incidence of end stage knee osteoarthritis in clinical trials: data from the osteoarthritis initiative. Semin Arthritis Rheum. 2019;49(1):3–8.
51. Food and Drug Administration. Guidance for Industry on clinical development programs for drugs, devices and biological products intended for the treatment of osteoarthritis (OA), 1999.
52. Montjean R, Escaich S, Paolini R, et al. REG-O3 chimeric peptide combining growth hormone and somatostatin sequences improves joint function and prevents cartilage degradation in rat model of traumatic knee osteoarthritis. PLoS One. 2020;15(4):e0231240.
53. Li C, Zheng Z, Ha P, et al. Neural EGFL like 1 as a potential pro-chondrogenic, anti-inflammatory dual-functional disease-modifying osteoarthritis drug. Biomaterials. 2020 Jan;226:119541.
54. Wang G, Bi L, Li X, et al. Maintenance of effect of duloxetine in Chinese patients with pain due to osteoarthritis: 13-week open-label extension data. BMC Musculoskelet Disord. 2019;20(1):174.
55. Arendt-Nielsen L, Nie H, Laursen MB, et al. Sensitization in patients with painful knee osteoarthritis. Pain. 2010;149(3):573–81.
56. Bajaj P, Bajaj P, Graven-Nielsen T, Arendt-Nielsen L. Osteoarthritis and its association with muscle hyperalgesia: an experimental controlled study. Pain. 2001;93(2):107–14.
57. Kidd BL. Osteoarthritis and joint pain. Pain. 2006;123(1–2):6–9.
58. Havelin J, Imbert I, Cormier J, Allen J, Porreca F, King T. Central sensitization and neuropathic features of ongoing pain in a rat model of advanced osteoarthritis. J Pain. 2016;17(3):374–82.
59. Chappell AS, Ossanna MJ, Liu-Seifert H, et al. Duloxetine, a centrally acting analgesic, in the treatment of patients with osteoarthritis knee pain: a 13-week, randomized, placebo-controlled trial. Pain. 2009;146(3):253–60.
60. Chappell AS, Desaiah D, Liu-Seifert H, et al. A double-blind, randomized, placebo-controlled study of the efficacy and safety of duloxetine for the treatment of chronic pain due to osteoarthritis of the knee. Pain Pract. 2011;11(1):33–41.
61. Enteshari-Moghaddam A, Azami A, Isazadehfar K, Mohebbi H, Habibzadeh A, Jahanpanah P. Efficacy of duloxetine and gabapentin in pain reduction in patients with knee osteoarthritis. Clin Rheumatol. 2019;38(10):2873–80.
62. Chen L, Gong M, Liu G, Xing F, Liu J, Xiang Z. Efficacy and tolerability of duloxetine in patients with knee osteoarthritis: a meta-analysis of randomised controlled trials. Intern Med J. 2019;49(12):1514–23.
63. Itoh N, Tsuji T, Ishida M, Ochiai T, Konno S, Uchio Y. Efficacy of duloxetine for multisite pain in patients with knee pain due to osteoarthritis: an exploratory post hoc analysis of a Japanese phase 3 randomized study. J Orthop Sci. 2021;26(1):141–8.
64. Hochberg MC, Altman RD, April KT, et al. American College of Rheumatology 2012 recommendations for the use of nonpharmacologic and pharmacologic therapies in osteoarthritis of the hand, hip, and knee. Arthritis Care Res (Hoboken). 2012;64(4):465–74.
65. Jevsevar DS. Treatment of osteoarthritis of the knee: evidence-based guideline, 2nd edition. J Am Acad Orthop Surg. 2013;21(9):571–6.
66. McAlindon TE, Bannuru RR, Sullivan MC, et al. OARSI guidelines for the non-surgical management of knee osteoarthritis. Osteoarthr Cartil. 2014;22(3):363–88.
67. Surveillance report 2017 – Osteoarthritis: care and management (2014) NICE guideline CG177 [Internet]. London: National Institute for Health and Care Excellence (UK); 2017.
68. Kolasinski SL, Neogi T, Hochberg MC, et al. 2019 American College of Rheumatology/arthritis foundation guideline for the management of osteoarthritis of the hand, hip, and knee. Arthritis Care Res (Hoboken). 2020;72(2):149–62.
69. Bannuru RR, Osani MC, Vaysbrot EE, et al. OARSI guidelines for the non-surgical management of knee, hip, and polyarticular osteoarthritis. Osteoarthr Cartil. 2019;27(11):1578–89.

70. Bruyère O, Honvo G, Veronese N, et al. An updated algorithm recommendation for the management of knee osteoarthritis from the European Society for Clinical and Economic Aspects of Osteoporosis, Osteoarthritis and Musculoskeletal Diseases (ESCEO). Semin Arthritis Rheum. 2019:1–14.
71. Guyatt GH, Oxman AD, Vist GE, Kunz R, Falck-Ytter Y, Alonso-Coello P, et al. GRADE: an emerging consensus on rating quality of evidence and strength of recommendations. BMJ. 2008;336(7650):924.
72. da Costa BR, Reichenbach S, Keller N, Nartey L, Wandel S, Juni P, et al. Effectiveness of non-steroidal anti-inflammatory drugs for the treatment of pain in knee and hip osteoarthritis: a network meta-analysis. Lancet. 2017;390(10090):e21–33.
73. Feeley BT, Gallo RA, Sherman S, Williams RJ. Management of osteoarthritis of the knee in the active patient. J Am Acad Orthop Surg. 2010;18(7):406–16.
74. National Institute for Health and Clinical Excellence. National Collaborating Centre for Chronic Conditions Osteoarthritis: national clinical guideline for care and management in adults. London: NICE; 2008.
75. Losina E, Weinstein AM, Reichmann WM, et al. Lifetime risk and age at diagnosis of symptomatic knee osteoarthritis in the US. Arthritis Care Res (Hoboken). 2013;65(5):703–11.
76. Khanna V, Sharma R. Incidence of primary osteoarthritis knee below 40 years of age and its etiological factors: OPD survey of 200 knee pain patients. Indian J Orthop. 2019;5(1):88–94.
77. Conrozier T. How to treat osteoarthritis in obese patients? Curr Rheumatol Rev. 2020;16(2):99–104.
78. Blagojevic M, Jinks C, Jeffery A, Jordan KP. Risk factors for onset of osteoarthritis of the knee in older adults: a systematic review and meta-analysis. Osteoarthr Cartil. 2010;18(1):24–33.
79. Galuska DA, Will JC, Serdula MK, Ford ES. Are health care professionals advising obese patients to lose weight? JAMA. 1999;282(16):1576–8.
80. Bray GA. A guide to obesity and the metabolic syndrome. Orlando, FL: CRC Press; 2011.
81. Torgerson JS, Hauptman J, Boldrin MN, Sjöström L. XENical in the prevention of diabetes in obese subjects (XENDOS) study: a randomized study of orlistat as an adjunct to lifestyle changes for the prevention of type 2 diabetes in obese patients. Diabetes Care. 2004;27(1):155–61.
82. LiverTox: Clinical and Research Information on Drug-Induced Liver Injury [Internet]. Bethesda (MD): National Institute of Diabetes and Digestive and Kidney Diseases; 2012
83. Bray GA, Hollander P, Klein S, et al. A 6-month randomized, placebo-controlled, dose-ranging trial of topiramate for weight loss in obesity. Obes Res. 2003;11(6):722–33.
84. Smith SM, Meyer M, Trinkley KE. Phentermine/topiramate for the treatment of obesity. Ann Pharmacother. 2013;47(3):340–9.
85. Astrup A, Rössner S, Van Gaal L, et al. Effects of liraglutide in the treatment of obesity: a randomised, double-blind, placebo-controlled study. Lancet. 2009;374(9701):1606–16.
86. McKinley TO, Borrelli J Jr, D'Lima DD, Furman BD, Giannoudis PV. Basic science of intra-articular fractures and posttraumatic osteoarthritis. J Orthop Trauma. 2010;24(9):567–70.
87. Schmal H, Marintschev I, Salzmann GM. Current status of anti-inflammatory therapy for posttraumatic osteoarthritis. Acta Orthop Belg. 2016; 82(3):427–39.
88. Scott CEH, MacDonald DJ, Howie CR. 'Worse than death' and waiting for a joint arthroplasty. Bone Joint J. 2019;101(8):941–50.
89. Li CS, Karlsson J, Winemaker M, Sancheti P, Bhandari M. Orthopedic surgeons feel that there is a treatment gap in management of early OA: international survey. Knee Surg Sports Traumatol Arthrosc. 2014;22(2):363–78.
90. Jung SY, Jang EJ, Nam SW, et al. Comparative effectiveness of oral pharmacologic interventions for knee osteoarthritis: a network meta-analysis. Mod Rheumatol. 2018;28(6):1021–8.
91. Higuera CA, Elsharkawy K, Klika AK, Brocone M, Barsoum WK. 2010 Mid-America orthopaedic association physician in training award: predictors of early adverse outcomes after knee and hip arthroplasty in geriatric patients. Clin Orthop Relat Res. 2011;469(5):1391–400.
92. Wongrakpanich S, Wongrakpanich A, Melhado K, Rangaswami J. A comprehensive review of non-steroidal anti-inflammatory drug use in the elderly. Aging Dis. 2018;9(1):143–50.
93. White WB, Kent J, Taylor A, Verburg KM, Lefkowith JB, Whelton A. Effects of celecoxib on ambulatory blood pressure in hypertensive patients on ACE inhibitors. Hypertension. 2002;39(4):929–34.
94. Bingham CO III, Sebba AI, Rubin BR, et al. Efficacy and safety of etoricoxib 30 mg and celecoxib 200 mg in the treatment of osteoarthritis in two identically designed, randomized, placebo-controlled, non-inferiority studies. Rheumatology (Oxford). 2007;46(3):496–507.
95. Mallen SR, Essex MN, Zhang R. Gastrointestinal tolerability of NSAIDs in elderly patients: a pooled analysis of 21 randomized clinical trials with celecoxib and nonselective NSAIDs. Curr Med Res Opin. 2011;27(7):1359–66.
96. Hunt RH, Barkun AN, Baron D, et al. Recommendations for the appropriate use of anti-inflammatory drugs in the era of the coxibs: defining the role of gastroprotective agents. Can J Gastroenterol. 2002;16(4):231–40.
97. Visser LE, Graatsma HH, Stricker BH. Contraindicated NSAIDs are frequently prescribed to elderly patients with peptic ulcer disease. Br J Clin Pharmacol. 2002;53(2):183–8.
98. Kent AP, Brueckmann M, Fraessdorf M, et al. Concomitant oral anticoagulant and nonsteroidal

anti-inflammatory drug therapy in patients with atrial fibrillation. J Am Coll Cardiol. 2018;72(3):255–67.

99. Baker M, Perazella MA. NSAIDs in CKD: are they safe? Am J Kidney Dis. 2020;76(4):546–57.
100. Nderitu P, Doos L, Jones PW, Davies SJ, Kadam UT. Non-steroidal anti-inflammatory drugs and chronic kidney disease progression: a systematic review. Fam Pract. 2013;30(3):247–55.
101. National Kidney Foundation. K/DOQI clinical practice guidelines for chronic kidney disease: evaluation, classification, and stratification. Am J Kidney Dis. 2002;39(2 Suppl 1):S1–266.
102. Zhan M, Doerfler RM, Xie D, et al. CRIC study investigators. Association of opioids and nonsteroidal anti-inflammatory drugs with outcomes in CKD: findings from the CRIC (Chronic Renal Insufficiency Cohort) Study. Am J Kidney Dis. 2020;76(2):184–93.
103. Meuwesen WP, du Plessis JM, Burger JR, Lubbe MS, Cockeran M. Prescribing patterns of non-steroidal anti-inflammatory drugs in chronic kidney disease patients in the South African private sector. Int J Clin Pharm. 2016;38(4):863–9.
104. Huang WN, Tso TK. Etoricoxib improves osteoarthritis pain relief, joint function, and quality of life in the extreme elderly. Bosn J Basic Med Sci. 2018;18(1):87–94.

10 Intra-articular Injection Therapy and Biologic Treatment

Seung-Suk Seo, In-Seung Lee, and Gi-Hun Lee

Abstract

Oral or parenteral administered drugs used to treat knee osteoarthritis (OA) enter the joint through complicated pharmacokinetic processes. Intra-articular (IA) injection therapy has a number of advantages over systemic administration such as bypassing this process and avoiding systemic adverse events. For IA injection therapy to work effectively, drugs must be injected accurately into the joints. Image guided injection using ultrasound is more useful than blind method for accurate IA injection. IA therapeutic agents for the treatment of knee OA include corticosteroids (CS), hyaluronic acid (HA), biologics. CS has a short-term effect on improving symptoms of knee OA, but HA has a relatively longer term effect. Biologic agents either target specific catabolic proinflammatory mediators or affect anabolism because OA results from an imbalance between catabolic and anabolic factors. Biologics used for treatment of knee OA are categorized into non-cellular or cell therapy. Non-cellular therapy includes human serum albumin, growth factors, cytokine antagonists. In particular, the recombinant human fibroblast growth factor 18 and the wnt receptor inhibitor have an anabolic effect. Cell therapy includes cell concentrates, mesenchymal stromal cells, and gene therapy. Recently, cell concentrates are commonly used for knee OA treatment as autologous point-of-care cell therapy regardless of its efficacy. Cell concentrates include stromal vascular fraction (SVF), bone marrow aspirate concentrate (BMAC), plasma rich platelet (PRP), and autologous protein solution. The therapeutic effects of PRP remain for more than 6 months, but effect size has not reached minimal clinical important difference. Mesenchymal stromal cells (MSCs) are grown from cell concentrates in vitro and separated with only cells with MSC characteristics. MSCs used in the treatment of knee OA include bone marrow-derived MSCs and adipose-derived MSCs. Despite the clinical potential of MSCs, clinical efficacy in knee OA treatment is limited. According to guidelines from non-profit organizations, PRP and MSC injections are strongly recommended against in patients with knee OA.

Keywords

Intra-articular injection · Pharmacokinetics
Ultrasound · Corticosteroid · Hyaluronic acid
Polydeoxyribonucleotide · Hypertonic dextrose · Biologics · Growth factors
Cytokine antagonists · Plasma rich platelet
Mesenchymal stromal cells

S.-S. Seo (✉) · I.-S. Lee · G.-H. Lee
Department of Orthopedics, Haeundae Bumin Hospital, Busan, South Korea
e-mail: seoss@bumin.co.kr

S.-S. Seo (ed.), *A Strategic Approach to Knee Arthritis Treatment*,
https://doi.org/10.1007/978-981-16-4217-3_10

10.1 Introduction

Osteoarthritis (OA) is defined as an irreversible and progressive damage to the articular cartilage of the knee. It was once known as a 'wear and tear' disease. However, complex interactions between aging, genetic, metabolic, biochemical, and biomechanical factors play an important role in the development of OA. Clinical manifestations of knee OA are pain, stiffness, joint swelling, and loss of motion. These symptoms can interfere with work and normal daily activities. The incidence of knee OA is increasing rapidly in the aging society. Knee OA produces a huge economic burden to society due to high prevalence and functional disabilities [1].

Current treatment for OA focuses on relieving symptoms and improving function. General guidelines for the management of knee OA mostly recommend a combination of non-pharmacological and pharmacological treatment [2]. Oral medications such as acetaminophen and nonsteroidal anti-inflammatory drugs (NSAIDs) are commonly used as pharmacological treatments. However, long-term use of oral medications has raised concerns about their risk/benefit ratio issues, especially for patients with cardiovascular, gastrointestinal, and metabolic comorbidities [3]. Intra-articular (IA) injections, such as a corticosteroid (CS) and hyaluronic acid (HA), may be used to treat knee OA after other conservative treatments have failed [4]. IA injection became popular in the late twentieth century since the introduction of IA CS. IA drug delivery might be the ideal mode of drug delivery for these patients because it has many advantages such as increased local bioavailability, reduced systemic exposure, and lower total drug cost [5].

Despite a number of advantages of IA drug delivery, there are many controversial issues regarding the safety and efficacy of IA injection procedure and drug delivery. The incidence of adverse events (AEs) attributable to IA therapies in knee OA is very low, furthermore, these events are rarely serious. Clinician can distinguish self-limited AEs, such as post-injection pain and swelling that are the most frequently reported AEs, from not self-limited AEs, such as septic arthritis that is rarely reported [6]. For a safe and accurate IA drug delivery, direct IA injection with a needle is most preferred. There is a question about the efficacy of IA injection therapy because IA injections itself have a strong placebo effect. The effect size of placebo injection is significantly greater than did oral or topical placebos [7]. IA-normal saline placebo injection yields a significant improvement in symptoms up to 6 months after the injection in knee OA [8]. This placebo effect might be caused by dilution and reduction of inflammatory mediators in the joint effusion, providing relief of perceived pain and subjective stiffness. As to the efficacy of IA drug, there are problems that need to be solved such as the number of injections, bioavailability of injection vehicle, effect size of injections, long-term efficacy, or exact mechanism of action because of a lack of science based evidence of IA injections for OA [9]. Despite various controversies over efficacy, IA injection treatments are still commonly used in clinical practice.

CS and HA injections have been attempted for decades to treat the symptoms of knee OA and its pros and cons are already well known [10]. Recently, there is a growing interest in the delivery of autologous blood products, recombinant proteins, particles, cells, and gene therapy vectors to diseased joints. Local delivery in this way is potentially safer, less expensive, and more effective than parenteral delivery. However, better drug formulations with longer lasting efficacy are needed to reduce the need for burdensome repeated injections of soluble therapeutic agents [11]. Many biologic agents, including non-cellular or cellular components, were introduced and investigated extensively for OA treatment since a decade ago. The efficacy of biological agents has yet to be proven, but some of these drugs are undergoing clinical research, producing promising results [5].

In this chapter, we briefly describe the pharmacokinetics of synovial joint and explain the injection technique to increase the accuracy of needle placement by manual or using imaging modalities. We also describe the mechanism of action of the IA therapeutic agents including biologics and discuss clinical studies that have investigated small molecule drug therapies and provide a high-level overview of biologics including cell-based therapies. Finally, we deliver an update on a critical assessment of some of the most anticipated and promising IA injection therapies of knee OA currently in clinical development.

10.2 Influx and Efflux of the Molecules in the Synovial Joint

The drug delivery via systemic administration is not efficient because the cartilage is an avascular tissue. When a therapeutic substance is administered through oral or parenteral, the substance does not reach the cartilage directly, instead, reaches the joint fluid through the capillary network and interstitial tissue in the synovial membrane and then diffused to the extracellular matrix (ECM) of the cartilage. In order to treat knee OA using certain therapeutic substances, the influx and efflux of the therapeutic substances or molecules, residence time within the joint, and diffusion in the ECM of the cartilage must be well understood.

In order for the molecules to enter the joint cavity from the synovial capillaries, the molecule must first pass through the walls of the capillaries and then through the ECM of synovial intima [12]. About 50% of synovial capillaries has a fenestration in the endothelial lining that is faced to the joint cavity. Such orientation facilitates the transport of molecules from these capillaries to synovial interstitium, vice versa. The synovial membrane is characterized by non-epithelial cells, wide intercellular gaps, no cell junctions, and no basement membrane [13]. The synovial membrane acts as a semipermeable membrane controlling molecular traffic into and out of the joint space. Furthermore, no basement membrane in the synovial layer facilitates molecular transport. The molecules exiting the blood vessels through the fenestration diffuse to synovial interstitium and then pass through the synovial membrane into the joint cavity. The factors determining the movement of the molecules are the pore size of the fenestration in the endothelium of the capillaries and the tight space of the synovial interstitial matrix. Small molecular weight (MW) compounds (MW <10 kDa) freely transport through passive diffusion. Because the fenestration in the endothelial lining of the capillaries roles as a size-dependent sieving effect, transportation of molecules from blood into synovial fluid is quantitatively related to molecular size. Therefore, relatively large molecules have different synovial fluid:serum concentration ratios compared to smaller molecules. For example, the concentration ratio of normal synovial fluid:serum for albumin (MW 67 kDa) is ~0.40; for the much larger molecules α2–macroglobulin (MW 820 kDa) is 0.03 [14]. In inflamed joint, capillary permeability increases, improving the entry of macromolecules into the joint space. Evidence indicating this effect can be found in the protein content of synovial fluid from patients with rheumatoid arthritis, which increases compared to healthy controls and significantly increases the ratio of large and small molecular components in rheumatoid arthritis samples [5, 14] (Fig. 10.1).

Molecules in synovial fluid are excreted through the vasculature and lymphatic system in synovium. Small molecules also leave via the vasculature whereas macromolecules such as proteins exit via the lymphatic system [15]. The residence time of molecules in the joint is affected by the rate at which they enter and exit the joint. Small molecules have short IA residence time because they easily enter and rapidly exit from the joint via the synovial capillaries. The entry of macromolecules into joints is constrained by a size-dependent sieving effect of the endothelial fenestration of capillaries. Although IA injection with macromolecules can bypass the capillary sieving effect, the IA residence time of macromolecules is typically a few hours or less because its removal from joints occurs via the lymphatic system regardless of its size. The half-lives of various substances reported are 1.23–13.1 h for albumin (MW 67 kDa), 0.35 h for lidocaine (MW 234 Da), and 26.3 h for hyaluronic acid (MW 3 × 10^6 Da). IA half-lives of NSAIDs were around 1.1–5.2 h and hydrocortisone at around 0.3–4.2 h [16].

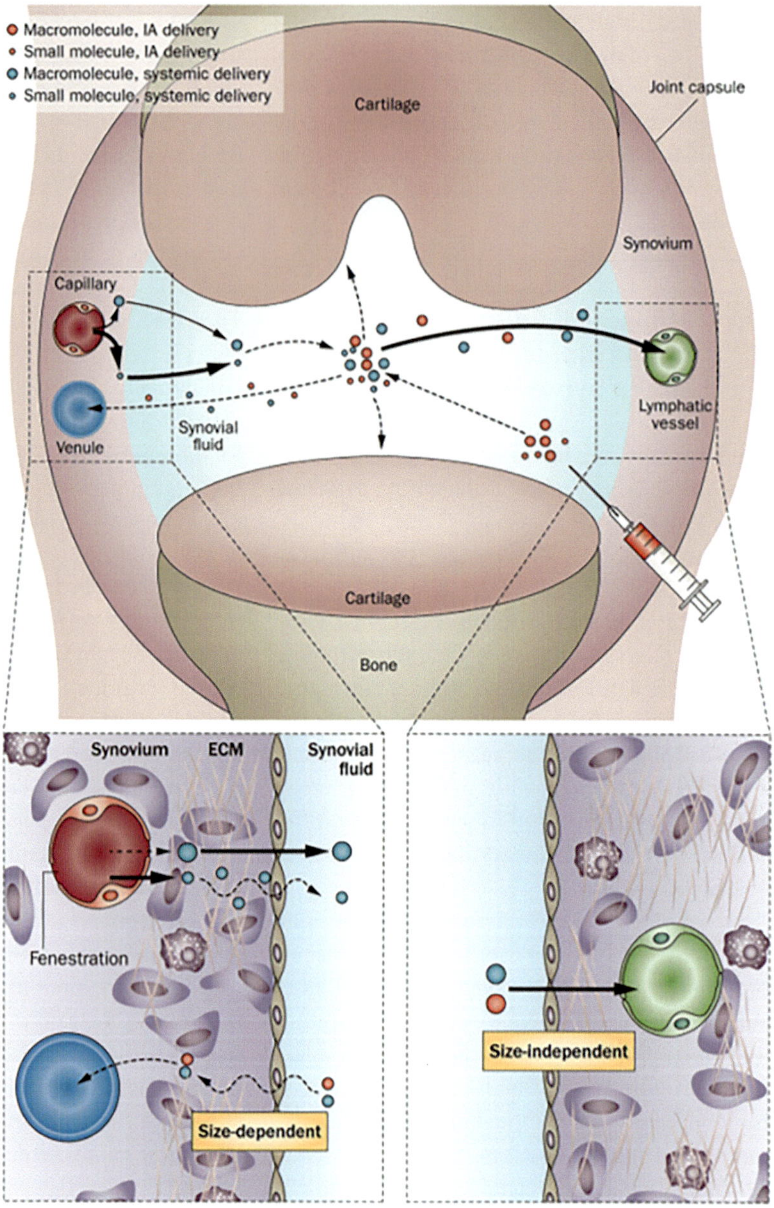

Fig. 10.1 Influx and efflux of the molecules in the synovial joint. Systematically administered molecules in the capillaries enter the joint cavity through capillary wall, extracellular matrix (ECM), and synovial membrane. Small molecules pass through capillary wall and synovium relatively easily but major resistance to their entry is the ECM of the synovial interstitium. Large molecules in the capillary are sieved by the fenestrated endothelium of the capillaries, which are obstacles to enter the joint cavity. Intra-articular injection is a way of circumventing this resistance. Molecules in synovial fluid are excreted through the vasculature and lymphatic system in synovium. Small molecules also leave via the vasculature whereas large molecules such as proteins exit via the lymphatic system. (Copyright permission: Nat. Rev. Rheumatol. Evans, 2013)

Likewise, the residence time of molecules is short regardless of its size. Furthermore, in case of joint inflammation, the residence time of molecules becomes shorter because of increased vascularity and lymphatic flow [17]. This short residence time of the molecules is a major barrier to successful therapy. The IA injected therapeutic drug must be maintained within the joint for sufficient time to work. To do so, it is necessary to develop various methods to increase the drug residence time.

10.3 Intra-articular Injection Technique

The IA injection of therapeutic agents is an attractive method for the local treatment of joint diseases. To achieve the maximal potential treatment, various therapeutic agents should be correctly delivered into the joint. It is important to position the needle precisely inside the joint in order to achieve sufficient therapeutic effect and reduce the AEs of the injection. Incorrect placement of the needle also causes more pain and discomfort to the patient during and after the procedure, which can have a negative influence on the efficacy of the product being injected [4]. Injection technique is a very important factor for accuracy of IA knee injection, especially in symptomatic knee OA with no effusion [4]. However, it is difficult to place accurately a needle into the IA space of the knee without effusion. Jones et al. [18] evaluated the accuracy of needle placement into the IA space of the knee in the absence of a joint effusion and reported that 39 (66%) of 59 knee joint injections were IA and almost one-third were extra-articular. If therapeutic materials are injected into extra-synovial tissue, it may result in either painful blockage of the injected material outflow or the development of acute pseudoseptic arthritis. Therefore, an accurate needle placement is very important for IA drug delivery for knee OA treatment. There are two techniques, such as blind (palpation guided or landmark guided) or image guided injection, for IA knee injection. Accurate IA knee injection is not easy for patients who have dry joint, especially obese and/or severe arthritic knees by blind technique. Various methods such as injection of contrast or air with radiography [19], ultrasonography (US)[20] or fluoroscopy [21], magnetic resonance imaging (MRI) [22], surgical confirmation of intra- or extra-articular placement of drugs [23] have been used to evaluate the accuracy of IA knee injection. The backflow technique is also a helpful method for confirmation of the IA placement of needle during injection that has an accuracy of about 97% [24]. However, because all of these techniques are influenced by observer error in the evaluation of images, there is no gold standard for evaluating the accuracy of IA knee injections. Accuracy is improved by fluoroscopic and US guided techniques, and these tools are particularly useful for treating joints that are difficult to access, such as obese or dry joint. In this section, we included all studies independently attempted to confirm IA placement, including successful aspiration of synovial fluid. Furthermore, the results on accuracy of the sites of injection were described by injection site and whether image guidance was used or not, and this review did not look separately at accuracy by image guided method.

10.3.1 Injection Techniques: Sites, Approaches

A number of IA injection sites have been proposed to maximize therapeutic benefits and avoid incorrect knee injection when performing IA knee injections using blind or image guided techniques. Injection "sites" refer to specific areas in the knee for needle entry, and injection "approaches" refer to techniques that deliver the needle, including angle of the needle or position of the knee. There are various approaches to the same injection site, and there is a lot of controversy over which area is the best injection area for accurate injection. In a systematic review, eight different knee injection sites were identified regardless of injection technique that were (1) anteromedial, (2) medial mid-patellar, (3) superomedial patellar, (4) anterolateral, (5) lateral mid-patellar, (6) superolateral patellar, (7) lateral suprapatellar bursa, and (8) infrapatellar [25]. Infrapatellar site will not be described due to lack of literatures (Fig. 10.2).

10.3.1.1 Anteromedial (AM)

For AM joint site, the needle is inserted into the portal formed by inferomedial patellar border, patellar tendon, and medial tibial plateau, directing the needle toward intercondylar notch with the knee flexed 30° [21] or 90° with the patient's leg hanging over the side of the examination table [23]. Accuracy rates of AM site in knee 30° and 90° flexion were 86% and 71%, respectively [26]. The use of the standard AM site may result in pain and potential harm with accidental injection into the cruciate ligaments, the ligamentum mucosum, or the fat pad.

10.3.1.2 Medial Mid-Patellar (MMP)

This technique is performed with the knee in extension. The patella is pulled medially or laterally, and a needle is advanced under the patella. Injection via the MMP approach is performed

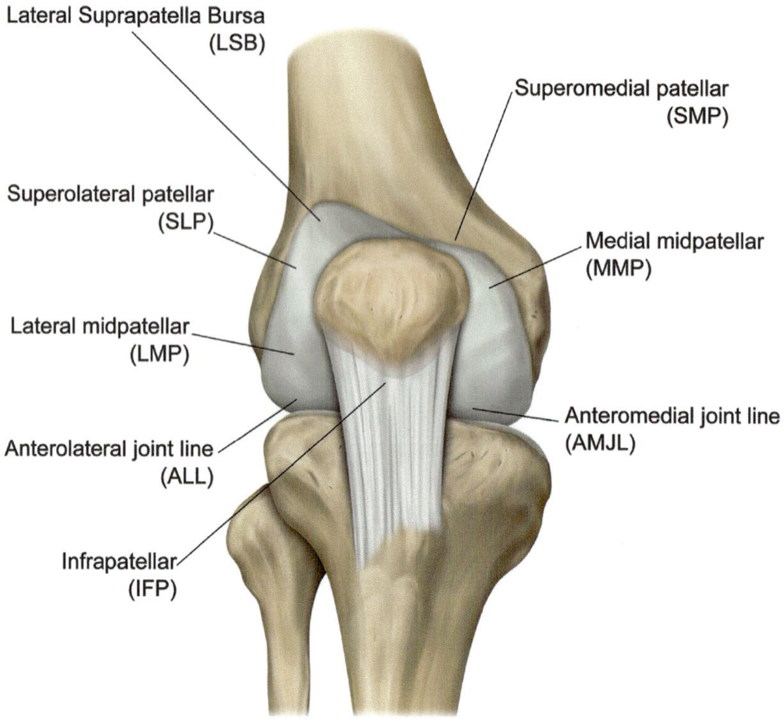

Fig. 10.2 Proposed intra-articular injection site

with the needle placed on the medial side of the knee joint under the middle of the patella (midpole) and directed towards the lateral patellar midpole [27]. The needles were inserted carefully to avoid injuring special structures such as the patella retinacula, periosteum, retropatella cartilage, and fat pad. MMP portal showed the least accuracy rate, which was 56% [23], 77.3% in blind injection [27], 75% in US guided injection [28].

10.3.1.3 Superomedial Patellar (SMP)

The SMP injection is performed by inserting a needle in a 45° cephalomedial to caudolateral direction between the femoral condyle and the lateral border of patella at the superior 1/3 margin of the patella with the knee extended. Gentle shaking of the patella will identify its border to facilitate the needle insertion. This portal provides 80% accuracy rate when using blind techniques [29].

10.3.1.4 Anterolateral (AL)

The standard AL injection was performed in the site formed by inferolateral patellar border, patellar tendon, and lateral tibial plateau with the patient sitting with the knees hanging freely over the side of the examination table and flexed to approximately 90°. However, there were several modified AL approaches regarding knee flexion degrees or needle direction. Different knee position had been proposed according to knee bending such as the knee flexed between 30° and 40° [21] or flexed to 90° [30] or full flexion ranging from 100° to 130° [31]. After palpation of the anatomic landmarks, the injection portal was selected one-fingerbreadth proximal to the tibial joint surface and one-fingerbreadth lateral to the patellar tendon. The needle was advanced obliquely toward the intercondylar notch or directing the needle toward medial femoral condyle. Accuracy rate of this approach was 71% [4], 85% [23], 97% [30], 97.1% [31]. These approaches are useful when the knee cannot be extended sufficiently, or when there is only a minimal amount of fluid in the knee joint. The AL site would provoke less pain as compared to the SL site [32]. The major problem with these approaches is that it is difficult to obtain fluid from the affected joint.

10.3.1.5 Lateral Mid-Patellar (LMP)

The LMP site is the most commonly utilized (64%) technique for knee arthrography among the North American radiologists [33]. For the LMP approach, the injection was made between patella and patellar groove at the mid lateral patellar junction with the knee extended. The needle was advanced transversely directing the needle at a 45° angle between the articular surfaces of the patellofemoral joint at the midpoint of the patella and pulled laterally [34]. Accuracy rate of the LMP approach was 55%–86%, that rate was directly proportional to severity of radiographic OA assessment [26], 76% [23], 91.5% [35], 93% [4]. The LMP has the advantage of allowing the needle to pass through the minimal soft tissue and reach the IA space. On the other hand, for those apprehensive individuals who involuntarily and forcefully contract the quadriceps muscles during a procedure, the elderly, individuals with knee contractures, the obese, large patellofemoral osteophytes, or wheelchair-bound individuals, the LMP approach can be difficult and/or inconvenient in these individuals. In addition, because less subcutaneous fat is transversed by the needle in the LMP portal, local AEs of injections may occur which can be easily observed, including visible ecchymosis, hematoma, and cutaneous atrophy or foreign body granuloma at the puncture site caused by reflux of CS or HA back through the needle tract [36].

10.3.1.6 Superolateral Patellar (SLP)

For the standard SLP approach, the patient is positioned supine on the examination table with the knee extended, and the patella and soft spot are palpated. The landmark is the intersection of the horizontal line from the upper border of the patella and another line crossing the lateral border of the patella. The needle was inserted in a 45° angle cephalolateral to caudomedial direction with parallel to the anterior femoral cortex. Accuracy rate of SLP site ranged from 55% to 100%, but the SLP approach resulted in the highest pooled accuracy rate of 91% (95% CI 84–99) among IA knee injection sites [37]. However, the SLP approach will not be suitable for several reasons: large osteophytes blocked the path for passage of the needle; the pain associated with patellar manipulation; determination of the configuration of bony landmarks is difficult, especially in obese patients.

10.3.1.7 Lateral Suprapatellar Bursa (LSB)

In the LSB approach, the needle is inserted from the superolateral aspect of patella, one-fingerbreadth above and one-fingerbreadth lateral to the patella with the knee extended [35, 38]. Accuracy rate of the LSB approach was 83.7% by blind and 96.0% by US guided injection [39], 82% by blind and 100% by US guided injection [40]. One of the advantages of an IA injection through the SB is that it reduces the risk of injuring other tissues in the knee joint [39]. When small effusions within the SB are detected, dynamic examination, such as isometric contraction of the quadriceps muscle or forced dorsiflexion of the foot with the knee extended, may be helpful. Quadriceps activation and hyperextension induce proximal shifting of fluid by displacing the Hoffa fat pad against the femoral condyles and tightening the posterior fascia.

10.3.2 Factors Related to Intra-articular Knee Accuracy

Accuracy of IA knee injections is affected by intrinsic factors such as obesity, severity of OA, presence or absence of joint effusion, etc. and external factors such as clinician's experience, site of needle insertion, and use of image guide. Accurate IA knee injection is not easy for patients who have dry joint, especially obese and/or severe arthritic knees. These intrinsic factors can not be modified when they first appear in the clinic, but extrinsic factors can be modified by clinician efforts.

In a systematic review with statistical pooling of accuracy rates, the SLP site resulted in high accuracy rates, with the highest pooled accuracy of 91% (95% CI 84–99%) and pooled accuracy rates for the LMP, AL, and AM site were 85% (95% CI 68–100%), 67% (95% CI 43–91%), and 72% (95% CI 65–78%), respectively [37]. This systematic review did not mention about guided injection data. The SLP site resulted in 100% accuracy rate, especially, in patient with effusion by blinded injection [19]. When attempting blind injection, SMP site (82%) had the highest injection accuracy among the three medial sites, followed by AM (74%) and MMP (64%), while SLP site (87%) had the greatest injection accuracy among the four lateral sites, followed by LMP (84%), LSB (83%), and AL (70%). When US guided injection was attempted, the accuracy was 100% on the SMP site and 86% on the MMP, which significantly increased the accuracy compared to the blind injection. Moreover, all four lateral sites (AL, LMP, SLP, and LSB) had 95–100% accuracy rate, when US guided injections were performed, and the best lateral site was still the SLP. The accuracy of medial sites was improved largely than the lateral sites by US guided injections. Therefore, US guided injections at MMP, SMP, LSB, and SLP sites were found to be significantly more accurate than their respective blinded injections. The experience of injector affected the accuracy rate of the blinded injections at the SLP site, which was 55% (95% CI 34–74) for the less experienced injector compared to 100% (95% CI 81–100) for the more experienced injector [38]. However, similar accuracy was found for less experienced junior clinicians and injectors when US guided injections were performed. When a research fellow performed the injections using US guided, accuracy rate of IA injection was 91% [41]. US guided has significantly improved the performance and effectiveness of the procedure, with a 43% decrease in pain associated with US guided procedures and a 26% increase in the proportion of treatment responses [40]. Accuracy is improved by US guided techniques that are particularly valuable for treating joints that are difficult to access, such as obese or dry joint.

10.3.3 Ultrasound Guided Injection Technique

Although the guideline of 2016 European League against Rheumatism (EULAR) recommends that IA injections using image guidance be used in specific situations but not routinely, IA injections using US have many advantages. US allows real-time monitoring during needle placement in a fast and less invasive manner without the risk of radiation exposure. In addition, a US machine is less expensive and widely available than a fluoroscopy or computed tomography/magnetic resonance scanner.

Choosing the right US device is important for accurate IA injection. In particular, appropriate transducers and ultrasonic frequency should be selected depending on the region of the musculoskeletal system. High frequency (7–15 MHz) line transducer is appropriate for the IA knee injection. This helps to obtain images of relatively superficial areas, such as knee joints, because of their low penetration and good resolution. Echogenicity refers to the ability to reflect a US wave. Each tissue type has a particular echogenicity in its normal state. Based on its echogenicity, a structure can be distinguished by hyperechoic (white on the screen), hypoechoic (gray on the screen), and anechoic (black on the screen). Bone appears anechoic or black on US and has a bright hyperechoic rim. Because the US beam cannot pass through the cortical bone, it casts an acoustic shadow underneath intensely hyperechoic bony structure. Articular cartilage appears grey or hypoechoic rim over a hyperechoic bony cortex. Blood vessels and joint fluid also appear anechoic. Muscles are hypoechoic with striate structure and fat is almost anechoic. Fascia/fascicles and other connective tissue appear as hyperechoic lines. Nerves appear hyperechoic with a stippled honeycomb pattern with hypo-anechoic fascia scattered between bright backgrounds. Tendons and ligaments appear hyperechoic, similar to the distal nerves. Tendons can be observed with characteristic striation in the long-axis view and are more *anisotropic* than nerves [42].

In order to inject needles accurately under US guided, meticulous manipulation of ultrasonic transducer is needed. To get a better image, clinician need to understand the angle of incidence. The angle of incidence is an angle that the US waves encounter a line perpendicular to the structure (Fig. 10.3). The closer the ultrasonic trans-

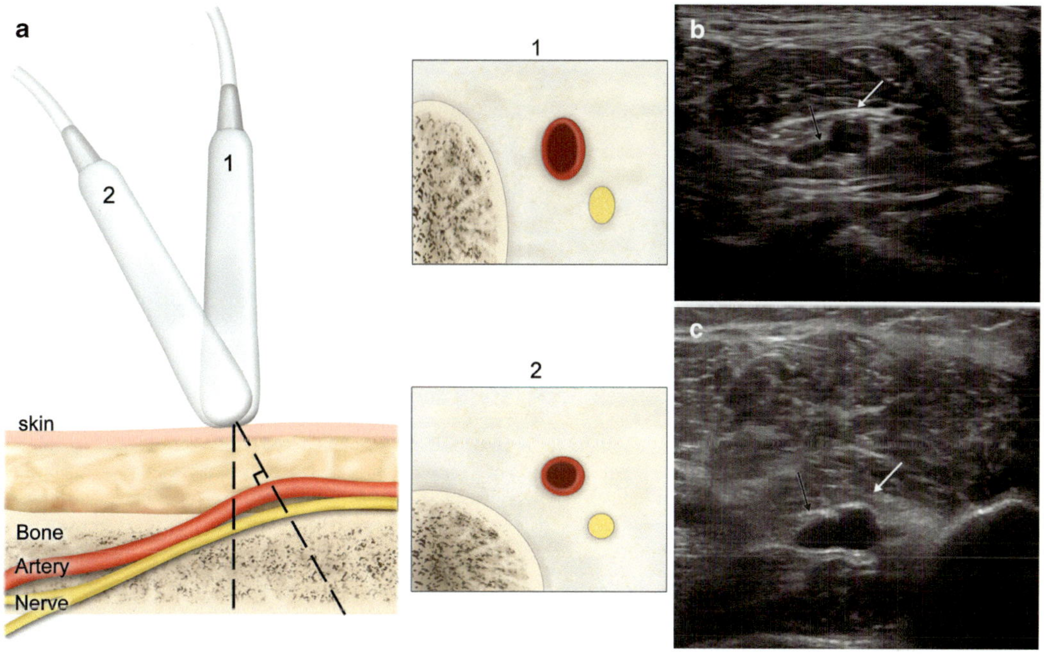

Fig. 10.3 Effects of the different angle of incidence. (**a**) Trajectory of US wave with probe 2 is more perpendicular to the surface of the artery and nerve. It shows more rounded and defined image of the artery and nerve than image obtained with probe1, of which US wave trajectory has a more parallel to the surface of object. (**b**) Oblique angle of incidence shows less defined image of anterior tibial artery (*white arrow*) and vein (*black arrow*). (**c**) Perpendicular angle of incidence shows a more round and defined image of the same vasculatures (Ultrasound photographs were provided in favor of Dr. BS Koo)

ducer and the surface of the object are to the perpendicular, the more US waves are reflected by the transducer to obtain a better image. Conversely, if the US waves become more parallel to the surface of the object, the image will have less definition. Better images can be obtained by adjusting the angle of incidence of the transducer with manipulation such as tilting or rotation. A close-to-perpendicular angle of incidence is also critical for better needle visualization during US guided needle insertion. To achieve better needle visualization, in addition to transducer manipulation, it is recommended to change the needle approach and advance more vertically to the US waves. Manipulating methods of ultrasonic transducers to obtain better images include pressure, alignment (sliding), rotation, and tilting [42].

US wave produces many responses, such as scatter reflection, transmission, refraction, and specular reflection, when traveling through tissue or materials. Scatter reflection is caused by the deflection of the US wave in several directions toward or away from the probe. Scattering occurs on small or irregular objects. Transmission refers to the continuing US wave through tissue away from the probe. Refraction is caused by when the US waves come into contact the interface between two mediums with different propagation velocities, the US wave is refracted bent depending upon the difference in velocities. Specular reflection is caused by reflection from a large, smooth surface such as a bone and returns the US wave toward the probe when it is perpendicular to the US beam [43]. As result, various kinds of artifacts can be seen on the monitor in addition to normal anatomy. Operators performing IA needle injection should discriminate and understand US artifacts such as reverberation, scattering, and acoustic shadowing caused by air bubble in the needle tip. Reverberation artifact is caused when a US beam encounters two strong parallel reflectors. This represents a linear density at the same interval representing multiple visualized needles

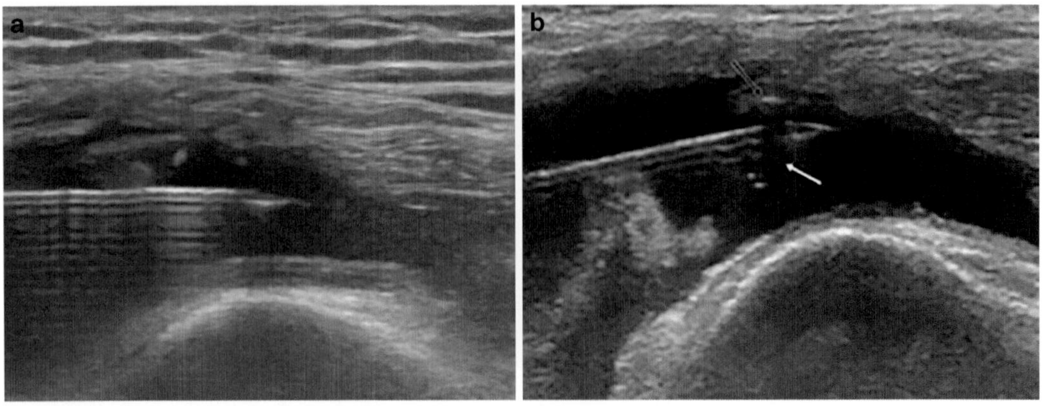

Fig. 10.4 US artifacts observed during needle insertion. (**a**) Reverberation artifact is that there are multiple needles visualized under the actual needle and equally spaced linear densities that represent ultrasound waves bouncing back and forth within the lumen of the needle. (**b**) A small amount of air (*black arrow*) serves as the perfect medium to generate an acoustic shadow (*white arrow*), as air does not conduct ultrasound. This image looks like the tip of needle is broken

under the actual needle. When the US energy returns to the probe to process finally, a duplicate image of the needle is displayed on the screen. This duplicate image appears deeper than the actual needle because more time has elapsed for the US energy to return to the probe. Because air does not conduct US, a small amount of air serves as the perfect medium for generating dropout shadow. The presence of an air bubble at the needle tip generated an acoustic shadow [44] (Fig. 10.4).

There are in-plane and out-of-plane methods for inserting needles into the joints under US guide. In-plane needle placement is a method that the needle can be seen on the US monitor in the long-axis view because long axis of the needle is located within the US scanning plane. Out-of-plane needle placement is a method that the long axis of the needle is directed at right angle to the scanning plane so the needle can be seen as a white dot of echo in the short-axis view (Fig. 10.5). The in-plane mode is a commonly preferred approach because it can visualize the entire needle. When performing needle insertion, especially with out-of-plane method, dynamic tilting or sliding of the transducer may help track the tip of the needle because the US beam has a very thin width of about 1 mm, so the needle can enter and exit viewing field even with subtle movements. Visualizing the tip of the needle is essential for accurate needle insertion. However, inexperienced operators often miss the tip of the needle or the entire needle from viewing field. In these instances, it is necessary to look at the probe again and re-align the needle to the US plane. If only the tip of the needle is out of sight, the operator can pull the needle back a little and try again with a slight reorientation [42].

There are several technical tips for enhancing needle placement under US guide. Use larger needles than smaller ones as possible. Large needles are more easily visualized. Direct the US beam perpendicular to the needle rather than parallel to it. Use styletted needles if possible, which decreases reverberation artifact. Fill the needle with a clear solution rather than air. Insert the needle with its bevel either pointing towards the US probe or away from it. The relatively rougher bevel results in more US scatter, enhancing the tip. Try to needle movement, which the needle is inserted in a short "in-and-out, side-to-side" motion causes deflection of the adjacent soft tissues and makes the trajectory of the needle more discernible. Use hydrolocation technique that injecting a small amount of a clear solution to the targeting site can enhance the visibility of the needle tip.

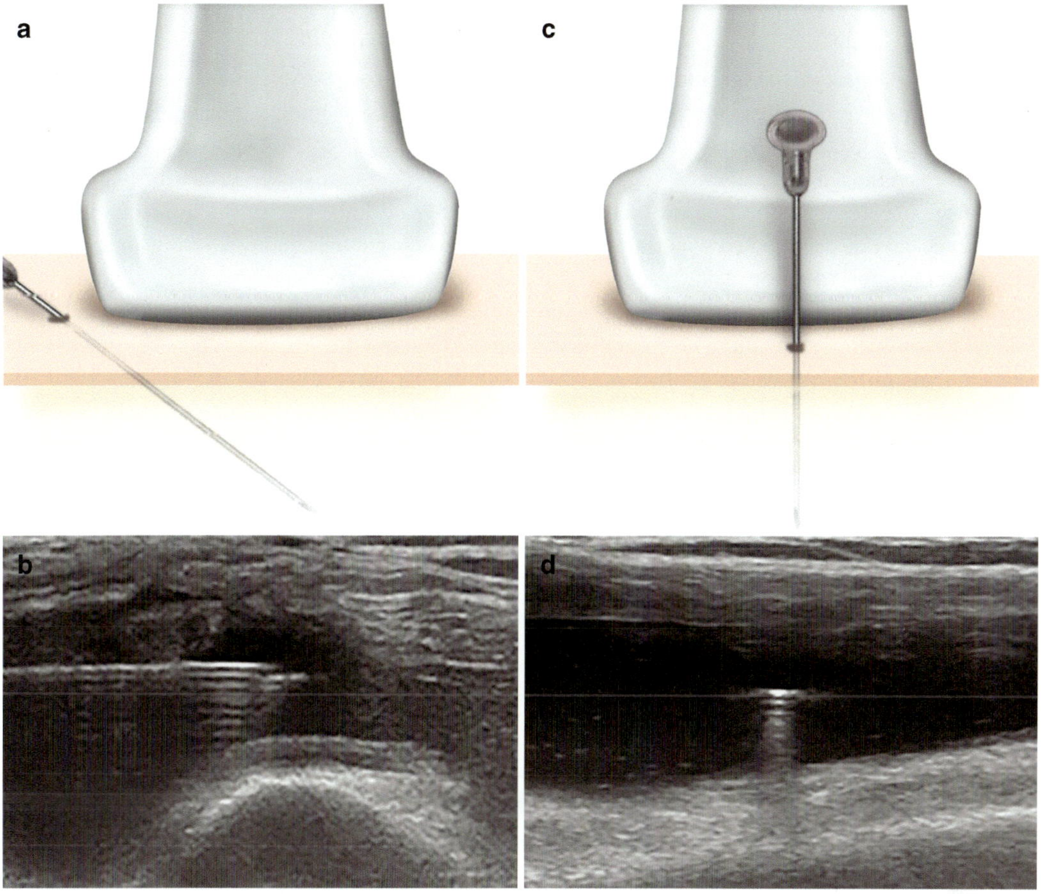

Fig. 10.5 Methods of needle insertion into joints under ultrasonic guide. (**a**) In-plane needle placement. Long axis of the needle is located within the US scanning plane. (**b**) Needle can be seen on the US monitor in the long-axis view. (**c**) Out-of-plane needle placement is a method that the long axis of the needle is directed at right angle to the scanning plane. (**d**) Needle can be seen as a white dot of echo in the short-axis view

10.3.4 Skin Preparation and Aseptic Technique, Choice of Needle, and Adverse Events

To reduce the risk of infection, IA injections should always be performed under sterile conditions using an aseptic technique. Povidone-iodine and/or alcohol was used to disinfect the skin around the injection portal. Operators should wear aseptic gloves and use sterilized gel for US probes. Only a sterilization wrap with pores to expose the applicable site might be needed during the procedure. Local anesthesia is usually not required before treatment, cooling spray or local anesthetic may be used for large and thick joints or pain sensitive areas or patients. In general, drug injection usually uses 22–25 gauge needles and 18–21 gauge thick needles for joint aspiration. No.25 gauge needle was occasionally used to decrease pain from injection. The length of the needle mostly chosen is regular-length (1.25 in and 1.5 in). When performing injection using the standard AM and AL site, the distance from the skin edge to the articular surface of the femoral condyle ranged from 4.5 cm to 5.5 cm (1.8 in to 2.2 in). The needle length of 2 inches is needed to clear the IA fat pad and reach the IA space in these sites [4]. Therefore, the length of the needle can be determined by measuring the expected distance of the injection path on the US or MRI, and it is necessary to prepare enough needle length to fit the path.

AEs from IA injection therapy may occur either by injection itself or by drugs used. If therapeutic materials are injected into extra-synovial tissue, such as the anterior fat pad and extra-synovial tissue layers, it may result in injection site pain due to painful blockage of the injected material outflow. HA injection might develop acute pseudoseptic arthritis. CS injection into extra-articular tissue produces skin hypopigmentation, atrophy of subcutaneous fat and muscle. Although there are relatively few AEs associated with IA injection of CSs or HAs, IA infections are serious AEs. Incidences of infection 1 in 3000 to 1 in 50,000 have been reported in association with IA CS injection. Although these rates are low, AEs of CSs, such as the increased cumulative risk of infection with repeat administration and concern about cartilage damage, create reluctance to inject CS into the joints too frequently. No rigid guidelines on this matter exist, but most practitioners are reluctant to inject a joint more than once every 3–6 months, unless delivering agents such as HA, which require multiple injections. Minor AEs include injection site pain (1 to 33%), local swelling (<1 to 30%), and local skin problems (3 to 21%). Pseudoseptic reactions can occur in 1 to 3%, usually after repeated multiple HA injections. It is characterized by joint inflammation and swelling not associated with joint infection [29]. According to a recent retrospective Danish study (n = 22,370), actual joint infections (septic arthritis) had a very low incidence (0.08%, 95% CI 0.03–0.12), and only 11 patients were diagnosed with septic arthritis (~1 in 2000 injections). Risk factors for this serious condition include old age, male, and pre-existing articular disease [30]. As the IA injection is an invasive procedure, there are absolute and relative contraindications. Absolute contraindications include known hypersensitivity to the injection, significant skin breakdown or osteochondral fracture at the injection site, bacteremia, osteomyelitis, sepsis, septic arthritis, periarticular conditions such as cellulitis, joint prosthesis, or uncontrolled coagulopathy. Relative contraindications are not clear, so they should be decided on a case-by-case basis [31].

10.4 Intra-articular Therapeutic Agents

Various kinds of materials have been developed as IA therapeutic agents for knee OA. CS and HA are most commonly used drugs for management of pain with knee OA failed to respond to non-pharmacologic treatment, NSAIDs or analgesics despite questions have been raised about the effectiveness. Standard IA treatment includes CS and HA, and its efficacy and AEs have been extensively investigated. Besides standard IA treatment, polydeoxyribonucleotide (PDRN) and hypertonic dextrose are frequently used for knee OA in the clinics. However, there are a few, low level clinical research with them for evaluating its efficacy of treatment of knee OA. OA results from an imbalance between catabolic and anabolic factors, and biologic agents either target specific catabolic proinflammatory mediators or affect anabolism more generally. Biologic agents show excellent clinical results in other rheumatic inflammatory diseases. There has been a lot of clinical research on biologic agents, assuming that biologic agents will have similar effects in the treatment of OA. Results of clinical studies did not support the routine use of biologic agents for OA management. However, there is still hope for biologic agents in the future treatment of OA [45]. Biologics have four sub-categories such as non-cellular therapeutics, expanded cell therapies, gene therapies, and point-of care autologous cell therapies [9].

10.4.1 Standard Intra-articular Treatments

10.4.1.1 Corticosteroids

Steroids have variable structures, functions, and sites of effect. Steroid molecules vary mainly due to changes in functional groups attached to their carbon rings. Human CSs are produced in the adrenal gland and have a wide range of physiologic effects. CSs can be classified as mineralocorticoids (e.g., aldosterone) that control water and electrolyte physiology and glucocorticoids (e.g., cortisol) that control metabolism and inflammation. CS-like molecules have been synthesized for use in drug therapy because of its powerful anti-inflammatory effects. The synthetic CSs are derivatives of prednisolone (an analogue of human cortisol). Methylprednisolone is the methyl derivative of prednisolone, whereas dexamethasone, betamethasone, and triamcinolone are all fluorinated derivatives of prednisolone [46]. Pharmacologic properties with anti-inflammatory effect can be improved through fluorination of CSs.

Action Mechanism CSs act directly on nuclear steroid receptors to regulate the rate of synthesis of mRNA and proteins. CSs have both anti-inflammatory and immunosuppressive effects, and CS's mechanisms of action are highly complex including changes in T and B cell functions, changes in white blood cell traffic, changes in levels of cytokines and enzymes, inhibition of phospholipase A2 and arachidonic acid metabolism [47]. This mechanism is largely divided into altered movement of leukocytes, altered function of leukocytes, reduced microvascular dilation and permeability in inflamed areas, and reduced prostaglandin synthesis. Leukocyte migration alteration occurs 4–6 h after drug administration and includes lymphocyte reduction, T-lymphocyte selective depletion, and inhibition of neutrophil and monocyte-macrophage accumulation in the inflammatory site. Leukocyte function alteration is associated with an immune response. This includes processes such as inhibition of lymphocyte proliferation and inhibition of T-lymphocyte mediated cytotoxicity. In addition, these inhibitory effects inhibit the release of interleukin-1, leukotrienes, and prostaglandins. The reduction of these inflammatory mediators often improves pain symptoms and increases the relative viscosity as the concentration of HA in the joint increases [48].

Composition, Pharmacodynamics, and Pharmacokinetics When a CS is injected into a joint, it is absorbed by synovial cells and then diffused into the blood and removed. The purpose of IA injection therapy is to achieve prolonged concentrations of CS in the synovial fluid and synovium. The duration and effectiveness of the drug depend on the anti-inflammatory potency, solubility, and dosage. Based on the chemical structure, the duration of effect should be inversely proportional to the solubility of the steroid. The less water soluble a CS is, the slower its onset and the longer its duration [49]. The CS formulations used for IA injection are microcrystalline suspensions of CS esters. When injected into the joint cavity, these esters are slowly hydrolyzed in synovial cells to form activated CSs. In this moment, if the solubility of esters is low, absorption in the synovial cell is delayed and the duration of the effect is increased [50]. The duration of the local effect of the drug is divided into short, intermediate, and long acting and is generally consistent with the anti-inflammatory effect. Several kinds of synthetic CS have been tried to improve the anti-inflammatory effect (Table 10.1). Triamcinolone acetate (TA) is completely absorbed from joint and can be detected in plasma for 2–6 weeks. Systemic TA absorption in plasma is relatively rapid after IA injection, the observed C_{max} of 11.06 ng/mL in plasma was reached at a median t_{max} of 6 h. The terminal $t_{½}$ varies between 3.0 and 6.4 days and MRT (mean residence time) is 2.5–4.3 days depending on the products and the dose [51, 52]. Triamcinolone hexacetonide (TH) is the least soluble injectable CS, which is absorbed from the joint completely over a period of 2–3 weeks. The terminal $t_{½}$ is 4.6 days and dose-independent, MRT is 6 and 6.1 days at a dose of 20 and 40 mg, respectively [51]. Betamethasone was investigated in plasma after the single IA injection, the terminal $t_{½}$ in plasma is 6.3 days, and MRT is 2.8 days [51]. FX006 is an extended-release (ER) IA formulation of TA (TA-ER) in 75:25 poly (lactic-co-glycolic acid) microspheres designed to maintain prolonged drug concentration in the joint [11]. Synovial fluid (SF) TA-ER concentrations were quantifiable through 12 weeks. SF TA-ER reached C_{max} 231.3 ng/mL at t_{max} 7 days. Plasma TA-ER reached C_{max} 0.97 ng/mL at t_{max} 7 h. The median $t_{½}$ was 14.5 days and MRT was 19 days [52]. By delaying the absorption of drugs, a significant

Table 10.1 Pharmacokinetics of intra-articular injectable corticosteroids

Corticosteroids	Intra-articular injection dosage	Pharmacokinetic parameters in plasma
Triamcinolone acetonide		$t_{½}$ 3.2–6.4d;
	10 mg[a] 20 mg[a] 40 mg[a]	MRT 3.2d, CL (L/h) 66.7, AUC (ng.d/ml) 6.5 MRT 4.3d, CL (L/h) 38.8, AUC (ng.d/ml) 22.4 MRT 3.9d, CL (L/h) 62.9, AUC (ng.d/ml) 26.8
	40 mg/1 ml[b]	C_{max} 11.06 ng/ml, t_{max} 6 h, $t_{½}$ 3.02d, MRT 2.5d, CL ([ml/h]/kg) 0.0000, AUC (pg.h/ml) 1248.9
Triamcinolone hexacetonide		$t_{½}$ 4.6d
	20 mg[a] 40 mg[a]	MRT 6.0d, CL (L/h) 75.0, AUC (ng.d/ml) 9.8 MRT 6.1d, CL (L/h) 67.5, AUC (ng.d/ml) 20.6.
Extended release microsphere-based formulation triamcinolone acetonide (FX006)	32 mg/4 ml[b]	C_{max} 0.97 ng/mL, t_{max} 7 h, $t_{½}$ 14.5d, MRT 19d, CL ([ml/h]/kg) 0.00012, AUC (pg.h/ml) 543,1
Betamethasone	7 mg[a]	$t_{½}$ 6.3d, MRT 2.8d, CL (L/h) 12.1, AUC 21.0 ng.d/ml

d day, *h* hour, C_{max} maximum concentration observed after drug administration, t_{max} median time to maximum concentration (C_{max}), $t_{½}$ the time takes for the plasma concentration to decrease by 50%, *MRT* mean residence time) arithmetic mean of the duration that a compound resides in the body before being eliminated, *CL* (total body or systemic clearance) rate of elimination from the body normalized to the concentration of the compound in plasma, *AUC* area under the curve

[a]Derendorf et al. [51]

[b]Kraus et al. [52]

pain improvement at 10 weeks and lower peak plasma concentration were reported using an ER microsphere-based formulation of TA (FX006 or Zilretta®) instead of a crystalline suspension formulation [52] (Table 10.1).

Choosing a Corticosteroid Preparation and Dose Several injectable CS preparations are commercially available. The choice is usually based on availability, cost, versatility, and pharmacokinetics. Methylprednisolone and triamcinolone are the two most common injectable CS used for knee OA. It is believed that more soluble preparations have a shorter duration of action than less soluble preparations. However, this may not always be the case. Research results on which CS preparation is effective in treating knee OA vary. Hepper et al. [53] reported that triamcinolone appeared to be more efficacious than either betamethasone or methylprednisolone. Pyne et al. [54] reported that triamcinolone was statistically more efficient in pain relief 3 weeks after injection than methylprednisolone, but its effect is lost by week 8. On the contrary, Yavuz et al. [55] stated that methylprednisolone was statistically more effective in relieving pain than triamcinolone until 6 weeks after injection. In another studies, comparing the efficacy of TH and methylprednisolone acetate (MA) injections in knee OA, both IA therapies have similar efficacy in relieving pain and improving function, and improvement in pain and function can be sustained for up to 24 weeks [56, 57]. From these clinical results, the effects of choice of CS preparation on the treatment of knee OA are not much different. Doses needed have not been systematically studied. One study showed that an 80 mg dose of TA had no additional benefit compared with 40 mg as treatment for knee arthritis [58]. Some general dosing guidelines and CSs preparations are provided in Table 10.2.

Procedural Precaution There are no contraindications to use of IA CS therapy. However, if there is infection in or around the joint, IA CS injection should be postponed. Other potential complication risk factors, such as allergy, coagulopathy/anticoagulant use, very poorly controlled diabetes, possible fracture, or uncooperative patient should be considered [49]. IA CSs for knee OA are mostly administered with local anesthetics (lidocaine or bupivacaine). There are concerns that the preservatives in some local

Table 10.2 Intra-articular corticosteroid injections

Corticosteroid	Generic name	Solubility	Duration of action (biologic half-life)	Serum half-life (min)	Concentration (mg/ml)	Equivalent dose[a] (mg)	Duration of action (days)	Usual dose for knee joint (mg)	Fluorinated
Hydrocortisone	Hydrocortisone acetate (HCA)	Relatively insoluble	Short (8–12 h)	90	25, 50	20	6	40–100	N
Methylprednisolone	Methylprednisolone acetate (Depo-Medrol)	Slightly soluble	Intermediate (12–36 h)	180	20, 40, 80	4	7	20–40	N
Prednisolone	Prednisolone tebutate (Hydeltra-TBA)	Slightly soluble	Intermediate (12–36 h)	200	20	5	10–15	20–30	N
	Prednisolone sodium phosphate (Hydeltrasol)	Soluble	NA	120–240	20	5	10	10–20	N
Triamcinolone	Triamcinolone acetonide (Kenalog-40)	Relatively insoluble	Intermediate (12–36 h)	88	20	4	14	20–40	Y
	Triamcinolone hexacetonide (Aristospan)	Relatively insoluble	Intermediate (12–36 h)	88	20	4	21	20–30	Y
Dexamethasone	Dexamethasone acetate (Decadron-LA)	Relatively insoluble	Long (36–72 h)	240	8	0.75	8	2–4	Y
	Dexamethasone sodium phosphate(Decadron)	Soluble	Short (8–12 h)	240	4	0.75	6	2–4	Y
Betamethasone	Betamethasone acetate and betamethasone sodium phosphate (Celestone Soluspan)	Mixed (slightly soluble)	Long (36–72 h)	100–300	6	0.6	9	6–12	Y

NA not available, *N* no, *Y* yes
[a]The amount equal to 5 mg of prednisolone

anesthetic preparations can cause aggregation when combined with other compounds. However, CS crystals do not aggregate or change particle size when mixed with local anesthetics [59]. Other concern is chondrotoxic effect of local anesthetics, which had been occurred after a single IA injection of 0.5% bupivacaine [60]. Rest and/or ice pack application for 24–48 h after IA CS injection are commonly advised because it helps delaying clearance of the agent from the joint space theoretically. One study reported that IA steroid injection into the knee joint followed by strict inpatient bed rest for 24 h results in a greater degree of clinical and serological improvement, compared to outpatient injections for up to 6 months [61]. But there is no strong evidence for non-weight bearing after IA CS injection of knee [62].

Efficacy and Clinical Guideline IA CS injection for symptomatic treatment of knee OA has been successfully used for over 60 years. However, questions about the efficacy of this treatment have been raised. This treatment could improve symptoms in a short period of time, but it did not help with the treatment of fundamental arthritic lesions. Moreover, this method masks the patient's pain, allowing them to resume activity, but it has the potential to cause further destruction to the joint. Several systematic reviews showed a short-term effect of IA CS injection for treatment for knee OA. There is evidence of pain reduction between 2 and 3 weeks, but a lack of evidence for efficacy in functional improvement. Longer term (from 4 weeks on) benefits have not been confirmed [63]. Up to 4 weeks after injection, IA CS appears to be relatively more effective for pain than IA HA. By week 4, both approaches have equal efficacy, but after week 8, HA has more effective. Understanding this tendency is useful to clinicians when treating knee OA [64]. IA CS injections were significantly and clinically efficacious at reducing knee OA pain for at least 1 week [53]. However, an updated meta-analysis study showed that, although IA CS injection seemed to offer small-to-moderate benefits over placebo for up to 6 weeks, it was unclear whether the difference was clinically important. The authors also concluded that there is no evidence that an effect remains 6 months after a CS injection [65]. Although the therapeutic effects from IA CSs are typically short-lived, a newly developed TA-ER is formulated in poly lactic-co-glycolic acid (PLGA) microspheres that slowly release TA in the synovium, enabling them to exist for a long time in the joint [66]. A single, 5 mL IA injection TA-ER 32 mg (Zilretta®) significantly improved pain, stiffness, and physical function in patients with knee OA compared to placebo over 24 weeks and reduced CS-related systemic AEs such as blood glucose elevation [67].

There are many factors affecting the response after IA CS injection. The presence of effusion, absence of synovitis, US guided injection, and greater symptoms at baseline may all improve the response to IA CS injection [68]. Clinical benefits of IA injections in patients with obesity and/or advanced arthritis are less predictable [69]. Compared with those who have mild joint damage, persons with more severe joint damage on either X-ray or MRI are less likely to respond to knee IA CS injection [70].

In 2013, American Academy Orthopaedic Surgeon (AAOS) guideline had published that there is inconclusive evidence (unable to recommend for or against) to support the use of IA CS injection for knee OA [71]. On the contrary, Osteoarthritis Research Society International (OARSI) guidelines showed that IA CS injections were appropriate and the quality of the evidence of its use was good [72]. Despite AAOS guideline for use of IA CS, many orthopedic surgeons have poor compliance to the guideline, resulting in lack of treatment consensus and continued use of modalities with no proven patient benefits [73]. Adherence to the recommendations contained within the AAOS guidelines was modest regardless of the Kellgren-Lawrence (KL) grade or history of treatment. IA injection with either CSs or HA was the most common intervention (32%) despite inconclusive to strong recommendation against their use [74]. A recently updated OARSI guidelines has published that IA CS injections are conditionally recommended for acute (1–2 weeks) and short-term (4–6 weeks) pain relief [75]. In 2019, European Society for Clinical and Economic Aspects of Osteoporosis, Osteoarthritis and Musculoskeletal Diseases (ESCEO) proposed a weak recommendation to the use of IA CSs, in the case of contraindications to NSAIDs, or if the patient is still symptomatic despite use of NSAIDs. IA CSs are more effective than IA HA in the first 2–4 weeks of treatment and its efficacy may be higher in patients with more severe pain [76]. IA CSs for knee OA are conditionally or weakly recommended for short-term effect for symptomatic treatment regarding recently updated guidelines, even though 2012 American College of Rheumatology (ACR) guidelines strongly recommended IA glucocorticoid injections for knee OA [2].

Adverse Events Local AEs to IA CSs are postinjection flares, infectious arthritis, subcutaneous lipoatrophy, and chondrolysis. The incidence of postinjection flares is about 2–6% of patients, which has been known as a result from chemical irritation of crystals including steroids suspension. Infectious arthritis is an uncommon complication of which incidences range from 1 in 3000 to 1 in 50,000. Symptoms of septic arthritis occur 3–4 days after injection, so they are distinguished from postinjection flare, where symptoms occur within 24 h of postinjection. Subcutaneous lipoatrophy is sometimes observed on extra-articular injection and may be more common with less soluble agents, such as the triamcinolone compounds. Cartilage destruction might occur after excessive use of IA CS injection, which is caused by the catabolic effect of the agent. Among patients with symptomatic knee OA, comparing IA triamcinolone and IA saline over 2 years, the group using IA triamcinolone had significant loss of cartilage volume compared to IA saline group, but there was no significant difference in knee pain [77]. However, no significant deleterious effects of the steroids on the anatomical joint structure were observed in patients receiving TA injections every 3 months for up to 2 years for knee OA [78].

Physicians commonly administer IA CS injections to patients who are candidates for total knee arthroplasty (TKA) but may be unaware of the potential long-term complications. The incidence of infection within 3 months and 6 months after TKA within 3 months of knee injection was significantly higher. Ipsilateral knee injection within 3 months prior to TKA is associated with a significant increase in infection [79]. Preoperative CS or HA injection 3 months before TKA increased the risk of periprosthetic joint infection [80]. Therefore, pre- and peri-operative IA CS injections might be associated with a higher incidence of postoperative periprosthetic infection, so caution is advised [81].

Systemic effects after IA CSs are uncommon. However, attention should be paid to the AEs of systemic absorption of CSs after injection. Typically, it can reduce the inflammatory response of other joints and inhibit the hypothalamic–pituitary axis. In one study, plasma cortisol was low 2 weeks after an IA injection of TH (20 mg) and 4 weeks after an injection of methylprednisolone acetate (40 mg) [82]. Systemic effects, such as flushing, CS-induced osteoporosis, myopathy are not a major concern in patients receiving reasonable numbers of IA CS injections. Although CSs can occasionally affect blood glucose level, diabetic patients who received IA injections of methylprednisolone acetate did not detect a significant effect on blood glucose levels [49].

10.4.1.2 Hyaluronic Acid

HA is a high MW molecule that naturally occurs within the cartilage and the synovial fluid. It is a linear glycosaminoglycan composed of repeating disaccharides of β-D-glucuronic acid and β-D-N-acetyl-glucosamine. In normal human synovial fluid, the MW of HA range from 6500 to 10,900 kDa, and the concentration is 2.5 to 4.0 mg/ml [83]. High molecular weight (HMW) HA has viscoelastic properties. It behaves as a viscous liquid at low shear rates (lubricant) and as an elastic solid at high shear rates (shock absorber). In OA, the MW of synovial fluid HA is reduced to 2700 to 4500 kDa and cleared at higher rates than normal. The average half-life of HA is about 20 h in the normal synovial joint, while this half-life is reduced to 11–12 h in the inflamed joint [84]. As a result, viscoelastic properties of the fluid in OA joint are decreased [85]. Exogenous IA HA is available as a treatment for the symptoms of knee OA because it helps to restore the viscoelasticity of the synovial fluid, which called viscosupplementation [86]. In the past, US Food and Drug Administration(FDA) approved injectable HA as medical device because of its viscosupplement effect. In Dec 2018, US FDA reclassified IA HA as drug because current published scientific literature supports that HA achieves its primary intended purpose of treatment through chemical action within the body.

Action Mechanism IA HA has not only mechanical role as viscosupplement, but also chemical role, which suppresses inflammation and promotes HA production. HA injected into the joint cavity restores the normal viscoelasticity of pathological SF, which called "viscosupplementation". Viscosupplements also have disease-modifying effects, such as reducing synovial inflammation, preventing cartilage erosion, and promoting IA HA production [87]. In addition to these roles, IA HA therapy produces anti-inflammatory effects through a multifactorial mechanism of action mediated through receptor-binding relationships with cluster determinant 44 (CD44), toll-like receptor 2 (TLR2) and 4 (TLR-4), intercellular adhesion molecule-1 (ICAM-1), and layilin (LAYN) cell surface receptors. HMW HA promotes anti-inflammatory responses inhibiting the expression of proinflammatory cytokines, matrix metalloproteinases, prostaglandins, and nitric oxide, whereas short HA oligosaccharides produce inflammatory reactions [88]. Also, other action mechanism of HA has been suggested that exogenous HA decreased joint pain by directly suppressing of nociceptors and reducing the synthesis of bradykinin and substance P [89].

Hyaluronic Acid Formulations for Intra-articular Injection Ideal injectable HA for knee OA is capable of recreating the full range of biological activities attributed to naturally occur HA. MW and concentration of HA should be considered before choosing HA formulation because it may be one of the most important differentiating characteristics between HA formulations. MW and concentration in the HA formulation is important for recreating the effects of endogenous HA for joint homeostasis. Exogenous HA of higher MW (>5 × 10^5 Da) may not only exert a greater protective effect but also encourage endogenous HA production. Also, higher HA concentration makes recreating the activities of endogenous HA and stimulating endogenous HA production [90]. There are several injectable HA formulations used for clinical use (Table 10.3). Each product differs in many characteristics, including source (rooster combs versus bacterial bio-fermentation using modified organisms), mean MW ranging from 500–6000 kDa, distribution of MW, structure of molecule (linear, cross-linked, or both), cross-linking method, concentration (0.8–30 mg/mL), injection dose (0.5–6.0 mL), number of injection [91]. Number of injection per treatment course varies from 1 to 5 injections per week according to the particular product being used. The number of injections is usually in accordance with the manufacturer's instructions. HA can also be injected repeatedly. Meta-analysis study showed that repeated IA injections of HA are effective and safe treatment for knee OA [92]. The US FDA has approved repeat courses of IA HA injection; however, many insurance plans require at least a 6-month interval between treatments [93]. Although cross-linked HA or HMW HA has been known for its effectiveness regarding improvement of pain and function, series of systematic and meta-analysis study did not show a superior effectiveness comparing to non-crosslinked HA or LMW HA [94–96]. There is no reliable evidence that any one brand of viscosupplement is superior to other brands.

Indications, Contraindications, and Adverse Events IA HA is FDA approved for the treatment of knee OA in patients who have failed conservative non-pharmaceutical therapy or simple pain medication. Patients with mild-to-moderate OA (grades 1–2) and those responding positively to the first injection were twice as likely to respond positively to the injection series. Patients

Table 10.3 Hyaluronate in healthy and osteoarthritis synovial joint and intra-articular hyaluronic acid injections approved by the FDA for knee OA

	Source(type)	Active ingredient	Molecular weight (×10^6 daltons)	Concentration (mg/mL)	Dose volume (mL)	Dose interval/ times
Hyaluronate in healthy synovial fluid	Natural		4.0–6.0			
Hyaluronate in OA synovial fluid	Natural		1.0–4.0			
Hyalgan	Rooster combs	Sodium hyaluronate	0.5–0.73	10	2	1 week /3 to 5
Supartz	Rooster combs	Sodium hyaluronate	0.6–1.2	10	2.5	1 week /5
Synvisc	Rooster combs	Cross-linked hylan G-F 20 (Hylan A&B)	6.0	8	2	1 week /3 to 4
Synvisc One	Rooster combs	Cross-linked hylan G-F 20 (Hylan A&B)	6.0	8	6	1
Orthovisc	Bacterial fermentation/ chemical modification	Sodium hyaluronate	1.1–2.9	15	2	1 week /3
Euflexxa	Bacterial fermentation	Sodium hyaluronate	2.4–3.6	10	2	1 week/3
Monovisc	Bacterial fermentation	Cross-linked sodium hyaluronate	1.0–2.9	20	4	1
Durolane	Bacterial fermentation	Cross-linked sodium hyaluronate	1.0	20	3	1

who did not show improvement by injection therapy were more likely to undergo arthroplasty [97]. However, patients 65 years of age or older and those with terminal stage of OA (complete loss of joint space) were less likely to get better with IA HA injections [98]. In addition, IA HA injections are less favorable for patients with significant inflammation or suspected synovitis and those with advanced patellofemoral OA with anterior knee pain tend to be less effective [99]. IA HA injection is contraindicated in patients with known hypersensitivity to hyaluronate products, patients with targeted knee or around infections, bacteremia patients, children, pregnant or lactating women [100].

Serious AEs after IA HA injection are rare but minor one is not uncommon. Minor AEs include pain at the injection site, local joint pain and swelling, and local skin reactions, which are usually subsided with rest, cold compression, or analgesics. More serious AEs are infectious arthritis and pseudoseptic arthritis. Joint infection after IA HA injections is rare. Pseudoseptic arthritis occurred in 1–3% of patients, which are clinically characterized by severe joint inflammation with pain and swelling occurring 24–72 h after an IA injection. These reactions usually occur after sensitization with the second or third injection of a series or with a repeat treatment course. Infectious arthritis and crystalline arthropathy are ruled out with a negative synovial fluid examination. Pseudoseptic arthritis is not self-limited, requiring treatment with NSAIDs or an IA steroid injection or arthroscopic debridement. The exact cause of pseudosepsis after HA injection is currently not well understood [84]. It seems to be occurred secondary to increased immunogenicity associated with the cross-linking process used in certain HA formulations. A meta-analysis of AEs showed that the frequency of flares of pain and swelling was higher after IA injections of hylan (chemically cross-linked HA molecules with average MW up to 23 x 10^6 Da, and resulting half-lives of 1.5–9 days) than after injections of the standard form of IA HA [94].

Efficacy and Clinical Guideline There have been several studies of the efficacy and safety of IA HA injection for knee OA over the past few decades. In a comparison of IA HA injection, oral NSAID treatment, and placebo, IA HA injection provided superior pain relief and functional improvement compared with placebo at 6-month follow-up [101]. Comparing to NSAIDs alone, patients treated with either HA supplementation alone or HA supplementation combined with NSAIDs had superior outcomes at 6-month follow-up [102]. In comparison with IA HA and CS injections, maximal benefit of steroids appeared more rapidly (within 2 weeks) but pain reduction and functional improvement were significantly better with HA supplementation during the 3- to 6-month follow-up period [103]. IA HA may delay the need for knee arthroplasty. The IA HA injection was associated with a longer time-to-knee arthroplasty of 8.7 months compared with the no IA HA injection [104]. In knee OA patients, the time-to-knee arthroplasty was increased by the dose of HA injections. Patients who did not receive HA injection underwent knee arthroplasty at an average of 0.7 years. In the patient group who received a single course of HA injection, the average time-to-knee arthroplasty was 1.4 years; patients who received 5 courses delayed knee arthroplasty by 3.6 years [105]. Furthermore, IA HA injection has beneficial effect on cartilage preservation. In patients with radiologically milder disease at baseline and receiving IA HA, the joint space narrowing was significantly reduced compared with placebo [106]. When IA HA was injected to patients with symptomatic OA of the knee for 6 months, the results of measuring cartilage volume and cartilage defect using MRI showed beneficial effects on knee cartilage preservation [107].

Despite numerous trials and meta-analyses, the effectiveness of IA HA injections in knee OA patients remains controversial and uncertain. Divine et al. [108] performed a systematic review of the five published meta-analyses and concluded that although they differ in several methods for determining individual trial quality, each of the five meta-analyses presented offers scientifically sound level 1 evidence to support the efficacy of HA use in select patients with OA. IA HA injections are effective at 4 weeks, peak effect at 8 weeks, and residues detected by 24 weeks. The maximum effect size is greater than the published effects of other OA pain relievers. Therefore, IA HA injections can be useful in certain clinical situations or combined with other therapies [109]. On the contrary, Rutjes et al. [94] concluded that the benefits of viscosupplement were small and clinically irrelevant and associated with an increased risk of serious AEs. Jevsevar et al. [96] concluded that the clinical significance of the results related to pain relief and functional improvement does not support the routine use of IA HA because patient benefit of IA HA was not clinically important when compared with IA saline solution injections used as a placebo. Meta-analyses assessing the efficacy of IA HA have had discordant findings because each review used different search strategies and selection criteria to identify trials for inclusion in the analysis [100].

Consistent with the contradictory meta-analyses, available guidelines also have conflicting recommendations, despite being based on the same research evidence. In the 2012 AAOS clinical practice guideline, it was determined that the evidence was inconclusive and a recommendation could not be made for or against the use of IA HA [71]. In 2019 ACR revised guideline, IA HA injections are conditionally recommended for knee OA patients when other alternatives have been depleted or have not provided satisfactory benefits [2]. The 2019 OARSI guidelines conditionally recommended IA HA for all patients at different stages of treatment depending on their comorbidity profiles. For example, in patients with knee OA who have no comorbidities, IA HA is recommended after failure to respond to core treatments, topical NSAIDs and oral NSAIDs (including COX2 inhibitors). IA HA may have beneficial effects after 12 weeks of treatment, and a long-term safety profile may be more favorable than repetitive IA CS [75]. The 2019 ESCEO working group gives a weak recommendation to the use of IA HA in patients who have contraindications to NSAIDs, or those who is still symptomatic despite the use of NSAIDs [76].

10.4.1.3 Hyaluronic Acid-Corticosteroid Combination

Both HA and CS IA injections have demonstrated therapeutic efficacy for knee OA. According to literature, CS injections relieve pain within 2–4 weeks after injection, but these effects decrease over time. On the other hand, HA injections take almost 2–3 months to induce pain relief, but these effects last longer [64]. Both of these treatments tend to be more popular, but show very different treatment trajectories [109]. Their combination in the management of OA symptoms may provide improved symptomatic relief for these patients, both early and late period. In a systematic review, the WOMAC pain score was further reduced at 2–4 weeks in the CS and HA combined group compared to the HA alone group. With a longer term follow-up, the WOMAC pain scores at 24–26 and 52 weeks also preferred the combined CS and HA groups over HA alone. There were no significant differences in treatment-related AEs [110]. Cingal® is an HA-TH combination drug. Comparing to HA and saline injection, the use of Cingal® IA injection provided better symptomatic relief than placebo, as measured by the WOMAC pain score at 26 weeks. At 1 and 3 weeks, Cingal® was significantly better than HA for most end-points but Cingal® and HA were similar in the 6–26 weeks. The incidence of related AEs has been reported as low [110].

10.4.2 Other IA Treatments Including Small Molecules

10.4.2.1 Polydeoxyribonucleotide (PDRN)

Polydeoxyribonucleotide (PDRN) is a linear polymer consisting of a mixture of double stranded deoxyribonucleotides with a chain length of 80–2200 base pairs and a MW ranging between 50 and 1500 kDa [111]. PDRN is commonly extracted from salmon trout gonads. PDRN was originally introduced to enhance wound regeneration in difficult wound problems. A pharmacokinetic profile of PDRN is that PDRN in plasma reached its peak level at ~1 h, half-life is ~3.5 h, and bioavailability is 80–90%. It is not metabolized by the liver but is degraded by unspecific plasma or membrane-bound DNA nucleases and is finally excreted through urine and, to a lesser extent, feces [112]. PDRN may be considered a pro-drug providing active deoxyribonucleotides that interact with purinergic receptors, such as adenosine A2A receptors (A2ARs). In addition, PDRN has been shown to act by promoting DNA synthesis or repairing and restoring cell proliferation and growth through the so-called salvage pathway that PDRN supplies cells with nucleotides and bases deriving from its degradation [111]. Polynucleotides are polymers that can bind to a large amount of water molecules, and by adjusting water molecules to form a 3-dimensional gel, when injected into the joint cavity, they provide moisture to the joint surface and can reshape the cartilage structure [113]. When PDRN is enzymatically decomposed, it releases water molecules and smaller-sized oligonucleotides to maintain moisture and viscoelasticity in the joint. In addition, PDRN protects basic fibroblast growth factor (bFGF) from oxidation at the storage site, inhibits proinflammatory factors (TNF-a, IL-6, HMGB-1) by activating the adenosine A2A receptor, and increases anti-inflammatory cytokine (IL-10) [114]. Therefore, PDRNs have therapeutic effects on chondrocytes by protecting cartilage because it can inhibit the degradation of proteoglycan [115]. From these scientific bases, IA PDRN injections to treat knee OA have been tried. However, there has been little known about what is effective PDRN formulations for relieving pain and function of knee OA. According to the literature, the number of injections of PDRN used to treat knee OA varies from 3 to 5 times a week, injected volume ranged from 2 to 3 ml and a concentration of PDRN ranged from 5.6 to 30 mg/ml [116].

In a randomized double-blind clinical trial (DB RCT), 5 weekly IA PDRN (2 ml, 20 mg/ml) injection showed better pain relief and KOOS scores improvement than IA HA injection at 3 months after the end of treatment [113]. Zazgyva et al. [117] conducted a study to assess the efficacy of IA injections of PDRN versus HA in knee OA. IA PDRN (2 ml) was injected 3 weekly and followed till 16 weeks post-injection. The symptomatic and functional improvements in PDRN injection were superior to those obtained by HA injection. Giarratana et al. [118] conducted a study to investigate the equivalence of IA PDRN compared to standard HA injection. IA PDRN (2 ml, 20 mg/ml) was injected 3 weekly and followed until 26 weeks post-injection. There was statistically significant improvement of pain and KOOS scores from baseline in both treatments. PDRN injection showed significant KOOS symptoms subscore after 2 weeks while the results with HA injection became significant only after 18 weeks. In comparison with IA HA injection alone, IA injection of HA combined with PDRN showed better outcomes in VAS, WOMAC, and KSS scores at study periods. Study drugs were injected 3 times per week in both groups. There were no AEs and any other complications [119]. In another comparison study, KSS total score showed significantly better results in a combination of PDRN(10 mg/ml) and HA (10 mg/ml) injection, 3 times per week, compared with HA (20 mg/ml) alone at each follow-up time. However, no significant differences were observed for the WOMAC score between groups [120].

10.4.2.2 Hypertonic Dextrose (Prolotherapy)

Prolotherapy, also known as proliferative therapy, or regeneration injection therapy, is a complementary injection treatment for musculoskeletal pains. Hypertonic dextrose with concentrations ranging from 12.5 to 25% is the most commonly injected solution among prolotherapy agents. In this treatment, appropriate amount of hypertonic dextrose is injected into the painful ligament, the attachment of the tendon, or into the joint cavity. The mechanism of action behind hypertonic dextrose injection is not completely understood. Hypertonic dextrose solutions dehydrate the cells at the injection site and create a local inflammatory cascade. This induces growth factor release, collagen deposition, granulocytes, and macrophages activity and promotes healing [121]. In addition, it stimulates fibroblast and vascular proliferation, causing local recovery to damaged tissues inside and outside of the joint, and contributing to joint stability by strengthening ligament. According to animal study, it is reported that cartilage specific anabolic growth is possible with IA dextrose injection [122]. Furthermore, chondrogenic effects were observed after prolotherapy with hypertonic dextrose injection in symptomatic severe knee OA patients [123]. Dextrose proliferant has been approved for injection by US FDA but not for prolotherapy; thus, it is currently used as an off-label substance in prolotherapy. There are some procedural precautions in prolotherapy. Patients received prolotherapy suffered from post-injection pain. Use of prescribed pre- and/or post-procedure opioid drug dramatically reduced injection-related pain. Patients with prolotherapy should not take NSAIDs because it interferes with healing process (inflammation).

Reeves et al. [124] conducted a DB RCT to investigate the efficacy of dextrose in knee OA patients with or without ACL laxity. The tibiofemoral joint was injected with 9 ml of 10% glucose 3 times bimonthly, and an additional 10% glucose was injected 3 times bimonthly in open-label fashion. They concluded that prolotherapy with 10% dextrose significantly improves knee OA clinically and statistically. Dumais et al. [125] performed randomized crossover study to assess the effectiveness of dextrose injection to improve pain and function in knee OA. 1 cc of 15% dextrose and 0.6% lidocaine were injected into 8 administration sites in the collateral ligaments and 5 cc of 20% dextrose and 0.5% lidocaine was also administered inside the knee joint. They concluded that dextrose injection significantly reduced symptoms and lasted more than 24 weeks. Rubago et al. [126] conducted a 3-arm, DB RCT to assess the efficacy of 25% dextrose injection for knee OA. Injections were given at 1, 5, and 9 weeks with optional sessions at 13 and 17 weeks. Patients were given an optional 5 mg oxycodone tablet 30 min prior to prolotherapy to relieve pain during injection. Extra-articular injections were performed to painful attachment site of tendon and ligament with up to 15 cutaneous punctures and total amount of 22.5 mL hypertonic dextrose were used. 6 mL was injected into the knee joint. WOMAC scores exceeded minimal clinically significant difference. There were no AEs. Sit et al. [127] have performed a systematic review with meta-analysis to comprehensive clinical evidence of the effectiveness of prolotherapy for knee OA. Prolotherapy is superior to exercise alone by the WOMAC scale. Overall, prolotherapy has clearly conferred beneficial effects on knee OA treatment.

Prolotherapy has long been used to treat musculoskeletal pain, but use in knee OA is relatively rare. There is a lack of scientific evidence to use prolotherapy generally in the treatment of knee OA. Therefore, various clinical studies regarding dextrose concentration and dose, number and duration of injection, and specific utility of intra- compared with extra-articular injections are needed in the future [127]. In 2019 ACR guideline, prolotherapy is conditionally recommended for knee OA patients [2]. A limited number of trials with a small number of participants have shown small effect sizes of prolotherapy in knee. Moreover, injection schedules, injection sites, and comparators have varied substantially between trials.

10.4.2.3 SM04690

Wnt is an extracellular secreted glycoprotein whose signals act on 19 Wnt genes and various Wnt receptors, regulating canonical β-catenin-dependent and non-canonical β-catenin-independent signaling pathways. Both pathways are associated with the occurrence and development of OA [128]. Excessive activation of β-catenin-dependent signaling pathways inhibits cartilage formation, while inhibition results in chondrogenesis. SM04690 is a new small molecule Wnt-β-catenin signaling pathway inhibitor with potential as a disease-modifying OA drug (DMOAD) [128]. Yazici et al. [129] reported a phase IIb study to assess the safety and efficacy of SM04690. Inclusion criteria was KL grades 2–3, and NRS range 4 and 8. A single 2 mL IA injection of SM04690 (0.03, 0.07, 0.15, 0.23 mg, respectively), vehicle placebo, or sham (dry needle only) were given. This study showed statistically significant improvements in the 0.07 mg and 0.23 mg dose groups compared to vehicle placebo for NRS score, WOMAC pain and physical function score, and patient global assessment.

10.4.2.4 CNTX-4975

Capsaicin is an agonist for the transient receptor potential cation channel subfamily V member 1 (TRPV1). TRPV1 is a non-specific cationic channel which is opened by heat, acids, and certain fatty acids [130]. This channel is selectively expressed at the ends of the nociceptors (pain sensory fibers) in the peripheral nervous system [131]. CNTX-4975 is a high-purity injectable trans-capsaicin that targets the capsaicin receptor (TRPV1). The analgesic effects of capsaicin-based treatments have been attributed to several different mechanisms (collectively referred to as the “defunctionalization” of nociceptive fibers), including the transient retraction of nerve fiber terminals [131]. Stevens et al. [132] reported a phase 2 DB RCT results. Patients ages 45–80 years who had moderate-to-severe OA were randomized into a single IA injection of placebo, CNTX-4975 0.5 mg, or CNTX-4975 1.0 mg. At week 12, injections of CNTX-4975 in the 0.5 mg and 1.0 mg groups showed a greater reduction in AUC for pain scores compared to placebo. At week 24, significant improvements were maintained in the 1.0 mg group. AEs were similar in both groups. CNTX-4975 has shown a dose-dependent improvement in pain of knee OA patients. CNTX-4975 1.0 mg was well tolerated, with a safety profile similar to that of the placebo throughout the study. In conclusion, CNTX-4975 1.0 mg significantly reduced OA knee pain for 24 weeks; CNTX-4975 0.5 mg significantly reduced pain at 12 weeks, but the effect was not clear at 24 weeks.

10.4.3 Biologic Treatments

Biologics are defined as any pharmaceutical drug product manufactured, extracted or semi-synthetic from biological sources. Different from totally synthesized pharmaceuticals, they include

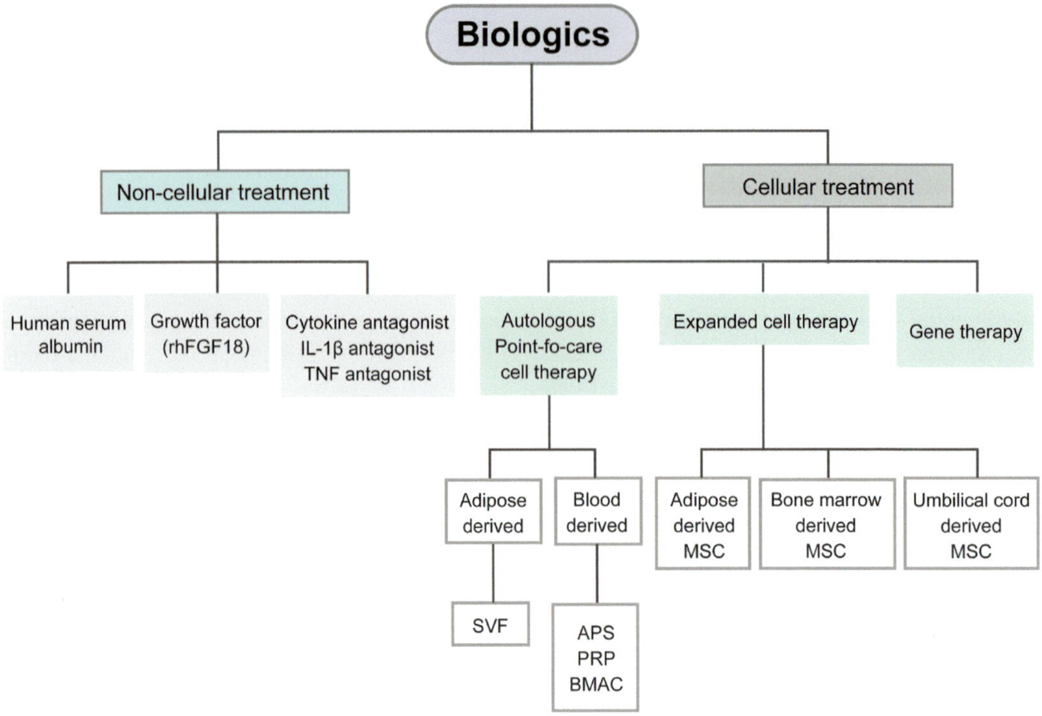

Fig. 10.6 Biologic treatments for knee osteoarthritis. Biologics for knee OA are categorized into non-cellular therapy or cell therapy. Non-cellular therapy includes human serum albumin, growth factors, cytokine antagonists. Cellular therapy includes cell concentrates as autologous point-of-care cell therapy, expanded cell therapy as mesenchymal stromal (or stem) cells, and gene therapy. *rhFGF* recombinant human fibroblast growth factor, *IL* interleukin, *TNF* tumor necrotizing factor, *APS* autologous protein solution, *BMAC* bone marrow aspirate concentrate, *MSC* mesenchymal stem/stromal cell, *PRP* platelet-rich plasma, *SVF* stromal vascular fraction

vaccines, whole blood and its components, allergens, somatic cells and tissues, gene therapies, recombinant therapeutic protein, and live medicines used in cell therapy. Biologics may consist glucoses, proteins, nucleic acids, or complex combinations of these substances, or may be living cells or tissues. Biologics have some promising applications to pain relief and healing of damaged tissues in many different areas of health and medical research [133]. OA is caused by an imbalance between anabolic and catabolic factors, and biologics target certain catabolic proinflammatory mediators or affect anabolism more generally. Moreover, biologic agents have dramatic effects in other inflammatory arthritis such as rheumatoid arthritis. Taking into consideration of this point, biologic agents are thought to have similar effects in treating OA [45]. Biologics used for treatment of knee OA are categorized into non-cellular therapy or cell therapy. Non-cellular therapy includes human serum albumin, growth factors, cytokine antagonists. Cell therapy includes cell concentrates as autologous point-of-care cell therapy, expanded cell therapy as mesenchymal stromal (or stem) cells (MSCs), and gene therapy. Cell therapies can be classified by the method used to produce them or by their relative heterogeneity compared with the source tissue [9] (Fig. 10.6).

10.4.3.1 Non-Cellular Therapy

Human Serum Albumin (LMWF-5A)

LMWF-5A (Ampion®) is an injectable, low MW fraction of 5% human serum albumin, of which constituent, aspartyl-alanyl diketopiperazine, modulated the inflammatory immune response in vitro through a molecular pathway implicated in T-lymphocyte anergy [134]. Comparing to saline injection, LMWF-5A injection group showed significantly better WOMAC pain scores at week 12 (estimated difference from control −0.25, $P = 0.004$). LMWF-5A effect on pain was more pronounced in severe knee OA patients. AEs were generally mild and similar in vehicle control group (47%) and LMWF-5A group (41%) [135]. Another RCT resulted that 71% of severe knee OA injected LMWF-5A met the OMERACT-OARSI responder criteria, exceeding the 30% threshold ($p < 0.001$) and at week 12, there were significantly more responders in the LMWF-5A group than saline control group (65% vs. 43%, $p < 0.001$). There were no reported drug-related serious AEs. Overall, the available data suggest that the short-term effects of LMWF-5A may be non-inferior (although not likely to be superior) to currently used IA treatment modalities. However, the long-term effects of LMWF-5A have not yet been determined [136].

Growth Factor Therapy

rhFGF18 (Sprifermin)

Sprifermin (recombinant human fibroblast growth factor 18; rhFGF18) specifically binds to fibroblast growth factor receptor 3 (FGFR-3) in cartilage and activates promoting chondrogenesis and cartilage matrix production in vitro. Post hoc analyses of the phase I data showed that the patellofemoral joint had less worsening from baseline to 12 months, and bone marrow lesions showed further improvement in the whole knee joint from 6 to 12 months [137]. A 5 years FGF-18 Osteoarthritis Randomized Trial with Administration of Repeated Doses (FORWARD) study was conducted with 40–85 years of symptomatic radiological knee OA patients were selected as eligible participants and KL grade 2 or 3. Five groups were randomized into IA injections of 100 μg of sprifermin every 6 or 12 months, 30 μg of sprifermin every 6 or 12 months, or placebo every 6 months. Each treatment consisted of weekly injections over 3 weeks. After 2 years, compared with placebo, there was a significant increase in total tibiofemoral cartilage thickness for 100 μg of sprifermin injection every 6 months group (0.05 mm) and every 12 months group (0.04 mm). There was no statistically significant difference in the mean absolute change from baseline in the total WOMAC score compared to placebo. Arthralgia was the most frequently reported AEs. Sprifermin is a potential anabolic IA disease-modifying OA drug but of uncertain clinical importance; the durability of response also was uncertain [138].

Cytokine Antagonist

Interleukin (IL)-1β Antagonist

IL-1β is a key mediator of the inflammation and catabolic processes that lead to cartilage degradation and destruction of joint tissues. It might directly mediate the erosive processes that lead to OA [139]. Systemic administration of IL-1 receptor antagonist (IL-1Ra), anakinra, may reduce joint inflammation and slow down the erosive process of the disease, such as rheumatoid arthritis. IA anakinra injection can have beneficial effects on symptoms and structural alterations in canine OA model [140]. In a randomized, multicenter, double-blind, placebo-controlled trial, pharmacokinetic profile of anakinra showed that the mean terminal half-life of it in serum after IA injection was ~4 h. The mean WOMAC score improvement from baseline to 4 weeks was not statistically different between the placebo group and injecting anakinra 50 or 150 mg group. Moreover, anakinra was well tolerated [141].

Tumor Necrotizing Factor (TNF) Antagonist

TNF is known to play an important role in cartilage matrix degradation in OA. It has the function of inducing the production of cytokines such as IL-6, matrix metalloproteinase and prostaglandins, and inhibiting the synthesis of proteoglycans and type II collagen [142]. Lindsley et al. [143] reported IA infliximab for knee OA showed significant improvement in the total WOMAC score by 8 weeks and baseline synovial cellularity and CRP also correlated with improvement. Comparing to single IA HA injection, single injection of IA etanercept in moderate-to-severe knee OA showed that VAS and WOMAC scores

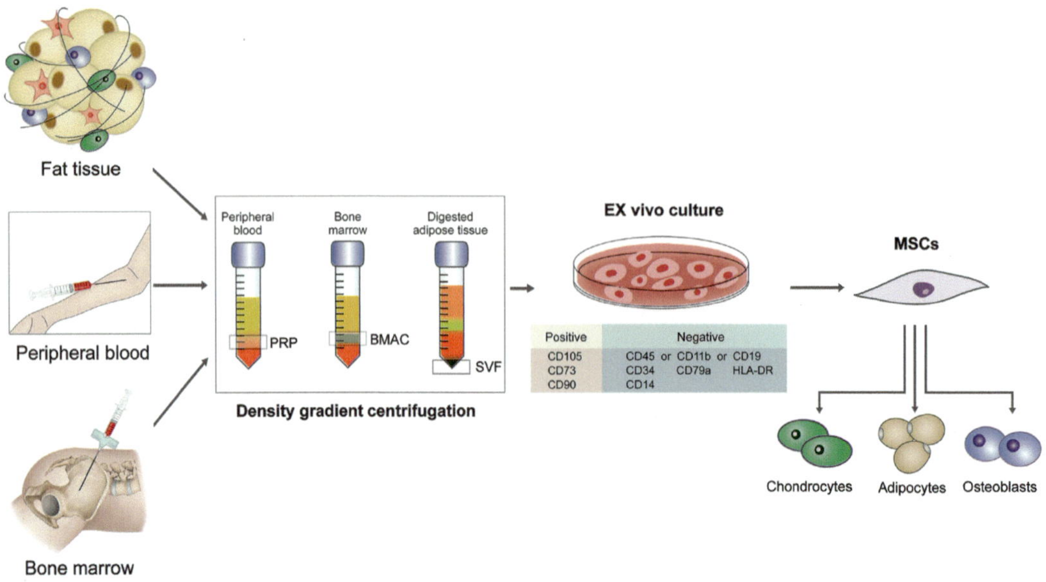

Fig. 10.7 Intra-articular cell therapies. Cell therapies can be classified by the method used to produce them or by their relative heterogeneity compared with the source tissue. Cellular therapy includes cell concentrates as autologous point-of-care cell therapy, expanded cell therapy as mesenchymal stromal (or stem) cells, and gene therapy. Autologous point-of-care cell therapies are heterogeneous mixtures containing cells (or cell products) that are derived from autologous blood, bone marrow, or adipose tissue. Expanded cell therapies are the cultivation and use of cells with MSC characteristics under ex vivo culture. MSCs must be plastic-adherent, express or lack specific cell surface markers, and be capable of trilineage differentiation into osteoblasts, adipocytes, and chondrocytes in vitro. *BMAC* bone marrow aspirate concentrate, *MSC* mesenchymal stem/stromal cell, *PRP* platelet-rich plasma, *SVF* stromal vascular fraction

did not differ significantly between groups, but significant pain relief was shown in the etanercept injection group at 1 and 2 weeks by VAS [144]. Single IA injection of 10 mg adalimumab compared to 25 mg single IA injection of HA in moderate-to-severe knee OA showed improvements in VAS and WOMAC scores [145]. In 2019 ACR guideline, TNF inhibitors and IL-1 receptor antagonists are strongly recommended against in knee OA patients [2]. Their efficacy was not proved and its risk was known.

10.4.3.2 Cellular Therapy

There has been many limitations in treating chronic diseases such as OA using standard drug. There have been attempts to overcome these limitations with regenerative medicine, such as cell therapy. Cell therapy is one of the fields of regenerative medicine, and there has been a lot of interest and research recently. However, cell therapy has a variety of unresolved issues in cell sources, manufacturing processes, administration methods, bioavailability, clinical results, etc. IA Cell therapy includes cell concentrates, MSCs, and gene therapy. Cell therapies can be classified by cell sources or by specific cell type from tissues or by cell processing methods [9] (Fig. 10.7). Cell sources maybe autologous avoiding immune response issues and disease transmission or allogeneic to eliminate donor-site morbidity and to maximize availability. Cells can be used as point-of care therapy with non- or minimal manipulated cell concentrates or as cell therapy with manipulated in ex vivo (expanded in culture) [146]. The most utilized IA injection cell therapies for knee OA include the use of concentrates of peripheral blood, bone marrow aspirate concentrates (BMAC), and stromal vascular fraction (SVF) from adipose tissue which comprise stem cells, growth factors, and cytokines. They can be obtained with minimal manipulation in the clinics, without the need to isolate and expand the cells, and immediately implanted in the patient as point-of-care cell therapies [146]. Because the number of MSCs extracted directly from tissues is too small to be used and it is difficult to distinguish MSCs, they are cultivated to distinguish cells with MSC characteristics and used for clinical use. Cell concentrates are the least processed and most heterogeneous therapies, whereas MSCs are the most processed and least heterogeneous. Within each treatment category, therapies (and the regulations that apply to clinical use) tend to differ significantly [9].

Stromal Vascular Fraction

Stromal vascular fractions (SVF) are derived from lipoaspirate and harvested with liposuction devices in the abdomen or flank under local anesthesia. The lipoaspirate is washed, processed with collagenases, and then placed into a centrifuge. Centrifugation allows for identification and collection of the SVF, which contains a heterogeneous cell population including MSCs, endothelial cells, and endothelial precursors. Alternative systems can use mechanical rather than enzymatic processes to break down adipose tissue or can use filtration rather than centrifugation to isolate the SVF. The resultant SVF ideally contains no adipocytes and has only low concentrations of leukocytes and extracellular matrix [147]. However, SVF is highly heterogeneous and only ~15–30% of the cellular content is stromal cells. Moreover, although adipose-derived stromal cells can be purified from SVF, be aware of the difference between SVF and adipose-derived stromal cells [148].

There are a few clinical research evaluating the efficacy of SVF on treatment for knee OA. Pak et al. [149] conducted a case series of treating knee OA patients with autologous adipose SVF and regenerating cartilage-like tissue. That showed the VAS, functional rating index (FRI), and ROM were improved and MRI evidence of cartilage regeneration was observed after 3 months. Koh et al. [150] conducted a case series for evaluating the effectiveness of SVF on knee OA using clinical outcome and second look arthroscopy. This study showed clinical parameters significantly improved at 2-year follow-up. Furthermore, 87.5% of elderly patients improved or maintained cartilage status at least 2 years postoperatively. Michalek et al. [151] performed a multicenter case-control study involving 1114 knee and hip OA patients from four different countries. The clinical outcomes such as pain, use of nonsteroidal analgesics, limping, joint movement and stiffness, all improved at 12 months after treatment. Garza et al. [152] performed a DB RCT for evaluating whether IA SVF injection improves knee OA symptom and this improvement would be dose dependent. They reported IA SVF injections can significantly decrease knee OA symptoms and pain for at least 12 months, dose dependently. There were no changes in cartilage thickness on MRI evaluation and no serious AEs occurred. However, one of the major drawbacks relating to autologous adipose SVF in the treatment of knee OA is the absence of accessibility of RCTs. Due to these limitations, despite successful results by these reports, it is not yet easily accepted as mainstream treatment [153].

Bone Marrow Aspirate Concentrate

Bone marrow aspirate (BMA) contains a mixture of cellular components including platelets, WBC, RBC, adipose cells, hematopoietic and non-hematopoietic precursors. Bone marrow aspirate concentrates (BMAC) is a centrifugation form of BMA and contains platelets, growth factors, and multipotent MSCs. However, multipotent MSCs in the BMAC comprise merely 0.001–0.01% of mononuclear cells within bone marrow aspirate. Numerous growth factors, such as TGF-β, PDGF, IL-1β, insulin growth factor-1 (IGF-1), fibroblast growth factor-18, bone morphogenetic protein-2 (BMP2) and BMP-7, have been identified in BMAC. BMA taken usually from the posterior iliac crest has the highest concentration of multipotent MSCs. The aspirate then undergoes centrifugation. After that, resultant concentrates were injected into the joint as a fluid or delivery of cells through an implantable scaffold. The wide variation in BMAC preparation protocols and lack of standardization methods make comparisons difficult because the true biological potential of each product in a patient is unknown [133].

Rodriguez-Fontan et al. [154] performed a case series to assess the clinical outcomes of IA injection of BMAC for the treatment of early knee OA. IA injections of BMAC for the treatment of early knee were safe and demonstrated satisfactory results in 63.2% of patients. Kim et al. [155] conducted a case series study evaluating the clinical efficacy of the IA injection of autologous BMAC with adipose tissue. This study showed improvement in the VAS pain scores, IKDC scores, Lysholm scores, and SF 36 at post-injection 12 months. The improvement of VAS pain score was less in grade IV OA patients, which means that BMAC is more effective in mild to moderate OA. Centeno et al. [156] reported improvement in Lower Extremity Functional Scale scores and lower mean NRS scores, and low rate of AEs in BMAC with and without adipose grafts. Addition of an adipose graft to the BMAC did not provide a detectible benefit over BMAC alone. Shapiro et al. [157] conducted a single-blind, saline injection placebo-controlled, RCT for evaluating the efficacy and safety of BMAC in knee OA. Their results showed that the VAS pain and OARSI Intermittent and Consistent Osteoarthritis Pain scores improved in both knees at 1 week, 3 and 6 months from baseline. However, there are no differences between BMAC and placebo injections. There were no serious AEs from the BMAC procedure. The same group of authors also conducted a DB RCT to evaluate cartilage appearance using MRI T2 quantitative mapping following these patients up to 12 months. No significant differences were found on T2 quantitative MRI mapping between the saline control and BMAC knees [158]. From these clinical studies, although the use of BMAC in the treatment of symptomatic OA demonstrates promising early clinical outcomes, no clear regenerative benefits have been showed to date.

Platelet-Rich Plasma

Platelets are small, nonnucleated cells in peripheral blood and its main function is a role in hemostasis. Platelets contain a number of proteins, cytokines, and other bioactive factors and normal platelet counts in blood range from 150,000 to 350,000/μL [159]. Plasma is the liquid part of the blood including clotting factors, other proteins, and ions. PRP, with a platelet concentration of at least 1,000,000 platelets/μL in 5 mL plasma, has a positive effect on tissue healing and regeneration. PRP includes a high concentration of platelets, which has more than 1100 proteins like growth factors. PRP increases growth factor concentration 3–5 times [160]. Platelets play an important role in the initiation of healing as they form scaffolds for the formation of clot, leading to the chemotaxis of appropriate cytokines. Platelet α-granules include growth factors and anti-inflammatory cytokines such as IGF-1, IGF-2, vascular endothelial growth factor, TGF-β, FGF, endothelial growth factor, and PDGF. These are released at the healing site and have been found to help promote the growth of autologous chondrocytes, MSCs, and extracellular matrix components like proteoglycans, type I and II collagen [161].

For PRP preparation, autologous venous blood was centrifuged to enrich platelets above the levels normally found in serum. Because the density of whole blood components is different, spinning the whole blood by density gradient centrifugation can separate each component into different layers: platelet-poor plasma, buffy coat, and RBCs. A buffy coat is located between the platelet-poor plasma and RBCs and it contains the highest concentration of platelets. PRP can be obtained in two forms: plasma based and buffy coat preparations. Plasma-based methods of PRP work to isolate only plasma and platelets while excluding leukocytes. The buffy coat-based method separates the platelet-poor plasma layer and the buffy coat layer, containing both white and red blood cells. The blood composition and humoral factors of PRP vary depending on the method used, and according to the leukocyte content, PRP is classified as pure PRP, leukocyte-poor PRP (LP-PRP), and leukocyte-rich PRP (LR-PRP) [162]. Although contrasting scientific evidence exists for PRP injections for knee OA from several studies, the efficacy of IA PRP injections has been widely reported. Dai et al. [163] conducted a meta-analysis to assess the efficacy and safety of PRP for symptomatic knee

OA. They reported PRP and HA had similar effects with regard to pain relief and functional improvement. However, at 12 months after injection, PRP had better pain and functional improvement than HA, and the improvement effect of WOMAC pain and functional score exceeded Minimal Clinically Important Difference (MCID) (−0.79 for WOMAC pain and −2.85 for WOMAC functional score). Compared to saline injection, PRP was more effective in pain and functional improvement at 6 and 12 months after injection, and the improvement effect of WOMAC pain and functional score exceeded MCID. PRP did not have a higher risk of AEs compared to HA and saline. Tang et al. [164] performed a meta-analysis study to evaluate the clinical efficacy of PRP injection compared with HA injection for knee OA. They concluded that IA PRP injection appeared to be more efficacious than HA injection for the treatment of knee OA in terms of short-term functional recovery. Moreover, PRP injection was superior to HA injection in terms of long-term pain relief and functional improvement. In addition, PRP injection did not increase the risk of AEs. The level of evidence was moderate or low due to the heterogeneity and/or study design limitations. So even though profits are conclusive, the degree of benefit must be studied. Filardo et al. [165] conducted a meta-analysis study to evaluate effectiveness of PRP injections for knee OA compared to placebo and other IA treatments. This study resulted in WOMAC score favored PRP, with a statistically and clinically significant difference versus placebo at 12 months follow-up ($P = 0.02$) and versus HA at 6 months ($P < 0.001$) and 12 months ($P < 0.001$) follow-ups. A clinically significant difference favoring PRP versus steroids was documented for VAS pain ($P < 0.001$), KOOS pain ($P < 0.001$), function in daily activities ($P = 0.001$), and quality of life ($P < 0.001$) at 6 months follow-up. However, superiority of PRP did not reach the MCID for all outcomes, and quality of evidence was low.

The different preparation of PRP leads to different concentrations of platelets, WBCs, and RBCs, which might affect clinical outcomes. Riboh et al. [166] performed a meta-analysis to compare the clinical outcomes between HA, LP-PRP, and LR-PRP for treatment of knee OA. The authors reported clearly better WOMAC scores in LP-PRP than the HA or placebo, but no such difference was observed with LR-PRP. Both PRP preparations resulted in higher incidences of AEs than HA but there was no difference in AEs between LP-PRP and LR-PRP. Belk et al. conducted a meta-analysis study to compare the efficacy of PRP and HA injections for the treatment of knee OA and evaluate the clinical outcomes according to leukocyte concentration. They concluded IA PRP injection showed better outcomes, such as WOMAC score, VAS and subjective IKDC score, at 11 months post-injection. Moreover, LP-PRP was associated with significantly better subjective IKDC scores versus LR-PRP.

The results of the meta-analysis studies show that the use of PRP can improve the short- and mid-term (6–12 months) pain scale over other IA treatments, such as HA injection. However, despite the apparent positive effects of PRP use, the methodological quality among studies is low, there is considerable heterogeneity between studies, and the diversity of PRP formulations confuses the clear demonstration of clinical efficacy [167]. Large-scale RCTs are needed to further evaluate the efficacy and duration of PRP treatment in patients with knee OA. The number and frequency of injections, the method of activation (for anticoagulant PRP), aspects of storage, plasma separation time, and concomitant therapy currently vary greatly from group to group and must be considered when planning or analyzing [168]. In 2019 OARSI and ACR guideline, IA PRP injection for knee OA is strongly recommended against because the quality of evidence supporting these treatments is extremely low, and there is a lot of the heterogeneity and lack of standardization in preparations [2, 75].

Autologous Protein Solution

An autologous protein solution (APS) is a kind of cell concentrates made from whole blood. The APS consists of WBCs which contain anti-inflammatory proteins, platelets which contain anabolic growth factors, and concentrated plasma that contains both. This solution produced by combination of WBCs, platelets, and concentrated plasma has properties of increased concentrations of anti-inflammatory cytokines and anabolic growth factors [169]. Conceptually, APS and LR-PRP are very similar. However, unlike traditional PRP systems, commercially available APS kit passes the concentrated plasma through a dried polyacrylamide gel that leads to a high level of anti-inflammatory cytokines while ensuring low levels of proinflammatory molecules, preferentially concentrates anti-inflammatory cytokines including IL-1 receptor antagonist and TNF receptor inhibitor [9]. Kon et al. [170] performed a multicenter, saline controlled, DB RCT to investigate if single IA injection of APS is able to reduce pain and improve function in knee OA. The results showed a statistically significant improvement in WOMAC pain score at 12 months for APS compared with placebo. However, improvements from baseline to 2 weeks and 1, 3, 6 months were similar between treatments. Additionally, this study failed to show any significant differences in VAS pain improvement between groups as primary outcome. The same group of authors also conducted 3 years follow-up study to investigate if the positive effects of APS, previously documented at 1 year in a clinical trial, last up to 3 years [171]. In the APS cohort, WOMAC pain improved from 11.5 to 4.3 at 1 year and to 5.7 at 3 years ($P < 0.0001$ vs baseline). The APS cohort also showed a statistically significant improvement in its KOOS pain score from 39 to 70 at 1 year and to 64 at 3 years ($P < 0.0001$ vs baseline) and VAS pain scores from 5.5 to 2.6 at 1 year and to 3.4 at 3 years ($P = 0.0184$ vs baseline). However, VAS pain score significantly worsened from 12 to 36 months ($P = 0.0411$). MRI Osteoarthritis Knee Score findings showed no statistically significant differences. Patients with better cartilage had greater WOMAC pain improvement when their baseline scores were worse, whereas the trend was reversed for patients with cartilage loss at baseline. IA injection of APS for mild to moderate knee OA was safe, and significant pain improvement was documented 3 years after a single injection.

Mesenchymal Stromal (or Stem) Cells

MSC is defined when it has the following cellular characteristics: First, MSC must be plastic-adherent when maintained under standard culture conditions. Second, MSC must express specific cell surface marker. Third, MSC must be differentiated into osteoblasts, adipose cells, and chondroblasts in vitro [172]. There have been many controversies about the action mechanism of MSCs in vivo if regenerative process occurs either by implanted MSC differentiation or by endocrine and paracrine activity on host cells, or both [173]. Although the in vivo mechanisms of MSCs are still unclear, the release of chemical mediators is thought to be important [174]. Exogenously administered MSCs induce to produce soluble growth factors and cytokines in the injury site and exert immunomodulatory, anti-inflammatory, and nourishing (regenerative) effects on the patient's resident stem cells to form the new tissue [175].

MSC can be obtained from any tissue, autogenous or allogenic source. Autogenous BMAC or SVF is most commonly used for injectable MSCs in knee OA, that components are heterogeneous. MSC proportion in BMAC or SVF is very low, for example, 0.001%–0.01% of mononuclear cells within BMAC and ~15–30% within SVF. Therefore, ex vivo isolation and expansion of cell concentrates might be needed to obtain clinically useful amount of MSCs. However, ex vivo expanded cell therapy might increase the risk of AEs. Although no major AEs have been reported on IA MSCs injection for knee OA, malignant transformation remains a potential risk for ex vivo expanded cell therapy [176]. Ex vivo expanded MSCs are classed as drugs that require government regulatory approval before clinical application. Although minimally manipulated cell product such as BMAC or SVF might contain MSCs, they might claim to be exempt from government regulation as point-of-care therapy. Autologous point-of-care cell therapy should not be confused with true MSC therapies because they tend to include more heterogeneous cells than those in true MSC therapies and have effects which are not mainly attributed to their pharmacological immunomodulatory and/or immunosuppressive capacity or differentiation potential [9]. In this section, only clinical research results on IA injection therapy for knee OA using ex vivo expanded MSCs will be reviewed. Recently, many clinical studies have been carried out in the hope that MSCs will heal damaged tissues. In spite of hopeful expectations, RCT studies are rare and the results of those studies have not reached MCID. In 2019 OARSI and ACR guideline, IA MSCs injection for knee OA is strongly recommended against because the quality of evidence supporting of these treatments is extremely low, and there is a lot of the heterogeneity and lack of standardization in preparations [2, 75].

Bone Marrow-Derived Mesenchymal Stromal Cells

Soler Rich et al. [177] conducted a case series to assess the efficacy and safety of autologous expanded BM-MSCs for KL 2–4 knee OA. This study showed the IA infusion of a dose of 40×10^6 expanded BM-MSC suspended in an 8 mL solution of Ringer-lactate and albumin has no local or systemic AEs and can significantly improve symptoms due to joint inflammation in a short period of time. Also, there is a report that the OA cartilage tissue evaluated through T2 mapping MRI was improved. Soler R et al. [178] reported a phase I–II trial using ex vivo expanded autologous MSCs for the treatment of KL 2–3 knee OA. Patients were injected with 10 mL of saline solution supplemented with 2% human serum albumin suspended with 40×10^6 expanded BM-MSC and followed up to 12 months post-injection. There were few reported AEs (mild joint and low back pain). Pain intensity was decreased since day 8 after the injection, which was maintained after 12 months. The SF-36 showed improvement in parameters including joint pain and physical function at month 12. Moreover, T2 mapping MRI showed cartilage regeneration in all patients 12 months after treatment. Emadedin et al. [179] performed a randomized, triple-blind, placebo-controlled phase 1/2 clinical trial to evaluate the safety and efficacy of IA implantations of autologous BM-MSCs in patients with knee OA. 43 patients enrolled this study and study group were injected with 40×10^6 ex vivo expanded MSCs in 5 ml saline supplemented with 2% human serum albumin and followed up for 6 months after the implantations. Patients who injected MSC had significantly improved in overall WOMAC scores, WOMAC pain and function subscales, and pain-free walking distance compared to those who received placebo. There were no major AEs attributed to the MSC treatment.

Doyle et al. [180] reported a narrative review that evaluated the efficacy of IA injections of BM-MSCs for the treatment of knee OA. This study showed clinical applications of IA injections of BM-MSCs are steadily increasing, with most studies demonstrating a decrease in poor cartilage index, improvements in pain, function and Quality of Life (QoL); with moderate-to-high level evidence regarding safety for therapeutic administration. A moderate number of cells (40×10^6) were identified as most likely to achieve optimal responses in individuals with KL grade ≥ 2 knee OA. However, low confidence in clinical efficacy remains due to a plethora of heterogenous methodologies used, resulting in need for comparative RCT.

Adipose-Derived Mesenchymal Stromal Cells (AD-MSCs)

Jo et al. [181] conducted a case series clinical trial to assess the mid-term safety and efficacy of AD-MSCs for knee OA. Patients in each group received low-dose (1.0×10^7 cells), mid-dose (5.0×10^7 cells), and high dose (1.0×10^8 cells) injections and followed up to 2 years post-injection. IA injections of autologous AD-MSCs improved knee functional scores as measured by WOMAC, KSS, and KOOS and decreased VAS pain scores for up to 2 years in all cell dosage groups. However, statistical significance was mainly seen in the high-dose group. Clinical outcomes tended to be worsen after 1 year in the low-dose and medium-dose groups, while lasting up to 2 years in the high-dose groups. The structural outcomes evaluated by MRI showed similar patterns. There were no treatment-related AEs during the 2-year period. Freitag et al. [182] reported an RCT to evaluate the efficacy of autologous AD-MSC on pain, function, and disease modification in knee OA. 30 participants were randomly divided into three groups. Two groups received IA AD-MSC injection consisting of either a single (100×10^7 cells) or two injections (100×10^7 cells at baseline and 6 months). The third group served as a control group, with only conservative treatment. Both treatment groups showed clinically significant pain and functional improvement at 12 months. Radiological analysis with MRI showed modification of disease progression. 2 IA injections of AD-MSCs at 6-month intervals achieved more consistent OA stabilization than single injection. Lee et al. [183] conducted a Phase IIb, saline controlled, RCT to evaluate the efficacy and safety of a single IA injection of AD-MSCs for knee OA patients. Patients received a single injection of 1×10^8 cells of ADMSCs in 3 mL of saline and followed up to 6 months. This study resulted in a significant improvement in WOMAC scores at 6 months with a single injection of AD-MSC. No serious AEs were observed in both groups during follow-up period. When measured by MRI, cartilage defects at 6 months after injection were not significantly changed in AD-MSC group, whereas defects increased in control group. Song et al. [184] reported a randomized phase I/IIa clinical trial with a 96-week follow-up to evaluate the safety and therapeutic potential of different dose and repeated injection of AD-MSCs in patients with knee OA. 18 participants were divided into three dose groups: the low-, mid-, and high-dose group (1×10^7, 2×10^7 and 5×10^7 cells, respectively), injected three times and followed up for 96 weeks. They concluded IA injections of AD-MSCs reduced pain, improved function and cartilage volume without treatment-related AEs. Also, this improvement was more pronounced when repeated injections were combined with a 5×10^7 cell dose.

Human Umbilical Cord Blood-Derived Mesenchymal Stem Cells

MSCs can be separated from umbilical cord Wharton's jelly, perivascular tissue, and blood using various techniques. Those cells are characterized by phenotypic similarities with BM-MSCs but their differentiation into the osteogenic and chondrogenic lineage is not as consistent as for BM-MSCs [185]. Human umbilical cord blood-derived mesenchymal stem cells (hUCB-MSCs) have biological benefits such as longer culture, large-scale expansion, retardation of senescence, and high anti-inflammatory effect compared to bone marrow or adipose tissue [186]. Park et al. [187] reported 7 years of follow-up case series study. The stem cell-based medicinal product (a composite of culture-expanded allogeneic hUCB-MSCs and HA hydrogel [Cartistem]) was surgically applied to the lesion site, not IA injection. The improved clinical results were stable for 7 years follow-up period. The histological findings at 1 year showed hyaline-like cartilage. Regenerated cartilage maintained persistence on MRI at 3 years. Mata et al. [188] conducted a controlled randomized phase I/II trial to evaluate the safety and efficacy of the IA injection of single or repeated allergenic hUCB-MSCs in knee OA. Patients with symptomatic knee OA were randomized to receive HA at baseline and 6 months, single-dose (20×10^6) hUCB-MSC at baseline, or repeated hUCB-MSC doses at baseline and 6 months ($20 \times 10^6 \times 2$: MSC-2) and followed up for 12 months. No severe AEs were reported. Only MSC-treated patients experienced significant pain relief and functional improvements from baseline ($p = 0.001$). At 12 months, WOMAC pain subscale significantly decreased in the MSC-2-treated group as compared with the HA group. For total WOMAC score, MSC-2 was lower than HA at 12 months. No differences in MRI Osteoarthritis Knee scores were detected. The author concluded repeated UC-MSC therapy is safer and better than active comparator in knee OA at 1 year follow-up.

Gene Therapy

Gene transfer has been performed in two ways, directly in vivo injection into the joint or cell harvesting from the patient, ex vivo exposure to vectors and return of modified cells to the joint. Gene therapy with genes encoding cartilage growth factor and anti-inflammatory cytokines is effective in treating OA [146]. TissueGene-C (TG-C) was developed as a cell-based growth factor expression strategy and contains human alloge-

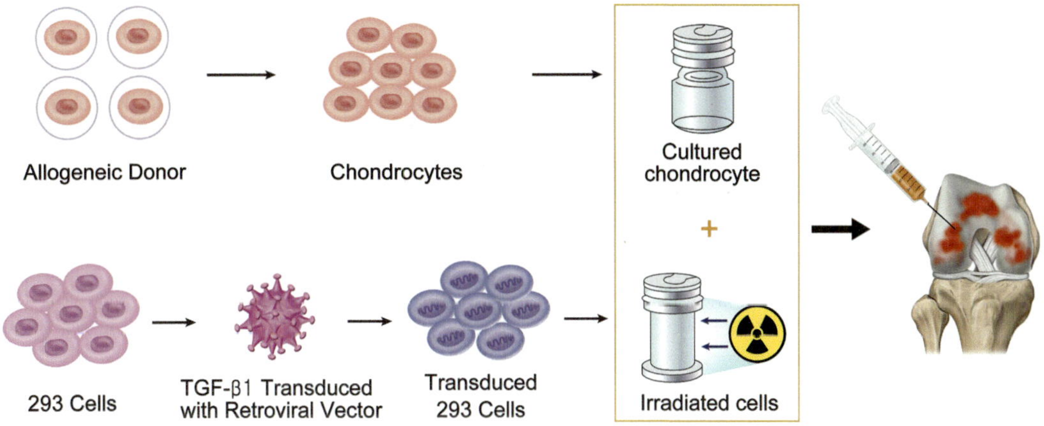

Fig. 10.8 Schematic process for gene therapy with TissueGene-C. Gene therapies with genes encoding for chondrogenic growth factors and anti-inflammatory cytokines are of interest to treat OA. TissueGene-C (TG-C) was developed as a cell-based growth factor expression strategy and involves a 3:1 ratio of human allogeneic chondrocytes and genetically modified 293 cells engineered to express TGF-b1. TGF-b1 expressing cells were irradiated with a low dose of gamma-ray so that they could not proliferate within the knee joint after injection. TG-C was administered by a single intra-articular injection. *TGF* transforming growth factor

neic chondrocytes and genetically modified chondrocytes engineered to express TGF-b1 in a 3:1 ratio. TGF-b1 expressing cells were irradiated with low-dose gamma rays to prevent proliferation within the knee joint after injection. TG-C was administered by a single IA injection [189] (Fig. 10.8). Cherian et al. [190] conducted a phase II randomized study to evaluate the efficacy and safety of genetically engineered allogeneic human chondrocytes expressing TGF-b1 in KL 3 knee OA patients. Improvement of IKDC subjective or VAS scores showed statistically significant differences at 12 weeks, 52 weeks and overall. Kim et al. [189] reported a multicenter, DB, phase III clinical trial to access the efficacy and safety of gene therapy in knee OA. In this study, 163 patients with KL grade III OA were randomly assigned to receive a single IA injection of TG-C or saline. TG-C showed statistically significant improvements over placebo in total IKDC scores and individual categories, VAS scores at 26, 39, and 52 weeks. Patients treated with TG-C were not statistically significant, but tended to have thicker cartilage and slower growth of the subchondral bone surface area in the joint ($p > 0.05$). There were minor AEs in the TG-C group, such as peripheral edema (9%), joint pain (8%), joint swelling (6%), and injection site pain (5%). Lee et al. [191] reported a phase II study to determine the 24 months efficacy and safety of genetically engineered allogeneic human chondrocytes expressing TGF-β1 in patients with KL III knee OA. 102 patients were 2:1 randomized to TG-C at a dose of 3.0×10^7 cells, or placebo injection. There were significant improvements in the IKDC and VAS scores in the TG-C cohort, comparing with the placebo cohort at 12, 52, 72, and 104 weeks ($p < 0.05$). MRI at 12 months after treatment showed fewer findings of cartilage damage, infrapatellar fat pad synovitis, and effusion synovitis in the TG-C cohort. No severe AEs were observed. Common AEs were arthralgia, inflammation, and effusion of joint which were similar between both cohorts. Although TG-C has a long-term safety issues due to viral transfected cells, TG-C appears to be an effective modality for the treatment of KL grade III knee OA, so far.

10.4.4 Summary

Articular cartilage is avascular structure. Oral or parenteral administered drugs used to treat knee OA must go through complicated processes, such as the drug passing through the wall of capillaries, then diffusing to the synovial interstitium, and then passing through the synovial membrane into the joint cavity. In this process, drugs with low MW enter the joint relatively easily, but high MW makes it difficult to enter the joint due to the capillary sieving effect. IA injection therapy has the advantage of bypassing this process and avoiding systemic AEs of drugs by oral or parenteral administration. In addition, the low MW drugs in the joints are absorbed through veins and the large through lymphatics. In case of joint inflammation, the residence time of drugs becomes shorter because of increased vascularity and lymphatic flow. In OA treatment, it is important to maintain the IA concentration of the therapeutic drug for enhancing its efficacy.

For IA injection therapy to work effectively, drugs must be injected accurately into the joints. This is because if a drug is injected into an extra-synovial area, the effect of the drug not only decreases but also the discomfort of the patient increases. Image guided injection using US is more useful than blind method for accurate IA injection. US images of anatomical structures around the joints should be understood when attempting IA injections under US guidance, and the ultrasonic artifact produced by needles should be differentiated.

There are CSs and HAs in the standard therapeutic agents used for IA injections. CS is effective in improving symptoms of knee OA because it has a strong anti-inflammatory effect, but the duration of the effect is only 4 weeks or less. However, systemic and local AEs such as articular cartilage destruction should be considered. According to the guideline of the non-profit organizations, IA CS injection recommends limited use in treating symptomatic knee OA that do not respond to non-pharmacological or pharmacologic treatment. HA not only acts as a viscosupplement that increases the viscosity of the synovial fluid but also has some anti-inflammatory effects. HA relieves symptoms over 3–6 months after injection, which is relatively longer than CS. However, most non-profit organization guideline does not recommend IA HA injection or recommends limited use in treating knee arthritis with symptoms that do not respond to non-pharmacological or pharmacologic treatment. Although PDRN or hypertonic dextrose injection is known to help wound healing and tissue regeneration, much research is still needed to prove a clinical efficacy in the treatment of knee OA. Recently, small molecule drug therapy for treatment of knee OA has been introduced. SM04690 is a novel small molecule Wnt-β-catenin signaling pathway inhibitor, which has potential as a disease-modifying OA drug (DMOAD). CNTX-4975 is an injectable, high-purity trans-capsaicin targeted the capsaicin receptor (TRPV1), which has a potent analgesic effect.

OA results from an imbalance between catabolic and anabolic factors, and biologic agents either target specific catabolic proinflammatory mediators or affect anabolism. Attempts to treat knee OA with biologics have been made relatively recently. Biologics used for treatment of knee OA are categorized into non-cellular therapy or cell therapy. Non-cellular therapy includes human serum albumin, growth factors, cytokine antagonists. In particular, the rhFGF 18 and the Wnt receptor inhibitor have an anabolic effect, drawing attention for their role as DMOAD along with the symptom improvements. However, non-cellular therapeutic agents of various substances are not yet widely used in clinical practice because of lacking of sound scientific evidence. Cell therapy includes cell concentrates, MSCs, and gene therapy. Although the composition of cell concentrates is heterogenous, it has recently drawn much attention as a kind of autologous point-of-care cell therapy, with the advantage of less government regulation because it can be extracted through minimal manipulation and injected into the patient immediately. SVF is a cell concentrate extracted from adipose tissue and has advantages as 15–30% of the extracted cells consist of stromal cells. The therapeutic effect of SVF in knee OA has shown good results in several studies but has not reached MICD. BMAC is a cell concentrates derived from bone marrow, and only 0.001%–0.01% of the cells extracted contain stromal cells. There is little research on the therapeutic effect of BMAC in knee OA. PRP is cell concentrates separated from blood. PRP is a plasma that contains high content of platelets. Platelet α-granules contain a variety of growth factors and anti-inflammatory cytokines, which help wound healing and regeneration. The therapeutic effect using PRP in knee OA is known to be maintained for 6–12 months, but the efficacy does not reach MCID. MSCs have cellular characteristics such as plastic-adherent, express or lack specific cell surface markers and be capable of trilineage differentiation into osteoblasts, adipocytes, and chondrocytes in vitro. MSCs are grown from cell concentrates in vitro and separated with only cells with MSCs characteristics and used to treat knee OA. Government regulation is needed in its use because the cell's properties change in this process and in vitro manipulation is required. MSCs used in the treatment of knee OA include bone marrow-derived MSCs and adipose-derived MSCs. Despite the possibility of tissue healing and regeneration in MSCs, clinical efficacy in knee OA treatment is limited. According to 2019 OARSI and ACR guideline, PRP and MSCs injections are strongly recommended against in patients with knee OA because the evidence in support of these treatments is of extremely low quality and there is a lot of heterogeneity and lack of standardization in preparations of PRP and MSCs.

References

1. Silverwood V, Blagojevic-Bucknall M, Jinks C, Jordan J, Protheroe J, Jordan K. Current evidence on risk factors for knee osteoarthritis in older adults: a systematic review and meta-analysis. Osteoarthr Cartil. 2015;23(4):507–15.
2. Kolasinski SL, Neogi T, Hochberg MC, Oatis C, Guyatt G, Block J, et al. 2019 American College of Rheumatology/Arthritis Foundation guideline for the management of osteoarthritis of the hand, hip, and knee. Arthritis Rheumatol. 2020;72(2):220–33.
3. Nahhas CR, Fuller BC, Hannon CP, Gerlinger TL, Nam D, Della Valle CJ. Which nonsurgical treatments do patients believe are most effective for hip and knee arthritis? J Am Acad Orthop Surg. 2020;4(5):e20.
4. Jackson DW, Evans NA, Thomas BM. Accuracy of needle placement into the intra-articular space of the knee. J Bone Joint Surg Am. 2002;84(9):1522–7.
5. Evans CH, Kraus VB, Setton LA. Progress in intra-articular therapy. Nat Rev Rheumatol. 2014;10(1):11.
6. Nguyen C, Rannou F. The safety of intra-articular injections for the treatment of knee osteoarthritis: a critical narrative review. Expert Opin Drug Saf. 2017;16(8):897–902.
7. Bannuru RR, McAlindon TE, Sullivan MC, Wong JB, Kent DM, Schmid CH. Effectiveness and implications of alternative placebo treatments: a systematic review and network meta-analysis of osteoarthritis trials. Ann Intern Med. 2015;163(5):365–72.
8. Saltzman BM, Leroux T, Meyer MA, Basques BA, Chahal J, Bach BR Jr, et al. The therapeutic effect of intra-articular normal saline injections for knee osteoarthritis: a meta-analysis of evidence level 1 studies. Am J Sports Med. 2017;45(11):2647–53.
9. Jones IA, Togashi R, Wilson ML, Heckmann N, Vangsness CT. Intra-articular treatment options for knee osteoarthritis. Nat Rev Rheumatol. 2019;15(2):77–90.
10. Paoloni M, Bernetti A, Belelli A, Brignoli O, Buoso S, Caputi AP, et al. Appropriateness of clinical and organizational criteria for intra-articular injection therapies in osteoarthritis: a Delphi method consensus initiative among experts in Italy. Ann Ist Super Sanita. 2015;51:131–8.
11. Oo WM, Liu X, Hunter DJ. Pharmacodynamics, efficacy, safety and administration of intra-articular therapies for knee osteoarthritis. Expert Opin Drug Metab Toxicol. 2019;15(12):1021–32.
12. Simkin PA, Pizzorno JE. Synovial permeability in rheumatoid arthritis. Arthritis Rheum. 1979;22(7):689–96.
13. Knight A, Levick J. Morphometry of the ultrastructure of the blood-joint barrier in the rabbit knee. Q J Exp Physiol. 1984;69(2):271–88.
14. Kushner I, Somerville JA. Permeability of human synovial membrane to plasma proteins. Relationship to molecular size and inflammation. Arthritis Rheum. 1971;14(5):560–70.
15. Simkin PA. Synovial perfusion and synovial fluid solutes. Ann Rheum Dis. 1995;54(5):424.
16. Larsen C, Østergaard J, Larsen SW, Jensen H, Jacobsen S, Lindegaard C, et al. Intra-articular depot formulation principles: role in the management of postoperative pain and arthritic disorders. J Pharm Sci. 2008;97(11):4622–54.
17. Scanzello CR, Goldring SR. The role of synovitis in osteoarthritis pathogenesis. Bone. 2012;51(2):249–57.
18. Jones A, Regan M, Ledingham J, Pattrick M, Manhire A, Doherty M. Importance of placement of intra-articular steroid injections. BMJ. 1993;307(6915):1329–30. https://doi.org/10.1136/bmj.307.6915.1329.
19. Glattes RC, Spindler KP, Blanchard GM, Rohmiller MT, McCarty EC, Block J. A simple, accurate method to confirm placement of intra-articular knee injection. Am J Sports Med. 2004;32(4):1029–31.

20. Qvistgaard E, Kristoffersen H, Terslev L, Danneskiold-Samsøe B, Torp-Pedersen S, Bliddal H. Guidance by ultrasound of intra-articular injections in the knee and hip joints. Osteoarthr Cartil. 2001;9(6):512–7.
21. Waddell D, Estey D, Bricker D, Marsala A. Viscosupplementation under fluoroscopic control. Am J Sports Med. 2001;3(4):327–241. 9
22. Tarhan S, Unlu Z. Magnetic resonance imaging and ultrasonographic evaluation of the patients with knee osteoarthritis: a comparative study. Clin Rheumatol. 2003;22(3):181–8.
23. Esenyel C, Demirhan M, Esenyel M, Sonmez M, Kahraman S, Senel B, et al. Comparison of four different intra-articular injection sites in the knee: a cadaver study. Knee Surg Sports Traumatol Arthrosc. 2007;15(5):573–7.
24. Luc M, Pham T, Chagnaud C, Lafforgue P, Legre V. Placement of intra-articular injection verified by the backflow technique. Osteoarthr Cartil. 2006;14(7):714–6.
25. Maricar N, Parkes MJ, Callaghan MJ, Felson DT, O'Neill TW. Where and how to inject the knee—a systematic review. Semin Arthritis Rheum. 2013;43(2):195–203.
26. Toda Y, Tsukimura N. A comparison of intra-articular hyaluronan injection accuracy rates between three approaches based on radiographic severity of knee osteoarthritis. Osteoarthr Cartil. 2008;16(9):980–5.
27. Im SH, Lee SC, Park YB, Cho S-R, Kim JC. Feasibility of sonography for intra-articular injections in the knee through a medial patellar portal. J Ultrasound Med. 2009;28(11):1465–70.
28. Park Y, Lee SC, Nam H-S, Lee J, Nam SH. Comparison of sonographically guided intra-articular injections at 3 different sites of the knee. J Ultrasound Med. 2011;30(12):1669–76.
29. Myung JS, Lee JW, Lee JY, Choi J-Y, Kim SH, Jun WS, et al. Usefulness of fluoroscopy-guided intra-articular injection of the knee. J Korean Radiol Soc. 2007;56(6):563–7.
30. Chavez-Chiang CE, Sibbitt WL, Band PA, Chavez-Chiang NR, DeLea SL, Bankhurst AD. The highly accurate anteriolateral portal for injecting the knee. Sports Med Arthros Rehabil Ther Technol. 2011;3(1):6.
31. Hussein M. An accurate full-flexion anterolateral portal for needle placement in the knee joint with dry osteoarthritis. J Am Acad Orthop Surg. 2017;25(7):e131–e7. https://doi.org/10.5435/jaaos-d-16-00338.
32. Lee SY, Gn KK, Chung BJ, Lee SW, Kim TK. Anterolateral portal is less painful than superolateral portal in knee intra-articular injection. Knee Surg Relat Res. 2015;27(4):228–32. https://doi.org/10.5792/ksrr.2015.27.4.228.
33. Shortt CP, Morrison WB, Roberts CC, Deely DM, Gopez AG, Zoga AC. Shoulder, hip, and knee arthrography needle placement using fluoroscopic guidance: practice patterns of musculoskeletal radiologists in North America. Skelet Radiol. 2009;38(4):377–85.
34. Douglas RJ. Aspiration and injection of the knee joint: approach portal. Knee Surg Relat Res. 2014;26(1):1.
35. Telikicherla M, Kamath SU. Accuracy of needle placement into the intra-articular space of the knee in osteoarthritis patients for viscosupplementation. J Clin Diagn Res. 2016;10(2):RC15.
36. Chavez-Chiang NR, Sibbitt WL, Band PA, DeLea SL, Park KS, Bankhurst AD. The outcomes and cost-effectiveness of intraarticular injection of the rheumatoid knee. Rheumatol Int. 2012;32(2):513–8.
37. Hermans J, Bierma-Zeinstra SM, Bos PK, Verhaar JA, Reijman M. The most accurate approach for intra-articular needle placement in the knee joint: a systematic review. Semin Arthritis Rheum. 2011;41:106–15.
38. Curtiss HM, Finnoff JT, Peck E, Hollman J, Muir J, Smith J. Accuracy of ultrasound-guided and palpation-guided knee injections by an experienced and less-experienced injector using a superolateral approach: a cadaveric study. PM&R. 2011;3(6):507–15.
39. Bum Park Y, Ah Choi W, Kim YK, Chul Lee S, Hae LJ. Accuracy of blind versus ultrasound-guided suprapatellar bursal injection. J Clin Ultrasound. 2012;40(1):20–5.
40. Sibbitt W Jr, Kettwich L, Band P, Chavez-Chiang N, DeLea S, Haseler L, et al. Does ultrasound guidance improve the outcomes of arthrocentesis and corticosteroid injection of the knee? Scand J Rheumatol. 2012;41(1):66–72.
41. Cunnington J, Marshall N, Hide G, Bracewell C, Isaacs J, Platt P, et al. A randomized, double-blind, controlled study of ultrasound-guided corticosteroid injection into the joint of patients with inflammatory arthritis. Arthritis Rheum. 2010;62(7):1862–9.
42. Ihnatsenka B, Boezaart AP. Ultrasound: basic understanding and learning the language. Int J Shoulder Surg. 2010;4(3):55.
43. Sites BD, Brull R, Chan VW, Spence BC, Gallagher J, Beach ML, et al. Artifacts and pitfall errors associated with ultrasound-guided regional anesthesia: Part I: Understanding the basic principles of ultrasound physics and machine operations. Reg Anesth Pain Med. 2007;32(5):412–8.
44. Sites BD, Brull R, Chan VW, Spence BC, Gallagher J, Beach ML, et al. Artifacts and pitfall errors associated with ultrasound-guided regional anesthesia: part II: a pictorial approach to understanding and avoidance. Reg Anesth Pain Med. 2007;32(5):419–33.
45. Chevalier X, Eymard F, Richette P. Biologic agents in osteoarthritis: hopes and disappointments. Nat Rev Rheumatol. 2013;9(7):400.
46. MacMahon PJ, Eustace SJ, Kavanagh EC. Injectable corticosteroid and local anesthetic preparations: a review for radiologists. Radiology. 2009;252(3):647–61. https://doi.org/10.1148/radiol.2523081929.

47. Creamer P. Intra-articular corticosteroid injections in osteoarthritis: do they work and if so, how? Ann Rheum Dis. 1997;56(11):634–5.
48. Pekarek B, Osher L, Buck S, Bowen M. Intra-articular corticosteroid injections: a critical literature review with up-to-date findings. Foot. 2011;21(2):66–70.
49. Schumacher HR, Chen LX. Injectable corticosteroids in treatment of arthritis of the knee. Am J Sports Med. 2005;118(11):1208–14.
50. Østergaard M, Halberg P. Intra-articular corticosteroids in arthritic disease. BioDrugs. 1998;9(2):95 103.
51. Derendorf H, Möllmann H, Grüner A, Haack D, Gyselby G. Pharmacokinetics and pharmacodynamics of glucocorticoid suspensions after intra-articular administration. Clin Pharmacol Ther. 1986;39(3):313–7.
52. Kraus V, Conaghan P, Aazami H, Mehra P, Kivitz A, Lufkin J, et al. Synovial and systemic pharmacokinetics (PK) of triamcinolone acetonide (TA) following intra-articular (IA) injection of an extended-release microsphere-based formulation (FX006) or standard crystalline suspension in patients with knee osteoarthritis (OA). Osteoarthr Cartil. 2018;26(1):34–42.
53. Hepper CT, Halvorson JJ, Duncan ST, Gregory AJ, Dunn WR, Spindler KP. The efficacy and duration of intra-articular corticosteroid injection for knee osteoarthritis: a systematic review of level I studies. J Am Acad Orthop Surg. 2009;17(10):638–46.
54. Pyne D, Ioannou Y, Mootoo R, Bhanji A. Intra-articular steroids in knee osteoarthritis: a comparative study of triamcinolone hexacetonide and methylprednisolone acetate. Clin Rheumatol. 2004;23(2):116–20.
55. Yavuz U, Sökücü S, Albayrak A, Öztürk K. Efficacy comparisons of the intraarticular steroidal agents in the patients with knee osteoarthritis. Rheumatol Int. 2012;32(11):3391–6.
56. Lomonte ABV, de Morais MGV, de Carvalho LO, de Freitas Zerbini CA. Efficacy of triamcinolone hexacetonide versus methylprednisolone acetate intraarticular injections in knee osteoarthritis: a randomized, double-blinded, 24-week study. J Rheumatol. 2015;42(9):1677–84.
57. Buyuk AF, Kilinc E, Camurcu IY, Camur S, Ucpunar H, Kara A. Compared efficacy of intra-articular injection of methylprednisolone and triamcinolone. Acta Ortop Bras. 2017;25(5):206–8.
58. Popma JW, Snel FW, Haagsma CJ, Brummelhuis-Visser P, Oldenhof HG, van der Palen J, et al. Comparison of 2 dosages of intraarticular triamcinolone for the treatment of knee arthritis: results of a 12-week randomized controlled clinical trial. J Rheumatol. 2015;42(10):1865–8.
59. Benzon Honorio T, Chew T-L, McCarthy Robert J, Benzon Hubert A, Walega DR. Comparison of the particle sizes of different steroids and the effect of dilution: a review of the relative neurotoxicities of the steroids. Anesthesiology. 2007;106(2):331–8. https://doi.org/10.1097/00000542-200702000-00022.
60. Chu CR, Coyle CH, Chu CT, Szczodry M, Seshadri V, Karpie JC, et al. In vivo effects of single intra-articular injection of 0.5% bupivacaine on articular cartilage. J Bone Joint Surg Am. 2010;92(3):599–608.
61. Chakravarty K, Pharoah P, Scott D. A randomized controlled study of post-injection rest following intra-articular steroid therapy for knee synovitis. Rheumatology. 1994;33(5):464–8.
62. Charalambous C, Paschalides C, Sadiq S, Tryfonides M, Hirst P, Paul A. Weight bearing following intra-articular steroid injection of the knee: survey of current practice and review of the available evidence. Rheumatol Int. 2002;22(5):185–7.
63. Bellamy N, Campbell J, Welch V, Gee TL, Bourne R, Wells GA. Intraarticular corticosteroid for treatment of osteoarthritis of the knee. Cochrane Database Syst Rev. 2006;2
64. Bannuru RR, Natov NS, Obadan IE, Price LL, Schmid CH, McAlindon TE. Therapeutic trajectory of hyaluronic acid versus corticosteroids in the treatment of knee osteoarthritis: a systematic review and meta-analysis. Arthritis Care Res. 2009;61(12):1704–11.
65. Jüni P, Hari R, Rutjes AW, Fischer R, Silletta MG, Reichenbach S, et al. Intra-articular corticosteroid for knee osteoarthritis. Cochrane Database Syst Rev. 2015;10
66. Paik J, Duggan ST, Keam SJ. Triamcinolone acetonide extended-release: a review in osteoarthritis pain of the knee. Drugs. 2019;79(4):455–62.
67. Conaghan PG, Hunter DJ, Cohen SB, Kraus VB, Berenbaum F, Lieberman JR, et al. Effects of a single intra-articular injection of a microsphere formulation of triamcinolone acetonide on knee osteoarthritis pain: a double-blinded, randomized, placebo-controlled, multinational study. J Bone Joint Surg Am. 2018;100(8):666.
68. Maricar N, Callaghan MJ, Felson DT, O'Neill TW. Predictors of response to intra-articular steroid injections in knee osteoarthritis—a systematic review. Rheumatology. 2013;52(6):1022–32.
69. Matzkin EG, Curry EJ, Kong Q, Rogers MJ, Henry M, Smith EL. Efficacy and treatment response of intra-articular corticosteroid injections in patients with symptomatic knee osteoarthritis. J Am Acad Orthop Surg. 2017;25(10):703–14.
70. Maricar N, Parkes MJ, Callaghan MJ, Hutchinson CE, Gait AD, Hodgson R, et al. Structural predictors of response to intra-articular steroid injection in symptomatic knee osteoarthritis. Arthritis Res Ther. 2017;19(1):88.
71. Jevsevar DS, Brown GA, Jones DL, Matzkin EG, Manner PA, Mooar P, et al. the American Academy of Orthopaedic Surgeons evidence-based guideline on: treatment of osteoarthritis of the knee, 2nd edition. J Bone Joint Surg Am. 2013;95(20):1885–6.

72. McAlindon TE, Bannuru RR, Sullivan M, Arden N, Berenbaum F, Bierma-Zeinstra S, et al. OARSI guidelines for the non-surgical management of knee osteoarthritis. Osteoarthr Cartil. 2014;22(3):363–88.
73. Carlson VR, Ong AC, Orozco FR, Hernandez VH, Lutz RW, Post ZD. Compliance with the AAOS guidelines for treatment of osteoarthritis of the knee: a survey of the American Association of Hip and Knee Surgeons. J Am Acad Orthop Surg. 2018;26(3):103–7. https://doi.org/10.5435/jaaos-d-17-00164.
74. Meiyappan KP, Cote MP, Bozic KJ, Halawi MJ. Adherence to the American Academy of Orthopaedic Surgeons clinical practice guidelines for nonoperative management of knee osteoarthritis. J Arthroplast. 2020;35(2):347–52.
75. Bannuru RR, Osani M, Vaysbrot E, Arden N, Bennell K, Bierma-Zeinstra S, et al. OARSI guidelines for the non-surgical management of knee, hip, and polyarticular osteoarthritis. Osteoarthr Cartil. 2019;27(11):1578–89.
76. Bruyère O, Honvo G, Veronese N, Arden NK, Branco J, Curtis EM, et al. An updated algorithm recommendation for the management of knee osteoarthritis from the European Society for Clinical and Economic Aspects of Osteoporosis, Osteoarthritis and Musculoskeletal Diseases (ESCEO). Semin Arthritis Rheum. 2019;49(3):337–50.
77. McAlindon TE, LaValley MP, Harvey WF, Price LL, Driban JB, Zhang M, et al. Effect of intra-articular triamcinolone vs saline on knee cartilage volume and pain in patients with knee osteoarthritis: a randomized clinical trial. JAMA. 2017;317(19):1967–75.
78. Raynauld JP, Buckland-Wright C, Ward R, Choquette D, Haraoui B, Martel-Pelletier J, et al. Safety and efficacy of long-term intraarticular steroid injections in osteoarthritis of the knee: a randomized, double-blind, placebo-controlled trial. Arthritis Rheum. 2003;48(2):370–7.
79. Cancienne JM, Werner BC, Luetkemeyer LM, Browne JA. Does timing of previous intra-articular steroid injection affect the post-operative rate of infection in total knee arthroplasty? J Arthroplast. 2015;30(11):1879–82.
80. Richardson SS, Schairer WW, Sculco TP, Sculco PK. Comparison of infection risk with corticosteroid or hyaluronic acid injection prior to total knee arthroplasty. J Bone Joint Surg Am. 2019;101(2):112–8.
81. McGarry JG, Daruwalla ZJ. The efficacy, accuracy and complications of corticosteroid injections of the knee joint. Knee Surg Sports Traumatol Arthrosc. 2011;19(10):1649–54.
82. Bird HA, Ring EF, Bacon PA. A thermographic and clinical comparison of three intra-articular steroid preparations in rheumatoid arthritis. Ann Rheum Dis. 1979;38(1):36–9.
83. Balazs EA, Watson D, Duff IF, Roseman S. Hyaluronic acid in synovial fluid. I. Molecular parameters of hyaluronic acid in normal and arthritic human fluids. Arthritis Rheum. 1967;10(4):357–76.
84. Strauss EJ, Hart JA, Miller MD, Altman RD, Rosen JE. Hyaluronic acid viscosupplementation and osteoarthritis: current uses and future directions. Am J Sports Med. 2009;37(8):1636–44.
85. Balazs EA, Denlinger JL. Viscosupplementation: a new concept in the treatment of osteoarthritis. J Rheumatol Suppl. 1993;39:3–9.
86. Rydell N, Balazs EA. Effect of intra-articular injection of hyaluronic acid on the clinical symptoms of osteoarthritis and on granulation tissue formation. Clin Orthop Relat Res. 1971;80:25–32.
87. Scale D, Wobig M, Wolpert W. Viscosupplementation of osteoarthritic knees with hylan: a treatment schedule study. Curr Ther Res. 1994;55(3):220–32.
88. Altman R, Bedi A, Manjoo A, Niazi F, Shaw P, Mease P. Anti-inflammatory effects of intra-articular hyaluronic acid: a systematic review. Cartilage. 2019;10(1):43–52.
89. Moreland LW. Intra-articular hyaluronan (hyaluronic acid) and hylans for the treatment of osteoarthritis: mechanisms of action. Arthritis Res Ther. 2003;5(2):54.
90. Smith MM, Ghosh P. The synthesis of hyaluronic acid by human synovial fibroblasts is influenced by the nature of the hyaluronate in the extracellular environment. Rheumatol Int. 1987;7(3):113–22.
91. Bowman S, Awad ME, Hamrick MW, Hunter M, Fulzele S. Recent advances in hyaluronic acid based therapy for osteoarthritis. Clin Transl Med. 2018;7(1):6.
92. Altman R, Hackel J, Niazi F, Shaw P, Nicholls M. Efficacy and safety of repeated courses of hyaluronic acid injections for knee osteoarthritis: a systematic review. Semin Arthritis Rheum. 2018;48(2):186–75.
93. Brockmeier SF, Shaffer BS. Viscosupplementation therapy for osteoarthritis. Sports Med Arthrosc Rev. 2006;14(3):155–62.
94. Reichenbach S, Blank S, Rutjes AW, Shang A, King EA, Dieppe PA, et al. Hylan versus hyaluronic acid for osteoarthritis of the knee: a systematic review and meta-analysis. Arthritis Care Res. 2007;57(8):1410–8.
95. Rutjes AW, Jüni P, da Costa BR, Trelle S, Nüesch E, Reichenbach S. Viscosupplementation for osteoarthritis of the knee: a systematic review and meta-analysis. Ann Intern Med. 2012;157(3):180–91.
96. Jevsevar D, Donnelly P, Brown GA, Cummins DS. Viscosupplementation for osteoarthritis of the knee: a systematic review of the evidence. J Bone Joint Surg Am. 2015;97(24):2047–60.
97. Bowman EN, Hallock JD, Throckmorton TW, Azar FM. Hyaluronic acid injections for osteoarthritis of the knee: predictors of successful treatment. Int Orthop. 2018;42(4):733–40.
98. Wang C-T, Lin J, Chang C-J, Lin Y-T, Hou S-M. Therapeutic effects of hyaluronic acid on osteoarthritis of the knee: a meta-analysis of randomized controlled trials. J Bone Joint Surg Am. 2004;86(3):538–45.

99. Levy DM, Petersen KA, Vaught MS, Christian DR, Cole BJ. Injections for knee osteoarthritis: corticosteroids, viscosupplementation, platelet-rich plasma, and autologous stem cells. Arthroscopy. 2018;34(5):1730–43.
100. Hunter DJ. Viscosupplementation for osteoarthritis of the knee. N Engl J Med. 2015;372(11):1040–7.
101. Altman R. Intra-articular sodium hyaluronate (Hyalgan®) in the treatment of patients with osteoarthritis of the knee: a randomized clinical trial. J Rheumatol. 1998;25:2203–12.
102. Adams ME, Atkinson MH, Lussier AJ, Schulz JI, Siminovitch KA, Wade JP, et al. The role of viscosupplementation with hylan GF 20 (Synvisc®) in the treatment of osteoarthritis of the knee: a Canadian multicenter trial comparing hylan GF 20 alone, hylan GF 20 with non-steroidal anti-inflammatory drugs (NSAIDs) and NSAIDs alone. Osteoarthr Cartil. 1995;3(4):213–25.
103. Caborn D, Rush J, Lanzer W, Parenti D, Murray C, Group SS. A randomized, single-blind comparison of the efficacy and tolerability of hylan GF 20 and triamcinolone hexacetonide in patients with osteoarthritis of the knee. J Rheumatol. 2004;31(2):333–43.
104. Ong KL, Anderson AF, Niazi F, Fierlinger AL, Kurtz SM, Altman RD. Hyaluronic acid injections in medicare knee osteoarthritis patients are associated with longer time to knee arthroplasty. J Arthroplast. 2016;31(8):1667–73.
105. Altman R, Lim S, Steen RG, Dasa V. Hyaluronic acid injections are associated with delay of total knee replacement surgery in patients with knee osteoarthritis: evidence from a large US health claims database. PLoS One. 2015;10(12):e0145776.
106. Jubb R, Piva S, Beinat L, Dacre J, Gishen P. A one year, randomised, placebo (saline) controlled clinical trial of 500-730 kDa sodium hyaluronate (Hyalgan) on the radiological change in osteoarthritis of the knee. Int J Clin Pract. 2003;57(6):467.
107. Wang Y, Hall S, Hanna F, Wluka AE, Grant G, Marks P, et al. Effects of Hylan GF 20 supplementation on cartilage preservation detected by magnetic resonance imaging in osteoarthritis of the knee: a two-year single-blind clinical trial. BMC Musculoskelet Disord. 2011;12(1):195.
108. Divine JG, Zazulak BT, Hewett TE. Viscosupplementation for knee osteoarthritis: a systematic review. Clin Orthop Relat Res. 2007;455:113–22.
109. Bannuru R, Natov N, Dasi U, Schmid C, McAlindon T. Therapeutic trajectory following intra-articular hyaluronic acid injection in knee osteoarthritis–meta-analysis. Osteoarthr Cartil. 2011;19(6):611–9.
110. Smith C, Patel R, Vannabouathong C, Sales B, Rabinovich A, McCormack R, et al. Combined intra-articular injection of corticosteroid and hyaluronic acid reduces pain compared to hyaluronic acid alone in the treatment of knee osteoarthritis. Knee Surg Sports Traumatol Arthrosc. 2019;27(6):1974–83.
111. Colangelo MT, Galli C, Guizzardi S. The effects of polydeoxyribonucleotide on wound healing and tissue regeneration: a systematic review of the literature. Regen Med. 2020; https://doi.org/10.2217/rme-2019-0118.
112. Squadrito F, Bitto A, Irrera N, Pizzino G, Pallio G, Minutoli L, et al. Pharmacological activity and clinical use of PDRN. Front Pharmacol. 2017;8:224.
113. Vanelli R, Costa P, Rossi SM, Benazzo F. Efficacy of intra-articular polynucleotides in the treatment of knee osteoarthritis: a randomized, double-blind clinical trial. Knee Surg Sports Traumatol Arthrosc. 2010;18(7):901–7. https://doi.org/10.1007/s00167-009-1039-y.
114. Bitto A, Polito F, Irrera N, D'Ascola A, Avenoso A, Nastasi G, et al. Polydeoxyribonucleotide reduces cytokine production and the severity of collagen-induced arthritis by stimulation of adenosine A((2)A) receptor. Arthritis Rheum. 2011;63(11):3364–71. https://doi.org/10.1002/art.30538.
115. Gennero L, Denysenko T, Calisti GF, Vercelli A, Vercelli CM, Amedeo S, et al. Protective effects of polydeoxyribonucleotides on cartilage degradation in experimental cultures. Cell Biochem Funct. 2013;31(3):214–27. https://doi.org/10.1002/cbf.2875.
116. Kim MS, Cho RK, In Y. The efficacy and safety of polydeoxyribonucleotide for the treatment of knee osteoarthritis: Systematic review and meta-analysis of randomized controlled trials. Medicine. 2019;98(39):e17386.
117. Zazgyva A, Gergely I, Russu OM, Roman C, Pop TS. Polynucleotides versus sodium hyaluronate in the local treatment of knee osteoarthritis. Acta Medica Transilvanica. 2013;2(2):260–3.
118. Giarratana LS, Marelli BM, Crapanzano C, De Martinis SE, Gala L, Ferraro M, et al. A randomized double-blind clinical trial on the treatment of knee osteoarthritis: the efficacy of polynucleotides compared to standard hyaluronian viscosupplementation. Knee. 2014;21(3):661–8.
119. Yoon S, Kang JJ, Kim J, Park S, Kim JM. Efficacy and safety of intra-articular injections of hyaluronic acid combined with polydeoxyribonucleotide in the treatment of knee osteoarthritis. Ann Rehabil Med. 2019;43(2):204.
120. Dallari D, Sabbioni G, Del Piccolo N, Carubbi C, Veronesi F, Torricelli P, et al. Efficacy of intra-articular polynucleotides associated with hyaluronic acid versus hyaluronic acid alone in the treatment of knee osteoarthritis: a randomized, double-blind, controlled clinical trial. Clin J Sport Med. 2018;30(1):1–7.
121. Hauser RA, Lackner JB, Steilen-Matias D, Harris DK. A systematic review of dextrose prolotherapy for chronic musculoskeletal pain. Clin Med Insights Arthritis Musculoskelet Disord. 2016;9:139–59. https://doi.org/10.4137/CMAMD.S39160.
122. Park Y-S, Lim S-W, Lee I-H, Lee T-J, Kim J-S, Han JS. Intra-articular injection of a nutritive mixture

solution protects articular cartilage from osteoarthritic progression induced by anterior cruciate ligament transection in mature rabbits: a randomized controlled trial. Arthritis Res Ther. 2007;9(1):R8.
123. Topol GA, Podesta LA, Reeves KD, Giraldo MM, Johnson LL, Grasso R, et al. Chondrogenic effect of intra-articular hypertonic-dextrose (prolotherapy) in severe knee osteoarthritis. PM&R. 2016;8(11):1072–82.
124. Reeves KD, Hassanein K. Randomized prospective double-blind placebo-controlled study of dextrose prolotherapy for knee osteoarthritis with or without ACL laxity. Altern Ther Health Med. 2000;6(2):68–80.
125. Dumais R, Benoit C, Dumais A, Babin L, Bordage R, de Arcos C, et al. Effect of regenerative injection therapy on function and pain in patients with knee osteoarthritis: a randomized crossover study. Pain Med. 2012;13(8):990–9.
126. Rabago D, Zgierska A, Fortney L, Kijowski R, Mundt M, Ryan M, et al. Hypertonic dextrose injections (prolotherapy) for knee osteoarthritis: results of a single-arm uncontrolled study with 1-year follow-up. J Altern Complement Med. 2012;18(4):408–14.
127. Sit RW, Chung VC, Reeves KD, Rabago D, Chan KK, Chan DC, et al. Hypertonic dextrose injections (prolotherapy) in the treatment of symptomatic knee osteoarthritis: a systematic review and meta-analysis. Sci Rep. 2016;6:25247.
128. Wang Y, Fan X, Xing L, Tian F. Wnt signaling: a promising target for osteoarthritis therapy. Cell Commun Signal. 2019;17(1):1–14.
129. Yazici Y, Mcalindon T, Gibofsky A, Lane N, Lattermann C, Skrepnik N, et al. THU0458 Efficacy and safety from a phase 2B trial of SM04690, a novel intra-articular wnt pathway inhibitor for the treatment of osteoarthritis of the knee. BMJ. 2019:591–19.
130. Tominaga M, Caterina MJ, Malmberg AB, Rosen TA, Gilbert H, Skinner K, et al. The cloned capsaicin receptor integrates multiple pain-producing stimuli. Neuron. 1998;21(3):531–43.
131. Simone DA, Nolano M, Johnson T, Wendelschafer-Crabb G, Kennedy WR. Intradermal injection of capsaicin in humans produces degeneration and subsequent reinnervation of epidermal nerve fibers: correlation with sensory function. J Neurosci. 1998;18(21):8947–59.
132. Stevens RM, Ervin J, Nezzer J, Nieves Y, Guedes K, Burges R, et al. Randomized, double-blind, placebo-controlled trial of intraarticular trans-capsaicin for pain associated with osteoarthritis of the knee. Arthr Rheumatol. 2019;71(9):1524–33.
133. Cotter EJ, Frank RM, Mandelbaum B. Management of osteoarthritis-biological approaches: current concepts. J ISAKOS. 2020;5(1):27–31.
134. Shimonkevitz R, Thomas G, Slone DS, Craun M, Mains C, Bar-Or D. A diketopiperazine fragment of human serum albumin modulates T-lymphocyte cytokine production through rap1. J Trauma Acute Care Surg. 2008;64(1):35–41.
135. Bar-Or D, Salottolo KM, Loose H, Phillips MJ, McGrath B, Wei N, et al. A randomized clinical trial to evaluate two doses of an intra-articular injection of LMWF-5A in adults with pain due to osteoarthritis of the knee. PLoS One. 2014;9(2):e87910.
136. Salottolo K, Cole B, Bar-Or D. Intra-articular injection of the anti-inflammatory compound LMWF-5A in adults with severe osteoarthritis: a double-blind prospective randomized controlled multi-center safety and efficacy trial. Patient Saf Surg. 2018;12(1):11.
137. Roemer FW, Aydemir A, Lohmander S, Crema MD, Marra MD, Muurahainen N, et al. Structural effects of sprifermin in knee osteoarthritis: a post-hoc analysis on cartilage and non-cartilaginous tissue alterations in a randomized controlled trial. BMC Musculoskelet Disord. 2016;17(1):267.
138. Hochberg MC, Guermazi A, Guehring H, Aydemir A, Wax S, Fleuranceau-Morel P, et al. Effect of intra-articular Sprifermin vs placebo on femorotibial joint cartilage thickness in patients with osteoarthritis: the FORWARD randomized clinical trial. JAMA. 2019;322(14):1360–70.
139. Jacques C, Gosset M, Berenbaum F, Gabay C. The role of IL-1 and IL-1Ra in joint inflammation and cartilage degradation. Vitam Horm. 2006;74:371–403.
140. Caron JP, Fernandes JC, Martel-Pelletier J, Tardif G, Mineau F, Geng C, et al. Chondroprotective effect of intraarticular injections of interleukin-1 receptor antagonist in experimental osteoarthritis. Suppression of collagenase-1 expression. Arthritis Rheum. 1996;39(9):1535–44.
141. Chevalier X, Goupille P, Beaulieu A, Burch F, Bensen W, Conrozier T, et al. Intraarticular injection of anakinra in osteoarthritis of the knee: a multicenter, randomized, double-blind, placebo-controlled study. Arthritis Care Res. 2009;61(3):344–52.
142. Stannus O, Jones G, Cicuttini F, Parameswaran V, Quinn S, Burgess J, et al. Circulating levels of IL-6 and TNF-α are associated with knee radiographic osteoarthritis and knee cartilage loss in older adults. Osteoarthr Cartil. 2010;18(11):1441–7.
143. Lindsley H, Schue J, Tawfik O, Bolce R, Smith D, Hinson G, et al. FRI0304 treatment of knee osteoarthritis with intra-articular infliximab improves total womac score. High baseline levels of synovial cellularity predict improvement. Ann Rheum Dis. 2013;71(Suppl 3):417.
144. Ohtori S, Orita S, Yamauchi K, Eguchi Y, Ochiai N, Kishida S, et al. Efficacy of direct injection of etanercept into knee joints for pain in moderate and severe knee osteoarthritis. Yonsei Med J. 2015;56(5):1379–83.
145. Wang J. Efficacy and safety of adalimumab by intra-articular injection for moderate to severe knee osteoarthritis: an open-label randomized controlled trial. J Int Med Res. 2018;46(1):326–34.

146. Roseti L, Desando G, Cavallo C, Petretta M, Grigolo B. Articular cartilage regeneration in osteoarthritis. Cell. 2019;8(11):1305.
147. Aronowitz JA, Ellenhorn JDI. Adipose stromal vascular fraction isolation: a head-to-head comparison of four commercial cell separation systems. Plast Reconstr Surg. 2013;132(6):932e–9e. https://doi.org/10.1097/PRS.0b013e3182a80652.
148. Bourin P, Bunnell BA, Casteilla L, Dominici M, Katz AJ, March KL, et al. Stromal cells from the adipose tissue-derived stromal vascular fraction and culture expanded adipose tissue-derived stromal/stem cells: a joint statement of the International Federation for Adipose Therapeutics and Science (IFATS) and the International Society for Cellular Therapy (ISCT). Cytotherapy. 2013;15(6):641–8.
149. Pak J. Regeneration of human bones in hip osteonecrosis and human cartilage in knee osteoarthritis with autologous adipose-tissue-derived stem cells: a case series. J Med Case Rep. 2011;5(1):1–8.
150. Koh Y-G, Choi Y-J, Kwon S-K, Kim Y-S, Yeo J-E. Clinical results and second-look arthroscopic findings after treatment with adipose-derived stem cells for knee osteoarthritis. Knee Surg Sports Traumatol Arthrosc. 2015;23(5):1308–16.
151. Michalek J, Moster R, Lukac L, Proefrock K, Petrasovic M, Rybar J, et al. Autologous adipose tissue-derived stromal vascular fraction cells application in patients with osteoarthritis. Cell Transplant. 2015;20:1–36.
152. Garza JR, Campbell RE, Tjoumakaris FP, Freedman KB, Miller LS, Santa Maria D, et al. Clinical efficacy of intra-articular mesenchymal stromal cells for the treatment of knee osteoarthritis: a double-blinded prospective randomized controlled clinical trial. Am J Sports Med. 2020;48(3):588–98.
153. Pak J, Lee JH, Park KS, Park M, Kang L W, Lee SH. Current use of autologous adipose tissue-derived stromal vascular fraction cells for orthopedic applications. J Biomed Sci. 2017;24(1):9.
154. Rodriguez-Fontan F, Piuzzi NS, Kraeutler MJ, Pascual-Garrido C. Early clinical outcomes of intra-articular injections of bone marrow aspirate concentrate for the treatment of early osteoarthritis of the hip and knee: a cohort study. PM&R. 2018;10(12):1353–9.
155. Kim J-D, Lee GW, Jung GH, Kim CK, Kim T, Park JH, et al. Clinical outcome of autologous bone marrow aspirates concentrate (BMAC) injection in degenerative arthritis of the knee. Eur J Orthop Surg Traumatol. 2014;24(8):1505–11.
156. Centeno C, Pitts J, Al-Sayegh H, Freeman M. Efficacy of autologous bone marrow concentrate for knee osteoarthritis with and without adipose graft. Biomed Res Int. 2014;2014
157. Shapiro SA, Kazmerchak SE, Heckman MG, Zubair AC, O'Connor MI. A prospective, single-blind, placebo-controlled trial of bone marrow aspirate concentrate for knee osteoarthritis. Am J Sports Med. 2017;45(1):82–90.
158. Shapiro SA, Arthurs JR, Heckman MG, Bestic JM, Kazmerchak SE, Diehl NN, et al. Quantitative T2 MRI mapping and 12-month follow-up in a randomized, blinded, placebo controlled trial of bone marrow aspiration and concentration for osteoarthritis of the knees. Cartilage. 2019;10(4):432–43.
159. Senzel L, Gnatenko DV, Bahou WF. The platelet proteome. Curr Opin Hematol. 2009;16(5):329.
160. Foster TE, Puskas BL, Mandelbaum BR, Gerhardt MB, Rodeo SA. Platelet-rich plasma: from basic science to clinical applications. Am J Sports Med. 2009;37(11):2259–72.
161. Southworth TM, Naveen NB, Tauro TM, Leong NL, Cole BJ. The use of platelet-rich plasma in symptomatic knee osteoarthritis. J Knee Surg. 2019;32(01):037–45.
162. DeLong JM, Beitzel K, Mazzocca AD, Shepard D, Roller BL, Hanypsiak BT. Update on platelet-rich plasma. Curr Orthop Pract. 2011;22(6):514–23.
163. Dai W-L, Zhou A-G, Zhang H, Zhang J. Efficacy of platelet-rich plasma in the treatment of knee osteoarthritis: a meta-analysis of randomized controlled trials. Arthroscopy. 2017;33(3):659–70.e1.
164. Tang JZ, Nie MJ, Zhao JZ, Zhang GC, Zhang Q, Wang B. Platelet-rich plasma versus hyaluronic acid in the treatment of knee osteoarthritis: a meta-analysis. J Orthop Surg Res. 2020;15(1):403 https://doi.org/10.1186/s13018-020-01919-9.
165. Filardo G, Previtali D, Napoli F, Candrian C, Zaffagnini S, Grassi A. PRP injections for the treatment of knee osteoarthritis: a meta-analysis of randomized controlled trials. Cartilage. 2020;1947603520931170
166. Belk JW, Kraeutler MJ, Houck DA, Goodrich JA, Dragoo JL, McCarty EC. Platelet-rich plasma versus hyaluronic acid for knee osteoarthritis: a systematic review and meta-analysis of randomized controlled trials. Am J Sports Med. 2021;49(1):249–60.
167. Delanois RE, Etcheson JI, Sodhi N, Henn RF III, Gwam CU, George NE, et al. Biologic therapies for the treatment of knee osteoarthritis. J Arthroplast. 2019;34(4):801–13.
168. Kon E, Di Matteo B, Delgado D, Cole BJ, Dorotei A, Dragoo JL, et al. Platelet-rich plasma for the treatment of knee osteoarthritis: an expert opinion and proposal for a novel classification and coding system. Expert Opin Biol Ther. 2020:1–14.
169. O'Shaughnessey K, Matuska A, Hoeppner J, Farr J, Klaassen M, Kaeding C, et al. Autologous protein solution prepared from the blood of osteoarthritic patients contains an enhanced profile of anti-inflammatory cytokines and anabolic growth factors. J Orthop Res. 2014;32(10):1349–55.
170. Kon E, Engebretsen L, Verdonk P, Nehrer S, Filardo G. Clinical outcomes of knee osteoarthritis treated with an autologous protein solution injection: a 1-year pilot double-blinded randomized controlled trial. Am J Sports Med. 2018;46(1):171–80.
171. Kon E, Engebretsen L, Verdonk P, Nehrer S, Filardo G. Autologous protein solution injections for the

treatment of knee osteoarthritis: 3-year results. Am J Sports Med. 2020;48(11):2703–10.
172. Dominici M, Le Blanc K, Mueller I, Slaper-Cortenbach I, Marini F, Krause D, et al. Minimal criteria for defining multipotent mesenchymal stromal cells. The International Society for Cellular Therapy position statement. Cytotherapy. 2006;8(4):315–7.
173. Galipeau J, Krampera M. The challenge of defining mesenchymal stromal cell potency assays and their potential use as release criteria. Cytotherapy. 2015;17(2):125–7.
174. Stappenbeck TS, Miyoshi H. The role of stromal stem cells in tissue regeneration and wound repair. Science. 2009;324(5935):1666–9.
175. Caplan AI. Mesenchymal stem cells: time to change the name! Stem Cells Transl Med. 2017;6(6):1445–51.
176. Pas HI, Winters M, Haisma HJ, Koenis MJ, Tol JL, Moen MH. Stem cell injections in knee osteoarthritis: a systematic review of the literature. Br J Sports Med. 2017;51(15):1125–33.
177. Soler Rich R, Munar A, Soler Romagosa F, Peirau X, Huguet M, Alberca M, et al. Treatment of knee osteoarthritis with autologous expanded bone marrow mesenchymal stem cells: 50 cases clinical and MRI results at one year follow-up. J Stem Cell Res Ther. 2015;5(285):2.
178. Soler R, Orozco L, Munar A, Huguet M, López R, Vives J, et al. Final results of a phase I–II trial using ex vivo expanded autologous mesenchymal stromal cells for the treatment of osteoarthritis of the knee confirming safety and suggesting cartilage regeneration. Knee. 2016;23(4):647–54.
179. Emadedin M, Labibzadeh N, Liastani MG, Karimi A, Jaroughi N, Bolurieh T, et al. Intra-articular implantation of autologous bone marrow–derived mesenchymal stromal cells to treat knee osteoarthritis: a randomized, triple-blind, placebo-controlled phase 1/2 clinical trial. Cytotherapy. 2018;20(10):1238–46.
180. Doyle EC, Wragg NM, Wilson SL. Intraarticular injection of bone marrow-derived mesenchymal stem cells enhances regeneration in knee osteoarthritis. Knee Surg Sports Traumatol Arthrosc. 2020:1–16.
181. Jo CH, Chai JW, Jeong EC, Oh S, Shin JS, Shim H, et al. Intra-articular injection of mesenchymal stem cells for the treatment of osteoarthritis of the knee: a 2-year follow-up study. Am J Sports Med. 2017;45(12):2774–83.
182. Freitag J, Bates D, Wickham J, Shah K, Huguenin L, Tenen A, et al. Adipose-derived mesenchymal stem cell therapy in the treatment of knee osteoarthritis: a randomized controlled trial. Regen Med. 2019;14(3):213–30.
183. Lee WS, Kim HJ, Kim KI, Kim GB, Jin W. Intra-articular injection of autologous adipose tissue-derived mesenchymal stem cells for the treatment of knee osteoarthritis: a phase IIb, randomized, placebo-controlled clinical trial. Stem Cells Transl Med. 2019;8(6):504–11.
184. Song Y, Du H, Dai C, Zhang L, Li S, Hunter DJ, Lu L, Bao C. Human adipose-derived mesenchymal stem cells for osteoarthritis: a pilot study with long-term follow-up and repeated injections. Regenerative medicine. 2018;13(3):295–307.
185. Klontzas ME, Kenanidis EI, Heliotis M, Tsiridis E, Mantalaris A. Bone and cartilage regeneration with the use of umbilical cord mesenchymal stem cells. Expert Opin Biol Ther. 2015;15(11):1541–52.
186. Jin HJ, Bae YK, Kim M, Kwon S-J, Jeon HB, Choi SJ, et al. Comparative analysis of human mesenchymal stem cells from bone marrow, adipose tissue, and umbilical cord blood as sources of cell therapy. Int J Mol Sci. 2013;14(9):17986–8001.
187. Park YB, Ha CW, Lee CH, Yoon YC, Park YG. Cartilage regeneration in osteoarthritic patients by a composite of allogeneic umbilical cord blood-derived mesenchymal stem cells and hyaluronate hydrogel: results from a clinical trial for safety and proof-of-concept with 7 years of extended follow-up. Stem Cells Transl Med. 2017;6(2):613–21.
188. Matas J, Orrego M, Amenabar D, Infante C, Tapia-Limonchi R, Cadiz MI, et al. Umbilical cord-derived mesenchymal stromal cells (MSCs) for knee osteoarthritis: repeated MSC dosing is superior to a single MSC dose and to hyaluronic acid in a controlled randomized phase I/II trial. Stem Cells Transl Med. 2019;8(3):215–24.
189. Kim M-K, Ha C-W, In Y, Cho S-D, Choi E-S, Ha J-K, et al. A multicenter, double-blind, phase III clinical trial to evaluate the efficacy and safety of a cell and gene therapy in knee osteoarthritis patients. Hum Gene Ther Clin Dev. 2018;29(1):48–59.
190. Cherian J, Parvizi J, Bramlet D, Lee K, Romness D, Mont M. Preliminary results of a phase II randomized study to determine the efficacy and safety of genetically engineered allogeneic human chondrocytes expressing TGF-β1 in patients with grade 3 chronic degenerative joint disease of the knee. Osteoarthr Cartil. 2015;23(12):2109–18.
191. Lee B, Parvizi J, Bramlet D, Romness DW, Guermazi A, Noh M, et al. Results of a phase ii study to determine the efficacy and safety of genetically engineered allogeneic human chondrocytes expressing TGF-β1. J Knee Surg. 2020;33(02):167–72.

11 Arthroscopic Treatment

Lih Wang and HyunHo Kim

Abstract

Since the mid-1980s, arthroscopy has become the preferred procedure with evidence of multiple advantages over open surgical procedures when indicated. In the treatment of degenerative arthritis of the knee, surgical interventions can be applied to patients who are refractory to conservative treatment. Surgical treatments mainly include osteotomy that restores the mechanical axis of the lower extremity and knee arthroplasty, but arthroscopic lavage and debridement are the most widely used surgical methods. Until the end of the twentieth century, a large number of studies reported that arthroscopy generally resulted in less pain and postoperative swelling than open procedures, and reduced the risk of complications such as infection and joint stiffness, allowing patients to return to their normal daily activities sooner. Arthroscopic management for osteoarthritis (OA) of the knee includes arthroscopic lavage and debridement, partial meniscectomy, removal of loose bodies or osteophytes, chondroplasty, and microfracture. However, since a prospective randomized comparative study reported that the group with arthroscopic surgery showed no difference in therapeutic efficacy compared to the group without arthroscopic procedures, there is a controversy over the treatment efficacy of arthroscopic management in patients with knee OA. Arthroscopic management alone is not recommended for patients with degenerative arthritis of the knee, excluding those with surgical indications including mechanical symptoms such as meniscal tears or recent traumatic injuries. For successful treatment, accurate clinical diagnosis is needed based on a detailed medical inquiry, symptoms, and signs through physical examination, and radiographs. It is also important for surgeons to understand the benefits of surgery and the impact of surgery on disease progression.

Keywords

Knee · Osteoarthritis · Arthroscopy Debridement · Menisectomy · Chondroplasty

11.1 Introduction

Osteoarthritis (OA) of the knee can cause joint pain, effusion, osteophyte formation, contracture, and degenerative tear of the meniscus [1]. Conservative treatment, arthroscopic debridement, realignment osteotomy, and arthroplasty can be options for treatment of OA, and when

L. Wang (✉) · H. Kim
Department of Orthopedics, College of Medicine, Dong-A University, Busan, South Korea
e-mail: libi33@dau.ac.kr

S.-S. Seo (ed.), *A Strategic Approach to Knee Arthritis Treatment*,
https://doi.org/10.1007/978-981-16-4217-3_11

conservative treatment fails, arthroscopic management may be considered before joint replacement. Arthroscopic management for the treatment of OA of the knee has been widely performed because it has many advantages since mid-1980 [2]. Arthroscopy offers several advantages, with minimally invasive procedures, decrease complications like infection and arthrofibrosis. As a result, patients tend to heal faster and return to normal activity and work sooner [3].

In 1990, Burks reported that the arthroscopy of the OA of the knee is to allow identification and treatment of a local lesion while preserving the joint, which is accepted by most authors [4]. Arthroscopic management for OA of the knee includes lavage, debridement, partial meniscectomy, chondroplasty, synovectomy, removal of loose body or osteophytes, and adhesiolysis. However, publications in the last 20 years have brought into question the role of arthroscopic management in the setting of knee OA. But, arthroscopic management is an attractive alternative for early OA with no malalignment of the lower extremity as it reduces the degree of surgical insult and postoperative rehabilitation with the hope of delay arthroplasty.

11.2 Surgical Method

Arthroscopic management for the treatment of OA of the knee mainly includes arthroscopic debridement and meniscectomy and arthroscopic treatment of chondral defects.

11.2.1 Arthroscopic Treatment for Degenerative Lesions of the Knee

11.2.1.1 Arthroscopic Lavage and Debridement

Arthroscopic lavage and debridement are operative treatments for OA. Lavage is a procedure in which intra-articular fluid is aspirated and the joint is washed out, removing inflammatory mediators, debris, or small loose bodies from the osteoarthritic knee. Articular debridement involves the removal of cartilage or meniscal fragments but also can include cartilage abrasion, excision of osteophytes, and synovectomy. Debridement is intended to improve symptoms and joint function in patients with mechanical symptoms such as locking or catching of the knee (Table 11.1). Because lavage and debridement are often performed at the same time, it is difficult to attribute the success or failure of arthroscopy to a specific procedure.

Magnuson described the debridement of the knee joint for OA first in 1974 [5]. This procedure is known as "House cleaning." He described that removal of all mechanically irritating products of OA renders the patient symptoms free. The procedure was performed through an extensive arthrotomy which included meniscectomy, synovectomy, osteophytes resection, and decortication of bone including multiple drill holes [6]. Jackson suggested that the irrigation of joint is of benefit in the management of the OA of the knee [7]. In 1981, arthroscopic debridement was first introduced for the treatment of OA of the knee by Sprague [8]. Arthroscopic lavage and debridement remove particulates such as cartilage fragments (Fig. 11.1), meniscus, and offending osteophyte and reduce synovitis. Arthroscopic lavage of the joint was considered helpful by washing out proteolytic enzymes and loose bodies in the joint that cause symptoms. Currently, this management has been used for short-term symptom relief although its long-term efficacy is unsatisfactory [9, 10]. These techniques could temporarily improve pain or symptoms, they cannot cease the disease progression. Besides some authors indicated that aggressive debridement of tissue may aggravate the patient's problem [11].

Table 11.1 Ideal candidate for arthroscopic debridement

Ideal candidate for arthroscopic debridement
• Normally aligned knee
• Mild osteoarthritis
• Displaced meniscus tear
• Mechanical symptoms such as locking
• Increasing pain
• No bone marrow lesions

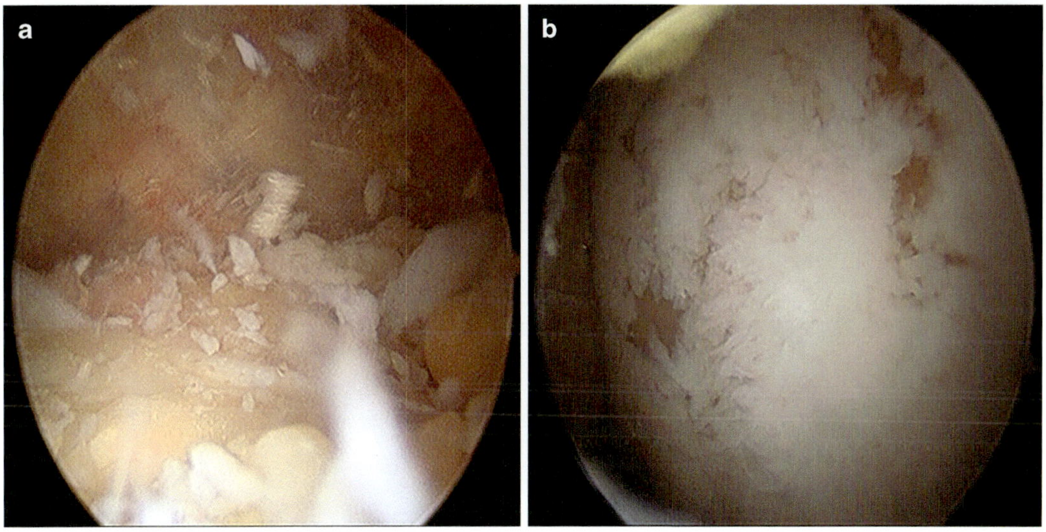

Fig. 11.1 Arthroscopic findings of the arthritic knee. Small particulate cartilage debris in the suprapatellar pouch (**a**), and chondral erosion and focal bony eburnation of the medial femoral condyle (**b**)

11.2.1.2 Meniscectomy

Partial meniscectomy attempts to debride the unstable degenerative tear in order to create a stable tear or a smooth rim of the remaining meniscus. The surgeon is tasked to remove the meniscal tear while simultaneously maintaining as much healthy meniscus as possible. When degenerative lesions are found, the surgeon must decide whether to surgically remove the lesions or not and determine the extent of resection. If a degenerative lesion is suspected to be fraying of the free edge of the lateral meniscus, it is left untreated because degenerative tears of the lateral meniscus can be asymptomatic. It is particularly important to consider the association of arthroscopic findings of degenerative lesions with clinical symptoms in every patient. Degenerative change in the medial meniscus is more broadly excised than in the lateral meniscus. This is because the severity and extent of fraying of the free edge of the medial meniscus is often worse and broader compared to that of the lateral meniscus, the injured medial meniscus can be more easily pinched between the femorotibial joint of the knee. When the distance from the free edge to the capsular margin of the medial meniscal tear increases, the torn meniscus stimulates the joint pain and tenderness. These cases often require partial or subtotal meniscectomy (Fig. 11.2).

It is also important to identify the causes of degenerative changes in the meniscus. If a patient has angular deformity such as genu varum, partial meniscectomy alone cannot solve problems. The presence of cartilage injuries caused by malfunctioning and instability of the anterior cruciate ligament (ACL) may require ACL reconstruction. Surgeons should be well aware that the associated lesion is a key factor that determines the outcome of meniscectomy especially in the treatment of degenerative meniscal tears.

Degenerative tears of meniscus can occur secondary to arthritis and it is important to determine whether the symptoms are due to OA itself or the tear of the meniscus. Partial meniscectomy in osteoarthritic patients with a documented tear and mechanical symptoms appears to be an effective procedure for the relief of pain at short-term follow-up. However, as the severity of OA increases, the results become less favorable. After a partial meniscectomy, the load on the joint of knee may increase by 45%, and it can accelerate the progression of OA and make joint replacement surgery necessary.

Pearse and Craig [12] reported that partial meniscectomy did not hasten the progression

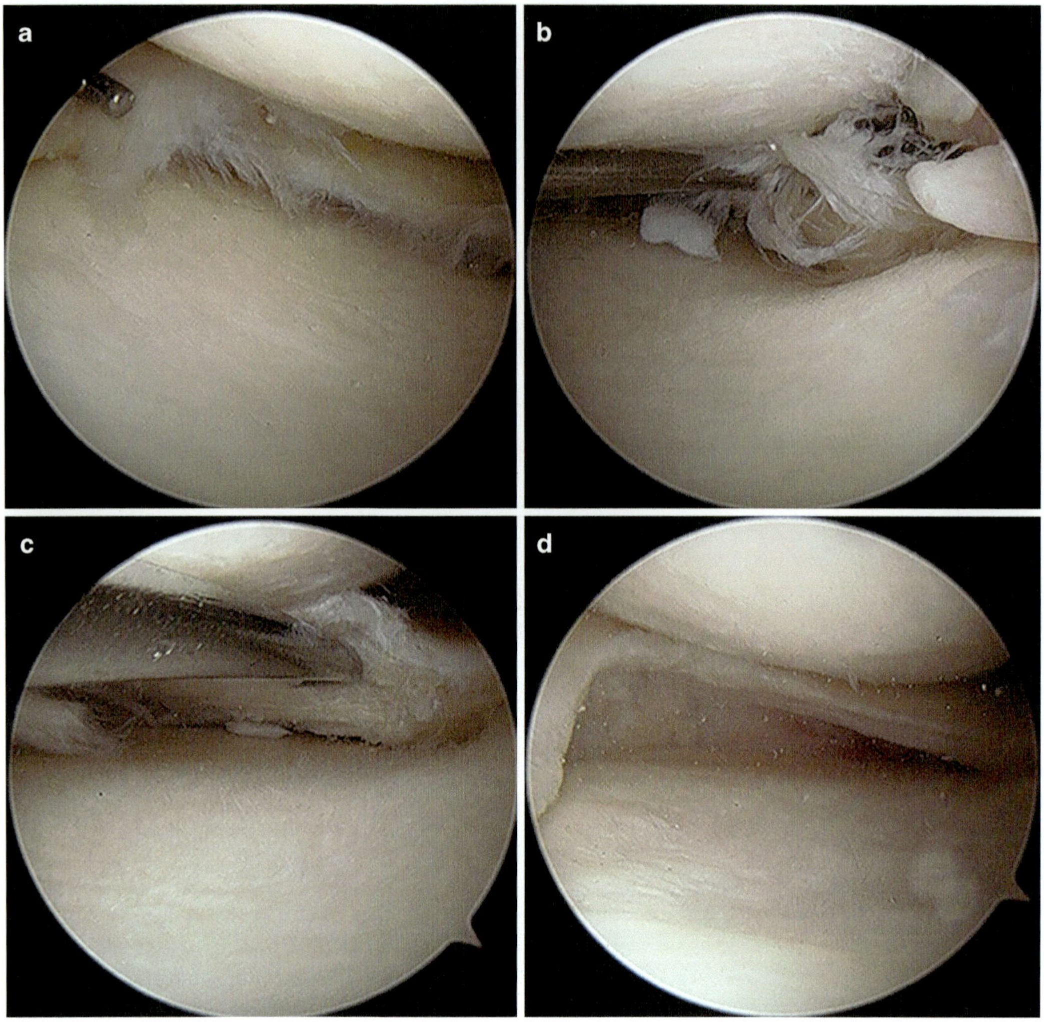

Fig. 11.2 Arthroscopic findings of the degenerative tear of the medial meniscus. Fraying fragments in the mid-body (**a**) and in the posterior horn (**b**) are pinched between the femur and tibia during the knee motion. The meniscal tears extended from the free edge to the capsular margin produce the joint line pain and tenderness (**c**), and these cases require partial or subtotal meniscectomy (**d**)

of OA. On the contrary, Rangger et al. [13] addressed that OA progressed after an average follow-up of 53.5 months in 38% of patients with a medial meniscus tear and 24% of patients with lateral meniscus tear among 284 patients after arthroscopic partial meniscectomy. A number of studies suggested that partial meniscectomy would be more effective for an early stage of OA rather than for advanced stage OA. Lotke et al. [14] reviewed 101 patients who underwent medial meniscectomy, and favorable postoperative results were obtained in 90% of patients with normal conditions, whereas only in 21% of patients with moderate-to-severe knee OA. They concluded that the preoperative severity of OA is an important prognostic factor in meniscectomy, and suggested that accurately identifying the major causes of symptoms was important in elderly patients. McBride et al. [15] concluded that the presence of preoperative degenerative changes affects postoperative results and Crevoisier et al. [16] reported that preoperative cartilage degeneration had more influence on the treatment outcome than age. Bonamo et al. [17]

performed partial meniscectomy without any treatment for articular cartilage on 118 patients and reported that the poor prognostic factors were female gender, ≥60 years of age, and pre-existing degenerative change. Bin et al. [18] examined 68 patients with Outerbridge grade IV OA who underwent arthroscopic medial meniscectomy. They reported the mean VAS decreased from 7.1 preoperation to 2.9 postoperation, and the mean Lysholm score increased from 65.7 to 82 ($P < 0.05$). Four patients (5.9%) underwent total knee arthroplasty at a mean of 49.8 months indicating that partial meniscectomy could improve meniscal tear symptoms in grade IV patients and delay TKA. Partial meniscectomy could not prevent further progression of degenerative changes in patients with OA, especially when pain or mechanical symptoms caused by unstable meniscal tissue were present. However, this procedure can be helpful in short-term symptom relief and performing additional surgery in the future.

11.2.1.3 Osteophyte Excision

The clinical symptoms of osteophyte vary depending on the site of the knee joint. According to the onset area of osteophyte, common symptoms are extension lag in the anterior intercondylar area, and capsular stretching and synovitis, resembling the symptoms of meniscal tears, during flexion/extension in the femoral condyle and tibial plateau. Osteophytes on the patellar apex are mainly characterized by patellofemoral joint pain and often associated with crepitation. Osteophytes can be sometimes asymptomatic. The presence of symptoms is a clear indication for surgical resection of osteophyte. Since osteophytes tend to recur, surgical removal is considered symptomatic treatment. Osteophytes on the patellar apex should be only excised when their presence severely damages the articular cartilage of the femoral trochlear (Fig. 11.3) or interferes with performing arthroscopic procedures. For osteophytes at the patellofemoral joint, conservative treatment such as quadriceps stretching exercise should be initially carried out for symptom relief in early stages with mild symptoms.

Osteophytes are the most common radiographic findings in OA. Since cartilage does not have nociceptive fibers, it has not been clarified yet whether the exact cause of local pain in arthritis is osteophytes. Cicuttini et al. [19] investigated the influence of joint space narrowing and osteophytes on the knee joint and reported that the presence of osteophytes was the more accu-

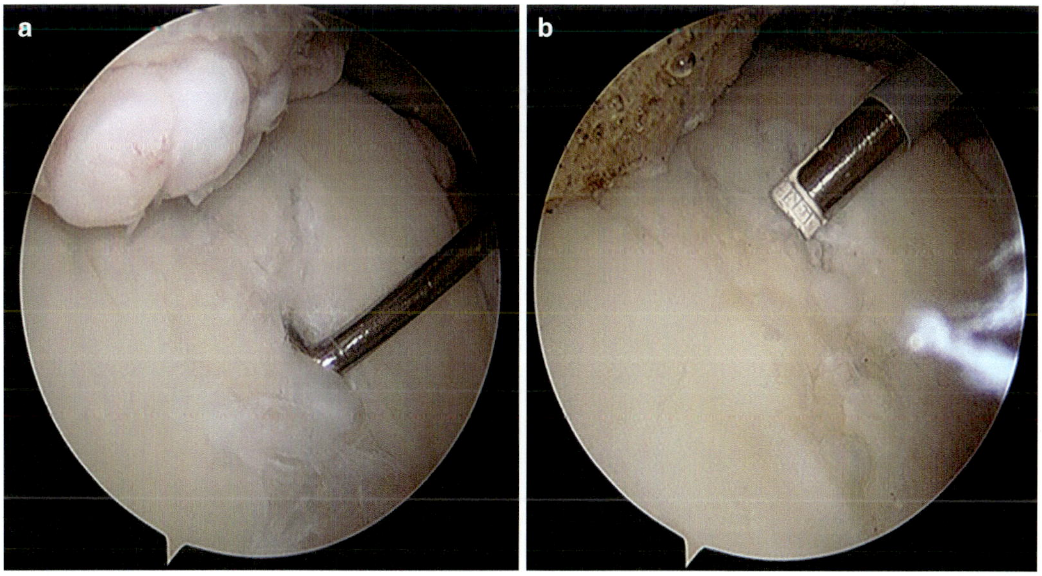

Fig. 11.3 Arthroscopic findings of the patellofemoral joint. When a large osteophyte is present on the patellar apex and articular cartilage damage of the femoral trochlear (**a**), osteophyte resection and chondroplasty can be performed (**b**)

rate predictor of knee pain, but did not clarify whether osteophyte itself was the cause of pain. Sengupta et al. [20] reported that high-signal osteophytes detected on MRI are not associated with the presence of pain, pain severity, or the self-reported location of pain. But, Ozdemir et al. [21] founded that the size, location, and direction of osteophytes and the joint space narrowing were correlated with the range of motion of the knee in patients with longstanding knee pain with radiographic OA. Fond et al. [22] and Steadman et al. [23] reported satisfactory results of excision of osteophytes, which was the cause of flexion contracture. When osteophytes are the primary cause for knee pain or limited range of motion (ROM), osteophyte excision can be considered.

11.2.2 Arthroscopic Treatment for Articular Cartilage Defects

Abrasion arthroplasty, microfracture, and chondroplasty can be performed for the treatment of osteochondral lesions. These surgical techniques expose the defect to the subchondral bone marrow and promote fibrous cartilage healing and include abrasion arthroplasty and microfracture. Although some authors have reported short-term symptom relief, evidence of efficacy have not been clearly established. Previous literature has shown that patient choice of surgery is important and efficacy decreases significantly with age. Autologous chondrocyte implantation, osteochondral autograft, periosteal or perichondral graft are extensive procedures and not applicable to patients with advanced OA.

11.2.2.1 Abrasion Arthroplasty and Drilling

In 1986, Johnson described the pathologic perspective of arthroscopic abrasion arthroplasty and observed that intracortical defects created in a sclerotic lesion without penetration of the subchondral bone uncovered small blood vessels [24]. Necrosis progresses on the hardened surface of the subchondral bone caused by complete articular cartilage loss and subchondral bone exposure, and this leads to the formation of local new blood vessels. Abrasion arthroplasty and arthroscopic drilling are performed by drilling a 1–2 mm deep canal in the exposed subchondral bone using a burr to stimulate hemorrhage and fibrocartilage response in which the formation of a blood clot will turn to a fibrous repair tissue for reconstruction of the defect site of articular cartilage. This arthroscopy-assisted cartilage regeneration procedure can be easily performed, but regenerated fibrocartilage has a limited capacity for intrinsic functions. Fibrocartilage is inferior to hyaline cartilage because it can easily break down by containing significantly less proteoglycan and is susceptible to wear with time. This fibrocartilage tissue has a weak and uneven surface, mechanically inferior to loading, thereby can result in poor mid- and long-term follow-up outcomes [25]. The premise underlying the potential success of this technique is that exposed sclerotic bone in the degenerative knee joint has a significant blood supply less than 1 mm below its surface. Superficial abrasion results in fibrocartilaginous healing without extensive disruption of the integrity of the bone. However, an overly aggressive abrasion can violate the subchondral bone plate and destabilize the joint, resulting in the distortion of the mechanical axis. In the malaligned knee, intra-articular debridement or abrasion arthroplasty is not recommended as an isolated procedure in light of the altered biomechanical forces and the fact that the original hyaline cartilage deteriorated under these same forces [26].

11.2.2.2 Microfracture

The microfracture procedure is done arthroscopically. The surgeon visually assesses the defect and performs the procedure using special instruments that are inserted through three small incisions on the knee. After assessing the cartilage damage, any unstable cartilage is removed from the exposed bone. The surrounding rim of the remaining articular cartilage is also checked for loose or marginally attached cartilage. This loose cartilage is also removed so that there is a stable edge of cartilage surrounding the defect.

The process of thoroughly cleaning and preparing the defect is essential for optimum results. After debridement of damaged cartilage tissue from the lesion, 3–4 holes/cm^2 at a depth of 4 mm are created using a microfracture awl in the exposed subchondral bone (Fig. 11.4). Bone marrow cells and blood from the holes combine to form a "super clot" that completely covers the damaged area. This marrow-rich clot is the basis for the new tissue formation. The microfracture technique produces a rough bone surface that the clot adheres to more easily.

The microfracture technique was first introduced by Steadman and founded based on similar methods of abrasion and drilling. According to Steadman et al. [27], the benefits of an awl are that it minimizes the risk of thermal necrosis of the subchondral bone, well maintains the subchondral bone shape, and facilitates clot formation by creating a rough surface on the subchondral bone. Their microfracture results showed that 75% of patients were improved at 3- to 5-year follow-up. In 1994, Rodrigo addressed that microfracture improved the restoration of cartilage defects with the use of the continuous passive motion following microfracture and non-weight bearing for 6–8 weeks [28]. However, this outcome of defects treated with microfracture alone was not compared with that of debridement only. The clinical outcome was less satisfactory in older adults with symptomatic knee OA or extensive lesions in the bone cartilage. Contraindications to microfracture include no maintenance of fibrocartilage clots following microfracture due to severe degenerative changes and thinning of the surrounding cartilage in the defect site and old age of 60–65 years.

Along with recent advances of biomaterials developed, autologous matrix-induced chondrogenesis (AMIC) technique is integrated with microfracture. The aim of the AMIC is to gain mechanical stability by attaching biomaterials to the site of microfracture in order to preserve multiple functions of bone marrow mesenchymal stem cells in fibrin clots initially formed as much as possible in the lesion area. Biomaterials maintain stability until newly formed cartilage tissues stabilize and naturally degrade and dissolve in the body after completing their tasks. A variety of biomaterials have been introduced. However, further studies on the efficacy of those biomaterials are warranted.

11.2.2.3 Laser and Thermal Chondroplasty

The goal of arthroscopic chondroplasty is to remove the cartilage lesions for prevention of further mechanical damage of remaining cartilage layers, instead of facilitating the regeneration of articular cartilage. The use of rotary mechanical debrider or hand instruments increases the risk of rough articulation surfaces or removal of excess cartilage [29]. Laser chondroplasty has been used to modify these

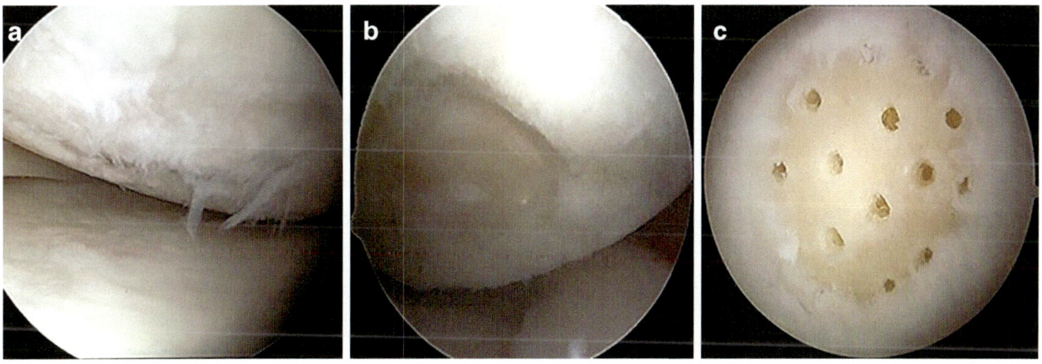

Fig. 11.4 Articular cartilage lesion of the medial femoral condyle is seen (**a**). Any unstable cartilage is removed and a subchondral bone is exposed (**b**). After debridement of a damaged cartilage tissue from the lesion, multiple holes in the exposed subchondral bone are created using a microfracture awl (**c**)

disadvantages. However, this technique is also limitedly used due to high cost and the risk of osteonecrosis caused by subchondral penetration [30, 31]. In recent years, radiofrequency (RF) is used in smoothing and stabilizing the lesions of the articular cartilage, and radiofrequency generators are economic heat sources with a reported high degree of safety [31, 32]. Two types of RF probes have been developed: monopolar and bipolar. Monopolar RFE passes from the tip of the probe, through the tissues, to a distantly placed skin electrode. This energy is rapidly dissipated because of the resistance of the tissues encountered. Bipolar RF causes an effect solely around the tip and energy arcs to a second electrode contained on the probe.

Kaplan and Uribe [32] reported that viable chondrocytes were left in the treated cartilage without any alterations in collagen or microstructure after chondroplasty using bipolar radiofrequency in vitro. Turner et al. [33], demonstrated that a smoother surface with chondrocyte viability resulted when a bipolar thermal probe was used compared with a traditional mechanical shaver in vivo in a sheep model. Kaab et al. [34] described that the use of radiofrequency resulted in damage to normal cartilage 24 weeks after application in their animal model. Hogan and Diduch [35] reported a case of progressive articular cartilage loss following radiofrequency treatment of a partial-thickness lesion. Likewise, the outcomes of radiofrequency treatment may vary depending on energy level, delivery time, clinical state of lesion, and electrode type, and consensus on treatment efficacy and complications has not yet been reached. When applying thermal chondroplasty, caution is warranted especially with thermal injury in normal surrounding articular cartilage and temperature rise within the intra-articular joint. The optimum surgical technique is now better understood, and refinement in probe design seems likely to herald further improvement. Research suggesting fewer immediate side effects from the use of this technology is encouraging, but the quality of evidence about efficacy and safety remains low.

11.3 Clinical Outcomes of Arthroscopic Management in Knee Arthritis

In the pathophysiology of OA, the cause of knee pain has not yet been fully understood. However, the main mechanism of pain has been explained due to synovial inflammation that occurs when cartilage chips and floating fragments of the meniscus by wear are released and wedged into the synovial fluid and phagocytosed by synovial cells. Moreover, irregularity of the cartilage by wear of the hyaline cartilage and meniscus tear may cause joint discomfort and even limited mechanical movement including a range of motion. The theoretical basis for arthroscopic treatment of OA is eliminating contributing factors of symptoms including removal of loose bodies or floating debris, removal of excess synovial fluid, meniscectomy, management of cartilage breakdown, and others. On the contrary, the primary reason for remaining skeptical about whether the procedure is effective in the treatment of OA is that because the hyaline cartilage tissue possesses no ability to regenerate. Even though cartilage regeneration is carried out with various procedures, cartilage regeneration may fail or restoration of the normal knee function by regenerated fibrocartilage is almost impossible [36].

Until 2002, no randomized comparative study on the efficacy of arthroscopic surgery and non-surgical procedure in the management of knee OA has been conducted in a strict and proper manner. Chang et al. [37] performed a randomized comparative study on arthroscopic surgery and percutaneous needle washing in 32 cases with OA. Many cohort studies have been performed to assess arthroscopic lavage and debridement and arthroscopic partial meniscectomy in symptomatic meniscal tears, but findings from these studies cannot be generalized because of a lack of statistical control [38, 39].

In 2002, Moseley et al. [40] carried out a randomized controlled trial to verify the efficacy of arthroscopic surgery for knee OA as a blind test in subjects and examiners. Over 2 years, investigators observed and compared the three groups of arthroscopic lavage, arthroscopic debridement, and placebo arthroscopy in 180 cases with knee OA between 1995 and 1998. All three groups showed early pain relief. The reduced pain persisted for 2 years without a difference. Therefore, they concluded that arthroscopic debridement and lavage were no better than placebo arthroscopy in the treatment of OA. Kirkley et al. [41] performed a randomized controlled study to compare the clinical results of patients between the two groups of rehabilitation therapy alone, and arthroscopic debridement combined with rehabilitation therapy. They reported that symptom improvement was better in the group with early arthroscopic management, but no difference was shown 3 months after the start of treatment. In addition, there was no difference in pain and functional assessment between the two groups. These findings demonstrated that arthroscopic debridement was no better than nonsurgical intervention in the treatment of OA. However, these previous studies of Moseley and Kirkley were limited in that they did not assess the clinical outcomes of patients with advanced stages of OA.

Herrlin et al. [42] conducted a randomized comparative study to evaluate treatment efficacy by comparing the two groups of exercise training alone and partial meniscectomy combined with exercise training in 96 patients aged 45–64 years with a diagnosis of a meniscal tear on MRI and a complaint of knee pain. No difference was found in pain and functional aspects between the two groups. The treatment plan was changed to surgical procedures in 30% of patients with persistent pain despite nonsurgical interventions, and their clinical outcomes were similar to those of the patients who received initial surgical treatment. Therefore, this previous study has recommended surgical treatment for patients who were refractory to initial conservative treatment and having symptoms of knee OA associated with a meniscal tear. In the MeTeOR trial [43] and a previous study of Yim et al. [44], arthroscopic and nonsurgical treatments were randomly performed on symptomatic patients with a meniscal tear. Comparable to the findings of Herrlin et al. [42], no difference was present in pain and functional scores during the follow-up between the two groups. In particular, rates of conversion to surgical treatment due to persisting pain after conservative treatment in those two previous studies were lower than the study of Herrlin et al. [42]. According to the reports of Potts et al. [45] and Kim et al. [46], even though arthroscopic surgery of the knee has been increasingly performed in the US and other countries, arthroscopy for knee OA has decreased since 2002 after Moseley et al. reported their surgical outcomes.

In 2007, the National Institute for Clinical Excellence (NICE) provided guidelines for arthroscopic treatment of OA of the knee. The selection of proper patient was emphasized because its efficacy is controversial and the procedure was recommended for the knees with locking associated with intra-articular loose bodies or meniscus tears [47]. The American Association of Orthopedic Surgery (AAOS) provided OA treatment guidelines, arthroscopy with lavage and/or debridement is not recommended in patient with a primary diagnosis of symptomatic OA of the knee (strength of recommendation: strong). And arthroscopic partial meniscectomy is unable to be recommended for or against in patients with OA with a torn meniscus (strength of recommendation: inconclusive) [48]. Several studies have discussed the indications for arthroscopic debridement including joint effusion, localized joint line tenderness, mechanical symptoms such as catching or locking, aggravation of symptoms related to acute trauma, intra-articular loose body, early-stage degenerative arthritis without malalignment, and multiple or large-sized osteophytes [49–54]. The prognostic factors include clinical symptoms in the affected joint, mechanical symptoms, duration of morbidity, presence of a meniscal tear, ROM, lower limb alignment, joint space narrowing, age, weight, and smoking. Favorable and unfavorable prognostic factors are listed in Table 11.2.

Table 11.2 Prognostic factors of arthroscopic debridement for knee osteoarthritis

Variable	Favorable	Unfavorable
Age	<40 years	>75 years
Compartment	Medial, single compartmental	Tricompartmental, lateral, tibial
Joint space preservation	>5 mm	<5 mm
Alignment	Neutral	Valgus
Duration of symptoms	<6 month	>1 year
Weight	Localized	Diffuse
Effusion	Present	Absent

The patient should be fully aware that the goal of arthroscopic treatment is not to cure the disorder but to relieve pain. Arthroscopic treatment can contribute to symptomatic improvement in patients with advanced OA if severe acute pain related to catching or locking occurs in the affected compartment, symptoms related to meniscal tear, loose body, or an articular cartilage flap exist in an intact compartment, or patellofemoral impingement, loss of extension, bursitis, synovitis, intra-articular ligament damage, which is caused by a large-sized osteophyte is present.

11.4 Summary

The efficacy of arthroscopic treatment for knee OA can be limited by the progressive condition of OA which aggravates over time. Arthroscopic debridement should be carefully considered in cases of a failure in symptom relief after sufficiently applying nonsurgical interventions, instead of performing it as a primary treatment in asymptomatic patients with knee OA. Patient selection of treatment options is considerably important in the successful treatment of knee OA. The indications for arthroscopic management include acute trauma, effusion, loose bodies, mechanical symptoms, and early degenerative change. However, the clinical outcomes are not promising in patients with advanced OA, malalignment, ligamentous instability, and contracture. For the achievement of successful treatment results, accurate clinical diagnosis is crucial based on symptoms and signs through physical examination, and weight-bearing radiographs. Furthermore, arthroscopic surgery can produce short-term symptomatic improvement and be helpful for patients who want to postpone total knee arthroplasty. Both surgeons and patients should understand the implications of the surgery that it has no long-term efficacy and cannot alter the progression of OA.

References

1. Felson DT. Osteoarthritis of the knee. N Engl J Med. 2006;354(8):841–8.
2. Bigony L. Arthroscopic surgery: a historical perspective. Orthop Nurs. 2008;27(6):349–54.
3. Treuting R. Minimally invasive orthopedic surgery: arthroscopy. Ochsner J. 2000;2(3):158–63.
4. Burks RT. Arthroscopy and degenerative arthritis of the knee: a review of the literature. Arthroscopy. 1990;6(1):43–7.
5. Magnuson PB. The classic: joint debridement: surgical treatment of degenerative arthritis. Clin Orthop Relat Res. 1974;101:4–12.
6. Schonholtz G. Arthroscopic debridement of the knee joint. Orthop Clin North Am. 1989;20(2):257–63.
7. Jackson RW. The role of arthroscopy in the management of the arthritic knee. Clin Orthop Relat Res. 1974;101:28–35.
8. Sprague NF. Arthroscopic debridement for degenerative knee joint disease. Clin Orthop Relat Res. 1981;160:118–23.
9. Livesley P, Doherty M, Needoff M, Moulton A. Arthroscopic lavage of osteoarthritic knees. J Bone Joint Surg Br. 1991;73(6):922–6.
10. Edelson R, Burks RT, Bloebaum RD. Short-term effects of knee washout for osteoarthritis. Am J Sports Med. 1995;23(3):345–9.
11. Goldman RT, Scuderi GR, Kelly MA. Arthroscopic treatment of the degenerative knee in older athletes. Clin Sports Med. 1997;16(1):51–68.
12. Pearse EO, Craig DM. Partial meniscectomy in the presence of severe osteoarthritis does not hasten the symptomatic progression of osteoarthritis. Arthroscopy. 2003;19(9):963–8.

13. Rangger C, Klestil T, Gloetzer W, Kemmler G, Benedetto KP. Osteoarthritis after arthroscopic partial meniscectomy. Am J Sports Med. 1995;23(2):240–4.
14. Lotke PA, Lefkoe R, Ecker M. Late results following medial meniscectomy in an older population. J Bone Joint Surg Am. 1981;63(1):115–9.
15. McBride GG, Constine RM, Hofmann A, Carson R. Arthroscopic partial medial meniscectomy in the older patient. J Bone Joint Surg Am. 1984;66(4):547–51.
16. Crevoisier X, Munzinger U, Drobny T. Arthroscopic partial meniscectomy in patients over 70 years of age. Arthroscopy. 2001;17(7):732–6.
17. Bonamo JJ, Kessler KJ, Noah J. Arthroscopic meniscectomy in patients over the age of 40. Am J Sports Med. 1992;20(4):422–9.
18. Bin S-I, Lee S H, Kim C-W, Kim T-H, Lee D-H. Results of arthroscopic medial meniscectomy in patients with grade IV osteoarthritis of the medial compartment. Arthroscopy. 2008;24(3):264–8.
19. Cicuttini FM, Baker J, Hart DJ, Spector TD. Association of pain with radiological changes in different compartments and views of the knee joint. Osteoarthr Cartil. 1996;4(2):143–7.
20. Sengupta M, Zhang Y, Niu J, Guermazi A, Grigorian M, Gale D, et al. High signal in knee osteophytes is not associated with knee pain. Osteoarthr Cartil. 2006;14(5):413–7.
21. Ozdemir F, Tukenmez O, Kokino S, Turan FN. How do marginal osteophytes, joint space narrowing and range of motion affect each other in patients with knee osteoarthritis. Rheumatol Int. 2006;26(6):516.
22. Fond J, Rodin D, Ahmad S, Nirschl RP. Arthroscopic debridement for the treatment of osteoarthritis of the knee: 2-and 5-year results. Arthroscopy. 2002;18(8):829–34.
23. Steadman JR, Ramappa AJ, Maxwell RB, Briggs KK. An arthroscopic treatment regimen for osteoarthritis of the knee. Arthroscopy. 2007;23(9):948–55.
24. Johnson LL. Arthroscopic abrasion arthroplasty historical and pathologic perspective: present status. Arthroscopy. 1986;2(1):54–69.
25. Bert J. Role of abrasion arthroplasty and debridement in the management of osteoarthritis of the knee. Rheum Dis Clin N Am. 1993;19(3):725–39.
26. Rand J. Arthroscopy and articular cartilage defects. Contemp Orthop. 1985;11:13–30.
27. Steadman JR, Rodkey WG, Singleton SB, Briggs KK. Microfracture technique forfull-thickness chondral defects: technique and clinical results. Oper Tech Orthop. 1997;7(4):300–4.
28. Rodrigo J. Improvement of full-thickness chondral defect healing in the human knee after debridement and microfracture using continuous passive motion. Am J Knee Surg. 1994;7:109–16.
29. Jackson RW. Arthroscopic surgery and a new classification system. Am J Knee Surg. 1998;11(1):51–4.
30. Grifka J, Boenke S, Schreiner C, Löhnert J. Significance of laser treatment in arthroscopic therapy of degenerative gonarthritis. Knee Surg Sports Traumatol Arthrosc. 1994;2(2):88–93.
31. Garino JP, Lotke PA, Sapega AA, Reilly PJ, Esterhai JL Jr. Osteonecrosis of the knee following laser-assisted arthroscopic surgery: a report of six cases. Arthroscopy. 1995;11(4):467–74.
32. Kaplan L, Uribe JW, Sasken H, Markarian G. The acute effects of radiofrequency energy in articular cartilage: an in vitro study. Arthroscopy. 2000;16(1):2–5.
33. Turner AS, Tippett JW, Powers BE, Dewell RD, Mallinckrodt CH. Radiofrequency (electrosurgical) ablation of articular cartilage: a study in sheep. Arthroscopy. 1998;14(6):585–91.
34. Kääb MJ, Bail HJ, Rotter A, Mainil-Varlet P, Apgwynn I, Weiler A. Monopolar radiofrequency treatment of partial-thickness cartilage defects in the sheep knee joint leads to extended cartilage injury. Am J Sports Med. 2005;33(10):1472–8.
35. Hogan CJ, Diduch DR. Progressive articular cartilage loss following radiofrequency treatment of a partial-thickness lesion. Arthroscopy. 2001;17(6):1–4.
36. Siparsky P, Ryzewicz M, Peterson B, Bartz R. Arthroscopic treatment of osteoarthritis of the knee: are there any evidence-based indications? Clin Orthop Relat Res. 2007;455:107–12.
37. Chang RW, Falconer J, David Stulberg S, Arnold WJ, Manheim LM, Dyer AR. A randomized, controlled trial of arthroscopic surgery versus closed-needle joint lavage for patients with osteoarthritis of the knee. Arthritis Rheum. 1993;36(3):289–96.
38. Gross DE, Brenner SL, Esformes I, Gross ML. Arthroscopic treatment of degenerative joint disease of the knee. Orthopedics. 1991;14(12):1317–21.
39. Baumgaertner MR, Cannon W Jr, Vittori JM, Schmidt ES, Maurer RC. Arthroscopic debridement of the arthritic knee. Clin Orthop Relat Res. 1990;253:197–202.
40. Moseley JB, O'Malley K, Petersen NJ, Menke TJ, Brody BA, Kuykendall DH, et al. A controlled trial of arthroscopic surgery for osteoarthritis of the knee. N Engl J Med. 2002;347(2):81–8.
41. Kirkley A, Birmingham TB, Litchfield RB, Giffin JR, Willits KR, Wong CJ, et al. A randomized trial of arthroscopic surgery for osteoarthritis of the knee. N Engl J Med. 2008;359(11):1097–107.
42. Herrlin S, Hållander M, Wange P, Weidenhielm L, Werner S. Arthroscopic or conservative treatment of degenerative medial meniscal tears: a prospective randomised trial. Knee Surg Sports Traumatol Arthrosc. 2007;15(4):393–401.
43. Katz JN, Brophy RH, Chaisson CE, De Chaves L, Cole BJ, Dahm DL, et al. Surgery versus physical therapy for a meniscal tear and osteoarthritis. N Engl J Med. 2013;368(18):1675–84.
44. Yim J-H, Seon J-K, Song E-K, Choi J-I, Kim M-C, Lee K-B, et al. A comparative study of meniscectomy and nonoperative treatment for degenerative horizontal tears of the medial meniscus. Am J Sports Med. 2013;41(7):1565–70.

45. Potts A, Harrast JJ, Harner CD, Miniaci A, Jones MH. Practice patterns for arthroscopy of osteoarthritis of the knee in the United States. Am J Sports Med. 2012;40(6):1247–51.
46. Kim S, Bosque J, Meehan JP, Jamali A, Marder R. Increase in outpatient knee arthroscopy in the United States: a comparison of National Surveys of Ambulatory Surgery, 1996 and 2006. J Bone Joint Surg Am. 2011;93(11):994–1000.
47. NICE Guidance. Arthroscopic knee washout, with or without debridement, for the treatment of osteoarthritis (Interventional procedures guidance), 2007. www.nice.org.uk/guidance/ipg230
48. Jevsevar DS. Treatment of osteoarthritis of the knee: evidence-based guideline. J Am Acad Orthop Surg. 2013;21(9):571–6.
49. Aaron RK, Skolnick AH, Reinert SE, Ciombor DM. Arthroscopic debridement for osteoarthritis of the knee. J Bone Joint Surg Am. 2006;88(5):936–43.
50. Stuart MJ, Lubowitz JH. What, if any, are the indications for arthroscopic debridement of the osteoarthritic knee? Arthroscopy. 2006;22(3):238–9.
51. Spahn G, Mückley T, Kahl E, Hofmann GO. Factors affecting the outcome of arthroscopy in medial-compartment osteoarthritis of the knee. Arthroscopy. 2006;22(11):1233–40.
52. Dearing J, Nutton RW. Evidence based factors influencing outcome of arthroscopy in osteoarthritis of the knee. Knee. 2008;15(3):159–63.
53. Howell SM. The role of arthroscopy in treating osteoarthritis of the knee in the older patient. Orthopedics. 2010;33(9):652.
54. Sgaglione NA, Chen E, Bert JM, Amendola A, Bugbee WD. Current strategies for nonsurgical, arthroscopic, and minimally invasive surgical treatment of knee cartilage pathology. Instr Course Lect. 2010;59:157–80.

Osteotomy Around Knee

12

Sang Won Moon and Young-Kyoung Min

Abstract

Osteotomy around the knee was mainly performed to correct bone deformity of the knee in children, but after that, it began to be applied to the treatment of arthritis. It was performed in osteoarthritis patients with varus or valgus deformity, and the concept of delaying degenerative changes in joints was established by realigning the lower extremities through osteotomy. Closing wedge osteotomy, which was performed at the proximal tibial ridge including fibular osteotomy, was first started, later developed into open wedge osteotomy. It also evolved from uniplane osteotomy to biplane osteotomy. As high tibia osteotomy (HTO) was applied to the treatment for deformed knees due to osteoarthritis, the incidence of osteotomy surgery increased. However, it was found that there are cases where it is difficult to treat with only HTO. Distal femoral osteotomy (DFO) was performed and this problem could be resolved. Like HTO, DFO has evolved from uniplane osteotomy to biplane osteotomy. There was a time when the interest in osteotomy declined as the artificial joint replacement surgery reported good results. However, in young, active patients with osteoarthritis, the results of artificial joint replacement were poor. Therefore, a new treatment was needed to be applied to them. Osteotomy is beginning to be used in young and active patients with osteoarthritis. As the fixation devices used in osteotomy were developed, surgical techniques were established. As the osteotomy was properly performed according to the preoperative plan, it was established as an effective treatment, especially for young and active osteoarthritis patients.

Keywords

Tibia · Femur · Osteotomy · HTO · DFO Uniplane · Biplane · Closing wedge osteotomy · Open wedge osteotomy · Varus deformity · Valgus deformity

12.1 History of Osteotomy

The concept of deformity correction for bones began in the era of Hippocratic (460–370 BC) using the Hippocratic Scamnum, a traction device used to fix bones [1]. Osteotomy to correct bone deformity around the knee is known to have started from the seventeenth century, and it has developed with the advancement of anesthesia technology, blood transfusion, aseptic equip-

S. W. Moon (✉)
Department of Orthopedics, Inje University Haeundae Paik Hospital, Busan, South Korea
e-mail: moonsw@inje.ac.kr

Y.-K. Min
Department of Orthopedics, Busan Medical Center, Busan, South Korea

S.-S. Seo (ed.), *A Strategic Approach to Knee Arthritis Treatment*,
https://doi.org/10.1007/978-981-16-4217-3_12

ment, and imaging equipment from the nineteenth century [1, 2]. Until then, it was mainly performed in diseases such as severe valgus knee, post-traumatic deformity, rickets, or other structural deformities [3]. Medial open wedge high tibia osteotomy (HTO) was first described by Lexer [4] in 1931 and Brett [5] in 1935. In 1961, Jackson and Waugh [6] published an HTO on knee osteoarthritis (OA) with valgus or varus deformity. For the first time, they published radiographic evidence of realignment and union and quantified the correction obtained after osteotomy around the knee at an average follow-up of 31 months. In France, Debeyre and Patte [7] first described an open medial HTO in 1961. In 1964, Gariepy [8] of Canada introduced the transfibular lateral closing wedge HTO in the proximal to the tibial tubercle, and the concept of delaying the degenerative change of the joint was established by realignment by HTO. Coventry [9] used Gariepy's osteotomy method to perform a closed wedge-shaped valgus osteotomy including a fibular osteotomy at the proximal tibial ridge. Early weight-bearing and range of motion were possible using one or two staples. This is also the most widely known technique. His rationale was that osteotomy should be performed near the area where the deformity has occurred, and should mainly include the cancellous bone where the union progresses faster and that the quadriceps muscle should be allowed to pull the osteotomy to encourage union. As the locking plate for solid fixation developed, the complications of failure to fix after osteotomy decreased [10]. However, as the results of total knee replacement arthroplasty (TKA) improved, interest in osteotomy, which had relatively poor treatment results compared to TKA, gradually decreased [11–14]. As the age at which TKA was performed gradually decreased, TKA began to be applied to young and active patients as well. However, the clinical outcomes and long-term survival rate of TKA were poor in young and active patients with knee OA. Therefore, alternative methods are needed for young and active patients with knee OA [15, 16]. As an alternative, osteotomy began to be used in young and active patients with knee OA. Osteotomy has been established as an effective treatment for young and active patients through appropriate patient selection, accurate preoperative planning, the establishment of surgical techniques, and development of fixation devices [17].

12.2 Alignment of Low Extremity

The weight-bearing line (Mikulicz line, mechanical axis) of the lower extremity is a straight line connecting the center point of the femoral head to the center point of the talar dome in the full length anteroposterior (AP) radiograph of the lower extremity in the standing position and passes through the center point of the tibia normally [18]. This line is known to pass through the center of the knee, and there are still controversies about the center of the knee, but generally, this line passes through the medial spine of the tibia. In addition, the knee joint line in the coronal plane has an obliquity with a high lateral side and a low medial side. For this reason, the medial compartment of the knee is loaded with 65%, and the lateral compartment is loaded with 35% [19]. As result, the progression of osteoarthritis tends to be faster in the medial compartment than in the lateral compartment [20]. Since the distance between the two hip joints is wider than the distance between the knee joints, the mechanical axis of the lower extremities represents varus 3 degrees with respect to the line perpendicular to the ground [21–23]. The case where the mechanical axis of the lower limb passes through the medial side without passing through the center of the knee joint is called the mechanical varus alignment, and the case that passes through the lateral side is called the mechanical valgus alignment. Varus deformity further increases the load on the medial compartment, and valgus deformity further increases the load on the lateral compartment [18, 24] (Fig. 12.1). The mechanical axis of the femur is a line connecting the center of the femoral head to the center of the intercondylar fossa, and the mechanical axis of the tibia is a line connecting the center of the tibial plateau to the center of the tibial ankle joint [25]. The anatomical axes of the femur and tibia are the axes of

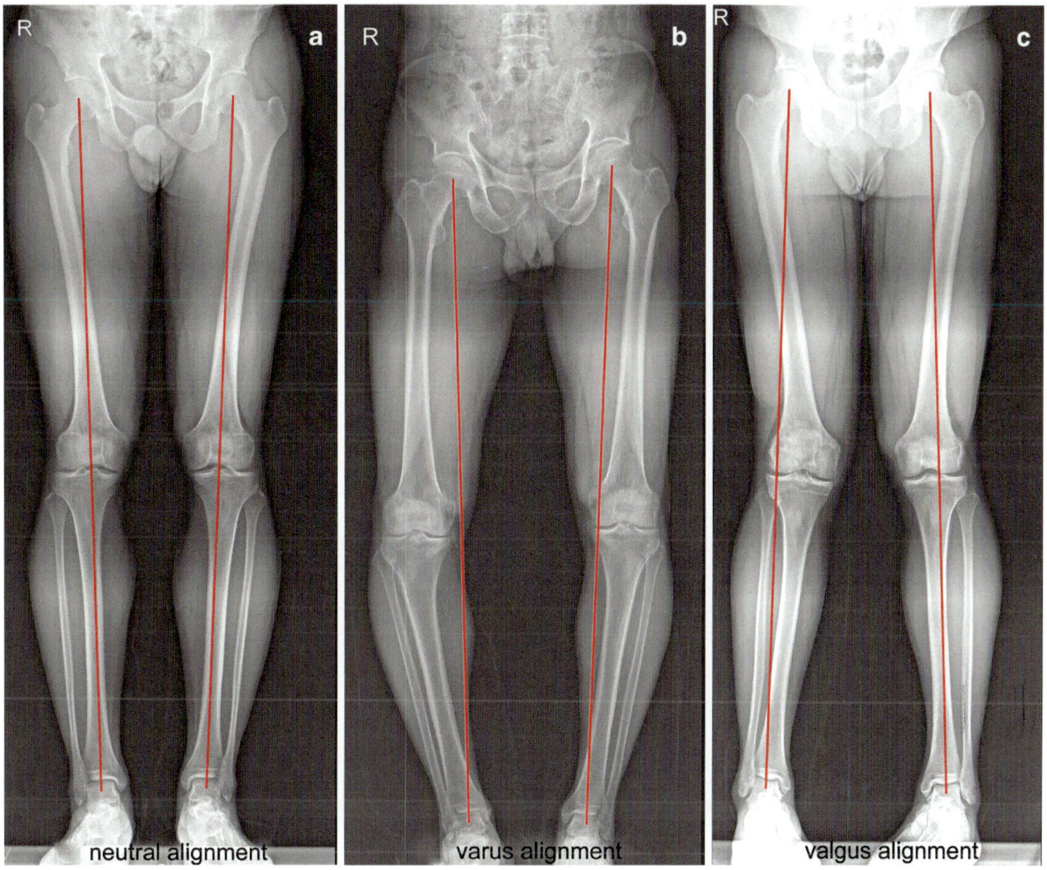

Fig. 12.1 Alignments of low extremity. (**a**) Neutral alignment. (**b**) Varus alignment. (**c**) Valgus alignment

the femur and tibial shaft, respectively, and constitute an average of 6 degrees of valgus. The mechanical axes of the femur are deviated in an average angle of 6 degrees from the anatomical axis of femur, and the mechanical and anatomical axes of the tibia are almost identical [26]. The mechanical lateral distal femoral angle (mLDFA), which is the lateral angle formed between the line mechanical axis line of the femur and a line connecting the articular surface of the medial and lateral condyle of the distal, is about 88 degrees on average (85–90) [27]. The mechanical medial proximal tibial angle (mMPTA) formed by the tibial plateau line and the mechanical axis of the tibia normally averages 87 degrees (85–90) [13, 28] (Fig. 12.2).

Applying the center of rotation of angulation, that is, the CORA concept defined by Dror Paley [29], to the mechanical axis, it played a decisive role in determining the location of the deformity, the degree of deformity, and the direction in which correction is required. If mLDFA is less than 85 degrees, it means that there is distal femur valgus deformity, and if it is greater than 90 degrees, it means that there is distal femur varus deformity. MPTA is an angle opposite to mLDFA, so if it is less than 85 degrees, it means proximal tibia varus deformity, and if it is greater than 90 degrees, it means proximal tibia valgus deformity (Fig. 12.3) When using the CORA concept, sometimes the deformity source is the opposite. If osteotomy surgery is performed without checking the deformity source, this can make another malalignment. This leads to a new deformity called joint line obliquity, leading to early failure [30]. Varus deformity further increases the load on the medial compartment, and valgus deformity further increases the load

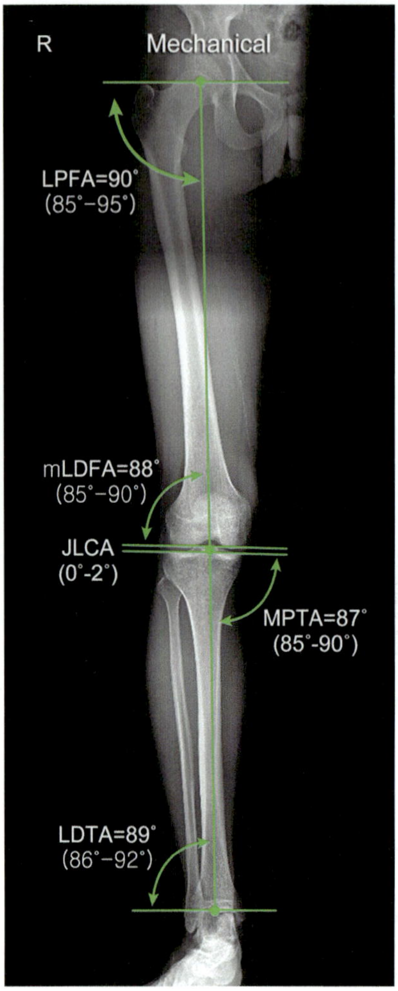

Fig. 12.2 Normal physiologic axes and angles of the lower extremities: The physiologic axes and angles have an abnormal value in the malalignment of the lower extremities. *LPFA* lateral proximal femoral angle, *mLDFA* mechanical lateral distal femoral angle, *JLCA* joint line convergence angle, *MPTA* medial proximal tibial angle, *LDTA* lateral distal tibial angle

on the lateral compartment. In addition to the pathological deformity in the frontal plane, constitutional deformity that is not pathological is also common [31]. According to a study conducted in Europe, 32% of males and 17% of females have constitutional varus of 3 degrees or more, and this needs to be considered [32, 33].

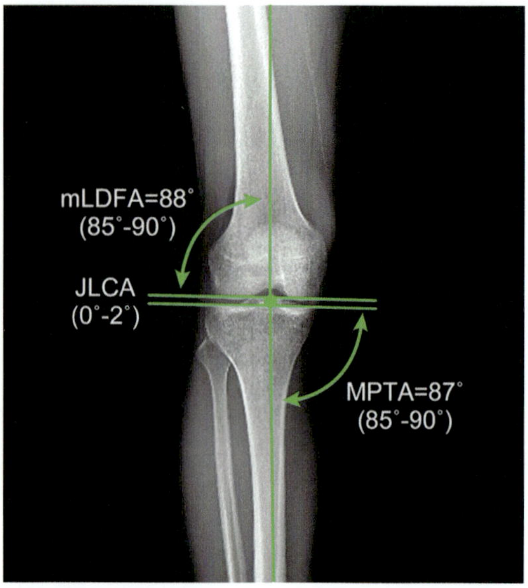

Fig. 12.3 Normal physiologic axes and angles of the knee. *mLDFA* mechanical lateral distal femoral angle, *JLCA* joint line convergence angle, *MPTA* medial proximal tibial angle

12.3 Effect of Varus or Valgus Alignment on Load in the Knee

The knee joint is located between the hip joint and the ankle joint, and the weight-bearing line by gravity normally passes through the center of the joint. If the alignment of the lower limbs is out of the normal range, an excessive load is induced in a specific compartment of the knee joint, resulting in pain and deterioration of function, as well as degenerative changes [34]. Chronic overload acting on the medial or lateral compartment of the knee causes damage to the articular cartilage. This is well known not only in biomechanical studies but also in several clinical studies [2, 35–37]. The purpose of osteotomy around the knee is to correct abnormal lower limb alignment between the femur and tibia to reduce chronic overload and to transfer the weight load of the arthritic compartment to a healthy joint surface. It is also to delay the conversion to TKA by slowing the progression of arthritis of the knee joint [38].

12.4 Preoperative Planning

In order to obtain successful results, a thorough medical history, preoperative examination, and accurate surgical planning are essential. Before surgery, the range of motion of the joint should be measured and the location of the pain should be checked, and instability should be evaluated through a varus-valgus stress test and anteroposterior stress test. The patient's gait should be evaluated, and the presence of varus thrust gait in the standing phase, quadriceps avoid gait, and recurvatum should be checked. As a basic examination, a teleradiography or both lower leg scanogram must be included for the evaluation of lower limb alignment with the knee joint fully extended. At this time, alignment of the lower limbs is important, and in general, the position of the foot should be slightly inwardly rotated and the patellar should be located in the center of the femur with weight-bearing of both lower limbs [39, 40]. In addition, for the evaluation of arthritis, both weight-bearing anterior-posterior (AP) and true lateral X-ray, and 45-degree flexion both weight-bearing AP (so-called, Rosenberg view) and patella axial view, should be taken [41]. The height of the patella can be evaluated using the Insall–Salvati, Blackburne–Peel, and Carton–Deschamps indexes on a true lateral X ray, and tibial tubercle osteotomy may be accompanied in cases of high patella [42]. The degree of laxity of the medial and lateral collateral ligament and the thickness of cartilage can be estimated through varus-valgus stress X-ray, and this is reflected in the surgical plan [43, 44]. Through magnetic resonance imaging, it is possible to evaluate the thickness of the cartilage and the presence of concomitant damage to the meniscus, the condition of the anterior and posterior cruciate ligament, the condition of the subchondral bone, bone necrosis, and the degree of femoral-patella arthritis. In addition, it is necessary to plan the surgery in consideration of not only the frontal alignment of the entire lower limb but also the torsional alignment and the dynamic force when walking.

In general, HTO is selected for varus deformity, which accounts for most of the knee joint deformity, and DFO is selected for relatively rare knee valgus deformity [28, 45]. However, if the corrective angle is too large or the tibia and femur are both deformed, and either the HTO or the DFO cannot obtain adequate correction, a double level osteotomy (DLO) can also be considered [18, 46].

12.5 High Tibia Osteotomy (HTO)

HTO is one of the surgical treatment methods performed in patients with early or mid-stage knee osteoarthritis confined to the medial compartment with varus deformity. HTO is a surgical method to reduce excessive weight load in the lesion by correcting the mechanical axis of patients with degenerative changes in the knee joint and malalignment of the lower extremities.

The purpose of HTO is, first, to correct the abnormal alignment of the lower extremities formed by the femur and tibia due to degenerative changes in the articular cartilage to transfer the weight load of the medial compartment to the lateral healthy compartment. Second, it is to delay the transition to TKA by slowing the progression of arthritis in the medial compartment of the knee joint [21]. With the recent development of TKA, the implementation of HTO is on the decline, but it is clear that HTO can provide favorable treatment results through appropriate patient selection, accurate surgical planning, and various surgical techniques [19]. Therefore, patient selection in consideration of the extent of joint cartilage damage and the patient's age, correct preoperative planning, and accurate surgical techniques are essential factors for a successful outcome.

HTO can be divided into lateral closed wedge osteotomy and medial open wedge osteotomy. The lateral closed wedge osteotomy and the medial open wedge osteotomy have opposite advantages and disadvantages. The advantages of lateral closed wedge osteotomy are as follows: (1) Bone union is relatively fast, allowing early walking. (2) The initial stability is excellent because the contraction of the quadriceps muscle acts as a compression force. (3) Patellar baja is relatively rare. (4) No bone graft or bone substitute is required. (5) The frequency of loss of correction angle is small. The disadvantages of lateral closed wedge osteotomy are as follows; (1) The length of the lower limb on the side to be corrected decreases. (2) It is difficult to obtain accurate correction. (3) Fibula osteotomy or tibiofibular separation is additionally required. (4) The technique is relatively difficult. (5) There is a possibility of nerve injury. (6) Bone defect is large when conversion to TKA [47]. The advantage of lateral closed wedge osteotomy is the disadvantage of medial open wedge osteotomy, and the disadvantage of lateral closed wedge osteotomy is the advantage of medial open wedge osteotomy. The advantages of medial open wedge osteotomy are as follows; (1) The length of the side to be corrected increases. (2) It is easy to obtain accurate corrections. (3) No fibular osteotomy or fibular separation is required. (4) The operation time is shortened due to its ease of operation. (5) No need for dissection of peroneal nerve, so there is less possibility of nerve injury. The disadvantages of medial open wedge osteotomy are as follows; (1) A bone graft or bone substitute is required. (2) Bone union is slower than closed osteotomy. (3) Patellar baja is relatively common [48–51].

It is necessary to understand the advantages and disadvantages of lateral closed wedge osteotomy and medial open wedge osteotomy and to select an appropriate surgical method according to the doctor's skill level and the patient's characteristics. Recently, medial open wedge osteotomy is more common than lateral closed wedge osteotomy, and the surgical plan and technique will be described focusing on medial open wedge osteotomy.

12.5.1 Indications and Contraindications

The selection of the appropriate patient is a very important factor in the success of the osteotomy. The indication for open wedge HTO is a patient under the age of 65 with osteoarthritis confined to the medial compartment with varus deformity of 3 degrees or more. The range of motion of the joint should be preserved. However, some degree of limitation of knee motion, such as flexion contracture is 15 degrees or less, flexion is 90 degrees or more, are accepted for surgical indications [2]. It also shows good results in cases with medial osteonecrosis, osteochondritis dissecans, and radial type rupture of the posterior horn of the medial meniscus [51]. Contraindications that do not show a good prognosis after surgery include severe medial osteoarthritis (Kellgren–Lawrence classification group 4), when the correction angle is more than 20°, the knee flexion contracture is more than 15°, osteoarthritis of the preceding lateral compartment, lateral subluxation of the tibia, and arthritis caused by inflammatory arthritis such as rheumatoid arthritis [52, 53].

12.5.2 Comparison of Indications Between HTO and Unicondylar Knee Arthroplasty (UKA)

Patients with varus deformity of 3 degrees or more and symptoms of the medial compartment osteoarthritis can be classified into two kinds of knee osteoarthritis phenotype. First, when at least one of LDFA or MPTA is out of the normal range, the joint line congruence angle is normal in early arthritis, or the joint line congruence angle is abnormal in advanced arthritis. Second, there is varus deformity and symptoms in the medial compartment, but LDFA and MPTA are normal, and joint line congruence angle is abnormal due to complete loss of articular cartilage or intra-articular lesions such as post-meniscectomy status. HTO is appropriate for the first case of varus deformity due to bone deformity, and the resulting medial compartment symptom. UKA is more suitable for the second case of varus deformity as an intra-articular lesion without bone deformities.

It is also reported that the tibia bone varus angle (TBVA) is 5 degrees or more as an HTO indication [54–56]. TBVA is the angle formed by the line connecting the center of the tibial spine and the point midway proximal tibia epiphysis and the tibia mechanical axis on the knee AP radiograph [55]. However, poor intra-observer reproducibility and low inter-observer agreement are reported due to the limitation of TBVA that it is difficult to accurately distinguish old epiphyseal growth plates [57, 58]. Therefore, TBVA assessment is not appropriate to assess tibia bone deformity [57].

12.5.3 Patients Selection

12.5.3.1 Age

There is still no consensus on the outcome of HTO according to patient age. There are some reports that the 10-year survival rate decreases when the patient is older than 65 years of age [16, 59–61], but there are also reports that age does not affect the survival rate [62, 63]. In general, surgeons tend to believe that the failure rate will be higher in the older patient group, so it appears to be narrowing the indications. As such, it is considered that it is more important to consider the physiological age rather than the actual age when determining the indication of age because the results vary according to the authors.

12.5.3.2 Activity

HTO guarantees the higher degree of activity after correction in patients with single compartment osteoarthritis [64, 65]. Fu et al. [66] reported that it was possible to walk faster after surgery in the HTO group than in the UKA group. Of course, there is a disadvantage in that the HTO group must undergo a longer rehabilitation period [67]. In contrast, in the case of joint replacement surgery, moderate activity is possible, and in patients with high activity, the longevity of the prosthesis may be shortened and the reoperation rate may increase [2].

12.5.3.3 Grade of Osteoarthritis

In HTO, the degree of medial compartment osteoarthritis is one of the important factors influencing the postoperative outcome. When cartilage damage is limited to the medial compartment, good results can be expected after surgery, but in severe osteoarthritis, the medial pain may persist even after surgery [16, 68]. In particular, cases with patellofemoral arthritis or progression to triple compartment osteoarthritis are contraindicated in HTO [53, 69, 70]. According to the classification of osteoarthritis proposed by Ahlbäck [71], the results were not good for grade 3 or higher [72, 73], and better results for grade 0 [74]. MRI may be performed in patients with medial compartment arthritis to identify cartilage damage and other concomitant disorders and to evaluate lateral compartment cartilage damage [75, 76].

12.5.3.4 Range of Motion

Before performing HTO surgery, the patient's range of motion should be examined. Berman et al. [77] reported that postoperative results were poor when the preoperative range of motion was less than 90 degrees. Akizuki et al. [78] reported that the range of motion before surgery was 100 degrees as a reference point for good results after surgery. Patients with osteoarthritis have flexion contracture, and HTO can correct flexion contracture less than 15 degrees. However, if there is a flexion contracture of 15 degrees or more, it is difficult to expect satisfactory surgical results after surgery because the posterior tibial slope change after HTO adversely affects the anterior and posterior cruciate ligament [79, 80].

12.5.3.5 Knee Instability

Since there may be cases of alignment abnormalities accompanied by knee instability, it is necessary to examine the ligament condition before performing HTO. Changes in the posterior tibial slope can affect preoperative planning and postoperative outcomes depending on the range of motion and the anterior and posterior cruciate ligament condition [81, 82]. That is, the increase of the posterior tibial slope caused by the medial open wedge HTO may result in a decrease in hyperextension and a decrease in posterior instability (increase in flexion contracture and an increase in anterior instability) [83, 84]. Conversely, the decrease of the posterior tibial slope by the closed wedge HTO can lead to an increase in hyperextension and an increase in posterior instability reduction in flexion contracture and reduction in anterior instability [85]. In the case of chronic anterior cruciate ligament injury and varus deformity, only HTO or combined anterior cruciate ligament reconstruction can be performed, which is determined by considering the patient's age and activity [17, 86, 87]. If there is only posterior cruciate ligament injury or chronic posterolateral instability is accompanied by damage to the posterior lateral structure, only HTO should be performed first. If the instability persists after surgery, consider performing posterior cruciate ligament and posterolateral structure reconstruction [17, 88].

12.5.3.6 Body Mass Index (BMI)

Flecher et al. [15] reported that when the body mass index (BMI) is less than 30 kg/m^2, the results after HTO are better. Giagounidis and Sell [89] reported that if the BMI is 10% higher than normal, the postoperative pain-free period is 5 years, and if the body mass index is lower than normal 10%, the postoperative pain-free period is 7.8 years. On the contrary, Naudie et al. [90] reported that patients with a BMI of less than 25 kg/m^2 had worse results after HTO, which argued that the lighter people were more active and put more load on the osteotomy site. As such, the debate on the incidence of weight and OA is still ongoing, but it is known that in general, obese patients place more load on the knee joint.

12.5.4 Ideal Correction Angle

The correction goals and preoperative planning methods of varus deformity vary from author to author. Coventry et al. [45] suggested that the anatomical femoral tibial angle should be overcorrected to 8 degree valgus, and Hernigou et al. [91] suggested that the mechanical axis should be corrected to 3–6 degree valgus. Fujisawa et al. [23] reported that the postoperative mechanical axis should pass 60%–70% from the medial side of the tibial plateau. Miniaci et al. [92] reported that it should pass 60%–70% of the tibial plateau, and Dugdale et al. [43] reported that it should pass through 62% of the tibial plateau. This was the same as the location mentioned by Fujisawa et al. [23]. The results of this study later became the gold standard for calibration targets under the name of Fujisawa point-62% from the tibia medial side. Afterward, recognizing the limitations of the Fujisawa point, the researchers began to look more closely at the results of the correction angle. In a study through gait analysis, Prodromos et al. [93] reported that even if the same correction angle was obtained after surgery, the adductor moment of the knee joint was different for each patient, and the loss of correction increased when the moment was large. Even after HTO surgery, patients with high adduction moments tended to get worse and more varus deformity before surgery. Therefore, dynamic loading such as gait analysis as well as static alignment should be considered in HTO surgery.

There are still controversies about the ideal corrective goal for reducing pain, restoring function, and prolonged knee use after surgery. Hernigou et al. [91], in a retrospective analysis of the 93 knees, found that the results deteriorated significantly from 7 years after surgery. However, patients with a hip–knee–ankle angle of 183–186 degrees (mechanical axis valgus 3–6) reported better results in long-term follow-up. Jakob and Jacobi [94] reported that the degree of correction should be adjusted according to the cartilage thickness of the medial compartment. If one-third of the medial cartilage is damaged, the mechanical axis should pass 10%–15% outward from the center of the tibial plateau, 20%–25% when two-third of the medial cartilage is damaged, and if all medial cartilage was damaged, it was reported that the 30%–35% point should be passed. In general, many studies to date have recommended correction in the range of 5 to 16 degrees valgus [95–98]. However, there are studies showing that there is no correlation between the degree of valgus and the improvement of symptoms after surgery [99, 100]. Several studies have also reported that lateral compartment degeneration progresses even with mild overcorrection [91, 101]. However, most authors generally agree that the ideal correction goal is in the range of 3–8 valgus [45, 96, 98, 101]. In summary, postoperative clinical results are considered to be good if the mechanical axis is 3–5° valgus or a weight-bearing line is positioned at 62%–65% in the lower extremities orthoscanogram after HTO.

12.5.5 Preoperative Correction Plan in Coronal Plane

1. Miniaci method: Draw a line so that the postoperative corrective line goes from the center of the femoral head to the ankle joint while passing the tibial plateau to the desired weight-bearing position by the operator. (Line A). Draw a line from the hinge point of the HTO to the center of the ankle joint (Line B), and draw a line where Line A intersects at the hinge point (Line C). At this time, it is important to note that the lengths of Line B and Line C must be the same. If they are not the same, a slight difference in angle may occur. The angle between Line B and Line C is the corrective angle planned by the Miniaci method [92] (Fig. 12.4).
2. Dugdale method: Draw a line from the center of the femoral head to the point of 62.5% of the tibial plateau (Line A). Next, draw a line from the center of the ankle joint to 62.5% of the tibial plateau (Line B). The angle between Line A and Line B is the corrective angle planned by the Dugdale method [43] (Fig. 12.5).
3. Weight-bearing scanography method: Take a weight-bearing scanogram and print it in actual size. After cutting the part to be osteotomy, draw a line and rotate it between 62% and 65% so that the weight-bearing target point is passed. The degree of correction can be planned by directly measuring the size of the osteotomy part using a ruler [102] (Fig. 12.6).
4. Method of checking lower limb alignment during surgery: During the operation, it is necessary to check whether the lower limb alignment is corrected according to the preoperative plan. In order to check the alignment of the lower extremities during surgery, a method using a cable or rod is classically used, but there are problems in accuracy and reproducibility [103]. Computer-assisted orthopedic surgery (CAOS) or navigation system, which is recently used to increase the accuracy, precision, and reproducibility of surgery, provides information on the anatomical position

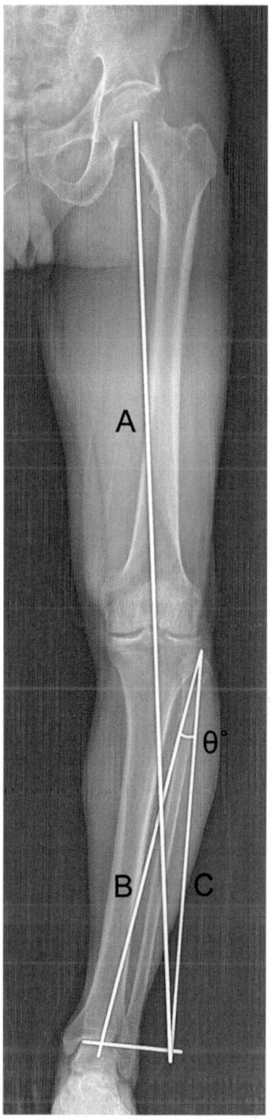

Fig. 12.4 Miniaci method: Line A represents the planned weight-bearing line for the postoperative correction extending from the center of the hip to about 62% of the tibial plateau width. Line B connects the osteotomy hinge point with the center of the ankle. Line C connects the osteotomy hinge point with the arc intersection of Line A. The θ angle formed by Lines B and C is the planned correction angle

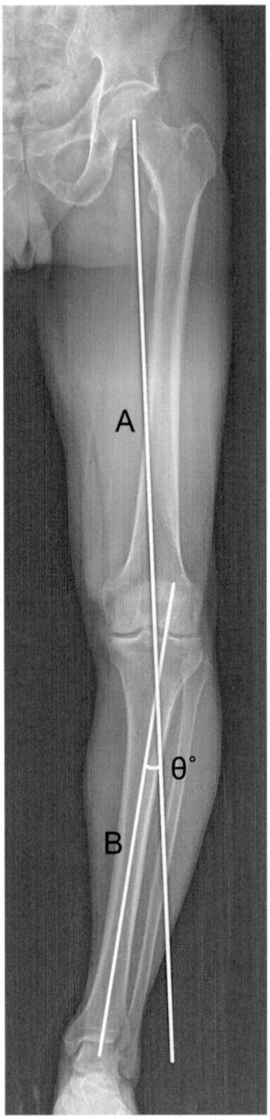

Fig. 12.5 Dugdale method: Line A is drawn from the center of the femoral head to 62.5% of the tibial width. Line B is drawn from the center of the talus to the 62% coordinate. The θ angle formed by these two lines is the correction angle

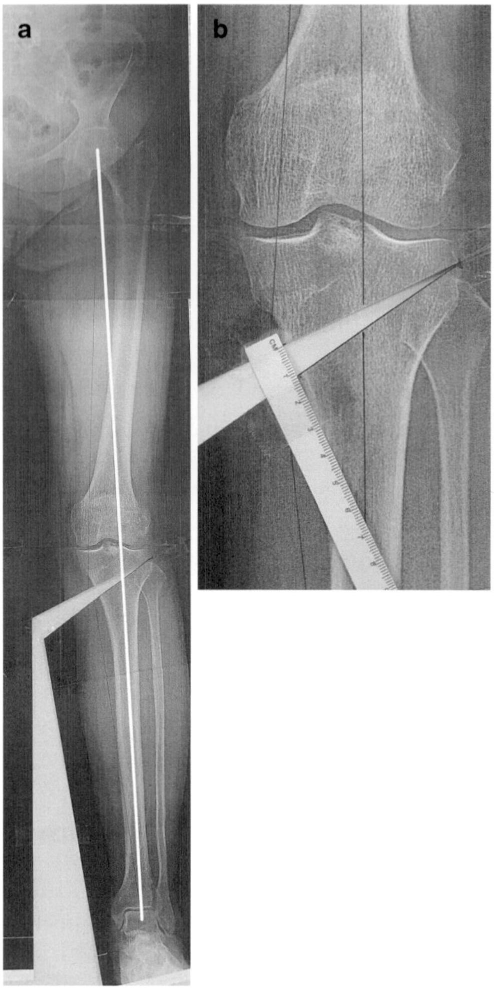

Fig. 12.6 Printed weight-bearing scenography measure method: A template was cut through the osteotomy site, and the osteotomy site was opened until the weight-bearing line passed through the 62%

in real time during surgery to determine the desired correction angle. There is an advantage of being able to obtain more accurately, reducing error ranges and outliers, and improving correction precision [102, 104]. Limb alignment assessment using a navigation system is performed under anesthesia in the supine position. Therefore, there is an angle discrepancy of limb alignment between supine and standing positions. Additional studies and long-term follow-up are needed for clinical results.

5. Trigonometric data: Hernigou et al. [105] used trigonometric data to transform the correction angle into the height or distance of the osteotomy gap, that is, mm.

12.5.6 Preoperative Correction Plan in the Sagittal Plane

When the posterior tibial slope angle is increased, flexion contracture occurs and the anterior subluxation of the tibia and the tension of the anterior cruciate ligament are increased, thereby reducing the posterior subluxation of the tibia that occurs when the posterior cruciate ligament is defective [81]. Conversely, when the posterior tibial slope angle decreases, hyperextension occurs and the posterior subluxation and tension of the posterior cruciate ligament increase, thereby reducing the anterior subluxation of the tibia that occurs when an anterior cruciate ligament is defective [82]. That is, it should be considered that the knee joint deformities such as flexion contracture and hyperextension could be corrected by adjusting the posterior tibial slope angle. However, if the posterior tibial slope angle increases by more than 10 degrees, the force applied to the anterior cruciate ligament increases more than three times, so care should be taken [106]. In the case of open HTO, the posterior tibial slope angle tends to increase by 3 degrees. In chronic posterior cruciate ligament injury, an increase in posterior tibial slope angle may be helpful. Conversely, in closed HTO, the posterior tibial slope angle tends to decrease by about 3 degrees. Reduction of the posterior tibial slope angle may be helpful in chronic anterior cruciate ligament injury [52].

Several studies have been conducted to find the cause of unintended change in tibial sagittal plane slope after medial open wedge HTO [44, 107, 108]. Known causes are incomplete posterior cut [44], improper gap ratio [108], and inappropriate hinge position [107]. Therefore, in order to prevent unintended change in tibial sagittal plane slope after medial open wedge HTO surgery, a complete posterior cut, proper gap ratio (open the anterior and posterior of the osteotomy site to about 2:3), and a true lateral hinge position are required [83, 84]. It is also important to make sagittal osteotomy inclination parallel to the native tibial sagittal plane slope [109]. In the process of spreading the osteotomy site using a spreader, a change in the tibial sagittal plane slope may be caused by the position of the spreader. In general, the spreader should be placed in the posterior of the osteotomy site. At this time, if the spreader is located at the posteromedial corner, the plate position may be located somewhat anterior. If the spreader is placed in the anterior of the osteotomy site to place the plate in the posterior, the tibial sagittal plane slope may increase.

12.5.7 Surgical Technique

12.5.7.1 Approach

The patient is placed in a supine position on a radiolucent surgical table. Placing a radiopaque label on the femoral head prior to the orthopedic drape helps to evaluate the mechanical axis of the lower limb during surgery. Anatomical landmarks such as the medial joint line and the proximal boundary of pes anserinus, superficial MCL, and tibial tubercle are drawn on the skin in a 30–45 degree knee flexion. After making a longitudinal incision of about 5–6 cm on the medial surface of the patellar tendon and the middle of the tibia posterior boundary, the subpatellar branch of the saphenous nerve is preserved. After exposing pes anserinus, make an incision at the attachment and pull it posteromedially. Pes anserinus can be operated while preserving, but it is better to remove it as it may cause tendinitis and flexion contracture due to friction with the metal plate if it is sutured after fixing the metal plate. There are two methods of partially dissecting the superficial medial collateral ligament, the first is to check the medial collateral ligament and then transection parallel to the articular surface at the osteotomy position, and the second is to reduce the pressure on the joint surface by detaching the medial collateral ligament from the distal attachment site. Among them, the method of transection of the ligaments has good visibility during surgery [50].

12.5.7.2 Single Plane Osteotomy Technique of Tibia

Before starting the osteotomy, a long tongue retractor should be used to protect the neurovascular structures at the posterior. Two guide pins must be inserted, and the insertion position of the pin is the most important. Before pin insertion, the knee joint must be slightly flexed so that the knee joint can be observed in parallel with a radiograph. Guide pin insertion begins at the metaphyseal flare, which is located 3 cm below the articular surface. The metaphyseal flare coincides with the patellar tendon attachment site and is formed parallel to the joint line, so the osteotomy is performed by palpating it. First, insert the front K-wire toward the "safe zone." The "Safe Zone" is the space between the tip of the fibula and the circumference line of the fibula head. There is a joint capsule on the outside, which can prevent dislocation due to fracture of the lateral cortex [110]. The second K-wire is inserted parallel to the first K-wire and parallel to the posterior slope angle, and the surface connecting the two K-wires becomes the cutting surface for the osteotomy. Insert an oscillating saw under the two guide pins (approximately 50%–60% of the osteotomy surface is with an oscillating saw, and then, carefully but sufficiently perform the osteotomy using an osteotomy). Osteotomy is completed by spreading the cutting area using 3 or 4 chisels. The important thing at this time is that osteotomy should be performed with about 5–10 mm of the lateral cortex remaining during the osteotomy. Insert the first chisel 5–10 mm from the end of the lateral cortex. The second chisel is inserted along the first chisel, and the third chisel is inserted between the first and second. Carefully apply valgus force to open the osteotomy surface and insert the bone spreader deeply into the osteotomy surface. Insert the driver into the bone spreader, turn it slowly clockwise, and check the alignment and correction of the lower extremities using fluoroscopy. There are several ways to maintain the osteotomy surface. The first is to use a metal block, the second is to use a distractor, the third is to use a tricortical iliac bone graft, and the last is to use a synthetic bone block. These are useful methods for maintaining the osteotomy spacing before inserting the metal plate. The distractor should be opened 1–2 mm wider than the planned value, and if it is opened more than 10 mm, it must be opened carefully to prevent lateral cortical fracture, and use a metal block or bone block is advantageous to fix it.

12.5.7.3 Dual-Plane Osteotomy Technique of Tibia

After exposing the insertion site of the patella tendon, the knee is flexed 90 degrees. The course of the osteotomy running from the front to the top is marked with an electric cautery, and the saw cut ending behind the patellar tendon attachment is raised at an angle of 110 degrees from the horizontal line to prepare for dual-plane osteotomy. After exposing the medial cortex of the tibia, drill two guide pins in the direction of the osteotomy line at about 4 cm below the joint surface. The posterior pin is inserted into the cranial border of pes anserinus just in front of the posterior tibial ridge, and the second pin is inserted 2 cm anteriorly parallel to the first pin. The pin must stop exactly in the lateral cortex. The depth of the resection should be 5–10 mm from the lateral cortex to leave the hinge of the lateral cortex, and the tibial tubercle should have a width of 15–20 mm or more. Horizontal osteotomy is performed with an oscillating saw with a rail under the two guide pins, and the posteromedial cortex of the tibia is completely osteotomized. At this time, the anatomical structure on the posterior side of the tibia is protected with a long nose Hohmann retractor, and irrigation is performed during saw cutting to continuously cool the saw blade and proceed slowly with very little pressure. When the posterior two-third of the tibia is sufficiently osteotomized, the anterior ascending saw cut is performed by changing to a narrow saw blade, and complete osteotomy including the lateral cortex is performed. After performing the osteotomy of the medial cortex, the saw blade faces the coronal surface, and when a double plane is cut, bones meet between the two surfaces of the anterior osteotomy to increase the stability of the sagittal plane after surgery.

12.5.7.4 Insertion and Fixation of Metal Plates

In a single plane osteotomy, three locking screws can be fixed to the proximal part of the osteotomy, and due to this, a somewhat weak fixation force can be assisted to endure axial compression using a metal block or a bone block. First, check the position of the metal plate using fluoroscopy, and adjust the position of the metal plate as necessary. When the metal plate is fixed to the bone, the locking screw is inserted in the proximal part of the osteotomy to fix it first, with the knee gently overextended to prevent an increase in the posterior slope angle of the knee joint. And then, the ankle is internally rotated to fix the metal screw at the distal part of the osteotomy to prevent external rotation of the lower limb. Finally, if a metal block is used, fix the screw connected to the metal block. For rigid fixation during single plane osteotomy, fix the proximal metal screw and fix only the near cortex with a drill bit in the hole at the bottom of the distal part, or temporarily fix it using K-wire, and then the gap between the metal plate and the bone can be narrowed by inserting a compression screw just below the osteotomy site. At this step, care must be taken not to overcompression when using a compression screw. Afterwards, the locking screw is fixed to the distal cortical bone in the remaining locking screw hole, and the previously inserted compression screw is also fixed again with the locking screw. The dual-plane osteotomy is a technique that can insert four locking screws in the proximal part, so it has the advantage of obtaining sufficient fixing power. The plate in the form of a locking-compression plate is rigid, and it is designed to be compression fixed. Compression fixation is useful when there is a Takeuchi type 1 lateral cortical fracture, and when the fracture line is located in the "safe zone," it is not necessary to use a compression screw [111]. Even if the fracture line is not observed, if compression fixation is performed when the gap between the plate and the bone is greater than 4 mm, a Takeuchi type 2 lateral cortical fracture may occur. During dual-plane osteotomy, fix the proximal locking screw for rigid fixation, then temporarily fix only the near cortex with a drill bit in the lowermost hole in the distal part, and then fix the compression screw just below the osteotomy. Afterwards, the locking screw is fixed to the distal cortical bone in the remaining locking screw hole, and the previously inserted compression screw is also fixed again with the locking screw. The recently developed metal plate is an anatomically designed metal plate that gives a posterior inclination and allows a little more bending when viewed from the side, so that it can be applied close to a bone. If the metal plate is firmly fixed, bone graft is not required even if the osteotomy space is about 12–14 mm. If the osteotomy gap is larger than this, an autogenous bone graft may be performed at the osteotomy gaps to promote mechanical support and bone union, and allogeneic cancellous bones and artificial bones may be used [15].

12.5.7.5 Rehabilitation

It is recommended to apply an ice pack immediately after surgery and to use an intermittent venous compression pump at the beginning. On the first day after surgery, dressing is performed to see the state of the soft tissue, and if the fixation is appropriate in the open HTO, wear an HTO brace with crutches from the first day and start walking with a weight of about 15–20 kg. However, weight-bearing walking may be delayed depending on the presence or absence of a fracture or the degree of fixation of the metal plate during surgery. For 1 week of surgery, start the 0° 90° joint movement using the HTO brace and gradually progress to full weight bearing over the next 4–6 weeks. Up to 12 weeks after that, increase weight bearing without braces. Since the results of surgery may vary depending on the patient, it is necessary to evaluate whether the correction is well maintained until 6 months after surgery by taking a basic radiographic examination and a full-length radiographic image of the lower extremity [112].

12.5.7.6 Complications

The most important thing after surgery is to prevent recurrence of deformity, and the most common cause of recurrence is a fracture of the lateral cortical bone that acts as a hinge. The prognosis can be predicted by the Takeuchi classification, and osteotomy line targeting the "safe zone" is an important surgical method to prevent lateral hinge fracture [110, 111]. Also, the most dangerous complication of open HTO is posterior popliteal artery and nerve damage [113]. To prevent this, as described above, the use of a saw should be performed up to 50%–60% of the osteotomy surface, and then osteotome should be used, and when posterolateral cortex osteotomy, an osteotomy protector such as a long nose Hohmann retractor should be used to protect the arteries and nerves. Soft tissue swelling and lymphedema may occur after surgery, and anti-inflammatory drugs, manual lymphatic drainage, and intermittent venous compression pumps can be applied. In the case of deep vein thrombosis or pulmonary embolism, medical treatment is required. Compartment syndrome may occur due to an increase in compartment pressure after surgery, and if there are imminent symptoms such as swelling of the lower extremities, abnormal sensations, and severe pain, early evaluation of clinical symptoms and compartment pressure is necessary. Diastolic blood pressure and blood pressure of compartment pressure when the difference is less than 30 mmHg, it can be strongly suspected and is an adaptation for emergency fascia incision. If the infection is strongly suspected after surgery, early marginal resection and antibiotics are required. In addition, a delayed union of the osteotomy may be suspected if continuous pain is accompanied during walking even at 6–9 weeks postoperatively, and fine movement of the lateral cortex of the osteotomy can be observed on the radiograph. About 0.7%–4.4% of complications such as delayed union and nonunion after open HTO have been reported [114]. In this case, bone graft or metal plate reapply should be considered. Autogenous bone graft should be considered for large correction angles (14 mm or more) because the possibility of nonunion is reduced during autologous bone graft.

12.5.7.7 Results

Darees et al. [115] performed medial open HTO in 51 patients using Tomofix™ locking plate (Synthes, Oberdorf, Switzerland) without void filling. An average of 10 years was observed, and finally, 48 patients were evaluated. Average HKA was 172 ± 3.18° (165–178°) before surgery, 181 ± 1.18° (176–185°) immediately after surgery, 181 ± 1.60° (176–185°) 2 years after surgery, 181 ± 1.60° (176–185°) 10 years after surgery ±1.60° (176–185°). The 10-year survival rate was 88% (95% CI: 81–98%). Complications occurred in four cases (8%). There were three cases within 2 years after surgery, two nonunions and one infection. And about 10 years after the operation, one infection occurred. Jin et al. [116] analyzed the results after medial open wedge HTO in 339 patients. Follow-up was observed for at least 5 years, and the average follow-up period was 9.6 years. Average HKA was from 7.2° of varus before surgery to 3.4° of valgus for 1 year after surgery and was maintained until 10 years after surgery. The 5-year survival rate was 96.8%, the 10-year survival rate was 87.1%, and the 13-year survival rate was 85.3%. The authors report that medial open wedge HTO is an effective treatment that provides acceptable survival rates and satisfactory outcomes in relatively young and active patients with osteoarthritis and varus deformity. Hantes et al. [117] performed medial open wedge high tibial osteotomy in 20 patients under 45 years of age. The mean mechanical tibiofemoral angle (mTFA) was 5.8 ± 2.4° before surgery, 2.5 ± 1.9° immediately after surgery, and 2.2 ± 1.7° at the last follow-up. The average survival rate was 95% at 12.3 years follow-up.

12.6 Distal Femoral Osteotomy (DFO)

The valgus deformity of the knee joint is less frequent than the varus deformity, and the biomechanical characteristics are also different from the varus knee. Usually, the valgus knee is a congenital origin with a superolateral tilt of the tibia. Acquired, it is often caused by lateral meniscus resection or trauma. Varus deformities mostly occur in the proximal tibia, while valgus deformities mostly occur in the distal femur. Just as varus deformity can be treated with HTO, DFO can be applied to valgus deformity. However, even if there is a valgus deformity, it must be corrected as HTO if the deformity occurs at the proximal tibia. The surgical method such as HTO or DFO should not be determined according to the deformity type, whether it is valgus or varus, but the surgical site should be determined according to where the deformity occurred. DFO is a surgical method that relieves pain by moving the weight load of the lower limbs from the lateral side to medial side [18, 118]. DFO has the advantage of minimizing the relaxation of the medial collateral ligaments, so that the transcondylar line and the mechanical axis of the lower extremities become vertical by reducing the superolateral tilt of the joint after surgery [119, 120].

12.6.1 Indication and Contraindication

Indications for DFO include degenerative changes limited only to the lateral compartment of the knee joint, with valgus deformity of 12 degrees or more, inclination angle of the joint surface more than 10 degrees after correction, age of patients under 60 years old, rickets, renal dystrophy, polio, lateral osteochondritis in young patients, congenital valgus, recurrent dislocation of the patella with valgus, and valgus deformity due to other trauma or muscle neurological disease [70, 120, 121]. In addition, if there is no instability of the knee, and the range of motion before the surgery is more than 90 degrees, and the flexion contracture is less than 15 degrees, surgery can be performed [122]. The primary indication for DFO is degenerative arthritis and valgus deformity, which complains of severe pain, but recently, it is also performed together to obtain the best results after surgery such as ligament reconstruction, cartilage transplantation, or meniscus allograft. In the case of recurrent patellar dislocations, medial implications with DFO can correct excessive Q angle and prevent recurrence of the dislocation [123]. Absolute contraindications to surgery are cases of extensive and ambiguous knee joint pain, the main cause of the pain is in the patellofemoral joint, the meniscectomy of the medial compartment where the weight bearing is likely to be concentrated after osteotomy, and degenerative arthritis involving bilateral compartments. Infectious or inflammatory diseases of the knee joint, poor soft tissue at the surgical incision, and the inability of the patient to cooperate with surgery and rehabilitation [70, 122, 124]. Relative contraindications include the age of patients over 60 years old, knee range of motion less than 90 degrees, obesity, subluxation of the knee joint, and moderate ligament instability [70, 122]. If the patient's main symptom is pain in the femoral-tibial joint, even if the patient is accompanied by less than severe patellar arthritis, it is not contraindicated in surgery [122].

12.6.2 Preoperative Planning

Before surgery, a thorough medical history and physical examination should be performed. The patient's age, occupation and preoperative activity, and expected activity after surgery should be considered. Through interviews, patients should be informed in advance that a completely normal joint cannot be acquired even after a successful operation and that the degree of pain reduction is less and the time required for rehabilitation is longer compared to TKA. Through the physical examination, the patient's degree of obesity, soft tissue conditions around the knee joint, range of motion, knee instability, and ligaments are evaluated, and an appropriate surgical plan is established. If ligament instability is suspected, stress tests can be performed and ligament relaxation should be considered when determining the correction angle. Radiography is performed to accurately assess the area and extent of degenerative changes. Basically, the true anteroposterior and lateral X-ray of the knee joint should be taken, and the patellar axial view is performed. In addition, in order to evaluate the degenerative change and joint spacing change of both sides of the knee joint, the Rosenberg view of the knee joint flexed 45 degrees with the standing position and both lower extremities orthoscanogram to evaluate the physiological axis of the lower limb and to determine the correction angle are necessary.

How to determine the correction angle is controversial and there is no consensus yet. Depending on the authors, it is recommended that the mechanical axis of the lower extremities pass through the center of the knee joint after surgery, or the mechanical axis passes the medial side of the knee joint with a mechanical femoral-tibial angle of 1–3 degrees or an anatomical femoral-tibial angle of 6–10 degrees [70, 124–126]. Currently, the angle of correction is often determined so that the mechanical axis passes right inside the center of the knee joint or the medial side of the medial tibial spine [70, 124]. The correction angle can be determined through both lower extremities orthoscanogram. Draw the mechanical axis line AD from the center point A of the talus to the center point D of the femur head. Draw a new mechanical axis line C through the femur center point D and a new target line through the target point (most directly inside the tibia medial spine). Draw a line AE from the center point A of the talus to the endpoint E, where E is the same level as the center point D of the femur. Draw a line HD from point H to the center point D of the femur (mostly the lateral cortex of the supracondylar region) and draw the line HE from the hinge point H to E as well. The angle α between the line HE and line HD formed at this time becomes the size of the angle to be corrected. After β is the same size as α, the osteotomy can be performed by the amount of β produced [70, 124] (Fig. 12.7).

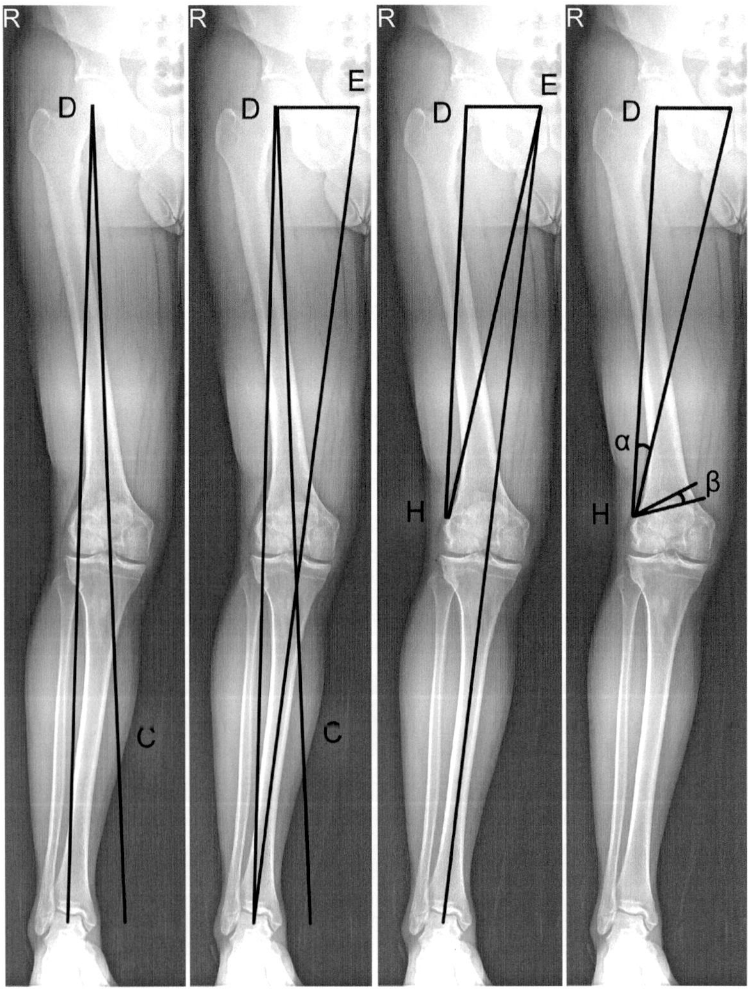

Fig. 12.7 Miniaci method: Line AD represents the weight-bearing line. Line C represents the planned weight-bearing line. Line AE intersects line C on tibia plateau. H is the hinge point. The angle α becomes the correction angle. If β is the same size as α, the osteotomy can be performed

12.6.3 Medial Closing Wedge Osteotomy

Medial closing wedge osteotomy is one of the most commonly used DFO methods. A surgical approach is performed from the medial side and then wedge osteotomy is performed to remove the bone and close the osteotomy site. Bone graft is not required and quick bone union can be obtained, but the shortening of the lower extremities may occur after surgery. Before performing an osteotomy with medial closed wedge osteotomy, arthroscopy is first performed to evaluate the condition of the knee joint. Surgery uses a slightly medial incision of the knee joint approximately 10–15 cm long from the joint line to the proximal portion of the distal femur. The fascia on the medial side of the distal femur is incised to expose the medial vastus and adductor tendon, detach from the medial intermuscular septum, and pull forward. If necessary, the medial patellofemoral ligament can be partially incised to expose the surgical site. Afterward, the musculoskeletal septum is incised, and a Hohmann retractor is inserted into the posterior of the femur to expose the femur medial condyle. To insert a guide pin, face the metal plate and mark the osteotomy site with an electrocautery device, and then insert the anterior K-wire obliquely in the lateral condyle direction starting from the osteotomy site. Insert the posterior K-wire parallel to the first k-wire. After that, measure the degree of bone to be removed using a ruler, and insert a K-wire so that the K-wires meet each other in the lateral cortex.

For uniplane osteotomy, osteotomized between the K-wires with a saw, and if there is 5 mm remaining from the lateral cortex, carefully perform the osteotomy using an osteotome. In order to remove the planned amount of femur and prevent lateral femoral fracture, multi-drilling was performed and then gradually applied varus force to complete the closed wedge DFO. The guide pins must be inserted with the same thickness on the front and bottom of the femur, so that the space behind the closed wedge osteotomy fits. If force is applied excessively, a surgical fracture occurs, so you can do it slowly and repeatedly with appropriate force. After performing a closed wedge osteotomy, press the sole of the foot with the operator's stomach (after weight-bearing) and check whether the desired correction is achieved. When fixing the metal plate, check that the metal pin does not enter the joint space. The principle of biplane osteotomy is to increase the fracture healing ability by expanding the osteotomy surface, but it has a disadvantage that the operation is difficult. In particular, the anterior femur in Asians is small, making it difficult to perform an osteotomy. However, since the contact area is large, it has an advantage for the bone union. First, a K-wire is inserted where the osteotomy is to be performed, and the target point is the same as for a single plane osteotomy. However, since one-third of the anterior thigh should be left like a roof, a K-wire is inserted into the area under two-third of the thickness of the femur, and osteotomy is performed. Use the smallest and thinnest saw to perform the osteotomy carefully. In particular, the saw should not damage the roof bone, and after the osteotomy of the lower femur is completed, the upper femur is cut with a thin saw in the 110° direction. After performing a closed wedge osteotomy, press the sole of the foot with the operator's stomach (after weight-bearing) and check whether the desired correction is achieved.

12.6.4 Rehabilitation

Depending on the operator, the duration and method of rehabilitation after surgery are somewhat different, but from 1 day after the surgery, range of motion exercise of the knee joint is allowed and toe-touch weight-bearing ambulation is performed using crutches for 2 weeks [125, 127]. From 2 weeks after surgery, start walking with partial weight as much as possible according to the patient's pain, and allow full weight-bearing walking when bone union at the osteotomy site is confirmed. Before the bone union is completed, since the osteotomy site is vulnerable to torsion force, care must be taken not to apply torsion force to the femur during the rehabilitation period.

12.6.5 Complications

Complications of surgery can be caused by a variety of causes, such as inappropriate patient selection, incorrect preoperative planning, problems with techniques, or postoperative rehabilitation. If the corrective angle before surgery is incorrectly planned, or if the correction is excessive due to improper correction during surgery, an excessive load is applied to the medial compartment and degenerative arthritis may also occur in the medial compartment. In case of insufficient correction, the planned movement of the mechanical axis before surgery is not performed properly and the patient's symptoms do not improve, resulting in failure of the surgery. It is very important to accurately establish a correction plan before surgery and to ensure that proper correction is made by fluoroscopy during surgery. In the case of partial detachment of the insertion portion of the medial patella-femoral ligament and the medial vastus muscle to expose the distal part of the femur, reconstruction can prevent patella instability or dislocation. When performing an osteotomy, care must be taken to prevent fracture by cutting to the opposite bone cortex, and if a fracture occurs, internal fixation using metal plates on both sides should be performed. There may be damage to the femoral nerve, sciatic nerve, or femoral vessel due to excessive traction or dissection during surgery, or direct damage during osteotomy [70, 121]. Therefore, in order to prevent nerve and blood vessel damage, it is necessary to carefully perform dissection, retractor position, and osteotomy during surgery. After surgery, a pad should be placed on the posterior of the knee joint or the knee joint should be fixed in a slightly flexed state to reduce the risk of peroneal nerve palsy. The occurrence of compartment syndrome after DFO is not common, but if overlooked, it can have serious consequences, so careful observation after surgery is required. Since hematoma formation is mostly caused by excessive bleeding, it is important to place a suction drainage tube at the surgical site to prevent blood from accumulating [70, 128]. If compartment syndrome occurs, immediate surgical hematoma removal and fascial dissection are performed. Deep infection at the surgical site is not common, but the incidence is high when using external fixators [128]. If antibiotics do not improve after starting administration, marginal debridement should be performed to remove necrotic and infected tissues, and removal of the fixator should be considered. In addition, after surgery, deep vein thrombosis or pulmonary embolism may occur, and knee joint stiffness may occur due to inappropriate rehabilitation [125]. In addition, delayed union or nonunion may occur at the osteotomy site, and broken off the internal fixator may occur, so care should be taken [122, 129].

12.6.6 Results

Several authors reported various results of DFO, and the choice of target patient, technique, and alignment of the lower limbs after surgery all affected the results. In the report of Backstein et al. [126], 40 cases of close osteotomy were followed up at 123 months, and functional improvement in 59% and survival rates of 82% after 10 years and 45% after 15 years were observed. Wang and Hsu [122] reported a functional improvement of 92% and a survival rate of 87% after performing a close osteotomy in 30 patients with valgus and lateral compartment arthritis of 12 degrees or more and observed for 99 months. Kosashvili et al. [130] performed closed osteotomy in 33 cases, and the average knee society score improved from 36.8 points to 77.5 points one year later, but reported a 48.5% failure rate after 15.6 years, requiring conversion to TKA in about half of the patients. Aglietti and Menchetti [131] reported that 18 patients with valgus knee were treated with DFO and followed up for 9 years with a success rate of 77%. Edgerton et al. [129] reported a success rate of 71% as a result of 8.3-year follow-up observation of 24 patients after surgery. Patients with degenerative changes confined to the lateral compartment showed a high success rate of 86%. Thein et al. [124] performed lateral open osteotomy in six patients with lateral compartment degenerative arthritis and followed up for 6.5 years. As a result of the study, symptoms improved in all patients, bone union was obtained, and additional surgery was not required. On the other hand, Nelson et al. [132] performed DFO in nine patients and observed that the average knee society score improved from 35 to 84 points and the range of motion from 81.8 to 105.9 degrees as a result of follow-up for 14 years. However, five patients converted to TKA due to persistent degenerative changes, and TKA was more difficult and poorer results due to the extra-articular deformity of the femur due to the previous osteotomy. Although the success rates of surgery reported by authors are all different, most of the authors emphasized that the selection of a patient group suitable for the indication is important for the success of surgery in common [28, 125, 131]. The alignment of the lower limbs after surgery is also an important factor influencing the patient's surgical outcome. According to Edgerton et al. [129], symptoms improved in 60% of patients when the valgus knee was not corrected after surgery, while in 77% of patients in the neutral or varus corrected group, symptoms improved.

12.7 Double Level Osteotomy (DLO)

In most cases of severe varus deformity of the knee, varus deformities of the proximal tibia and distal femur are present at the same time, rather than a varus deformity of the proximal tibia alone [133]. If the varus deformity accompanied by deformation in both the femur and tibia is corrected with only HTO, an excessive oblique joint line in the proximal tibia occurs. This increases the shear force exerted on the articular cartilage, and can cause subluxation of the distal femur and overloading of the joint capsule during weight-bearing [134, 135]. In addition, new deformities occur after HTO, which may make it difficult to convert to TKA [136–138]. And it is known that the distal femur varus deformity contributes to the recurrence of varus deformity after HTO [139]. The double osteotomy that can be considered in this case is to perform both HTO and DFO, which was first proposed by Benjamin et al. [140] DLO can simultaneously correct the varus deformity of the proximal tibia and distal femur to restore normal knee joint alignment and orientation as well as correcting the mechanical axis of the lower limb [135].

12.7.1 Indication

Surgery is performed in patients with severe varus malalignment with arthritis of the medial knee joint. When it is planned to perform medial open wedge HTO alone, DLO should be considered if MPTA >94° after surgery, or if mLDFA >90° and MPTA <87° in preoperative deformity analysis. If the MPTA is greater than 94° after the medial open wedge HTO, this means that excessive joint obliquity is made. Also, preoperative mLDFA >90° and MPTA <87° indicate that both the distal femur and the proximal tibia have varus deformities [141].

12.7.2 Preoperative Planning

A weight-bearing orthoscanogram is required for preoperative correction planning. Considering the deformation of the femur and tibia, it is decided whether the osteotomy is to be performed in an open type or a closed type in the femur and tibia respectively [141]. For deformity analysis using both lower leg scanogram, alignment assessing parameters such as joint angle of femur and tibia, joint line convergence angle, are evaluated, and the normal range of each parameter must be known. Miculicz lines are used to simulate load distribution in the knee. The knee joint line orientation, as well as the Miculicz line, must be considered when planning the osteotomy level. The weight-bearing orthoscanogram is printed in actual size, and the part to be osteotomy is cut and rotated so that the deformation of the femur and tibia is corrected and the lower limb alignment is restored, so that the degree of correction can be determined. Recently, digital radiography can be used to easily use digital planning using computer software. Although DLO's correction goal has not been established, considering that DLO is a surgery to restore normal knee joint alignment and orientation, authors aim for slightly valgus alignment (valgus 0.5–1 or 0–2) rather than overcorrection [133, 135].

12.7.3 Results

Babis et al. [142] applied the CORA concept and reported good results by performing double osteotomy in which both tibia and femur were osteotomized in complex deformity patients. Babis et al. [142] performed 29 DLO in 24 patients and reported that the cumulative survival rate was 95% in the mean follow-up period of 100 months, when severe pain complained after DLO or when the transition to TKA was defined as failure. Saragaglia et al. [141] also reported good results after performing double-level osteotomy in patients with osteoarthritis with severe varus. Nakayama et al. [135] studied 20 patients with a minimum follow-up period of 1 year after DLO and Schroter et al. [133] had an average follow-up period of 18 months after DLO in 24 patients, reported good clinical results avoiding excessive oblique joint line and restoring normal joint alignment and orientation.

12.8 Conclusion

Recent studies have shown similar results in open and closed wedge HTOs when skillfully performed with modern fixation techniques and appropriate angle corrections. The key to successful knee function after the osteotomy is to select the osteotomy site, location, and size well, and to provide proper alignment by preventing joint line obliquity or the creation of new deformities. There is still no consensus on the optimum angle of correction, but alignment must be tailored to the individual and the specific disease process. Therefore, for an unstable knee, a neutral alignment may be more appropriate than overcorrection. Osteotomy is ideally performed as a measure to prevent the progression of deformity and pathology in young active individuals in the early stages of OA, but it provides good results even when OA is somewhat advanced. Therefore, this allows TKA to be avoided at a young age, and TKA can be postponed until old age.

References

1. Griffiths DL, Brockbank W. Orthopaedic surgery in the 16. and 17. centuries; traction apparatus; the vidian pictures. J Bone Joint Surg Br. 1949;31B(2):313–7.
2. Lobenhoffer P, Van Heerwaarden RJ, Staubli AE. Osteotomies around the knee: indications-planning-surgical techniques using plate fixators. Thieme; 2011.
3. Pennington T. Osteotomy as an indicator of antiseptic surgical practice. Med Hist. 1994;38(2):178–88.
4. Lexer E. Die gesamte wiederherstellungs-chirurgie. Ja Barth; 1931.
5. Brett A. Operative correction of genu recurvatum. JBJS. 1935;17(4):984–9.
6. Jackson J, Waugh W. Tibial osteotomy for osteoarthritis of the knee. J Bone Joint Surg. 1961;43(4):746–51.
7. Debeyre J, Patte D. The place of corrective osteotomies in the treatment of gonarthrosis. Acta Orthop Belg. 1961;27:374.
8. Gariepy R. Genu varum treated by high tibial osteotomy. J Bone Joint Surg Br. 1964;46:783–4.
9. Coventry MB. Osteotomy of the upper portion of the tibia for degenerative arthritis of the knee. A preliminary report. J Bone Joint Surg Am. 1965;47:984–90.
10. Muller W, Jani L. Experiences with 75 high tibial osteotomies. Reconstr Surg Traumatol. 1971;12:53–63.
11. Amendola A, Panarella L. High tibial osteotomy for the treatment of unicompartmental arthritis of the knee. Orthop Clin North Am. 2005;36(4):497–504. https://doi.org/10.1016/j.ocl.2005.05.009.
12. Nagel A, Insall JN, Scuderi GR. Proximal tibial osteotomy. A subjective outcome study. J Bone Joint Surg Am. 1996;78(9):1353–8. https://doi.org/10.2106/00004623-199609000-00009.
13. Brinkman JM, Lobenhoffer P, Agneskirchner JD, Staubli AE, Wymenga AB, van Heerwaarden RJ. Osteotomies around the knee: patient selection, stability of fixation and bone healing in high tibial osteotomies. J Bone Joint Surg Br. 2008;90(12):1548–57. https://doi.org/10.1302/0301-620X.90B12.21198.

14. Ronn K, Reischl N, Gautier E, Jacobi M. Current surgical treatment of knee osteoarthritis. Arthritis. 2011;2011:454873. https://doi.org/10.1155/2011/454873.
15. Flecher X, Parratte S, Aubaniac JM, Argenson JN. A 12-28-year followup study of closing wedge high tibial osteotomy. Clin Orthop Relat Res. 2006;452:91–6. https://doi.org/10.1097/01.blo.0000229362.12244.f6.
16. Hui C, Salmon LJ, Kok A, Williams HA, Hockers N, van der Tempel WM, et al. Long-term survival of high tibial osteotomy for medial compartment osteoarthritis of the knee. Am J Sports Med. 2011;39(1):64–70. https://doi.org/10.1177/0363546510377445.
17. Badhe NP, Forster IW. High tibial osteotomy in knee instability: the rationale of treatment and early results. Knee Surg Sports Traumatol Arthrosc. 2002;10(1):38–43. https://doi.org/10.1007/s001670100244.
18. Yoo JD, Kim NK. Distal femoral varization osteotomy. J Korean Orthop Assoc. 2014;49(2):118–25.
19. Agneskirchner JD, Hurschler C, Wrann CD, Lobenhoffer P. The effects of valgus medial opening wedge high tibial osteotomy on articular cartilage pressure of the knee: a biomechanical study. Arthroscopy. 2007;23(8):852–61. https://doi.org/10.1016/j.arthro.2007.05.018.
20. Hsu RW, Himeno S, Coventry MB, Chao EY. Normal axial alignment of the lower extremity and load-bearing distribution at the knee. Clin Orthop Relat Res. 1990;255:215–27.
21. Moreland JR, Bassett LW, Hanker GJ. Radiographic analysis of the axial alignment of the lower extremity. J Bone Joint Surg Am. 1987;69(5):745–9.
22. Tetsworth K, Paley D. Malalignment and degenerative arthropathy. Orthop Clin North Am. 1994;25(3):367–77.
23. Fujisawa Y, Masuhara K, Shiomi S. The effect of high tibial osteotomy on osteoarthritis of the knee. An arthroscopic study of 54 knee joints. Orthop Clin North Am. 1979;10(3):585.
24. Kettelkamp DB, Wenger DR, Chao EY, Thompson C. Results of proximal tibial osteotomy. The effects of tibiofemoral angle, stance-phase flexion-extension, and medial-plateau force. J Bone Joint Surg Am. 1976;58(7):952–60.
25. Moore J, Mychaltchouk L, Lavoie F. Applicability of a modified angular correction measurement method for open-wedge high tibial osteotomy. Knee Surg Sports Traumatol Arthrosc. 2017;25(3):846–52. https://doi.org/10.1007/s00167-015-3954-4.
26. Pape D, Rupp S. Preoperative planning for high tibial osteotomies. Oper Tech Orthop. 2007;17(1):2–11.
27. Brown GA, Amendola A. Radiographic evaluation and preoperative planning for high tibial osteotomies. Oper Tech Sports Med. 2012;20(1):93–102.
28. Hunter DJ, Sharma L, Skaife T. Alignment and osteoarthritis of the knee. JBJS. 2009;91(Suppl_1):85–9.
29. Paley D, Herzenberg JE, Tetsworth K, McKie J, Bhave A. Deformity planning for frontal and sagittal plane corrective osteotomies. Orthop Clin N Am. 1994;25(3):425–66.
30. Smith J, Wilson A, Thomas N. Osteotomy around the knee: evolution, principles and results. Knee Surg Sports Traumatol Arthrosc. 2013;21(1):3–22.
31. Vanlommel L, Vanlommel J, Claes S, Bellemans J. Slight undercorrection following total knee arthroplasty results in superior clinical outcomes in varus knees. Knee Surg Sports Traumatol Arthrosc. 2013;21(10):2325–30.
32. Bellemans J, Colyn W, Vandenneucker H, Victor J. The Chitranjan Ranawat Award: is neutral mechanical alignment normal for all patients?: The concept of constitutional varus. Clin Orthop Relat Res. 2012;470(1):45–53.
33. Victor JM, Bassens D, Bellemans J, Gürsu S, Dhollander AA, Verdonk PC. Constitutional varus does not affect joint line orientation in the coronal plane. Clin Orthop Relat Res. 2014;472(1):98–104.
34. Nakagawa Y, Mukai S, Yabumoto H, Tarumi E, Nakamura T. Cartilage degeneration and alignment in severe varus knee osteoarthritis. Cartilage. 2015;6(4):208–15.
35. Heijink A, Gomoll AH, Madry H, Drobnič M, Filardo G, Espregueira-Mendes J, et al. Biomechanical considerations in the pathogenesis of osteoarthritis of the knee. Knee Surg Sports Traumatol Arthrosc. 2012;20(3):423–35.
36. Hirschmann MT, Schön S, Afifi FK, Amsler F, Rasch H, Friederich NF, et al. Assessment of loading history of compartments in the knee using bone SPECT/CT: a study combining alignment and 99mTc-HDP tracer uptake/distribution patterns. J Orthop Res. 2013;31(2):268–74.
37. Horisberger M, Fortuna R, Valderrabano V, Herzog W. Long-term repetitive mechanical loading of the knee joint by in vivo muscle stimulation accelerates cartilage degeneration and increases chondrocyte death in a rabbit model. Clin Biomech. 2013;28(5):536–43.
38. Mina C, Garrett WE Jr, Pietrobon R, Glisson R, Higgins L. High tibial osteotomy for unloading osteochondral defects in the medial compartment of the knee. Am J Sports Med. 2008;36(5):949–55.
39. Lee YS, Lee BK, Lee SH, Park HG, Jun D-S. Effect of foot rotation on the mechanical axis and correlation between knee and whole leg radiographs. Knee Surg Sports Traumatol Arthrosc. 2013;21(11):2542–7.
40. Lee YS, Lee BK, Kwon JH, Kim JI, Reyes FJV, Suh DW, et al. Serial assessment of weight-bearing lower extremity alignment radiographs after open-wedge high tibial osteotomy. Arthroscopy. 2014;30(3):319–25.
41. Sancheti P, Patil K, Gugale S, Shyam A. 6 How can preoperative planning prevent occurrence of a painful total knee replacement? The unhappy total knee replacement. Springer; 2015. p. 59–68.
42. Phillips C, Silver D, Schranz P, Mandalia V. The measurement of patellar height: a review of the methods of imaging. J Bone Joint Surg. 2010;92(8):1045–53.

43. Dugdale TW, Noyes FR, Styer D. Preoperative planning for high tibial osteotomy. The effect of lateral tibiofemoral separation and tibiofemoral length. Clin Orthop Relat Res. 1992;274:248–64.
44. Marti CB, Gautier E, Wachtl SW, Jakob RP. Accuracy of frontal and sagittal plane correction in open-wedge high tibial osteotomy. Arthroscopy. 2004;20(4):366–72.
45. Coventry MB, Ilstrup DM, Wallrichs SL. Proximal tibial osteotomy. A critical long-term study of eighty-seven cases. J Bone Joint Surg Am. 1993;75(2):196–201.
46. Leonardi F, Rivera F, Zorzan A, Ali SM. Bilateral double osteotomy in severe torsional malalignment syndrome: 16 years follow-up. J Orthop Traumatol. 2014;15(2):131–6.
47. Windsor R, Insall J, Vince K. Technical considerations of total knee arthroplasty after proximal tibial osteotomy. J Bone Joint Surg Am. 1988;70(4):547–55.
48. Gaasbeek RD, Welsing RT, Verdonschot N, Rijnberg WJ, van Loon CJ, van Kampen A. Accuracy and initial stability of open-and closed-wedge high tibial osteotomy: a cadaveric RSA study. Knee Surg Sports Traumatol Arthrosc. 2005;13(8):689–94.
49. Miller BS, Downie B, McDonough EB, Wojtys EM. Complications after medial opening wedge high tibial osteotomy. Arthroscopy. 2009;25(6):639–46.
50. Staubli AE, De Simoni C, Babst R, Lobenhoffer P. TomoFix: a new LCP-concept for open wedge osteotomy of the medial proximal tibia–early results in 92 cases. Injury. 2003;34:55–62.
51. Gomoll AH. High tibial osteotomy for the treatment of unicompartmental knee osteoarthritis: a review of the literature, indications, and technique. Phys Sportsmed. 2011;39(3):45–54.
52. Oh SM, Nha KW, Han JH. Opening Wedge High Tibia Osteotomy. J Korean Orthop Assoc. 2018;53(4):293–300.
53. Wright JM, Crockett HC, Slawski DP, Madsen MW, Windsor RE. High tibial osteotomy. JAAOS-J Am Acad Orthop Surg. 2005;13(4):279–89.
54. Niemeyer P, Schmal H, Hauschild O, von Heyden J, Südkamp NP, Köstler W. Open wedge osteotomy using an internal plate fixator in patients with medial-compartment gonarthritis and varus malalignment: 3-year results with regard to preoperative arthroscopic and radiographic findings. Arthroscopy. 2010;26(12):1607 16.
55. Bonnin M, Chambat P. Current status of valgus angle, tibial head closing wedge osteotomy in media gonarthrosis. Der Orthopade. 2004;33(2):135–42.
56. Jenny J, Tavan A, Jenny G, Kehr P. Long-term survival rate of tibial osteotomies for valgus gonarthrosis. Revue de chirurgie orthopedique et reparatrice de l'appareil moteur. 1998;84(4):350–7.
57. van Raaij TM, Takacs I, Reijman M, Verhaar JA. Varus inclination of the proximal tibia or the distal femur does not influence high tibial osteotomy outcome. Knee Surg Sports Traumatol Arthrosc. 2009;17(4):390–5.
58. Jenny J, Boéri C, Ballonzoli L, Meyer N. Difficulties and reproducibility of radiological measurement of the proximal tibial axis according to Lévigne. Revue de chirurgie orthopedique et reparatrice de l'appareil moteur. 2005;91(7):658.
59. Smith WB, Steinberg J, Scholtes S, Mcnamara IR. Medial compartment knee osteoarthritis: age-stratified cost-effectiveness of total knee arthroplasty, unicompartmental knee arthroplasty, and high tibial osteotomy. Knee Surg Sports Traumatol Arthrosc. 2017;25(3):924–33.
60. Kuwashima U, Okazaki K, Iwasaki K, Akasaki Y, Kawamura H, Mizu-uchi H, et al. Patient reported outcomes after high tibial osteotomy show comparable results at different ages in the mid-term to long-term follow-up. J Orthop Sci. 2019;24(5): 855–60.
61. Keenan O, Clement N, Nutton R, Keating J. Older age and female gender are independent predictors of early conversion to total knee arthroplasty after high tibial osteotomy. Knee. 2019;26(1):207–12.
62. Goshima K, Sawaguchi T, Sakagoshi D, Shigemoto K, Hatsuchi Y, Akahane M. Age does not affect the clinical and radiological outcomes after open-wedge high tibial osteotomy. Knee Surg Sports Traumatol Arthrosc. 2017;25(3):918–23.
63. Kohn L, Sauerschnig M, Iskansar S, Lorenz S, Meidinger G, Imhoff A, et al. Age does not influence the clinical outcome after high tibial osteotomy. Knee Surg Sports Traumatol Arthrosc. 2013;21(1):146–51.
64. Brosset T, Pasquier G, Migaud H, Gougeon F. Opening wedge high tibial osteotomy performed without filling the defect but with locking plate fixation (TomoFix™) and early weight-bearing: prospective evaluation of bone union, precision and maintenance of correction in 51 cases. Orthop Traumatol Surg Res. 2011;97(7):705–11.
65. Belsey J, Yasen SK, Jobson S, Faulkner J, Wilson AJ. Return to physical activity after high tibial osteotomy or unicompartmental knee arthroplasty: a systematic review and pooling data analysis. Am J Sports Med. 2021;49(5):1372–80.
66. Fu D, Li G, Chen K, Zhao Y, Hua Y, Cai Z. Comparison of high tibial osteotomy and unicompartmental knee arthroplasty in the treatment of unicompartmental osteoarthritis: a meta-analysis. J Arthroplast. 2013;28(5):759–65.
67. Nwachukwu BU, McCormick FM, Schairer WW, Frank RM, Provencher MT, Roche MW. Unicompartmental knee arthroplasty versus high tibial osteotomy: United States practice patterns for the surgical treatment of unicompartmental arthritis. J Arthroplast. 2014;29(8):1586–9.
68. Dowd G, Somayaji H, Uthukuri M. High tibial osteotomy for medial compartment osteoarthritis. Knee. 2006;13(2):87–92.

69. Kfuri M, Lobenhoffer P. High tibial osteotomy for the correction of varus knee deformity. J Knee Surg. 2017;30(05):409–20.
70. Lobenhoffer P. The rationale of osteotomy around the knee. J Knee Surg. 2017;30(05):386–92.
71. Ahlback S. Osteoarthrosis of the knee. A radiographic investigation. Acta Radiol. 1968;227:7–72.
72. Benzakour T, Hefti A, Lemseffer M, El Ahmadi JD, Bouyarmane H, Benzakour A. High tibial osteotomy for medial osteoarthritis of the knee: 15 years follow-up. Int Orthop. 2010;34(2):209–15.
73. Stukenborg-Colsman C, Wirth C, Lazovic D, Wefer A. High tibial osteotomy versus unicompartmental joint replacement in unicompartmental knee joint osteoarthritis:: 7–10-year follow-up prospective randomised study. Knee. 2001;8(3):187–94.
74. Floerkemeier S, Staubli AE, Schroeter S, Goldhahn S, Lobenhoffer P. Outcome after high tibial open-wedge osteotomy: a retrospective evaluation of 533 patients. Knee Surg Sports Traumatol Arthrosc. 2013;21(1):170–80.
75. Parker DA, Beatty KT, Giuffre B, Scholes CJ, Coolican MR. Articular cartilage changes in patients with osteoarthritis after osteotomy. Am J Sports Med. 2011;39(5):1039–45.
76. Zampogna B, Vasta S, Papalia R. Patient evaluation and indications for osteotomy around the knee. Clin Sports Med. 2019;38(3):305–15.
77. Berman AT, Bosacco SJ, Kirshner S, Avolio A Jr. Factors influencing long-term results in high tibial osteotomy. Clin Orthop Relat Res. 1991;272:192–8.
78. Akizuki S, Shibakawa A, Takizawa T, Yamazaki I, Horiuchi H. The long-term outcome of high tibial osteotomy: a ten-to 20-year follow-up. J Bone Joint Surg. 2008;90(5):592–6.
79. Jacobi M, Villa V, Reischl N, Demey G, Goy D, Neyret P, et al. Factors influencing posterior tibial slope and tibial rotation in opening wedge high tibial osteotomy. Knee Surg Sports Traumatol Arthrosc. 2015;23(9):2762–8.
80. Ozalay M, Ozkoc G, Circi E, Akpınar S, Hersekli MA, Uysal M, et al. The correlation of correction magnitude and tibial slope changes following open wedge high tibial osteotomy. Knee Surg Sports Traumatol Arthrosc. 2008;16(10):948–51.
81. Giffin JR, Vogrin TM, Zantop T, Woo SL, Harner CD. Effects of increasing tibial slope on the biomechanics of the knee. Am J Sports Med. 2004;32(2):376–82.
82. Dean CS, Liechti DJ, Chahla J, Moatshe G, LaPrade RF. Clinical outcomes of high tibial osteotomy for knee instability: a systematic review. Orthop J Sports Med. 2016;4(3):2325967116633419.
83. Chae DJ, Shetty GM, Lee DB, Choi HW, Han SB, Nha KW. Tibial slope and patellar height after opening wedge high tibia osteotomy using autologous tri-cortical iliac bone graft. Knee. 2008;15(2):128–33.
84. Ogawa H, Matsumoto K, Ogawa T, Takeuchi K, Akiyama H. Effect of wedge insertion angle on posterior tibial slope in medial opening wedge high tibial osteotomy. Orthop J Sports Med. 2016;4(2):2325967116630748.
85. Bae DK, Ko YW, Kim SJ, Baek JH, Song SJ. Computer-assisted navigation decreases the change in the tibial posterior slope angle after closed-wedge high tibial osteotomy. Knee Surg Sports Traumatol Arthrosc. 2016;24(11):3433–40.
86. Herman BV, Giffin JR. High tibial osteotomy in the ACL-deficient knee with medial compartment osteoarthritis. J Orthop Traumatol. 2016;17(3):277–85.
87. Lattermann C, Jakob R. High tibial osteotomy alone or combined with ligament reconstruction in anterior cruciate ligament-deficient knees. Knee Surg Sports Traumatol Arthrosc. 1996;4(1):32–8.
88. Petrigliano FA, Suero EM, Voos JE, Pearle AD, Allen AA. The effect of proximal tibial slope on dynamic stability testing of the posterior cruciate ligament–and posterolateral corner–deficient knee. Am J Sports Med. 2012;40(6):1322–8.
89. Giagounidis E, Sell S. High tibial osteotomy: factors influencing the duration of satisfactory function. Arch Orthop Trauma Surg. 1999;119(7–8):445–9.
90. Naudie D, Bourne RB, Rorabeck CH, Bourne TJ. The Install Award. Survivorship of the high tibial valgus osteotomy. A 10- to -22-year followup study. Clin Orthop Relat Res. 1999;367:18–27.
91. Hernigou P, Medevielle D, Debeyre J, Goutallier D. Proximal tibial osteotomy for osteoarthritis with varus deformity. A ten to thirteen-year follow-up study. The J Bone Joint Surg. 1987;69(3):332.
92. Miniaci A, Ballmer F, Ballmer P, Jakob R. Proximal tibial osteotomy. A new fixation device. Clin Orthop Relat Res. 1989;246:250–9.
93. Prodromos CC, Andriacchi T, Galante J. A relationship between gait and clinical changes following high tibial osteotomy. J Bone Joint Surg Am. 1985;67(8):1188–94.
94. Jakob R, Jacobi M. Closing wedge osteotomy of the tibial head in treatment of single compartment arthrosis. Der Orthopade. 2004;33(2):143.
95. Keene JS, Monson DK, Roberts JM, Dyreby JR. Evaluation of patients for high tibial osteotomy. Clin Orthop Relat Res. 1989;243:157–65.
96. Rinonapoli E, Mancini GB, Corvaglia A, Musiello S. Tibial osteotomy for varus gonarthrosis: a 10-to 21-year followup study. Clin Orthop Relat Res. 1998;353:185–93.
97. Valenti JR, Calvo R, Lopez R, Canadell J. Long term evaluation of high tibial valgus osteotomy. Int Orthop. 1990;14(4):347–9. https://doi.org/10.1007/BF00182642.
98. Yasuda K, Majima T, Tsuchida T, Kaneda K. A ten- to 15-year follow-up observation of high tibial osteotomy in medial compartment osteoarthrosis. Clin Orthop Relat Res. 1992;282:186–95.
99. Bhan S, Dave P. High valgus tibial osteotomy for osteoarthritis of the knee. Int Orthop. 1992;16(1):13–7.

100. Sundaram N, Hallett J, Sullivan M. Dome osteotomy of the tibia for osteoarthritis of the knee. J Bone Joint Surg. 1986;68(5):782–6.
101. Insall JN, Joseph D, Msika C. High tibial osteotomy for varus gonarthrosis. A long-term follow-up study. J Bone Joint Surg Am. 1984;66(7):1040–8.
102. Lee D-H, Han S-B, Oh K-J, Lee JS, Kwon J-H, Kim J-I, et al. The weight-bearing scanogram technique provides better coronal limb alignment than the navigation technique in open high tibial osteotomy. Knee. 2014;21(2):451–5.
103. Krettek C, Miclau T, Gru O, Schandelmaier P, Tscherne H. Intraoperative control of axes, rotation and length in femoral and tibial fractures technical note. Injury. 1998;29:29–39.
104. Reising K, Strohm PC, Hauschild O, Schmal H, Khattab M, Südkamp NP, et al. Computer-assisted navigation for the intraoperative assessment of lower limb alignment in high tibial osteotomy can avoid outliers compared with the conventional technique. Knee Surg Sports Traumatol Arthrosc. 2013;21(1):181–8.
105. Hernigou P, Ovadia H, Goutallier D. Mathematical modelling of open-wedge tibial osteotomy and correction tables. Revue de Chirurgie Orthopedique et Reparatrice de L'appareil moteur. 1992;78(4):258–63.
106. Dejour H, Bonnin M. Tibial translation after anterior cruciate ligament rupture. Two radiological tests compared. J Bone Joint Surg. 1994;76(5):745–9.
107. Moon SW, Park SH, Lee BH, Oh M, Chang M, Ahn JH, et al. The effect of hinge position on posterior tibial slope in medial open-wedge high tibial osteotomy. Arthroscopy. 2015;31(6):1128–33.
108. Noyes FR, Goebel SX, West J. Opening wedge tibial osteotomy: the 3-triangle method to correct axial alignment and tibial slope. Am J Sports Med. 2005;33(3):378–87.
109. Moon SW, Ryu JY, Lee S-J, Woo SW, Park SH, Choi Y. The effect of the sagittal plane osteotomy inclination on the posterior tibial slope in medial open wedge HTO: experimental study with a square column model. BMC Musculoskelet Disord. 2021;22(1):89. https://doi.org/10.1186/s12891-021-03951-0.
110. Han SB, Lee DH, Shetty GM, Chae DJ, Song JG, Nha KW. A "safe zone" in medial open-wedge high tibia osteotomy to prevent lateral cortex fracture. Knee Surg Sports Traumatol Arthrosc. 2013;21(1):90–5.
111. Takeuchi R, Ishikawa H, Kumagai K, Yamaguchi Y, Chiba N, Akamatsu Y, et al. Fractures around the lateral cortical hinge after a medial opening-wedge high tibial osteotomy: a new classification of lateral hinge fracture. Arthroscopy. 2012;28(1):85–94.
112. Rossi R, Bonasia DE, Amendola A. The role of high tibial osteotomy in the varus knee. J Am Acad Orthop Surg. 2011;19(10):590–9.
113. Shenoy PM, Oh HK, Choi JY, Yoo SH, Han SB, Yoon JR, et al. Pseudoaneurysm of the popliteal artery complicating medial opening wedge high tibial osteotomy. Orthopedics. 2009;32(6):442.
114. Spahn G. Complications in high tibial (medial opening wedge) osteotomy. Arch Orthop Trauma Surg. 2004;124(10):649–53.
115. Darees M, Putman S, Brosset T, Roumazeille T, Pasquier G, Migaud H. Opening-wedge high tibial osteotomy performed with locking plate fixation (TomoFix) and early weight-bearing but without filling the defect. A concise follow-up note of 48 cases at 10 years' follow-up. Orthop Traumatol Surg Res. 2018;104(4):477–80.
116. Jin C, Song E-K, Santoso A, Ingale PS, Choi I-S, Seon J-K. Survival and risk factor analysis of medial open wedge high tibial osteotomy for unicompartment knee osteoarthritis. Arthroscopy. 2020;36(2):535–43.
117. Hantes ME, Natsaridis P, Koutalos AA, Ono Y, Doxariotis N, Malizos KN. Satisfactory functional and radiological outcomes can be expected in young patients under 45 years old after open wedge high tibial osteotomy in a long-term follow-up. Knee Surg Sports Traumatol Arthrosc. 2018;26(11):3199–205.
118. Seo YR, Nha KW, Ha SS. Surgical technique for distal femur varization osteotomy. J Korean Orthop Assoc. 2018;53(4):301–6.
119. Learmonth I. A simple technique for varus supracondylar osteotomy in genu valgum. J Bone Joint Surg. 1990;72(2):235–7.
120. McDermott A, Finklestein J, Farine I, Boynton E, MacIntosh D, Gross A. Distal femoral varus osteotomy for valgus deformity of the knee. JBJS. 1988;70(1):110–6.
121. Gross AE, Hutchison CR. Realignment osteotomy of the knee—Part 1: distal femoral varus osteotomy for osteoarthritis of the Valgus knee. Oper Tech Sports Med. 2000;8(2):122–6.
122. Wang J-W, Hsu C-C. Distal femoral varus osteotomy for osteoarthritis of the knee. JBJS. 2005;87(1):127–33.
123. Shen HC, Chao KH, Huang GS, Pan RY, Lee CH. Combined proximal and distal realignment procedures to treat the habitual dislocation of the patella in adults. Am J Sports Med. 2007;35(12):2101–8. https://doi.org/10.1177/0363546507305014.
124. Thein R, Bronak S, Thein R, Haviv B. Distal femoral osteotomy for valgus arthritic knees. J Orthop Sci. 2012;17(6):745–9. https://doi.org/10.1007/s00776-012-0273-1.
125. Finkelstein JA, Gross AE, Davis A. Varus osteotomy of the distal part of the femur. A survivorship analysis. J Bone Joint Surg Am. 1996;78(9):1348–52. https://doi.org/10.2106/00004623-199609000-00008.
126. Backstein D, Morag G, Hanna S, Safir O, Gross A. Long-term follow-up of distal femoral varus osteotomy of the knee. J Arthroplast. 2007;22(4 Suppl 1):2–6. https://doi.org/10.1016/j.arth.2007.01.026.
127. Puddu G, Cipolla M, Cerullo G, Franco V, Giannì E. Which osteotomy for a valgus knee? Int Orthop. 2010;34(2):239–47.
128. Scott WN. Insall & Scott surgery of the knee E-book. Elsevier Health Sciences; 2011.

129. Edgerton BC, Mariani EM, Morrey BF. Distal femoral varus osteotomy for painful genu valgum. A five-to-11-year follow-up study. Clin Orthop Relat Res. 1993;288:263–9.
130. Kosashvili Y, Safir O, Gross A, Morag G, Lakstein D, Backstein D. Distal femoral varus osteotomy for lateral osteoarthritis of the knee: a minimum ten-year follow-up. Int Orthop. 2010;34(2):249–54.
131. Aglietti P, Menchetti P. Distal femoral varus osteotomy in the valgus osteoarthritic knee. Am J Knee Surg. 2000;13(2):89–95.
132. Nelson CL, Saleh KJ, Kassim RA, Windsor R, Haas S, Laskin R, et al. Total knee arthroplasty after varus osteotomy of the distal part of the femur. JBJS. 2003;85(6):1062–5.
133. Schröter S, Nakayama H, Yoshiya S, Stöckle U, Ateschrang A, Gruhn J. Development of the double level osteotomy in severe varus osteoarthritis showed good outcome by preventing oblique joint line. Arch Orthop Trauma Surg. 2019;139(4):519–27.
134. Nakayama H, Schröter S, Yamamoto C, Iseki T, Kanto R, Kurosaka K, et al. Large correction in opening wedge high tibial osteotomy with resultant joint-line obliquity induces excessive shear stress on the articular cartilage. Knee Surg Sports Traumatol Arthrosc. 2018;26(6):1873–8.
135. Nakayama H, Iseki T, Kanto R, Kambara S, Kanto M, Yoshiya S, et al. Physiologic knee joint alignment and orientation can be restored by the minimally invasive double level osteotomy for osteoarthritic knees with severe varus deformity. Knee Surg Sports Traumatol Arthrosc. 2020;28(3):742–50.
136. Hernigou P, Duffiet P, Julian D, Guissou I, Poignard A, Flouzat-Lachaniette CH. Outcome of total knee arthroplasty after high tibial osteotomy: does malalignment jeopardize the results when using a posterior-stabilized arthroplasty? HSS J. 2013;9(2):134–7. https://doi.org/10.1007/s11420-013-9344-x.
137. Preston S, Howard J, Naudie D, Somerville L, McAuley J. Total knee arthroplasty after high tibial osteotomy: no differences between medial and lateral osteotomy approaches. Clin Orthop Relat Res. 2014;472(1):105–10.
138. Ramappa M, Anand S, Jennings A. Total knee replacement following high tibial osteotomy versus total knee replacement without high tibial osteotomy: a systematic review and meta analysis. Arch Orthop Trauma Surg. 2013;133(11):1587–93. https://doi.org/10.1007/s00402-013-1838-y.
139. Terauchi M, Shirakura K, Katayama M, Higuchi H, Takagishi K, Kimura M. Varus inclination of the distal femur and high tibial osteotomy. J Bone Joint Surg. 2002;84(2):223–6.
140. Benjamin A. Double osteotomy for the painful knee in rheumatoid arthritis and osteoarthritis. J Bone Joint Surg. 1969;51(4):694–9.
141. Saragaglia D, Sigwalt L, Rubens-Duval B, Chedal-Bornu B, Pailhe R. Concept of combined femoral and tibial osteotomies. J Knee Surg. 2017;30(08):756–63.
142. Babis GC, An K-N, Chao EY, Rand JA, Sim FH. Double level osteotomy of the knee: a method to retain joint-line obliquity: clinical results. JBJS. 2002;84(8):1380–8.

Unicompartmental Knee Arthroplasty

13

SeungJoon Rhee

Abstract

Surgical treatment options for the unicompartmental femorotibial joint arthritis include cartilage transplantation, osteochondral auto- or allograft, high tibial osteotomy (HTO), and knee arthroplasty. Unicompartmental knee arthroplasty (UKA) selectively replaces one of the three compartments of the knee joint. The advantages of UKA are as follows: (1) Less skin incision and less bone resection than the total knee arthroplasty (TKA) can preserve more host tissue and more function, (2) Less hemorrhage can lower the transfusion requirement, (3) Excellent clinical results with better range of motion and earlier postoperative recovery than TKA can be expected, (4) Conversion to the TKA after failed UKA is easier than conversion to the TKA from the failed HTO or revision TKA after failed TKA. Disadvantages include narrow indication and difficult surgical technique with variable results depending on the implant design and operator's experience. Reports of the higher early failure rate over the TKA are another concern. The incidence of medial UKA comprises over 90% of the entire UKA, and lateral UKA comprises the rest 10%. Thus, in this chapter, the indications and contraindications, implant designs, surgical techniques, and clinical results with complications of the unicompartmental arthroplasty will be discussed in detail. The lateral UKA and patellofemoral arthroplasty will be described briefly after the medial UKA.

Keywords

Osteoarthritis · Unicompartmental Arthroplasty · Indications · Contraindications Implant designs · Surgical techniques Clinical results · Complications

13.1 Medial Unicompartmental Knee Arthroplasty

Unicompartmental knee arthroplasty (UKA) was first performed as a form of hemiarthroplasty to substitute tibial plateau in the 1950s by McKeever and MacIntosh [1]. In the early 1970s, fixed-bearing UKA became available in the market following the development of the femoral component and cement fixation technique by Marmor [2]. Mobile bearing UKA implant, the Oxford knee which adapted mobile congruous design polyethylene mimicking normal meniscal shape to reduce wear and loosening was developed by Goodfellow and O'Connor in 1978 [3]. In the early era of the UKA, high failure rate was

S. Rhee (✉)
Department of Orthopedics, Biomedical Research Institute, Pusan National University Hospital, Busan, South Korea
e-mail: pnuhosknee@pusan.ac.kr

S.-S. Seo (ed.), *A Strategic Approach to Knee Arthritis Treatment*,
https://doi.org/10.1007/978-981-16-4217-3_13

reported in relation to the implant designs, lack of surgical instruments, and errors in patient selection. Recently, however, strict surgical indication and continuing improvement in the implants and instruments have led to improved results. Especially, the minimally invasive surgical technique, which was introduced by Repicci in the late 1990s, has aroused unprecedented interests about UKA with expectations of better surgical results, and connected to the increasing usage [4]. The ratio of UKA to total knee arthroplasty (TKA) is showing an annual global increase of 8.1% in the USA (2005), 9.7% in Australia (2007), 7.0% in Sweden (2007) in 2000s despite lower than 5% in Korea [5, 6]. Most recent survey reported continuing increase in the incidence of UKA in the USA, Finland, New Zealand, and Norway, including Korea whereas the surgery is decreasing in Australia and Canada [7].

13.1.1 Indications and Contraindications

13.1.1.1 Indications

Degenerative arthritis restricted to one compartment of the knee joint is the main indicative disease of the UKA, and additional indications include posttraumatic arthritis, osteochondritis dissecans, and idiopathic osteonecrosis limited in epiphyseal to subchondral depth [8].

Conventional indication of UKA has been known as a relatively inactive patient whose age is over 60 years old and weighs under 180 lb. with over 90° knee range of motion and under 5° flexion contracture, under 15° angular deformity, and non-inflammatory arthritis [9]. However, many researchers owing to the development of surgical technique and instruments are extending the indication. Surgical indications of UKA has been considerably expanded to include the patients regardless of their age or activity or body weight though the difference in the permissible degree of varus deformity and flexion contracture between the fixed (15°) and mobile (10°) bearing implant [10, 11]. Recently, there are two major indications according to two age groups. One is a primary operation in the relatively younger and slim patients who are anticipating more than one arthroplasty in their life time, and the other is a time-saving, low-morbidity salvage surgery for the elderly whose survival is expected to be less than 10 years. Laskin et al. reported that 15% of the knees treated with TKA could have been treated using UKA [12]. Spontaneous osteonecrosis of knee (SPONK) lesion located shallower than the subchondral bone in the magnetic resonance imaging can be considered a good indication. Minimum requirement for knee range of motion is 90° and mechanical axis derangement should not exceed 5° varus or 10° valgus in the standing full length radiography. Femorotibial subluxation of more than 3 mm or impingement between the intercondylar notch and tibial eminence, which is called "kissing lesion," is not considered feasible for the UKA despite some good results from the experienced operators. Indication according to the patellar lesion is debatable, but in general, exposure of the patellar subchondral bone contraindicates the medial or lateral UKA whereas the lesion equivalent to chondromalacia is permissible for the operation.

13.1.1.2 Contraindications

Diagnosis of inflammatory arthritis including rheumatoid arthritis, progressed other compartment disease, ligamentous instability including the cruciate or collateral ligament injury, excessive angular deformity or severe flexion contracture, and less than 90° knee range of motion are contraindications of UKA [10, 11]. Dennis emphasized the importance of anterior cruciate ligament (ACL) in the UKA in their study, which reported accelerated wear in the anterior part of the implant caused by eccentric weight loading under attenuated and eventually malfunctioning ACL [13]. In the mechanical standpoint, Argenson concluded that ACL should be intact to maintain the normal function of the knee joint based on their videofluoroscopic findings which showed femoral roll back reaching −0.8 mm in the medial UKA and −2.5 mm in the lateral UKA [14]. Goodfellow reported ten times higher failure rate of the UKA in the insufficient or injured ACL [15]. Accordingly, instability in the anteroposterior or varus-valgus stress radiography contraindicates the UKA. Progressive disease characteristics of rheumatoid arthritis that manifest probable slackening of the ligamentous structures make the surgeons regard the disease and other compartment osteoarthritis as relative contraindications of UKA (Fig. 13.1).

13.1.1.3 Indications of UKA Versus High Tibial Osteotomy

Although high tibial osteotomy (HTO) has been preferred for the young and active osteoarthritic patients owing to the joint preserving characteristics of the surgery, there are also complications including the superficial wound infection, delayed union or nonunion, breakage of the fixative, and iatrogenic fractures after HTO. Moreover, rapid deterioration of the mid- to long-term survival after the fifth postoperative year and difficulty in the revision surgery after failed HTO raised recent tendency to perform UKA as an alternative surgical treatment for relatively young patients [16–20]. UKA has been performed in relatively thin and inactive patients between 60 and 80 years old conventionally. Higher early success rate and lower complication rate were reported regarding UKA. Despite the indications of the UKA and HTO are quite overlapping, it is a reasonable recommendation to perform UKA in patients with severe osteoarthritis of grade 3 or 4, and to perform HTO in patients with joint instability including ACL rupture or obvious tibia vara.

13.1.1.4 Indications of UKA Versus TKA

The top most advantage of the UKA over the TKA is the preservation of intact tissue. Normal knee joint kinematics and proprioception can be preserved by sparing the intact compartments and resecting less bone from the affected compartment while preserving ligament structures. Additionally, shorter operative time and lower morbidity contribute to the reduced hospital stay. McAuley et al. [21] mentioned that UKA is easier than TKA in the setting of revision surgery. On the other hand, demand for the surgical technique is higher with UKA than TKA owing to the narrower acceptable range of implant alignment which could be causing other compartment disease if malaligned. Patient age is an important factor in the selection of the appropriate surgical option [9]. It is reasonable that considering

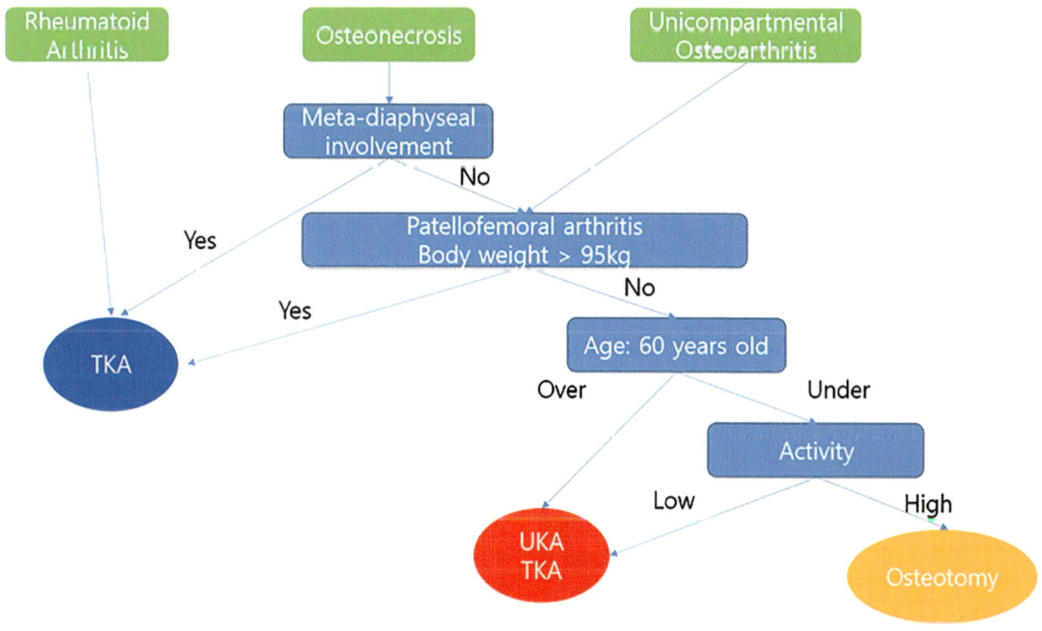

Fig. 13.1 Indication algorithm for unicompartmental knee arthroplasty

UKA in a young patient under 60 years old in whom more than one revision is expected in the life time, because the revision of UKA is relatively easier that the revision of TKA. In addition, in an elderly patient over 75 years old whose perioperative risk expected to be higher, UKA can be considered as a low-morbidity alternative for TKA. If the age of a patient falls within 60–75 years old and no more than single surgery is expected throughout one's life, TKA can be considered primarily depending on the better long-term survival. However, majority of researches report similar clinical results between the two surgical treatments. Nonetheless, it is a general opinion that UKA is functionally superior to TKA while TKA is prevailing in terms of implant survival. Newman [22] reported that UKA showed better functional results over TKA for at least 5 years after surgery.

13.1.2 Types of Implants

Implants for UKA can be roughly categorized into the mobile bearing type and the fixed-bearing type; mobile bearing type implant is further categorized as meniscal-bearing type and tracked-bearing type. The former permits unconstrained movement of the mobile polyethylene insert between the femoral and tibial metal component, and the latter permits anteroposterior movement of the mobile polyethylene insert. Fixed-bearing implant is further categorized into all-poly type with pure polyethylene tibial component and metal-backed type with metal tibial component and polyethylene insert [23–25].

Similar to TKA, it has been known that increasing conformity lead to more loosening and decreasing conformity lead to more wear in UKA. The flat-on-flat conformation of the femoral and tibial component will decrease the stress but cause edge-contact, whereas the round-on-round conformation raise concerns regarding the loosening owing to the restriction of motion. Higher wear rate was reported with the increased stress in the implants with round femoral component on the flat tibial component, which caused attenuation of the ACL and subsequent promotion of wear. Especially, the femoral posterior condyle and polyethylene insert have been transformed into relatively large posterior condylar radius and quite conforming insert shape to overcome the increased wear rate in small radius posterior condyle and flat polyethylene insert. Width of the femoral component has been widened to cover the resected femoral condylar surface without subsidence that occurred in the earlier designs with narrow femoral component width. Mobile bearing was developed to decrease the wear rate of the polyethylene in the conforming design. The advantages of mobile polyethylene bearing include decreased insert wear rate and decreased implant loosening related failure owing to the reduced contact stress per dimension by increased contact surface in the conforming design. Less bone resection required as a resurfacing concept is another advantage of mobile bearing design. However, demanding surgical technique and bearing dislocation are considered as disadvantages [25]. Fixed-bearing design, on the other hand, has been known to be vulnerable to insert wear and loosening of the tibial component until the era of the all-poly tibial component. With metal-backed tibial component with modularity, regularity of load bearing, easier cementing and easier polyethylene exchangeability are regarded as advantages of the fixed-bearing design [23] (Fig. 13.2).

13.1.2.1 Femoral Component

Femoral component design is differed by the width, condylar curvature, and the method to reinforce the implant fixation. Fixation devices including fins or pods or lugs increase fixation strength. Two lugs or metal bar or cruciform recess were devised to prevent rotation (Fig. 13.3).

13.1.2.2 Tibial Component

All-polyethylene tibial component was developed in the early era, and metal-backed tibial component and polyethylene insert were developed followingly. Metal-backed tibial baseplate has advantages in even load bearing and exchangeability of worn polyethylene insert while it has disadvantage such as use of thinner polyethylene

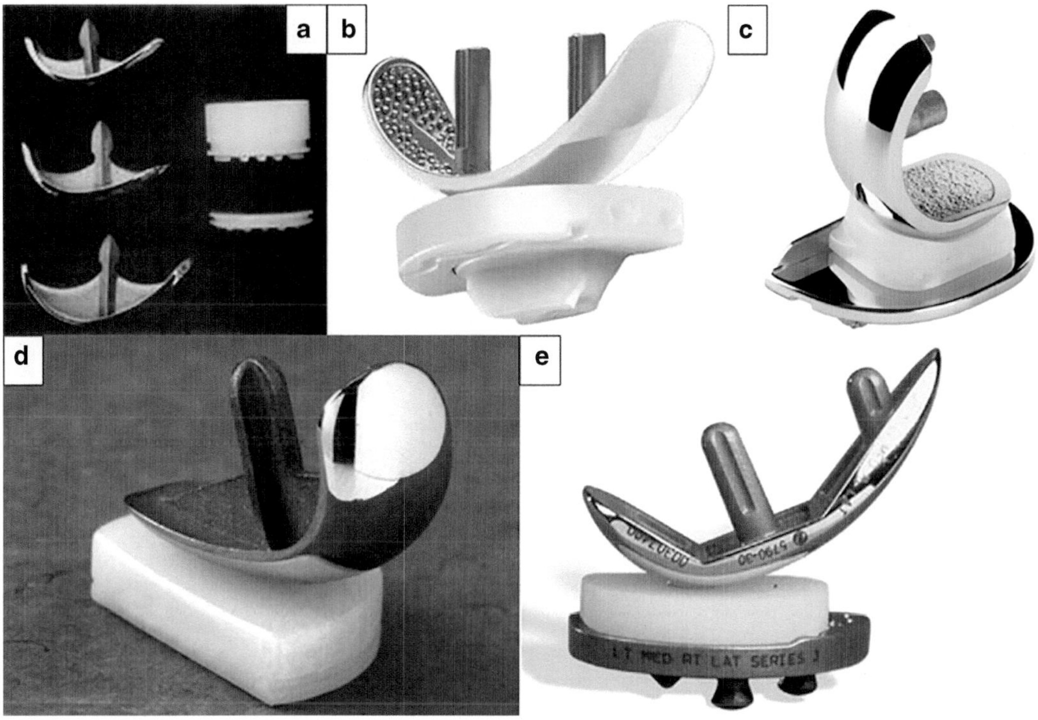

Fig. 13.2 Various unicompartmental knee arthroplasty implants. (**a**) Marmor (**b**) George sledge (**c**) Oxford (**d**) Repicci II (Biomet, Warsaw, Indiana, USA) Reproduced with permission. (**e**) Miller-Galante (Zimmer, Warsaw, Indiana, USA) Reproduced with permission

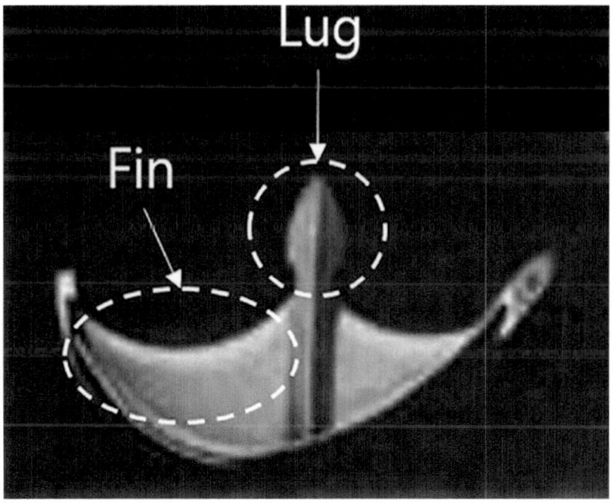

Fig. 13.3 Design elements to reinforce the femoral component fixation

insert. Despite the debates regarding pros and cons about the polyethylene insert, the thinnest part of the polyethylene should exceed 6 mm to minimize the wear rate. It is reported that thinner than 6 mm polyethylene is susceptible to wear and other compartment arthritis which is caused by the inflammation around the wear particle. Recent design transformation into the surface replacement implant and minimal bone resection is facing the problem of metal-backed polyethylene owing to the inevitably reduced polyethylene thickness (Fig. 13.4).

13.1.3 Surgical Principles and Techniques

While in the past, conventional approach of open knee arthrotomy was used to perform UKA, minimally invasive surgical technique is a dominant technique recently. The advantages of minimally invasive surgery include less discomfort, low morbidity, less pain, earlier recovery of range of motion and function with shorter hospitalization. On the other hand, risk of malalignment due to the

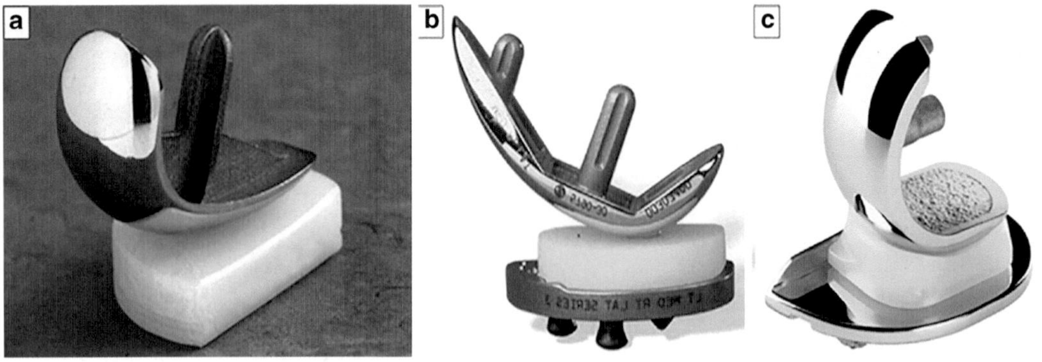

Fig. 13.4 Various types of tibial components. (**a**) Fixed-bearing all-polyethylene tibial component. (**b**) Fixed-bearing modular metal-backed tibial component. (**c**) Mobile-meniscal bearing tibial component

restricted visual field is regarded as disadvantage [26]. Numerous recent researches are reporting satisfactory implant alignment and clinical results in precisely performed minimally invasive UKAs.

The most important technical factors for the successful UKA are axial alignment, ligament balance, and fixation of the implant. Femorotibial alignment in the UKA is defined by the level of contact point between medial femoral condyle and tibial component. The alignment is known to be influenced by the design of implant, resection level of the proximal tibia, stability of ligament, degree of preoperative deformity, thickness of the polyethylene insert, and the operator's surgical technique. Therefore, all the efforts should be tried to achieve planned postoperative femorotibial alignment as possible by preparing proper implant to the patient condition and meticulous preoperative planning with intraoperative verification. Ligament balancing in the UKA is mainly achieved by changing the size and location of the implant, and excision of osteophyte. The primary objective in the ligament balancing is recovering normal soft tissue tension through the insertion of the size-matched implant without overly releasing the medial soft tissue sleeve. As for implant position, alignment in the coronal, sagittal, and axial plane with mediolateral position on the femoral condyles should be monitored for the femoral component. For the tibial component, mediolateral position on the tibial plateau, posterior tibial slope, and rotation in the axial plane should be monitored.

13.1.3.1 Approach

Minimally invasive surgery is recommendable while conventional approach for TKA is still in use. Repicci et al. insisted minimally invasive surgery to improve earlier recovery and functional rehabilitation by minimizing skin incision and soft tissue dissection. Frequent erroneous varus implantation in the early days has been improved with the help of improved surgical instruments, accumulated experiences, and computer assisted surgery.

For the medial UKA, about 7–8 cm longitudinal skin incision is performed from patellar superior pole proximally to the level of tibial tuberosity or 2 cm below the joint line distally, about 1 cm medially apart from the patellar tendon. Arthrotomy can be performed along the line of skin incision (Fig. 13.5). Lateral incision can be performed for the lateral UKA, alternatively midline skin incision can be performed considering the future TKA. During the arthrotomy along the skin incision line, care should be taken not to injure the ACL, medial collateral ligament, and anterior horn of the lateral meniscus. The conventional method everts the patella, but in the minimal invasive approach, the patella must be retracted medially or laterally and the quadriceps tendon should be preserved. Conversion to TKA should be considered if cruciate ligament deficiency or mediolateral instability or severe arthritis in the other compartment or patellofemoral compartment is observed during performing UKA. Degree of arthritic lesion in the other compartment should not exceed grade II for the femorotibial joint and grade IV for the patellofemoral joint.

13.1.3.2 Soft Tissue Preparation

Remove medial meniscus and remove osteophyte in the intercondylar notch and periphery of the tibia and femur. Removal of the medial tibial plateau edge osteophyte allows passive correction of varus deformity in the medial UKA (Fig. 13.6).

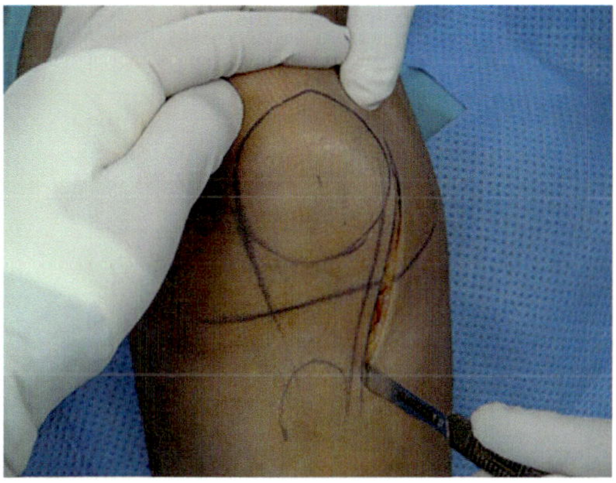

Fig. 13.5 Minimally invasive surgery (MIS) approach in unicompartmental arthroplasty (Courtesy of MH, Song)

Medial collateral ligament should be minimally released until the retractor can be inserted. TKA should be indicated in cases which require further relaxation of the medial collateral ligament. Overly releasing the medial collateral ligament can cause joint instability that promotes arthritis in the contralateral joint.

13.1.3.3 Bone Resection

There are two ways of bone resection. In femur-first technique, intramedullary cutting guide is utilized. Whereas in tibia-first technique, extramedullary cutting guide is utilized because the femoral resection is subject to the tibial resection level. Conservative bone resection should be performed to avoid overcorrection. Align the lower extremity in accordance with the mechanical alignment in extension and in a perpendicular angle between the femur and tibia in flexion. Some researchers reported that slight undercorrection was advantageous in unloading the lateral compartment which subjected to overload in 4–7 degree anatomical femorotibial alignment.

In the femur-first technique, reaming for the intramedullary guide begins right in front of the posterior cruciate ligament insertion in the fem-

Fig. 13.6 Influence of medial osteophyte to the ligament and medial sleeve of the joint capsule. (**a**) Medial osteophyte is tenting the medial collateral ligament. (**b**) Relaxation of the medial collateral ligament after the excision of the osteophyte

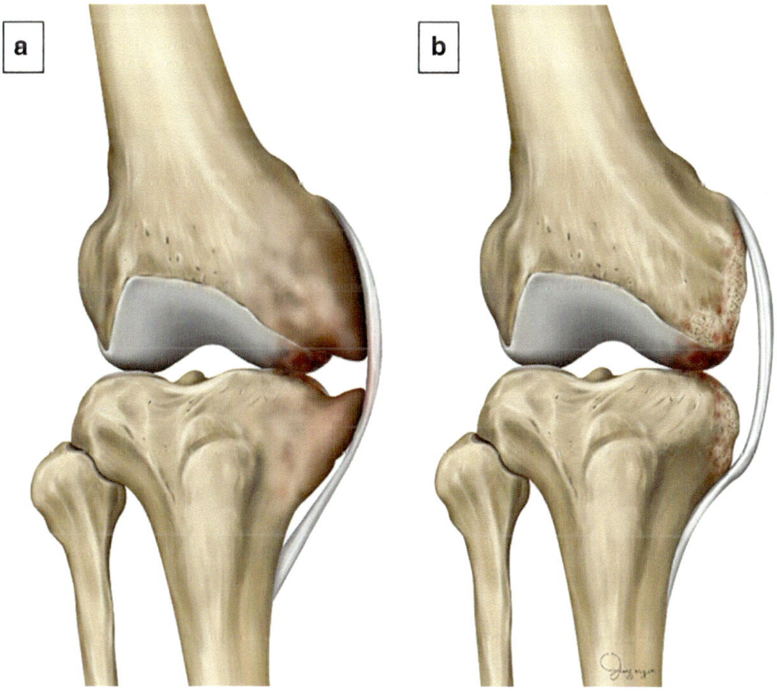

oral intercondylar notch. In 90° flexion of the knee, distal femoral cutting guide is assembled to the intramedullary guide and the cutting guide is fixed on the femur to parallel with tibial joint surface and to perpendiculate with tibial mechanical axis. Considering the preoperative planning, bone resection can be increased in millimeters until 6 mm, and additional 2 mm resection is permitted when the valgus angle exceeds 6 degree. This step enables expanding the extension gap and reducing valgus deformity without additional bone resection in the tibial side.

Posterior femoral condylar resection should be sufficient to ensure an affordable posterior compartment. Anteroposterior dimension of the distal femur after the bone cutting is an indicator for deciding the size of femoral component. It is recommended to select a femoral component size that spares peripheral margin of at least 1 mm thickness in the distal femoral condylar resection surface, preferably larger size in in-between sized bone. Accordingly, it is safer to attempt cutting with larger size resection guide ahead when the size is questionable. Inclination of the distal femoral resection should follow the natural posterior tibial slope. Size of the femoral component should be large enough to cover the anterior part of the resected bone surface to prevent impingement between the femoral articular cartilage and tibial component. Simultaneously, care should be taken to make a smooth transition from the anterior edge of the femoral component to the articular surface to allow an uninterrupted patellar tracking. Trial of the knee extension to verify the contact point between the femur and tibia or the "tide mark" which is formed by the border between subchondral bone and articular cartilage can be referenced intraoperatively to ensure the appropriate size of the femoral component (Fig. 13.7). In lateral unicompartmental arthroplasty, on the contrary, downsizing the femoral component is recommended to avoid the problems related to the patellofemoral joint.

In this stage, bone resection should be sufficient and well-positioned to prevent overhanging the femoral component which could interrupt patellar tracking. Resection of the chamfer and posterior condyle can be performed after the sizing while the chamfer resection can also be performed after the proximal tibial resection and soft tissue balancing. Femoral component should be located in the middle of condylar mediolateral dimension in the coronal plane and in the mid-point on the tibial anteroposterior dimension in extension in the sagittal plane. Errors in the positioning can cause impingement to the tibial spine or edge loading on the polyethylene. Marking the center of the femoral trial while gradually extending the knee from 90° to 60°, 30°, 0° helps to determine the best location of the femoral component. Rotational alignment is closely related to insert wear especially in UKA. Slight external rotation of the femoral component not exceeding 5° is recommended. Lug hole is drilled when the rotational alignment is determined. Some operators prefer multiple microdrilling to enhance the fixation on the sclerotic bone.

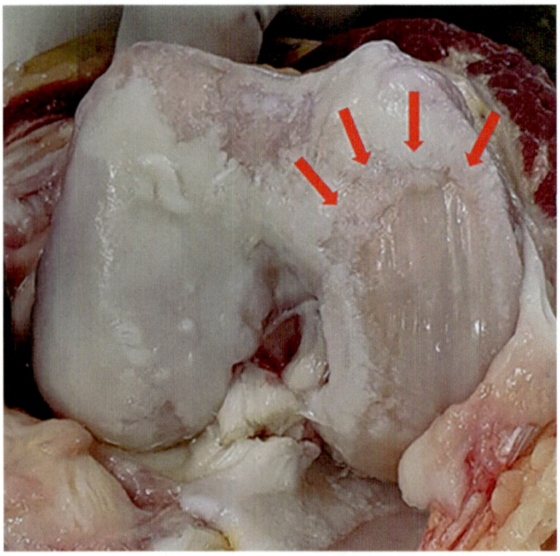

Fig. 13.7 Tide mark

Next, extramedullary guide is set for the tibial resection. Similar to TKA, the guide is located just medial to the tibial tuberosity proximally and on the center of the tibiotalar joint distally. Over-resection of the tibia should be avoided since the over-resection not only causes joint subluxation but also produces tibial plateau fracture. 2–3° under-correction which draw the mechanical axis into the point between medial tibial spine and middle of the tibial component is recommended

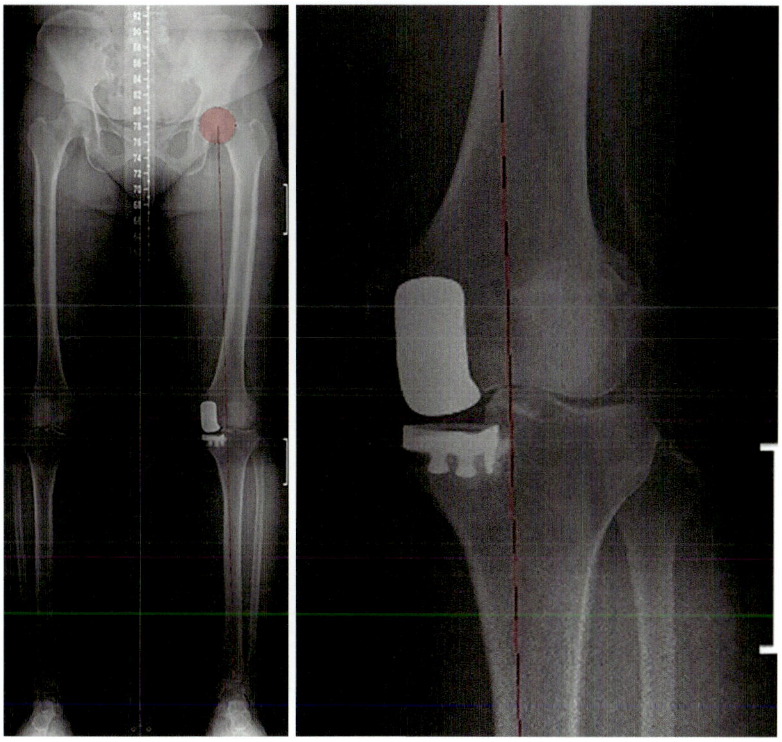

Fig. 13.8 Ideal position of the mechanical axis passage

despite the resection level differs among operators (Fig. 13.8). Remnant varus deformity exceeding 5° is related to a higher risk of rotational deformity and wear in the operated compartment. 3–5° posterior tibial slope is desirable even if 0–10° slope is permissible according to preoperative measurement. Depth of resection reaches the deepest level of subchondral bone in the most medial part and reaches 8–10 mm from the joint surface in the most lateral part. Vertical resection should be performed as close to the medial spine as possible while avoiding ACL injury.

The size of the tibial component can be selected independently from the femoral component, and selecting a larger size is recommended until the component does not make medial and posterior overhanging. Coronal alignment of the tibial component is verified in all-trial state as the tibial component to parallel the femoral component. Patellar should be reduced in position while the test is performed to avoid an inadvertent external rotation of the tibia. Pennington et al. [27] suggested that tibial component should be fixed in 10–15° internal rotation considering the screw-home movement in the lateral UKA. Malrotation possibly lead to quadriceps active tibial external rotation or tibial subluxation. In the mobile bearing design, an additional procedure to balance the flexion and extension gap is required. Procedures for implant fixation follow the determination of the rotational alignment.

In UKA, femorotibial alignment and knee range of motion should be examined in all-trial state to take into account polyethylene insert thickness, which is very crucial. Tibial component thickness including the insert thickness should reach the level of native tibial plateau. Ligament balance is examined by valgus stress test in full extension, 45° flexion, and 90° flexion, as the medial compartment feels not too tight and not too loose to exceed 2 mm distraction. Overly tight gap tends to subluxate tibia laterally and possibly promotes wear of the implant. Additional tibial resection should be considered if the knee tolerates less than 120° flexion. Any sign of ligament laxity or valgus/varus deformity dictates additional calibration in the tibial component thickness or tibial bone resection.

In the tibia-first resection technique, proximal tibia is resected initially using the extramedullary cutting guide, then the femur is resected considering extension gap which is measured using spacer block. In this technique, femoral resection level is about 2 mm shallower than the femur-first technique, and the joint can feel tight in flexion. Fitz et al. [28] recommended additional resection of the posterior femoral condyle than additional tibial resection in such situations.

Surgical Techniques in Mobile Bearing Design

Oxford Partial Knee Microplasty (Zimmer-Biomet, Warsaw, IN, USA), a mobile bearing unicompartmental knee design, microplasty begins with short oblique to longitudinal incision on the knee joint capsule running distally from 1 cm medial to the patellar superior pole. Following the arthrotomy, operator examines the status of intraarticular structures including the degree of articular cartilage injury, cruciate ligaments, and meniscus without dislocating the patella. Spoon instrument of an appropriate size is selected and used to measure the femoral component size and gap. Medial proximal tibia is resected after the selected spoon is connected to the tibial cutting guide using G-clamp. Then a femoral intramedullary cutting guide is inserted, and femoral peg hole is drilled following the linking between the intramedullary cutting guide and femoral drill guide. Resect femoral posterior condyle using posterior condylar cutting guide, and measure the flexion and extension gap using gauge. Approximate the flexion and extension gap by milling distal part of the femoral condyle as the difference between the two gaps. Verify stability, alignment, and insert thickness with trial inserts. After the tibial and femoral components are fixed on the bone using bone cement, mobile bearing is inserted, and smooth gliding in flexion and extension of the knee is confirmed before the closure of the operative field (Fig. 13.9).

Surgical Techniques in Fixed-Bearing Design

Minimally invasive approach is used for the fixed-bearing Zimmer Unicompartmental High Flex Knee System ((ZUK), Zimmer-Biomet, Warsaw, IN, USA). Skin incision is performed from the proximal and medial to the patella to 1 cm distal to the joint line, and joint capsule is incised along the line of skin incision. Medial tibial plateau resection using extramedullary cutting guide is first performed, and distal femoral resection is performed considering the gap formed by the medial tibial plateau resection. Flexion and extension gap is measured using a spacer block.

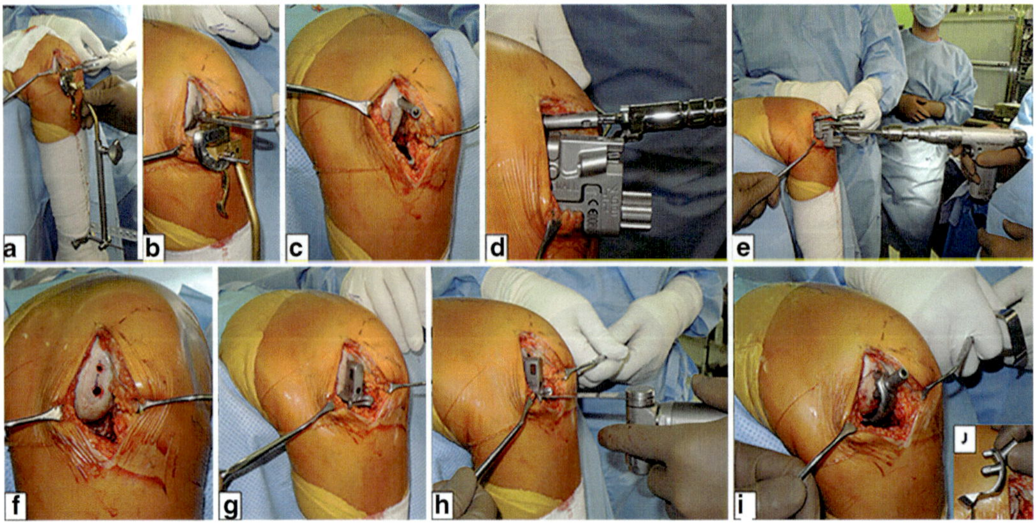

Fig. 13.9 Surgical technique of mobile bearing unicompartmental arthroplasty (Courtesy of KM, Jang)

Femoral posterior condyle and chamfer are resected using femoral size/finishing guide after ligament balancing. Confirm the gliding between the components and ligament balance using trial insert, then the components are fixed using bone cement, and polyethylene insert is inserted using an instrument. Capsular suture and skin suture are performed in knee joint flexion position (Fig. 13.10).

13.1.3.4 Fixation

Irrigate the joint space to remove hematoma and ground bone fragments then confirm the posterior condylar clearance. Pack dry gauze densely behind the posterior border of the proximal tibial cut surface and in front of the posterior capsule, and expose the space clearly with retractors to prevent the cement from isolation in the posterior space. It is a general recommendation that cementing tibia and femur sequentially. Overflowed cement in the posterior space should be removed through pulling out the packed gauze because the space cannot be visualized directly after the cementing and implantation. Spread less cement in the posterior part of the tibial component, and press posterior part ahead of the anterior part, then keep knee in extension until the cement consolidate to minimize the cement overflow in the posterior space. Cement in the tibial spine area should also be removed meticulously. Polyethylene is inserted following the completion of the femoral component, and alignment, stability, range of motion are again examined. If everything is confirmed well, insert drain as necessary and close the joint capsule and skin (Fig. 13.11).

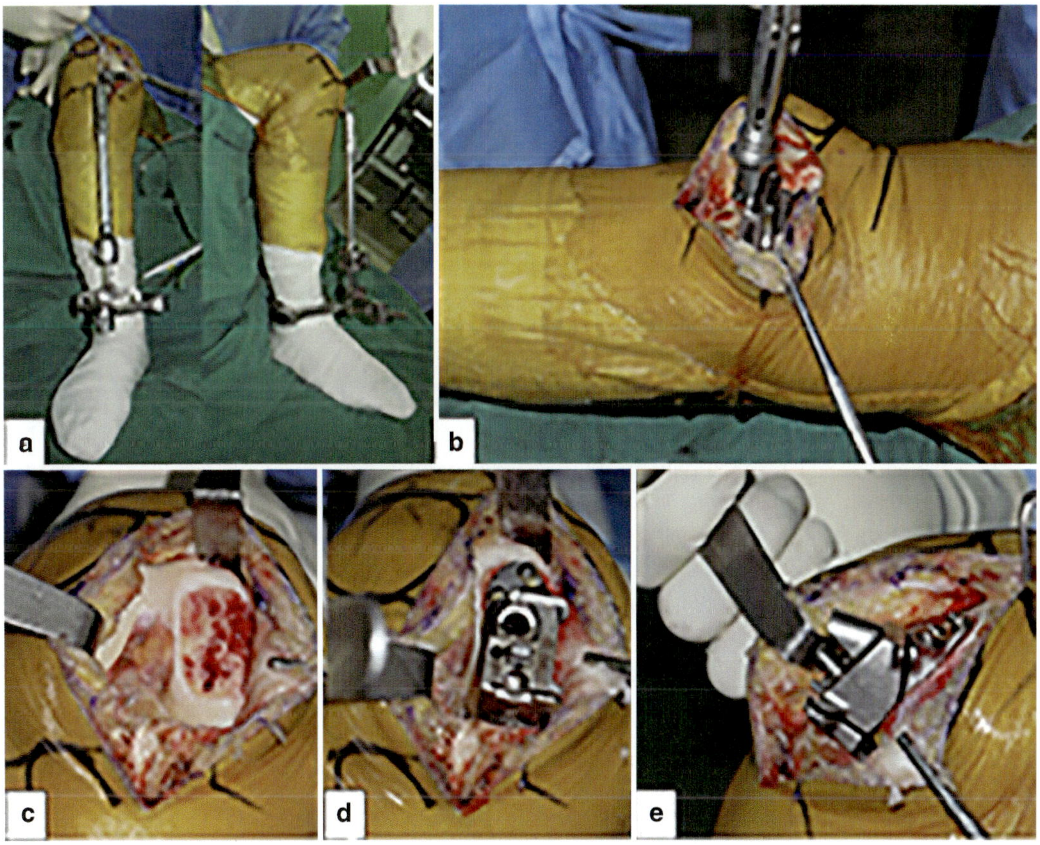

Fig. 13.10 Surgical technique of fixed-bearing unicompartmental arthroplasty arthroplasty. (**a**) Application of extramedullary cutting guide. Tibial cutting guide is placed in right angle to the mechanical axis of tibia in frontal plane and parallel to the tibial articular surface in sagittal plane. (**b**) Application of distal femoral cutting guide as space block technique. (**c**) Axial view of distal femoral cutting surface. Alignment of distal femoral cutting surface depends on the proximal tibial cutting surface. Axial (**d**) and lateral (**e**) view after application of femoral size/finishing guide

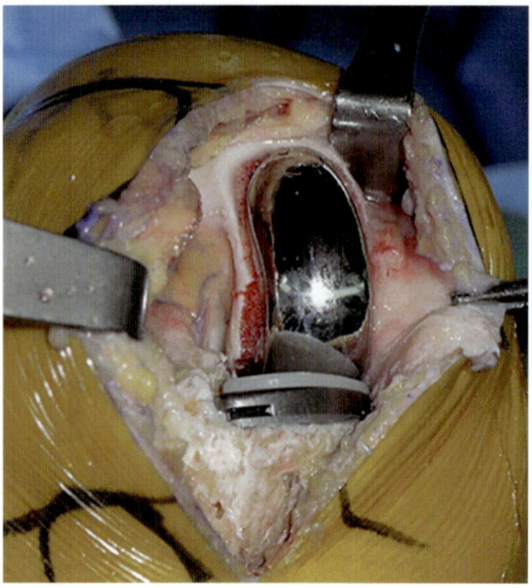

Fig. 13.11 Complete fixation of the implant

13.1.4 Postoperative Evaluation and Rehabilitation

Implant position is monitored using plain radiography. Mediolateral position, posterior tibial slope, axial rotation need to be assessed regarding the tibial component. The femoral component is also assessed for mediolateral position, coronal and sagittal plane alignment, and rotational alignment. As the position of tibial component center influences the position of other components, the tibial tray margin should coincide with posteromedial cortex of the proximal tibia. Tibial implant position in the coronal plane should be placed perpendicular to the mechanical axis of the tibia because more than 3–5° deviation to the mechanical axis produces poor outcomes. It is known that posterior slope of the tibial component is closely related to implant survival in the UKA so that the posterior slope should be less than 5–7° while restoring patients' native posterior tibial slope. On the other hand, axial rotation of the tibial component is known to be related to both patient satisfaction and implant survival. Grossly in extension, femoral component tends to look internally rotated relative to the tibial component about 15°. Center of the femoral component should coincide with the center of the tibial component, and coincide with the center of femoral condyle if the implantation was accurate. Coronal plane inclination of the femoral component should be perpendicular to the femoral mechanical axis, and sagittal position should align with the longitudinal axis of the femur.

Postoperative Care Postoperative recovery pace from UKA is nearly the same or slightly faster than TKA. Continuous passive motion can be initiated from the recovery room or 2–3 days after drain removal. Continuous passive motion begins from 30–40° with 10–20° increment daily until it reaches and maintains 90° flexion. Early active range of motion is also encouraged to achieve more than 90° flexion in one week. Practice of ambulation starts from the third postoperative day, and independent full weight bearing ambulation becomes possible at the second postoperative week with expectations of returning to normal activities of daily living at the sixth postoperative week.

13.1.5 Clinical Results

13.1.5.1 Functional Results

Numerous researchers reported excellent results regarding the pain reduction, restoration of range of motion, angular deformity correction, and subjective report outcomes after UKA. Since Kozinn and Scott reported excellent outcome could be expected in the strictly chosen patients who were older than 60 years old, most of the researchers agree to their opinion [10, 29, 30]. Recently, number of researchers is reporting good results which are comparable to TKA in younger patients despite there have been debates according to the researchers and implant designs regarding the results of UKA [6]. Fischer et al. [31] reported significant increase in UCLA physical activity score and 93% return to sports activity and activities of daily living in 18 month follow up after UKA.

13.1.5.2 Survival of Implant

In the early era of UKA, implant survival was unsatisfactory owing to the implant design, lack of surgical instrument, and errors in patient selection as Laskin et al. [12] reported 65% satisfaction rate in the 1970s and Insall et al. [32] reported 42% poor results. However, afterwards, reports of good results followed with careful patients section and developing surgical instruments and implant designs. Murray et al. [15] and Berger et al. [33] reported 98% 10-year survival rate in 1998, regarding Oxford mobile bearing design and Miller-Galante fixed bearing, respectively. Marmor et al. [2] reported 70% satisfaction rate and Scott et al. [23] reported 85% implant survival rate. Egidy et al. [34] reported a case of 31-year survival after Marmor unicompartmental knee arthroplasty. Argenson et al. [35] reported 92% excellent outcome with 94% 10-year survival rate.

Long-term survival rate of UKA is reported as 98% until 10 year, 93% until 15 year, 84% until 20 year, and 72% until 25 year recently [11, 36–38]. However, still there has been reports of varying 10-year survival rate ranging from 84% to 100% depending on implant design and surgeon so that the survival rate of UKA is known to be inferior to TKA [16, 39].

13.1.6 Complications, Causes of Failure, and Treatment

Postoperative complications of UKA include dislocation of mobile bearing, aseptic loosening of the implant, wear of polyethylene insert, periprosthetic fracture, progression of other compartment disease, infection, impingement of implant to bone, residual cement debris in the joint, joint stiffness, recurrent hemarthrosis, and persisting knee joint pain [40]. Early complications include deep vein thrombosis and infection with 0.1–0.7% incidence which is slightly lower than TKA. Intraoperative or postoperative tibial condylar fractures were also reported. Aseptic loosening, polyethylene wear, other compartment disease are important late complications. Radiographic analysis by zonal assessment is used for the diagnosis of loosening [41] (Fig. 13.12). Radiolucency exceeding 2 mm in each zone or cement breakage or gross subsidence of implant is considered a significant finding suspicious of implant loosening. As for the dislocation of mobile bearing, Gunther et al. [42, 43] reported higher incidence of bearing dislocation in lateral than medial unicompartmental arthroplasty presumably due to the overly relaxed lateral collateral ligament in flexed knee. They suggested lateral parapatellar approach, poplit-

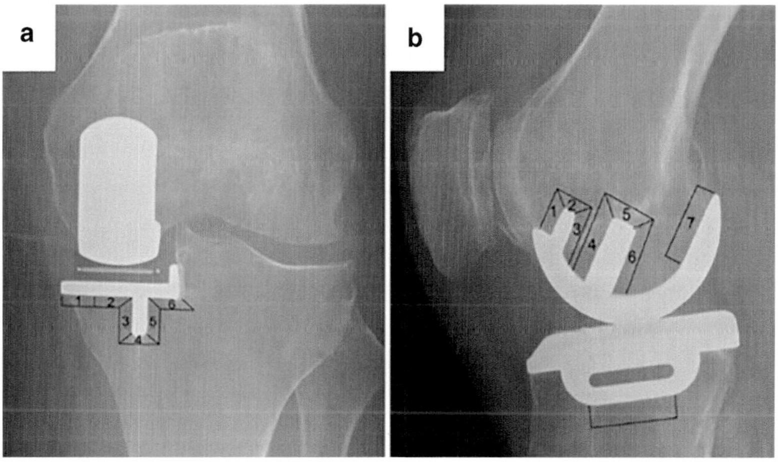

Fig. 13.12 Radiographic zones in unicompartmental knee arthroplasty (**a**. Anteroposterior radiograph, **b**. lateral radiograph) (Mohammad KSSTA, 2019)

eus tendon release with clearance of redundant posterolateral soft tissue, and meticulous balancing of flexion/extension gap to prevent the bearing dislocation in the lateral unicompartmental arthroplasty. Suboptimal pain relief can be caused by over-activity after the surgery, and pes anserinus bursitis accounts for about 10% of persisting pain. Topical injection of hydrocortisone mixed with local anesthetic agent often helps improving symptoms in such cases.

Large numbers of complications occur in the first and second postoperative period of UKA, and early failures are closely related to surgical technique. Experiences regarding the patient selection and surgical techniques are required to prevent such complications [44].

Treatment for the complications can be divided into revision operation and operations other than revision [40, 45]. Operative options other than revision include open or arthroscopic debridement, closed manipulation, ligament repair, open reduction, and internal fixation according to the complications. Revision surgery options include simple polyethylene insert exchange, revision to UKA, and conversion to TKA.

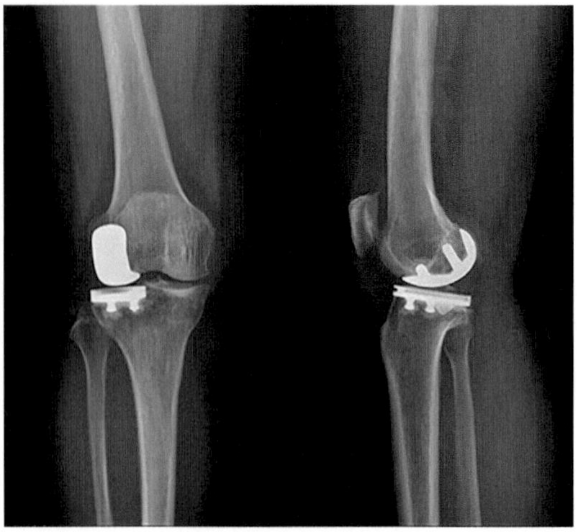

Fig. 13.13 Postoperative radiography of the lateral unicompartmental arthroplasty

13.2 Lateral Unicompartmental Knee Arthroplasty

Lateral compartmental arthritis of knee is uncommon than medial compartment arthritis and the treatment is yet challenging. Surgical treatment options for the lateral compartment arthritis include arthroscopic debridement, realignment osteotomy, lateral UKA, and TKA. Among the options, lateral UKA has advantages in earlier postoperative recovery, restoring normal knee kinematics while maintaining normal knee joint anatomy, and feasible revision surgery [46]. Surgical technique of lateral UKA is known to be complicated owing to a few anatomical and functional characteristics of the knee joint including unfamiliar surgical approach, relaxation of lateral ligament structure in flexed knee, and larger posterior movement of lateral femoral condyle than medial femoral condyle during knee flexion [47]. In general, fixed-bearing design is preferred in lateral UKA depending on the clinical results reporting better survival in fixed bearing than mobile bearing which are at risk of early failure related to bearing dislocation, in considerations on biomechanical behaviors of lateral compartment [48] (Fig. 13.13).

13.2.1 Indications and Contraindications

Indications of lateral UKA include osteoarthritis limited in the lateral compartment of the knee, osteonecrosis, and posttraumatic arthritis with intractable pain and severe loss of lateral joint space in radiography [48, 49]. Patient with intact ACL and less than 15° valgus deformity allowing 100° range of motion without fixed flexion contracture is a favorable indication. Age, body mass index, and activity are reported as no longer important considerations though those factors were considered for indication in the past. Diagnosis of inflammatory arthritis, coexisting medial compartment arthritis, and symptomatic patellofemoral arthritis are contraindication of lateral UKA. Insufficiencies in the cruciate or collateral ligaments, valgus deformity exceeding 15°, range of motion less than 100°, or existence of fixed flexion contracture are also contraindications. Specifically, lateral UKA should be avoided in a knee joint with fixed flexion contracture which necessitate soft tissue procedure, for the soft tissue release possibly cause femorotibial joint subluxation in coronal plane [49].

13.2.2 Clinical Results

Lateral UKA comprises 5–10% of UKA, so that reports regarding the clinical results are fairly insufficient than medial UKA [12, 46]. The report regarding lateral UKA in Korean population is much more rarer because the ratio of lateral compartment arthritis is much lower in Korean than Caucasian and lateral UKA is scarcely performed accordingly [50]. Most of the researchers reported good functional results regardless of the implant design though the rarity of the cases [46, 50–53].

Debates exist about the long-term survival of lateral UKA in relation to implant design. Regarding the mobile design, Gunther et al. [43] reported unsatisfactory results with 82% 5-year survival rate and 10% bearing dislocation rate in lateral UKA using Oxford phase 1 implant. Pandit et al. [54] reported 98% 4-year survival rate in domed tibial articular surface design which was developed to reduce mobile bearing dislocation and wear, which was improved from 82% survival rate of Oxford phase 1, 2 implant. In 2013, Altuntas et al. [53] reported 2 (3.1%) revision surgeries for each of instability and medial compartment pain in their minimum 2-year (mean 38 month) followed 64 domed lateral UKA.

Relatively better survival rate over mobile bearing lateral UKA has been reported by various researchers regarding fixed-bearing lateral UKA since Scott et al. [51] reported 83.3% postoperative 3.5-year survival rate in 1981. Argenson et al. [46] reported 92% 10-year survival rate and 84% 16-year survival rate. Servien et al. [55] reported 98% 10-year survival rate, and Lustig et al. [52] reported 94% 10-year survival rate and 91% 15-year survival rate in 2014 in all-poly fixed type lateral UKA.

13.2.3 Complications

Progression of arthritis to the other compartment, aseptic loosening of femoral or tibial component, implant breakage, periprosthetic fracture, valgus malalignment, dislocation or wear of polyethylene insert, deep infection, persisting pain, and knee joint stiffness can be considered complications of lateral UKA [48, 56]. Citak et al. [56] reported progression of other compartment disease including medial compartment or patellofemoral compartment (43%) and aseptic loosening (18.8%) as major reasons of failure.

13.3 Patellofemoral Arthroplasty

Disease of patellofemoral joint is known to be caused by unusual load transmission to the patellofemoral joint, and malalignment, dysplasia, instability, trauma, inflammatory arthritis, idiopathic osteoarthritis are known causes of patellofemoral arthritis [57]. Arthritis limited to patellofemoral joint can be initially treated with conservative treatment. In resistant cases, surgical treatments can be attempted. Realignment surgery can be considered in patellofemoral malalignment without severe arthritic change, in advanced patellofemoral arthritis, excision of the osteophyte, chondroplasty including drilling and abrasion arthroplasty, tibial tubercle advancement to reduce patellofemoral pressure, and resection arthroplasty can be considered. However, most of surgical options are performed for temporary improvement with ambiguous effectiveness. Moreover, some surgical options have clear limitations such as non-regeneration of cartilage in chondroplasty or deprivation of muscle strength and nutrition to the trochlea in resection arthroplasty. Osteochondral graft or chondrocyte implantation only can be considered in focal chondral defects. Therefore, patellofemoral arthroplasty was introduced as a solution for end-stage patellofemoral arthritis. The concept of patellofemoral arthroplasty was developed owing to the unnecessary resection of intact femorotibial joint in patients with limited patellofemoral arthritis who were once reported to underwent TKA in 3–5% of morbid population. Patellofemoral arthroplasty has advantages of less bone resection, earlier postoperative recovery and rehabilitation, biomechanical similarity to a normal knee joint owing to the preservation of femorotibial joint and cartilage as a salvage operation for patellofemoral arthritis which does not respond to conservative treatment [58].

13.3.1 Indications and Contraindications

Patellofemoral arthritis is indicated for osteoarthritis limited in patellofemoral compartment of knee joint, posttraumatic arthritis, advanced stage patellofemoral chondramalacia, and patellofemoral dysplasia. Also, it can be indicated for intractable anterior knee pain or posterior patellar pain which is debilitating activities of daily life. Functional disabilities including difficulties in stair climbing, prolonged sitting, standing from sitting position, and squatting, and previous history of patellar dislocation, fracture, failed surgical treatment are also considered good indications. Prerequisites for patellofemoral arthroplasty include intact cruciate ligaments and collateral ligaments with intact menisci. Regarding the optimal age, debates exist while some researchers insist no limitation others insist that patellofemoral arthroplasty should be performed in senile patients who are older than middle age. Lubinus et al. [59] and Arciero and Toomey [60] suggested patellofemoral arthroplasty is favorably indicated for elderly over 60 years old, whereas Lonner [61] and Blazina et al. [62] suggested patellofemoral arthroplasty for patients under 60 years old and TKA for older patients who are at higher risk of femorotibial arthritis progression. Contraindications of patellofemoral arthroplasty include diagnosis of inflammatory arthritis, osteoarthritis exceeding slight degree, advanced chondromalacia, and severe chondrocalcinosis. Flexion contracture, limitation of motion, malalignment or maltracking patella, Complex regional pain syndrome, infection, Q-angle exceeding 20°(female)/15°(male) are not indicated for patellofemoral arthroplasty. Laborer or athletes who are not willing to restrict their activity level are considered relative contraindications. Obese patient or patient with cruciate ligament insufficiency is at higher risk of failure even if one is not considered a contraindication of patellofemoral arthroplasty.

13.3.2 Designs

In the 1950s Mckeever developed implant for patellar replacement using Vitallium, however, as patellofemoral pain often arose from trochlear side, Bechtol, Aglietty, Lubinus, Richards et al. have developed modern implants replacing both patellar and trochlear side since the 1970s. Early implant designs with anatomically shaped trochlea and patella are categorized as first-generation designs. Trochlear component of the first-generation design had blunt curvature in the sagittal plane with short anterior flange, and narrow trochlear groove in the axial plane. This design was eventually abandoned due to high failure rate because the short anterior flange with blunt curvature tends to lift the anterior flange off from the anterior femoral cortex, and resulted in snapping and catching during knee motion. Moreover, narrow trochlear groove in the axial plane allowed narrow range of normal patellar tracking so that the design was susceptible to the maltracking. Anatomically shaped patella also served for another reason of maltracking for the patellar component failed to match individual variations of patella shape, which was even more difficult in knees with degenerative changes.

Therefore, recent second-generation implant designs have lengthened anterior flange and right-angled curvature in trochlear component, and broadened less constrained trochlea groove allowed better patellar tracking while avoiding impingement of notch to the ACL or proximal tibia. Patellar component, which could not be applied universally to all the patients, was also innovated to dome shape or mobile shape on the basis of biomechanics. Patellar component instability was reduced with the design renovation, and Lonner [63] reported 4% failure rate in second-generation designs versus 17% failure rate in first-generation implant designs.

In other words, implants for patellofemoral arthroplasty can be categorized into resurfacing (inlay) type and anterior cut (onlay) type according to the type of femoral trochlear component. Implant lays parallel with the slope of femoral trochlea in the femoral trochlear cartilage and condylar articular cartilage in resurfacing type implant. Lubinus, Blazina, Autocentric, and LCS are resurfacing type implants (Fig. 13.14). In anterior cut type implants, trochlear component is longer and broader than resurfacing implants and lays extending on the femur. Femoral bone resection is perpendicular to the anteroposterior axis of the femur, and implant seats in externally rotated position. Avon, Vanguard, Gender Solution are anterior cut type implants (Fig. 13.15).

In product-specific perspectives, Autocentric Patellofemoral Prosthesis (Medinov, Roanne, France), Lubinus (Link, Hamburg, Germany), Richards I (Smith&Nephew, Richards, Memphis TN) are categorized into first-generation designs which reported numerous complications related to their short anterior flange and narrow trochlear groove and blunt curvature. The products developed after them, including Richards II (Smith&Nephew, Richards, Memphis TN), Low Contact Stress Patellofemoral Joint (DePuy Orthopedics, Warsaw, IN), Natural—Knee II

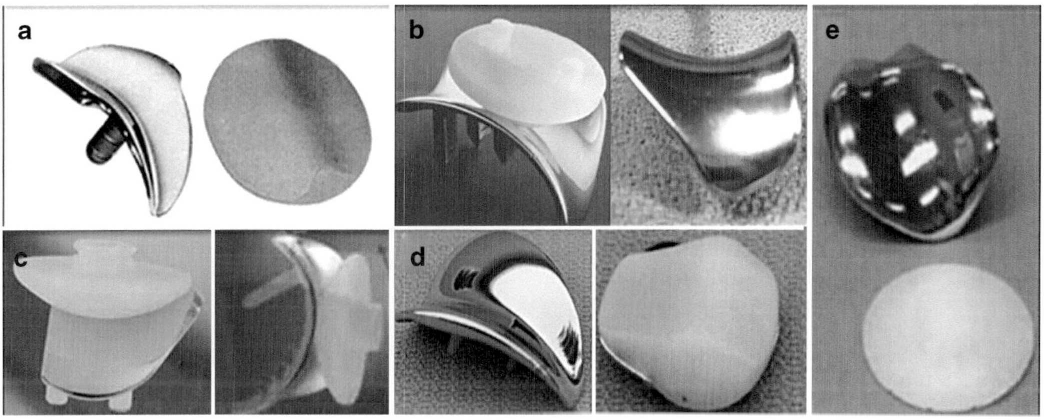

Fig. 13.14 Resurfacing type implants for patellofemoral arthroplasty (Inlay type implants): Richards III™ (**a**), Spherocentric™ (**b**), Autocentric™ (**c**), LCS™ (**d**), Lubinus™ (**e**). (Lustig OTSR, 2014)

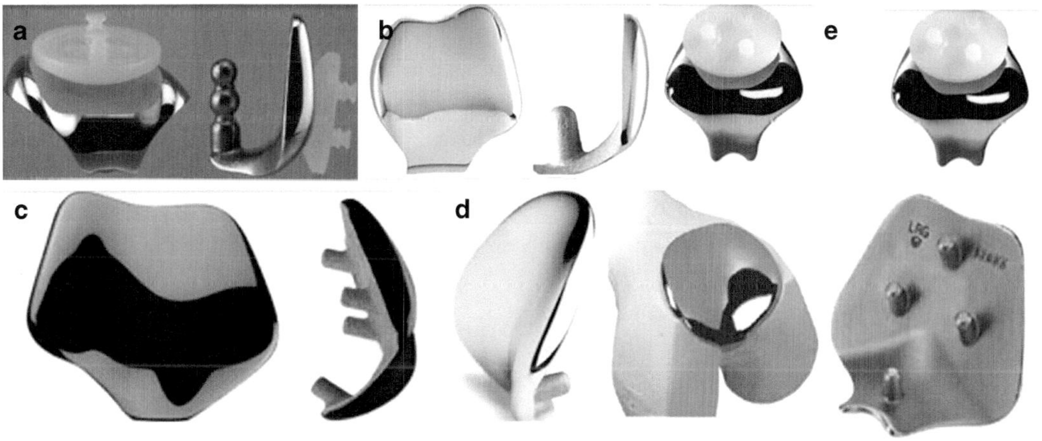

Fig. 13.15 Anterior cut type implants for patellofemoral arthroplasty (onlay type implants): Hermes™ (**a**), Vanguard™ (**b**), Journey Competitor™ (**c**), Gender™ (**d**), Avon™ (**e**). (Lustig OTSR, 2014)

Patellofemoral Jolnt (Zimmer, Warsaw, IN), and Avon (Stryker/Howmedica, Mahwah, NJ) are regarded as second-generation designs. Implant material is cobalt chromium for the trochlear component, and polyethylene in the patellar component [64].

13.3.3 Surgical Technique

Approach takes midline skin incision and paramedical arthrotomy or subvastus approach similar to TKA. Incision can be shortened distally as to allow patella eversion to inspect intraarticular structures, however patella is not necessary for every cases. Care should be taken to avoid harming the meniscus during the arthrotomy. It is recommended to perform TKA if the intraarticular findings are suggestive of inflammatory arthritis or chondrocalcinosis or advanced femorotibial joint degeneration. In the procedure to remove osteophyte, notchplasty to remove the osteophytes and smoothing around the notch is important.

For trochlear bone resection, there are some common surgical techniques despite product-specific procedures exist. First, externally rotate trochlear component 3–6° referencing from transcondylar axis or Whiteside's line or transepicondylar axis. Trochlear component can be located 11–12 mm laterally but should be in line with anatomical axis of the femur. Second, maximize trochlear coverage until it does not overhang. The edge of trochlear component should be located 3–5 mm proximal to femoral intercondylar notch to avoid the trochlear component overhanging the notch or trespassing the weight bearing surface and impinging to proximal tibia. Third, cling to the resurfacing concept and avoid excessive subchondral bone resection. Perform 3–4 mm anterior femoral resection along the anterior cortical level, and flush trochlear component to adjacent cartilage surface neither too proud nor too sunk.

Patellar replacement is identical to one in TKA. It is recommended to adjust the patellar thickness nearly identical to preoperative native patellar thickness and to medialize the patellar component while beveling the uncovered region of the patella. Specifically, patella baja should be avoided.

After bone resection, patellar tilt, subluxation, and catching should be examined during the patellar tracking in trial insert insertion state. Realignment procedures, lateral retinacular release, for instance, can be considered if needed. Generally speaking, contact of the patellar medial facet to the medial trochlea and medial femoral condyle through the entire range of motion using no thumb technique can be considered a good tracing. Fixation can be done with or without cement, but cemented fixation is desirable because loosening is frequent in cementless fixation. However, a few surgeons prefer cementless fixation for patellar component (Fig. 13.16).

Postoperative rehabilitation is a little faster or nearly similar to TKA. Immediate knee joint motion is allowed including CPM, and immediate tolerable weight bearing is also allowed.

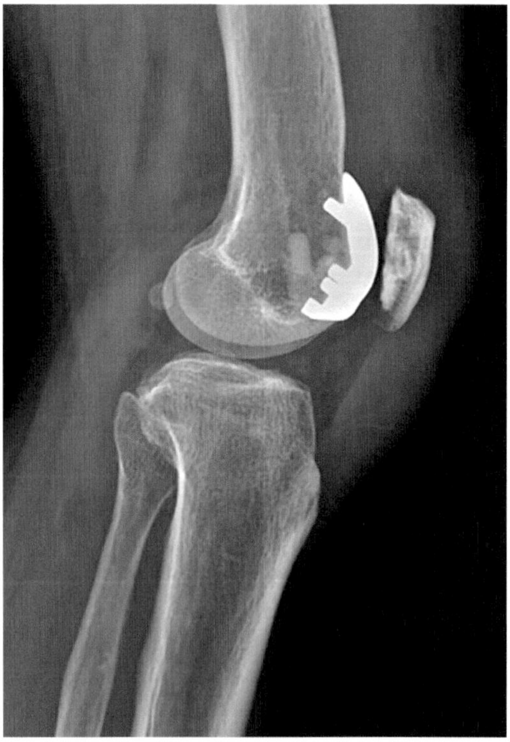

Fig. 13.16 Postoperative radiography of the patellofemoral arthroplasty (Courtesy of MH, Song)

13.3.4 Clinical Results

Isolated patellofemoral replacement raised interests following the reports of the first-generation implants' (Lubinus, Autocentric, Richards I) clinical results since the late 1970s. However, high early failure rate was reported owing to the problems in implant design and surgical technique. Patellofemoral replacement using second-generation implants (Avon, LCS, Richards 11) reported good result with decreased failure rate related to the implant factor though number of the cases was insufficient. Most recently, good results are expected with third-generation implants (Vanguard, Journey, Sigma) which were introduced as a "Bridging surgery" to delay the TKA in middle age patients.

Extremely various results were reported regarding patellofemoral arthroplasty. Numerous researches reported better than good results in 66–100% of cases in 3–17 year follow-up studies. Results of patellofemoral arthroplasty is closely related to implant design, patient factors, comorbidities, surgical technique, and fixation methods, of which implant design has the biggest impact. Australian National Joint Replacement Registry reported 5-year cumulative revision rate was 21.8% in inlay type implants and 9.9% in onlay type implants after patellofemoral arthro plasty [65]. Argenson et al. [66] reported satisfactory results in 84% of mid-term follow up and 58% 16-year survival rate. However, Tauro et al. [67] reported merely 45% success rate and 65% 8-year survival rate using Lubinus implant, which made them abandon this operation.

13.3.5 Complications

Early complications of patellofemoral arthroplasty include maltracking, catching or snapping, instability, extension lag, motion limitation, persisting pain or effusion, giving way, femorotibial arthritis. Late complications include aseptic loosening of femoral or patellar component, progression of other compartment disease, implant breakage, patellar instability. Among them, femorotibial arthritis is regarded as a major cause of onlay type implant failure, whereas instability is regarded as a major cause of inlay type implant failure. Patellar instability is known to be related to malpositioned implant and malaligned extensor mechanism.

13.4 Summary

UKA is a very effective surgical treatment option for degenerative arthritis involving one compartment of the knee joint. Despite the cases were decreased along the early era for the unsatisfactory results related to errors in patient selection, implant designs, lack of fine instruments, and demanding surgical technique, global number of UKA cases are increasing with excellent functional results and implant survival owing to the fine-tuned surgical indication, innovations in implant design, development of surgical instruments and techniques. Thorough understanding of UKA with appropriate patient selection, utilization of verified implant design, and precise surgical technique are requirements for a successful UKA.

References

1. MacIntosh DL, Hunter GA. The use of the hemiarthroplasty prosthesis for advanced osteoarthritis and rheumatoid arthritis of the knee. J Bone Joint Surg. 1972;54(2):244–55.
2. Marmor L. Marmor modular knee in unicompartmental disease. Minimum four-year follow-up. J Bone Joint Surg Am. 1979;61(3):347–53.
3. Goodfellow JW, O'Connor J. Clinical results of the Oxford knee. Surface arthroplasty of the tibiofemoral joint with a meniscal bearing prosthesis. Clin Orthop Relat Res. 1986;205:21–42.
4. Repicci JA, Hartman JF. Minimally invasive unicondylar knee arthroplasty for the treatment of unicompartmental osteoarthritis an outpatient arthritic bypass procedure. Orthop Clin North Am. 2004;35(2):201–16.
5. Riddle DL, Jiranek WA, McGlynn FJ. Yearly incidence of unicompartmental knee arthroplasty in the United States. J Arthroplast. 2008;23(3):408–12. https://doi.org/10.1016/j.arth.2007.04.012.
6. Dahl AW, Robertsson O, Lidgren L, Miller L, Davidson D, Graves S. Unicompartmental knee arthroplasty in patients aged less than 65. Acta Orthop. 2010;81(1):90–4. https://doi.org/10.3109/17453671003587150.

7. Ko YB, Gujarathi MR, Oh KJ. Outcome of unicompartmental knee arthroplasty: a systematic review of comparative studies between fixed and mobile bearings focusing on complications. Knee Surg Relat Res. 2015;27(3):141–8. https://doi.org/10.5792/ksrr.2015.27.3.141.
8. Jamali AA, Scott RD, Rubash HE, Freiberg AA. Unicompartmental knee arthroplasty: past, present, and future. Am J Orthop (Belle Mead NJ). 2009;38(1):17–23.
9. Berger RA, Della Valle CJ. Unicompartmental knee arthroplasty: indications, techniques, and results. Instr Course Lect. 2010;59:47–56.
10. Panni AS, Vasso M, Cerciello S, Felici A. Unicompartmental knee replacement provides early clinical and functional improvement stabilizing over time. Knee Surg Sports Traumatol Arthrosc. 2012;20(3):579–85. https://doi.org/10.1007/s00167-011-1613-y.
11. Pandit H, Hamilton TW, Jenkins C, Mellon SJ, Dodd CA, Murray DW. The clinical outcome of minimally invasive Phase 3 Oxford unicompartmental knee arthroplasty: a 15-year follow-up of 1000 UKAs. Bone Joint J. 2015;97-b(11):1493–500. https://doi.org/10.1302/0301-620x.97b11.35634.
12. Laskin RS. Unicompartmental knee replacement: some unanswered questions. Clin Orthop Relat Res. 2001;392:267–71.
13. Dennis D, Komistek R, Scuderi G, Argenson JN, Insall J, Mahfouz M, Aubaniac JM, Haas B. In vivo three-dimensional determination of kinematics for subjects with a normal knee or a unicompartmental or total knee replacement. J Bone Joint Surg Am. 2001;83-A(Suppl 2 Pt 2):104–15. https://doi.org/10.2106/00004623-200100022-00008.
14. Argenson JN, Komistek RD, Aubaniac JM, Dennis DA, Northcut EJ, Anderson DT, Agostini S. In vivo determination of knee kinematics for subjects implanted with a unicompartmental arthroplasty. J Arthroplast. 2002;17(8):1049–54. https://doi.org/10.1054/arth.2002.34527.
15. Murray DW, Goodfellow JW, O'Connor JJ. The Oxford medial unicompartmental arthroplasty: a ten-year survival study. J Bone Joint Surg. 1998;80(6):983–9. https://doi.org/10.1302/0301-620x.80b6.8177.
16. Dahl AW, Robertsson O, Lidgren L. Surgery for knee osteoarthritis in younger patients. Acta Orthop. 2010;81(2):161–4. https://doi.org/10.3109/17453670903413186.
17. Faour Martín O, Valverde García JA, Martín Ferrero M, Vega Castrillo A, Zuil Acosta P, Suárez De Puga CC. The young patient and the medial unicompartmental knee replacement. Acta Orthop Belg. 2015;81(2):283–8.
18. Kim KT, Lee S, Lee JS, Kang MS, Koo KH. Long-term clinical results of unicompartmental knee arthroplasty in patients younger than 60 years of age: minimum 10-year follow-up. Knee Surg Relat Res. 2018;30(1):28–33. https://doi.org/10.5792/ksrr.17.025.
19. Kim YJ, Kim BH, Yoo SH, Kang SW, Kwack CH, Song MH. Mid-term results of oxford medial unicompartmental knee arthroplasty in young asian patients less than 60 years of age: a minimum 5-year follow-up. Knee Surg Relat Res. 2017;29(2):122–8. https://doi.org/10.5792/ksrr.16.045.
20. Takeuchi R, Umemoto Y, Aratake M, Bito H, Saito I, Kumagai K, Sasaki Y, Akamatsu Y, Ishikawa H, Koshino T, Saito T. A mid term comparison of open wedge high tibial osteotomy vs unicompartmental knee arthroplasty for medial compartment osteoarthritis of the knee. J Orthop Surg Res. 2010;5(1):65. https://doi.org/10.1186/1749-799x-5-65.
21. McAuley JP, Engh GA, Ammeen DJ. Revision of failed unicompartmental knee arthroplasty. Clin Orthop Relat Res. 2001;392:279–82. https://doi.org/10.1097/00003086-200111000-00036.
22. Newman J, Pydisetty RV, Ackroyd C. Unicompartmental or total knee replacement: the 15-year results of a prospective randomised controlled trial. J Bone Joint Surg. 2009;91(1):52–7. https://doi.org/10.1302/0301-620X.91B1.20899.
23. Scott RD. Mobile-versus fixed-bearing unicompartmental knee arthroplasty. Instr Course Lect. 2010;59:57–60.
24. Peersman G, Stuyts B, Vandenlangenbergh T, Cartier P, Fennema P. Fixed-versus mobile-bearing UKA: a systematic review and meta-analysis. Knee Surg Sports Traumatol Arthrosc. 2015;23(11):3296–305. https://doi.org/10.1007/s00167-014-3131-1.
25. Emerson RH Jr. Unicompartmental mobile-bearing knee arthroplasty. Instr Course Lect. 2005;54:221–4.
26. Price AJ, Webb J, Topf H, Dodd CA, Goodfellow JW, Murray DW, Oxford H, Knee G. Rapid recovery after oxford unicompartmental arthroplasty through a short incision. J Arthroplast. 2001;16(8):970–6. https://doi.org/10.1054/arth.2001.25552.
27. Pennington DW, Swienckowski JJ, Lutes WB, Drake GN. Unicompartmental knee arthroplasty in patients sixty years of age or younger. J Bone Joint Surg Am. 2003;85(10):1968–73. https://doi.org/10.2106/00004623-200310000-00016.
28. Fitz W, Bliss R, Losina E. Current fit of medial and lateral unicompartmental knee arthroplasty. Acta Orthop Belg. 2013;79(2):191–6.
29. Saccomanni B. Unicompartmental knee arthroplasty: a review of literature. Clin Rheumatol. 2010;29(4):339–46. https://doi.org/10.1007/s10067-009-1354-1.
30. Kozinn SC, Scott R. Unicondylar knee arthroplasty. J Bone Joint Surg Am. 1989;71(1):145–50.
31. Fisher N, Agarwal M, Reuben SF, Johnson DS, Turner PG. Sporting and physical activity following Oxford medial unicompartmental knee arthroplasty. Knee. 2006;13(4):296–300. https://doi.org/10.1016/j.knee.2006.03.004.

32. Padgett DE, Stern SH, Insall JN. Revision total knee arthroplasty for failed unicompartmental replacement. J Bone Joint Surg Am. 1991;73(2):186–90.
33. Berger RA, Nedeff DD, Barden RM, Sheinkop MM, Jacobs JJ, Rosenberg AG, Galante JO. Unicompartmental knee arthroplasty. Clinical experience at 6- to 10-year followup. Clin Orthop Relat Res. 1999;367:50–60.
34. Egidy CC, Sherman SL, Macdessi SJ, Cross MB, Windsor RE. Long-term survivorship of a unicondylar knee replacement – a case report. Knee. 2012;19(6):944–7. https://doi.org/10.1016/j.knee.2012.03.015.
35. Argenson JN, Blanc G, Aubaniac JM, Parratte S. Modern unicompartmental knee arthroplasty with cement: a concise follow-up, at a mean of twenty years, of a previous report. J Bone Joint Surg Am. 2013;95(10):905–9. https://doi.org/10.2106/JBJS.L.00963.
36. Emerson RH, Alnachoukati O, Barrington J, Ennin K. The results of Oxford unicompartmental knee arthroplasty in the United States: a mean ten-year survival analysis. Bone Joint J. 2016;98-b(10 Supple B):34–40. https://doi.org/10.1302/0301-620x.98b10.bjj-2016-0480.r1.
37. Kim KT, Lee S, Kim JH, Hong SW, Jung WS, Shin WS. The survivorship and clinical results of minimally invasive unicompartmental knee arthroplasty at 10-year follow-up. Clin Orthop Surg. 2015;7(2):199–206. https://doi.org/10.4055/cios.2015.7.2.199.
38. Lim HC, Bae JH, Song SH, Kim SJ. Oxford phase 3 unicompartmental knee replacement in Korean patients. J Bone Joint Surg. 2012;94(8):1071–6. https://doi.org/10.1302/0301-620X.94B8.29372.
39. Lyons MC, MacDonald SJ, Somerville LE, Naudie DD, McCalden RW. Unicompartmental versus total knee arthroplasty database analysis: is there a winner? Clin Orthop Relat Res. 2012;470(1):84–90. https://doi.org/10.1007/s11999-011-2144-z.
40. Kim KT, Lee S, Lee JI, Kim JW. Analysis and treatment of complications after unicompartmental knee arthroplasty. Knee Surg Relat Res. 2016;28(1):46–54. https://doi.org/10.5792/ksrr.2016.28.1.46.
41. Mohammad HR, Kennedy JA, Mellon SJ, Judge A, Dodd CA, Murray DW. Ten-year clinical and radiographic results of 1000 cementless Oxford unicompartmental knee replacements. Knee Surg Sports Traumatol Arthrosc. 2020;28(5):1479–87. https://doi.org/10.1007/s00167-019-05544-w.
42. Kirschner S, Lutzner J, Fickert S, Gunther KP. Revision of unicompartmental knee arthroplasty. Der Orthopade. 2006;35(2):184–91. https://doi.org/10.1007/s00132-005-0910-x.
43. Gunther TV, Murray DW, Miller R, Wallace DA, Carr AJ, O'Connor JJ, McLardy-Smith P, Goodfellow JW. Lateral unicompartmental arthroplasty with the Oxford meniscal knee. Knee. 1996;3(1):33–9. https://doi.org/10.1016/0968-0160(96)00208-6.
44. Whiteside LA. Making your next unicompartmental knee arthroplasty last: three keys to success. J Arthroplast. 2005;20(4 Suppl 2):2–3. https://doi.org/10.1016/j.arth.2005.03.029.
45. Clark M, Campbell DG, Kiss G, Dobson PJ, Lewis PL. Reintervention after mobile-bearing Oxford unicompartmental knee arthroplasty. Clin Orthop Relat Res. 2010;468(2):576–80. https://doi.org/10.1007/s11999-009-1089-y.
46. Argenson JN, Parratte S, Bertani A, Flecher X, Aubaniac JM. Long-term results with a lateral unicondylar replacement. Clin Orthop Relat Res. 2008;466(11):2686–93. https://doi.org/10.1007/s11999-008-0351-z.
47. Ollivier M, Abdel MP, Parratte S, Argenson JN. Lateral unicondylar knee arthroplasty (UKA): contemporary indications, surgical technique, and results. Int Orthop. 2014;38(2):449–55. https://doi.org/10.1007/s00264-013-2222-9.
48. Lombardi AV Jr, Berend KR, Berend ME, Della Valle CJ, Engh GA, Fitz W, Hurst JM, Jinnah RH, Lonner JH, Macaulay WB, Repicci JA, Scuderi GR. Current controversies in partial knee arthroplasty. Instr Course Lect. 2012;61:347–81.
49. Heyse TJ, Tibesku CO. Lateral unicompartmental knee arthroplasty: a review. Arch Orthop Trauma Surg. 2010;130(12):1539–48. https://doi.org/10.1007/s00402-010-1137-9.
50. Kim KT, Lee S, Kim J, Kim JW, Kang MS. Clinical results of lateral unicompartmental knee arthroplasty: minimum 2-year follow-up. Clin Orthop Surg. 2016;8(4):386–92. https://doi.org/10.4055/cios.2016.8.4.386.
51. Scott RD, Santore RF. Unicondylar unicompartmental replacement for osteoarthritis of the knee. J Bone Joint Surg Am. 1981;63(4):536–44.
52. Lustig S, Lording T, Frank F, Debette C, Servien E, Neyret P. Progression of medial osteoarthritis and long term results of lateral unicompartmental arthroplasty: 10 to 18 year follow-up of 54 consecutive implants. Knee. 2014;21(Suppl 1):S26–32. https://doi.org/10.1016/s0968-0160(14)50006-3.
53. Altuntas AO, Alsop H, Cobb JP. Early results of a domed tibia, mobile bearing lateral unicompartmental knee arthroplasty from an independent centre. Knee. 2013;20(6):466–70. https://doi.org/10.1016/j.knee.2012.11.008.
54. Pandit H, Jenkins C, Beard DJ, Price AJ, Gill HS, Dodd CA, Murray DW. Mobile bearing dislocation in lateral unicompartmental knee replacement. Knee. 2010;17(6):392–7. https://doi.org/10.1016/j.knee.2009.10.007.
55. Servien E, Merini A, Lustig S, Neyret P. Lateral uni-compartmental knee replacement: current concepts and future directions. Knee Surg Sports Traumatol Arthrosc. 2013;21(11):2501–8. https://doi.org/10.1007/s00167-013-2585-x.
56. Citak M, Cross MB, Gehrke T, Dersch K, Kendoff D. Modes of failure and revision of failed lateral unicom-

partmental knee arthroplasties. Knee. 2015;22(4):338–40. https://doi.org/10.1016/j.knee.2015.03.008.
57. Starks I, Roberts S, White SH. The Avon patellofemoral joint replacement: independent assessment of early functional outcomes. J Bone Joint Surg. 2009;91(12):1579–82. https://doi.org/10.1302/0301-620X.91B12.23018.
58. Walker T, Perkinson B, Mihalko WM. Patellofemoral arthroplasty: the other unicompartmental knee replacement. Instr Course Lect. 2013;62:363–71.
59. Lubinus HH. Patella glide bearing total replacement. Orthopedics. 1979;2(2):119–27. https://doi.org/10.3928/0147-7447-19790301-03.
60. Arciero RA, Toomey HE. Patellofemoral arthroplasty. A three- to nine-year follow-up study. Clin Orthop Relat Res. 1988;236:60–71.
61. Lonner JH. Patellofemoral arthroplasty: pros, cons, and design considerations. Clin Orthop Relat Res. 2004;428:158–65.
62. Blazina ME, Fox JM, Del Pizzo W, Broukhim B, Ivey FM. Patellofemoral replacement. 1979. Clin Orthop Relat Res. 2005;436:3–6.
63. Lonner JH. Patellofemoral arthroplasty: an evolving science. Instr Course Lect. 2017;66:211–21.
64. Lustig S. Patellofemoral arthroplasty. Orthop Raumatol Surg Res. 2014;100(1 Suppl):S35–43. https://doi.org/10.1016/j.otsr.2013.06.013.
65. Scholes C, Ebrahimi M, Field C, Farah S, Kerr D, Kohan L. Minimally invasive inlay prosthesis unicompartmental knee arthroplasty for the treatment of unicompartmental osteoarthritis: a prospective observational cohort study with minimum 2-year outcomes and up to 14-year survival. J Knee Surg. 2019; https://doi.org/10.1055/s-0039-3400536.
66. Argenson JN, Flecher X, Parratte S, Aubaniac JM. Patellofemoral arthroplasty: an update. Clin Orthop Relat Res. 2005;440:50–3. https://doi.org/10.1097/01.blo.0000187061.27573.70.
67. Tauro B, Ackroyd CE, Newman JH, Shah NA. The Lubinus patellofemoral arthroplasty. A five- to ten-year prospective study. J Bone Joint Surg. 2001;83(5):696–701. https://doi.org/10.1302/0301-620x.83b5.11577.

Total Knee Arthroplasty

14

Chang-Wan Kim, Chang-Rack Lee, Young-Chae Seo, and Seung-Suk Seo

Abstract

Appropriate patient selection is necessary to achieve successful outcomes after total knee arthroplasty (TKAs). Indication for TKAs is an end-stage arthritis not responding to any other treatment. However, infected arthritis is absolute contraindication of TKA. In order to improve postoperative patient satisfaction and prevent complications, the patient's physical and mental health status besides knee condition should be assessed preoperatively. Materials used for prosthesis should be biologically inert. The type of the prosthesis is divided into CR or PS type depending on PCL retention and fixed or mobile type depending on the method of PE insert fixation. There is no significant difference in clinical outcomes or long-term survival rates based on prosthesis types. The basic principle of performing TKA is to obtain proper soft tissue balancing and restoration of lower limb alignment. In a practical way, mechanical alignment is the most widely used for restoration of limb alignment. Proper soft tissue balancing is also an important factor in the successful outcome of TKA. Therefore, it is necessary to understand the anatomy and function of various soft tissues around the knee. In addition, soft tissue release must be carried out meticulously and gradually to avoid over-release. The most widely used method for prosthesis fixation is cemented fixation. Postoperative management is also important for patient satisfaction and clinical outcomes. Failure to control pain after surgery has a great effect on patient dissatisfaction and function loss. Every effort should be made for decreasing the postoperative pain. Periprosthetic joint infection (PJI) is still the most common cause of failed TKAs. Prevention of PJI is important, but once it occurs, accurate diagnosis and prompt treatment are needed. TKA is a successful surgical method for patients with knee OA. Successful outcomes require proper patient selection, preoperative planning, meticulous surgical techniques, and postoperative planned management. Surgeons should do their best to give patients the best results.

Keywords

Knee · Osteoarthritis · Total knee arthroplasty Indication · Contraindications · Soft tissue balancing · Lower limb alignment Postoperative management · Type of prosthesis · Periprosthetic joint infection · Outcome

C.-W. Kim (✉) · C.-R. Lee · Y.-C. Seo
Department of Orthopedics, Inje University Busan Paik Hospital, Busan, South Korea
e-mail: kcw8737@paik.ac.kr; leechangrack@inje.ac.kr; 085241@paik.ac.kr

S.-S. Seo
Department of Orthopedics, Haeundae Bumin Hospital, Busan, South Korea
e-mail: seoss@bumin.co.kr

S.-S. Seo (ed.), *A Strategic Approach to Knee Arthritis Treatment*,
https://doi.org/10.1007/978-981-16-4217-3_14

14.1 Patient Selection

In order to establish an appropriate surgical plan for the patient before surgery, it is necessary to know in detail not only the patient's overall physical health but also the mental state, and based on this, preparations for postoperative treatment should be made. Since the patient's pathologic condition may put the patient at risk during and after surgery, the risk of surgery due to the patient's systemic condition should also be considered, along with benefits such as pain relief and function improvement. Although severe radiographic degenerative changes of knee joint provide important findings in the selection of indications for surgery, radiologic changes are not necessarily associated with clinical symptoms and functional impairment. Therefore, it is necessary to select the correct target group requiring TKA through a method that can systematically evaluate functional impairment and pain.

14.1.1 Social and Economic Conditions

Social and economic conditions of a patient are also important in determining whether to perform TKA. Social conditions include every factor such as the patient's family, surrounding environment, and the extent and scope of the patient's life activities; among other factors, the most important to consider is whether a person and an environment to care for the patient are well prepared. If education level is relatively low, if there are no guardians to take care of the patient, or if the patient needs to continue economic activity for a living, the postoperative result may not be favorable.

14.1.2 Mental Status

Mental status may be easily overlooked in decision of TKA, but it is very important. Patients seeking additional financial or emotional benefits from continued physical disability need a thorough preoperative examination and careful consideration as to whether to perform surgery. In case patients live with dementia or suffer from mental illness such as depression, mania, or schizophrenia, whether to have surgery must be consulted with a psychiatrist. Ellis et al. [1] found that the surgery itself helped to improve the knee functioning of patients with depression, panic, and anxiety; however, the patients were less satisfied with the surgical result. As a result, they recommended that all patients undergo a mental status examination prior to surgery. Weak-minded, dependent patients who have a low pain threshold and are sensitive and have a closed, antisocial personality are likely to have a unfavorable clinical outcome since they fail to establish a good relationship with their doctor after surgery, which makes rehabilitation treatment even harder.

14.1.3 Physical Condition

14.1.3.1 Age

In general, younger people tend to lead active lifestyle, and thus place more pressure on the knee joint, which shortens the longevity of implants, resulting in revision surgery. However, if patients are too old, the risk of anesthesia and postoperative complication increase and the clinical outcomes might be not good due to muscle weakness and deterioration of general health. Therefore, the surgery is appropriate for those in their 60s to 70s whose general condition is relatively good and less likely to perform a revision surgery caused by wear or loosening of implant. Nevertheless, TKA is not absolutely contraindicated in patients over the age of 80s without severe medical illness. As for adolescent patients, since they are growing teenagers, TKA is never indicated. In the case of those in their 20s to 40s, TKA is restrictively considered only when they suffer from very serious secondary OA or rheumatoid arthritis (RA).

14.1.3.2 Comorbid Medical Illness

Comorbid illness has a great influence on perioperative complications and clinical outcomes. Illnesses such as hypertension and diabetes are not contraindicated as they can be controlled to some extent before surgery. In case of cardiovascular or kidney disease, it should be ensured that the patient can tolerate the surgery, and even after the surgery, much attention should be paid to the selection of drugs. In particular, taking anticoagulants for cardiovascular disease may cause a lot of bleeding during perioperative period; therefore, it is necessary to make an appropriate pre- and postoperative plan in consultation with a cardiologist before surgery. As for kidney disease, care should be taken in the use of non-steroidal anti-inflammatory drugs (NSAIDs) due to occurrence of acute kidney injury after surgery. There are several methods for classifying a patient's status, which can be helpful in predicting operative risk. American Society of Anesthesiologists (ASA) provides a five-category classification ranging from a normal healthy patient to a patient who is not expected to survive beyond the next 24 hours regardless of surgery. Charlson Comorbidity Index is adapted to predict postoperative morbidity and major complications. Voskuijl et al. [2] reported that Charlson Comorbidity Index can be used to estimate the risk of readmission after surgery.

14.1.3.3 Obesity

Obesity is strongly associated with development of degenerative arthritis. In addition, obese patients who undergo surgery are at higher risk for surgical site infection and slower wound healing due to decreased blood flow in soft tissue. Moreover, many obese patients accompany diabetes, which further increases the risk of surgical site infections. Even though obese patients are not contraindicated from arthroplasty, much attention should be paid because TKA in obese patients is related to perioperative medical complications, intraoperative technical demands on the surgeon, and long-term outcomes. Foran et al. [3] reported that the long-term follow-up of the clinical outcomes of TKA performed in obese patients was poor and also showed higher rates of revision due to wear and loosening. Dewan et al. [4] reported that morbidly obese patients with a BMI of 40 or more may suffer from muscle weakness and abnormalities in the patella-femoral mechanism .

14.1.3.4 Condition of Muscle, Nerve, and Blood Vessel

It is necessary to evaluate the muscle strength or paralysis of the affected part. Generally, it is recommended that the muscle strength of the operated knee be Grade 4 or higher for arthroplasty. Parkinson's disease is often accompanied by loss of motor coordination, mental illness, and muscle tremor. Even though TKA in Parkinson's disease results in excellent pain relief and functional recovery, it is better not to perform surgery in the late stage of disease. The condition of blood vessels is as much important while it is generally overlooked. Patients with vascular diseases are highly likely to suffer from postoperative wound complications. Moreover, in severe cases, ischemic changes in the lower extremities may result in amputation or even death, thus, it is essential to check whether a patient has peripheral vascular disease. In addition, if a patient suffers from varicose veins or frequent edema in the lower extremities, accurate preoperative examination is required as the incidence of postoperative thrombosis is high.

14.1.4 Knee Joint Condition

14.1.4.1 Symptom

The first indication for TKA is uncontrolled pain not relieved even with conservative treatment [5]. Since pain is subjective, the degree of pain varies from person to person, and the degree of arthritis indicated on X-ray may not be corresponded with the pain perceived by each person. In this respect, if OA represented in the X-ray is corresponded with the symptoms of pain, it will be an indication for TKA; however, if actual pain is not much severe than OA on the X-ray, conservative treatment shall be primarily attempted. On the contrary, if arthritis accompanies much severe pain than which is indicated on the X-ray, attempts to find other causes of pain should be performed.

14.1.4.2 Dysfunction of Knee Joint

The second indication is the knee dysfunction. It is necessary to check ROM when evaluating the function of the knee, and if it is not possible, it can be estimated by asking the movements necessary for daily life. For example, how much patients can do in their daily life including whether they can walk, squat, or go up and down stairs, and at which point they feel pain or discomfort should be checked. If it is hardly possible to walk on flat ground due to severe muscle weakness, it is meaningless to undergo TKA. However, if it is only difficult to go up and down stairs or cane is required, or walking with a lot of shaking due to instability of the knee, TKA can be a possible option to consider.

14.1.4.3 Disease Type

Most common disease type need TKA is OA (primary or secondary). In addition, RA, other inflammatory arthritis, osteonecrosis, ankylosing spondylitis, and neuropathic arthritis are also included. Radiologic findings are very important in deciding TKA. Kellgren-Lawrence (KL) classification is useful to evaluate the severity of knee OA. According to the KL classification, Grade III is defined moderate and Grade IV is severe. TKA is usually indicated for KL grade IV OA. Though OA is not diagnosed on radiologic findings, if patients complain of continuous pain, other reasons may have caused such pain. In such cases, it is highly likely that the problem is an early degenerative lesion of the cartilage, or that there are abnormalities in the ligaments and soft tissues (Fig. 14.1).

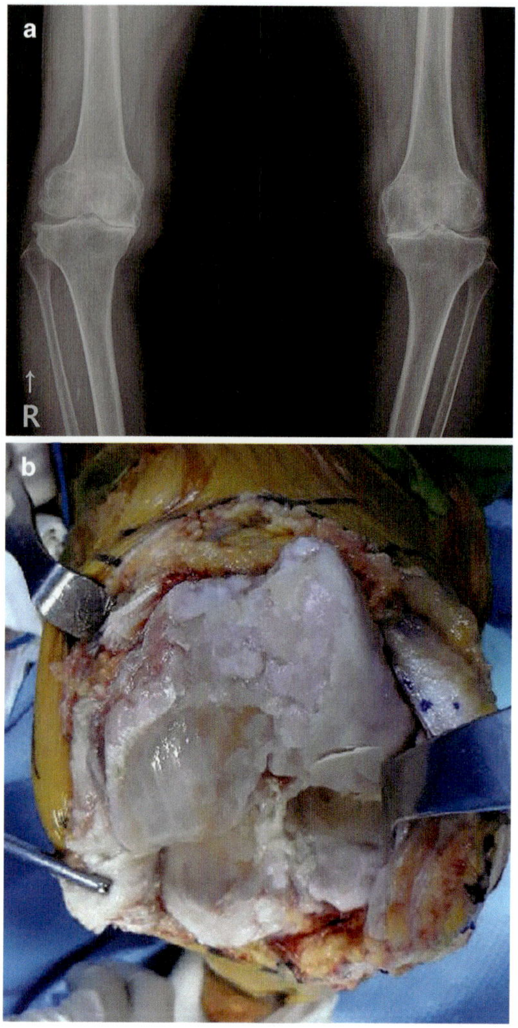

Fig. 14.1 Radiographic and surgical finding of severe OA. (**a**) KL grade IV OA changes were seen on standing AP radiograph, (**b**) Severe cartilage wear and osteophytes were found on intraoperative photo

RA of the knee joint is also a good indication for TKA. RA was once known as a risk factor for TKA as it accompanies comorbidity. Stundner et al. [5] compared postoperative problems in OA patients with RA patients and found that there were no other differences than an increase in infection risk and an increase in blood transfusion in RA. It is important to check prior to TKA in RA whether other joints have been affected. If other joints also need surgery, it is necessary to prioritize which to undergo surgery first. In addition, if the inflammatory reaction is severe, it is recommended to perform surgery after the acute phase subsided.

Surgical indications for osteonecrosis are when pain is very severe; more than half of the joint surface is invaded; the lesion is deep; and joint surface cracking and collapse is observed. On the other hand, when the necrosis does not exceed 1/2 of the joint surface and the lesion is not deep, it is advisable to consider conservative treatment. The secondary osteonecrosis shows a high rate of failure in TKA due to poor bone quality. Complications such as postoperative infection and aseptic loosening are likely to occur in the case of secondary osteonecrosis. According to a study by Mont et al. [6], 31 cases of TKA for steroid-induced osteonecrosis were performed, and about half were ended in failure, of which,

11 knees were reported for loosening and 3 knees were reported for infection.

14.1.5 Contraindications

14.1.5.1 Relative Contraindications

If there is a severe stiffness of the knee joint with ROM less than 50 degrees, a successful TKA is not easy due to shortening of the quadriceps muscles and fibrosis and contracture of the joint capsule. In addition, it may cause joint instability and neurological problems after TKA due to severe ligamentous imbalance and nerve stretching injury. Neuropathic arthritis is a destructive arthropathy where the joint has been damaged from repetitive trauma due to decreased sensation of pain. As for neuropathic arthritis, TKA itself is difficult, and even if it is performed, as there is no pain to protect the joint, the incidence of complications such as infection and periprosthetic fracture is high. TKA is relatively contraindicated when there is difficulty in walking due to muscle weakness caused by paralysis to the involved lower extremity. In the case of polio, in particular, TKA is technically difficult due to severe deformity of the knee joint such as external rotation of the tibia, valgus deformity and flexion contracture, and even after the surgery, the incidence of complications such as recurrence of instability or decreased function has been reported to be high.

14.1.5.2 Absolute Contraindications

Absolute contraindications for TKA include infection, severe soft tissue defects around knee joint, and severe peripheral vascular disease. In particular, it is an absolute contraindication to TKA where there is a possibility of acute joint infection. In case there was a prior infection, the surgery must be performed after ensuring that the infection has been completely cured. In addition, if there is a recent history of acupuncture or moxibustion, or if an intra-articular injection of steroid has been performed, it is advisable to perform the surgery after completely eliminating the possibility of infection.

14.2 Implant Options in Total Knee Arthroplasty

The degree of arthritis, joint deformity and laxity, and bone defects vary from patient to patient. In order to obtain a successful result in TKA, it is important to select the correct implant along with a close evaluation of the patient's status before surgery [7–9]. With the development of biomaterials, type of prosthesis and fixation method, the options available to surgeons are increasing. It is necessary for surgeon to carefully decide which implant to select for patient's better outcomes [10].

14.2.1 Implant Fixation

For TKA, implant fixation method is largely divided into cemented fixation and cementless fixation. A cemented fixation can be further divided into all cemented or hybrid fixation. All cemented fixation is a method that both the femur and tibia implants are fixed with cement. Hybrid fixation method is that the tibia implant is fixed with cement but the femur is not [8]. Recently, most of the patellar implants are made of PE, which utilizes cement fixation.

There are two major components of cement (polymethylmethacrylate (PMMA)): polymer powder and monomer liquid [11]. The monomer, a colorless liquid with a characteristic odor, is packaged in ampules. Methyl methacrylate comprises 97–99% of the liquid. *N*-dimethyl-*p*-toluidine acts as an activator, making up 0.4–2.8% by weight. Traces of hydroquinone (15–75 ppm) stabilize the monomer, preventing premature polymerization. The powder contributes to differences in properties. Microspheres of ground PMMA or copolymer contribute to 83–99% of the powder. The remaining components include a radiopacifier. Other additives to the powder may include antibiotics or dyes. PMMA powder has repeating carbon units and various lengths of chains. The longer the chain, the higher the molecular weight and the higher viscosity. Although the viscosity is not significantly related to the strength, if the viscosity is too low cement is difficult to handle, which is why a higher viscosity is currently preferred. When making cement, powder and liquid are mixed through four steps: mixing, waiting, working time, and hardening [10]. In order to obtain initial stability, the viscosity and timing of the cement paste are important; the time when cement does not stick with a finger is ideal [12]. Low-viscosity cements have longer sticky phases and shorter working phases. High-viscosity cements have long handling times and a short sticky phase. The advantage of cement fixation is that bleeding can be reduced, being useful when contact between instruments and bones is not consistent, and early weight bearing is possible because of its firm initial fixation. Although it is widely used in the elderly with severe osteoporosis or patients with RA, complications such as third-body wear, fat embolism, thermal necrosis may occur due to the use of cement, and the procedure may become more complicated when performing revision surgery [13].

Cementless fixation method was introduced in the 1980s to reduce complications related to cement. It was initially done by a porous coated type and press-fit type. Currently, most of them are porous coating types which facilitates bone ingrowth into the porous surface and then eventually fixed [14]. The advantage of cementless fixation is that the fixation is strong and permanent when intraosseous proliferation occurs, and bone loss is relatively small and complications due to the use of cement can be reduced during revision TKA. It is mainly recommended for young and active patients, but a sophisticated procedure is required to ensure good contact between the bone resection surface and the implant [15].

14.2.2 Biomaterials

14.2.2.1 Metals

Currently, the metals used in TKA are cobalt chrome alloy and titanium or zirconium. Metal substitutes must be biocompatible. It should not have any inflammatory or allergic reactions that can cause bone resorption, and not cause systemic reactions due to absorbed metal ions. In addition, there should be excellent durability, which depends on the fatigue strength and corrosion resistance [9, 16].

Cobalt Based Alloys

Cobalt chromium alloys are most commonly used material in manufacturing an artificial joint. It has excellent abrasion resistance and corrosion resistance, adequate biocompatibility, and generally exhibits satisfactory fatigue strength. Cobalt chromium alloy is widely used in femoral implants because it can be polished to a mirror like surface for articulation with polyethylene (PE), which decreased wear due to joint motion. When the surface of the cobalt chromium alloy is scratched, the wear of the PE increases [17–19]. Use of cobalt chromium tibial trays in comparison with titanium alloys produced a stress-shielding effect on the proximal tibia.

Titanium Based Alloys

Currently, most commonly used titanium based alloy in the field of orthopedic surgery is an aluminum-vanadium-titanium alloy called Ti-6Al-4V. It has excellent ductility and castability, and its modulus of elasticity is about 1/2 of that of cobalt chromium alloy, so that the force from the implant to the bone is well distributed, thereby reducing bone absorption. Ti-6Al-4V suffers from poor shear strength and poor surface wear properties in certain loading conditions. Therefore, titanium alloys are not used for femoral components because they have poor scratch resistance properties. In addition, fine particles of aluminum and vanadium caused by wear may cause toxicity in vivo [17, 20, 21]. Generally, titanium alloys are not good loading materials. Since it has low abrasion resistance and high coefficient of friction, titanium–titanium joint surfaces are not generally used, and their use as joint surfaces for ultra-high molecular weight polyethylene (UHMWPE) is limited. Cobalt alloys and ceramics are more suitable for joint surfaces than titanium alloys.

14.2.2.2 Ceramics

Ceramic materials produced from aluminum oxide and zirconium oxide have been mainly used for femoral component. Ceramic materials are formed by thermally driven oxidative process producing an articulating surface with ceramic properties on the metal implant. This surface is very smooth, and due to its smooth surface, the coefficient of friction is lower than that of the metal–PE interface, resulting in 3–16 times less occurrence of wear. Ceramics are much more resistant to compressive force than to tensile force. However, it is fragile and is hard so that it cannot withstand irregular impacts or loads [22].

14.2.2.3 Polyethylene (PE)

PE is made by polymerization of ethylene and has been used for a bearing surface for orthopedic implant. Initially, high molecular weight PE (HMWPE) was used, which contains substances that have the same chemical composition but differ in various molecular and microstructures. Currently, ultra-high molecular weight PE (UHMWPE), a molecular weight about 2–6 million, is widely used and has excellent impact strength, toughness, and wear-resistancy [23]. PE liner of TKA is more vulnerable to mechanical failure due to biomechanical and kinematic characteristics of knee joint. Recently Vitamin E containing PE was developed for decreasing oxidation and degradation of mechanical properties of PE.

14.2.3 Bearing Surfaces

There are many bearing surface options for TKA. Among them, cruciate retaining (CR type), cruciate sacrificing (CS type), and posterior stabilized (PS type) replacements have been commonly used. The bearing surface used in TKA was designed based on the kinematics of structures including the PCL. Therefore, it is important to understand the basic kinematics of the knee joint and the kinematics of TKA.

14.2.3.1 Kinematics

The knee is an unstable joint structure by nature in terms of the shape of the bone. The lateral tibia plateau is convex in the sagittal and coronal planes, and the medial tibial plateau is wider and concave than the lateral. Complex movement of rolling, sliding, and rotation occurs in normal knee. During the first 30 degree flexion of the knee, a rolling motion between the tibia and the femur occurs mainly, and after that, the PCL becomes tense and a sliding phenomenon, the so-called femoral roll back between the two joint surfaces, begins. The femoral roll back mechanism prevents the posterior tibia and femur from colliding during maximum flexion, allowing the knee to be bent up to 140 degrees at a normal knee. In the lateral tibial plateau, which has a convex surface than the medial one, a sliding motion occurs, causing the tibia to rotate internally to the femur while flexing the knee joint. The femoral roll back mechanism also increases the strength of the quadriceps muscle when flexing the knee by lengthening the moment arm to advance the pulling direction of the quadriceps muscle. Both CR type and the PS type TKA cannot reproduce normal knee kinematics because contact surface of native knee joint is significantly different from that of metal and PE in their biomechanical properties. Some authors suggested that it is impossible to preserve the intrinsic characteristics such as the length and tension of the PCL in TKA [24]. Dennis et al. [25] reported that the CR options showed a consistent anterior movement of the femur during knee flexion. The movement of femur in the opposite direction to the expected femoral roll back is called a paradoxical roll-forward.

14.2.3.2 Cruciate Retaining (CR or PCL Retaining) Type

Traditionally, flat tibial PE liner has been used for CR types, which theoretically allows intact PCL to occur natural femoral roll back during knee flexion. Theoretically, femoral roll back occurs more in CR type than PS type or CS type. Therefore, advocates of CR type insist it improves joint function, ROM, strength, and stability, reduces contact surface stress, and shows a more normal and efficient gait pattern, especially when climbing stairs [26]. Other advantages of the CR type include anteroposterior stability, improved proprioceptive sensation, good femoral roll back, increased abduction-adduction stability, and improved strength of quadriceps muscle which adds stability when going up and down stairs [27]. In addition, the angle of knee flexion is thought to be more increased and femoral bone to be more preserved compared to the PS type. Several designs of CR types have reported successful clinical outcome with a survival rate of more than 10–15 years over 95% [28–31]. In spite of these advantages, there were several disadvantages of CR types. PE insert in the early model of the CR type was thin and flat, so the load was excessively concentrated in one place, which produces an excessive PE wear. If the PCL is too tight, the femoral roll back would be excessive, and if it is too loose, the paradoxical femoral roll-forward may occur [32, 33]. If the PCL is not properly balanced when flexion or extension instability exists, the ligament may rupture later. In addition, the PCL rupture after CR TKA in inflammatory arthritis may lead to posterior instability.

14.2.3.3 Posterior Stabilized (PCL Substituting, PS) Type

The PCL is histologically not normal in patients with arthritis and significant degenerative changes were found in 63% of the PCL collected during surgery [34]. Montgomery et al. [27] reported that delayed rupture of the PCL occurs in the incidence of 2% after CR TKA, which may cause chronic instability, disabling pain, and revision TKA. To overcome the disadvantages of CR type, alternative bearing surface was introduced which substituted the PCL. Typical PS type TKA consists of a polyethylene tibial post that engages a cam on the femoral component, which is called cam-post design. PS type TKA is easy to correct the deformity and to obtain a joint compatibility, which can thereby reduce the wear of PE. It can also control the femoral roll back and show good clinical results regardless of technical differences among operators. Even with the severe deformity in sagittal or coronal plane, it can be easily corrected with PS type. In addition to this, there are several advantages of PS type TKA, such as technically easy surgery, kinematically reproducible femoral roll back mechanism, less PE wear, and easy correction of severe deformity. Disadvantages of PS type are dislocation of tibia post due to flexion gap imbalance, intercondylar fracture of the distal femur, patella fracture, patella clunk syndrome, and wear or fracture of the tibial post, etc. (Fig. 14.2).

14.2.3.4 Cruciate Sacrificing (CS) Type

CS type has no structure, such as cam-post, to complement the femoral roll back after removing the PCL. Shape of CS type is ultracongruent, deep dished anterior buildup appearance that reinforces the front of PE and deepens the articular surface of PE. The front side is reinforced with about 12.5 mm, while the lowest point (null point) of PE is located at about 4–6 mm posterior to form a ball-in-socket structure. By doing this, conformity can be increased and posterior stability can be obtained. The advantage of this design is that it can be used regardless of the preservation of the PCL and the anteroposterior mobility of the tibia and femur is kept constant, the bone loss is less than that of the PS type, and there is no wear or damage of the post. Parsley et al. [35] compared CS type with PS type, which showed a larger ROM in the PS group, but there was no difference in functional outcome (Fig. 14.3).

14.2.3.5 Varus-Valgus Constrained Prosthesis

The constrained condylar knee (CCK) or varus-valgus constrained (VVC) type implants have a larger and broader central post of tibial PE and a deep femoral box, which provide more inherent coronal plane stability than do PS prostheses. By this design characteristics, varus-valgus stability can be obtained, but since hyperextension cannot be controlled, it cannot be used for recurvatum deformity [36]. The CCK design can be used for revision surgery or for primary surgery in patients with unstable knee or extreme valgus deformity with medial collateral insufficiency [37].

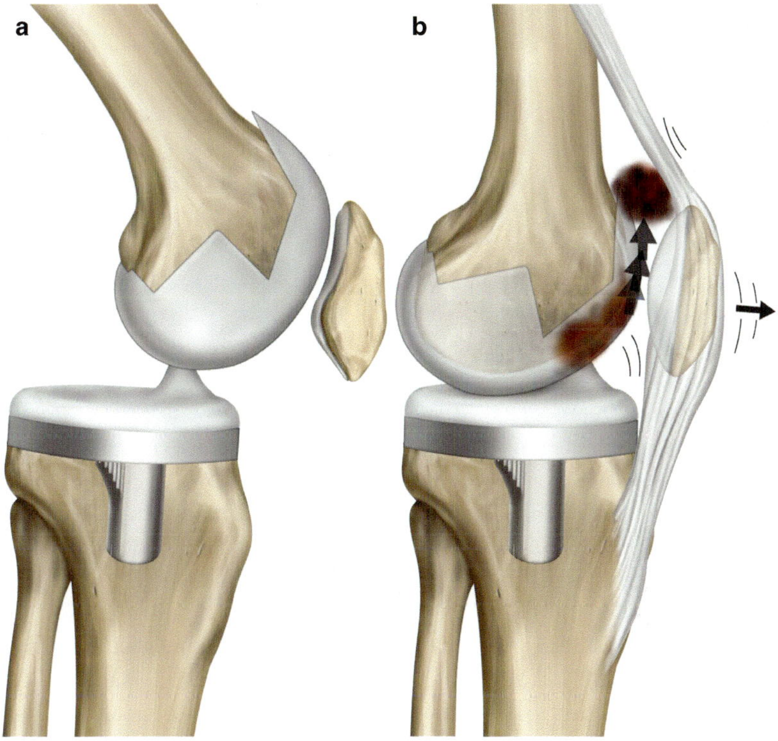

Fig. 14.2 Disadvantages of PS type TKA. (**a**) posterior dislocation of tibia in posterior stabilized knee might occurs in flexion instability, (**b**) patellar clunk syndrome. The scar tissue on the distal part of the quadriceps tendon falls into the intercondylar groove when the knee is flexed and then comes out when extended, causing pain and clunk sound

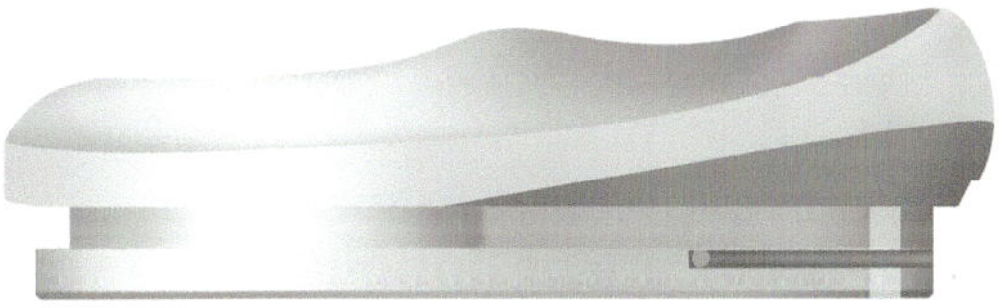

Fig. 14.3 Schematics of ultracongruent, deep dished anterior buildup PE prosthesis

14.2.3.6 Rotating Hinged Prosthesis

It is a fully constrained prosthesis. The tibial and femoral components of RH prosthesis are linked with an axle that restricts varus-valgus and translational stresses. RH prosthesis permits rotation of the tibial bearing around a yoke on the tibial platform to decrease the overall amount of constraint [37, 38]. It was designed for primary or revision option when there are severe bone defects, high degree ligament insufficiency, severe flexion and extension gap imbalance, and severe recurvatum deformity. It can also be used for limb salvage procedure after radical resection of tumor in the distal femur or proximal tibia [38].

14.2.4 Implant Design

14.2.4.1 Mobile Bearing Design

The concept of a mobile bearing is to permit unrestricted motion of PE between the femur and tibia while providing congruity of the joint surface. The main advantage is to reduce the contact stress between the components, and this type of joint surface minimizes wear and allows the movement of the PE insert to maintain joint motion and ligament function. Other advantages are that it reduces the contact stress on the joint surface, enables the rotational motion of the tibial PE when walking, and compensates for a small amount of rotational malalignment of the tibial base plate caused by the automatic alignment of the PE [39]. Even though the concept of dealing with the PE wear problem is attractive, there is no evidence of lowering the wear rate in the mobile bearing design in long-term follow-up studies. Furthermore, it cannot be said that it shows better results than fixed type design in terms of clinical prognosis and ROM [40, 41].

14.2.4.2 High Flexion Design

Knee ROM, especially knee flexion, is one of the most important factors determining success after TKA. However, knee flexion seldom exceeds 110–115° using conventional TKA design [42]. It has been tried to modify the femoral component design to enhance knee flexion after TKA. CR implant with high flexion design is usually not used because the PCL tension in CR type is occasionally inappropriate. The PS design is mostly used in high flexion design because the PE insert of PS type is more congruent and the post-cam is used to easily reproduce the femoral roll back. Disadvantages of high flexion design are high incidence of patellofemoral complication, the shear force to the femoral component increases due to the high flexion, which may lead to early loosening of the femoral prosthesis. Although some report the high flexion design showed better results in early ROM after surgery [43], others report that there was no significant difference in patient satisfaction and functional evaluation compared to the conventional design [44, 45].

14.2.5 Selection of Patellar Components

Patellar components can be classified according to their composition, fixing method, and placement and shape of the patella prosthesis. In terms of composition, it is classified into a metal-backed patella, which is an early design, and an all-PE type, which is mainly used in recent years. Metal-backed patella is rarely used nowadays because the thickness of PE is thin, which makes PE wear occur more easily. All-PE patella implant is usually fixed with cement, and there is a peg at the bottom to facilitate fixing. If there is one peg, the fixing force is weak and it can easily cause a patella fracture, so the 3 peg type is widely used. However, even in the 3 peg type, the peg may be damaged, so the connection part is improved to be thicker to withstand repeated shearing force. It can be classified by location into an onset type that is placed on a flatly excised patella and an inset type that is planted in the excised bone. The inset type is a dome shaped implant with one peg and was developed to thicken PE or to be used when there is a bone defect, but it is rarely used because of its complicated surgical technique and a risk of a patella fracture. Onset type is commonly used, but it has some disadvantages such as fragility to shearing force, possibility of patellar inclination, and that the fixed peg may be damaged [46, 47]. The shape is classified into circular shape, oval shape, and anatomical shape according to the shape of the dome. The circular shape itself does not have an axis for tracking, so it is easy to operate. Elliptical or ovoid shape is known to perform better sliding motion than the circular shape. However, if the axis is not aligned correctly, a patellar maltracking occurs. The anatomical type resembles the native patella in morphology closely, so theoretically the patellar tracking should be the best. However, it is a technically demanding procedure because the restoration of anatomical shape of patella is difficult. Other than that, there is a sombrero type, which is a variant of circular type, theoretically resistant to abrasion by thickening the edge [46, 47].

14.3 Preoperative Preparation and Patient Optimization

14.3.1 Medical Evaluation

The main purpose of preoperative medical evaluation is to apprehend surgery-related risks beforehand and minimize perioperative morbidity of the patient. Most of the patients receiving TKA are old aged peoples and are more likely to deteriorate cardiovascular and respiratory function. These patient groups are usually accompanied with hypertension, diabetes, and osteoporosis which all increase postoperative complication. Therefore, safety of the patient must be guaranteed after evaluation and treatment of preexisting conditions, supplementary tests for postoperative management, and cooperation with another medical department.

14.3.1.1 Cardiovascular Disease

Hypertension

Hypertension must be checked during preoperative interview and physical examination. Generally, in planned surgery such as TKA, hypertension lower than 180/110 mmHg does not increase risk of cardiovascular complication, and TKA can be performed while maintaining proper blood pressure before the surgery. However, patients with high blood pressure over 180/110 mmHg must be postponed of the surgery until it is downregulated. If hypertension is confirmed before surgery, other cardiovascular risk factors and hypertension medication prescription must be evaluated and appropriate medical consultation is needed. Β-blocker, among all antihypertensive medication, is used as drug of choice for hypertension as it reduces risk of cardiovascular complication and mortality, while it has a risk of postoperative atrial fibrillation. Diuretic, angiotensin converter enzyme inhibitor (ACEi), and angiotensin receptor blocker (ARB) can cause electrolyte imbalance and hypotension during the surgery, whose administration must be stopped on the day of surgery and be resumed after the patient has fully recovered [48].

Arrhythmia

Arrhythmia is an independent risk factor that increases risk of coronary artery disease before and after the surgery. Lately, as many patients with arrhythmia tend to have pacemakers or take anticoagulants, type and program of pacemaker must be checked before surgery, and the pacemaker mode must be changed after consultation with cardiologist. In general, when patients are dependent on pacemaker, it must be changed to non-synchronized mode and in those with implantable defibrillator, the program is recommended to be stopped. In addition, if the patient is taking anticoagulant, appropriate cessation period must be kept as it may interrupt hemostasis during perioperative periods [48].

Heart Failure

If there is a history of congestive heart failure, aggressive volume loading should be avoided perioperatively because of the possibility of pulmonary edema and peripheral edema.

14.3.1.2 Endocrine Disease

Diabetes Mellitus (DM)

Diabetes is commonly accompanied by other medical conditions like renal failure or chronic cardiac ischemia and peripheral circulatory disease. Moreover, diabetes causes problem in recovery of postoperative wound. No other special treatments are needed if the blood glucose is controlled at less than 200 mg/dl in fasting state and less than 7.0 HbA1c level before the surgery, but if not, the glucose must be controlled with preoperative insulin injection. In addition, diabetes patients also commonly have nephropathy, so NSAIDs use must be cautious in postoperative pain control [49].

Long-term Corticosteroids User

Most OA patients are taking various types of pain medication for long time. Especially, when taking steroids for long period, adrenal function is highly likely to be depressed, resulting in unstable blood pressure during the surgery. Therefore, adrenal insufficiency must be evaluated, and corticosteroids injection should be considered perioperatively. In TKA, 50–75 mg of hydrocortisone is to be administered on the day of surgery or daily administration after gradual attenuation for 1–2 days after 10–15 mg of methylprednisolone injection [50].

14.3.1.3 Chronic Renal Disease

Patients with chronic renal disease may show anemia, dysfunctional platelet, chronic metabolic acidosis, and electrolyte and calcium imbalance. Evaluating patients who are receiving dialysis for chronic renal disease must be cautious as it may increase myocardial enzymes. As NSAIDs have great impact on renal perfusion, patients with renal dysfunction must avoid them. Patients having dialysis must be conscious of volume loading, hypercalcemia, and acidosis [51].

14.3.1.4 Psychiatric Comorbidities

The prevalence of psychiatric disorders in patients undergoing TKA exceeded 20%, which is higher than that of the general population. Psychiatric comorbidities are associated with negative short-term and long-term outcomes after TKA, particularly for physical function, quality of life, patient satisfaction, as well as pain and the use of analgesic medication. Psychiatric comorbidities such as anxiety, depression, or somatization disorder should be evaluated before TKA [52].

14.3.2 Preoperative Preparation for Patients Taking Medications

14.3.2.1 Non-steroidal Anti-inflammatory Drugs

NSAIDs inhibit formation of platelet-derived thromboxane A2 with COX-1 inhibition and impede thromboxane-dependent platelet aggregation, increasing bleeding time. As such interaction is reversible, antithrombotic effect of NSAIDs is not occurred after drug cessation for 5 times the half-life (Table 14.1).

14.3.2.2 Antithrombotic Drug

People with senile medical diseases or history take antithrombotic medications such as aspirin, and recently, antithrombotic drugs are increasingly being used for preventive purposes even for those without symptoms [53]. It is recommended that preoperative use of aspirin must be ceased 7–10 days before surgery due to lifespan of hemoglobin [54]. But, a recent study showed low dose aspirin (100 mg) did not result in more blood loss [55]. In general, aspirin and clopidogrel bisulfate need to be stopped 7–10 days for restoring the anticoagulation effect. Patient taking both aspirin and clopidogrel bisulfate may be recommended to stop taking clopidogrel bisulfate 7–10 days and aspirin 5 days before surgery (Table 14.2).

14.3.2.3 Anti-rheumatic Drug

Anti-rheumatic drugs are metabolized through multiple pathways and have variable half-lives. Methotrexate metabolite is removed via renal excretion, and patients with deteriorated renal function may show bone marrow suppres-

Table 14.2 Typical antithrombotic drugs and recommended discontinuation days

Ingredient name	Product name	Number of days to stop
Apixaban	Eliquis	5
Aspirin	Aspirin Astrix	7
Aspirin + Clopidogrel	Clopirin	7
Cilostazol	Cilo V Plataal SR	3
Clopidogrel	Plateless Plavix	5
Ginko bliloba Ext	Ginexin F	1
Limaprost	Opalmon	1
Rivaroxaban	Xarelto	5
Warfarin sodium	Warfarin	5

Table 14.1 Half-life and preoperative treatment of commonly used NSAIDs

NSAIDs	Half-life (hr)	Preoperative treatment
Naproxen	12–15	Stop 4 days before surgery
Ibuprofen	1.8–2	Stop 1 day before surgery
Diclofenac	2	Stop 1 day before surgery
Nabumetone	23–24	Stop 5 days before surgery
Piroxicam	50	Stop 10 days before surgery

sion due to the toxic metabolite. Therefore, it is recommended to cease the drug for 1 week before and after surgery in healthy patients and 2 weeks in poor general condition patients [56]. Leflunomide has long half-life, it is generally recommended to be discontinued for 2 weeks before the surgery and resumed 3 days after the surgery. Sulfasalazine and azathioprine have relatively short half-life and are excreted via kidney. So they should be discontinued from 1 day before the surgery until third day after the surgery. Clinical data are insufficient, and anti-TNF-α agents must be discontinued 1 week before the surgery and resumed 10–14 days after the surgery, while IL-1 inhibitor is recommended to be discontinued 1–2 days before the surgery and resumed 10 days after the surgery [56].

14.3.3 Knee Specific Evaluation

14.3.3.1 Preoperative Examination

The patient must be inquired of level of pain and function of involved knee, past medical history and other comorbidity, and especially, it must be differentially diagnosed if it is vascular disease in lower limb or hip joint and spine disease. On physical examination, soft tissue status around knee, deformity and instability of the joint must be examined. ROM is generally measured in passive ROM. Patients with extension deficiency might be needed a different surgical method depending on its cause, whether it is due to flex ion contracture or extension lag. In addition, as strength of quadriceps muscle greatly affects prognosis, strength of quadriceps and hamstring muscle must be measured. Before TKA, infection risk must be assessed. If the surgery is performed with infection not only in knee but also remote part, the risk of periprosthetic deep infection is increased. Pulmonary or urinary tract infection, recent tooth extraction, intra-articular injection must be checked before the surgery, and any intra-articular injection or acupuncture is prohibited until the surgery.

14.3.3.2 Preoperative Radiologic and Other Examination

Radiographic examination is essential for preoperative planning of TKA. Radiographic view for TKA should include both knee standing AP, lateral, axial view and whole leg standing AP view. Prior to surgery, the degree of arthritis, ligamentous instability, intra-articular loose body, and size and location of the bone defect should be evaluated. Varus-valgus stress X-ray should be taken in case of ligamentous instability that might be needed a more constraint insert. If significant bone defect is observed, bone defect management should be planned. It is also necessary to predict the extent of bone resection during surgery, size and location of the implant by radiographs. Whole leg standing AP view is essential for assessing the alignment of the lower extremities and predicting the bone resection in advance to obtain satisfactory alignment of the lower extremities after TKA. Mechanical and anatomical axis of lower limb is also measured on whole leg standing AP view. CT and MRI are not always needed in TKA patients. However, CT scan is useful for evaluating rotational alignment and bone defect of the knee joint. MRI is helpful for evaluating the accompanying soft tissue problems or inflammatory disorder. If inflammatory arthritis is suspected, serologic examination and joint fluid analysis should be performed before the surgery.

14.4 Surgical Techniques

14.4.1 Innervation and Blood Supply

14.4.1.1 Blood Supply

The anterior part of the knee joint is composed of thin skin and incorrect incisions may cause would healing problems, which might lead to complications. The blood vessels on the anterior side of the knee are largely composed of external and internal blood vessels. The external blood vessels consist of branches originating from the descending genicular artery that arises from the superficial femoral artery just before it passes through the adductor hiatus, and the saphenous branch and articular branch are the main branches. These structures eventually supply the subcutaneous tissue and skin layer, thus highly influencing the wound healing. The internal blood vessels are composed of lateral superior genicular artery, medial superior genicular artery, lateral inferior genicular artery, and medial inferior genicular artery and are located under the deep fascia to form a ring around the patella. The external and internal blood vessels are interconnected via a perforating artery that penetrates the deep fascia (Fig. 14.4a, b). The descending genicular artery originates from the medial side running to the lateral side. For this reason, if the skin incision is performed from the medial side, it is highly likely that the external blood vessels will be damaged; therefore, it is better to perform the skin incision from the lateral side if possible (Fig. 14.5).

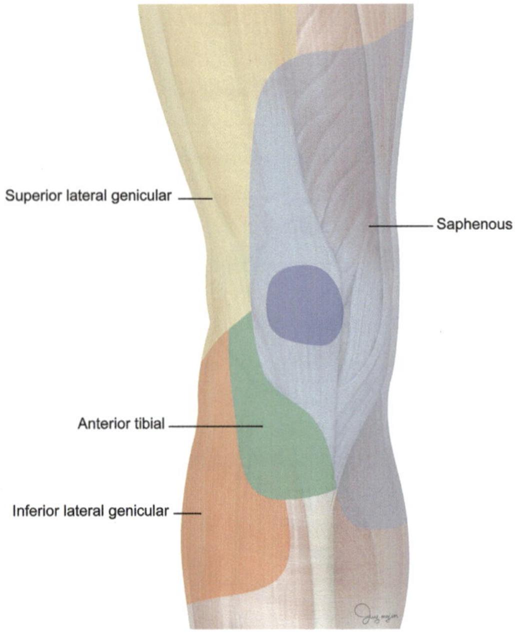

Fig. 14.5 The main vascular supply area of the epidermis of the right knee joint

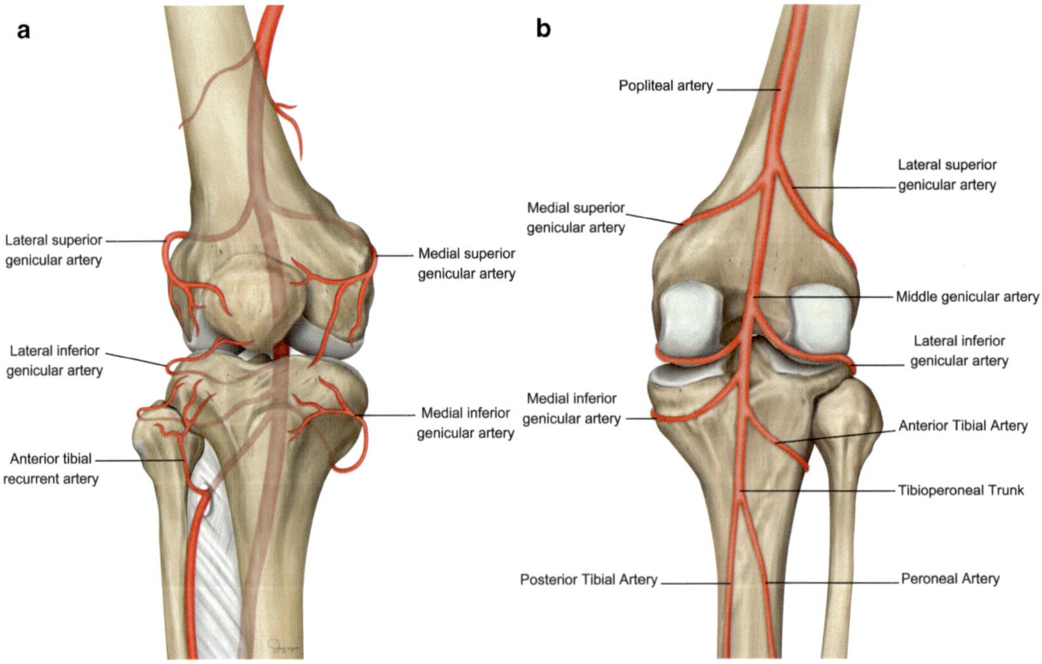

Fig. 14.4 Blood supply around knee joint. (**a**) view from anterior aspect, (**b**) view from posterior aspect

14.4.1.2 Nerve Innervation

After TKA, a significant number of patients complain of decreased sensation in the lateral region of the incision line. The nerves that innervate anterior knee joint are largely composed of four. In the femur, the medial cutaneous nerve of thigh and the intermediate cutaneous nerve of thigh run across from the medial part to the lateral part. In the tibia, the infrapatellar branch of saphenous nerve runs across from the medial to the lateral side. Lateral cutaneous nerve of calf, which is a branch of the common peroneal nerve innervates to the lateral side of knee joint. The longer the incision line to the upper part of the patella, the more likely it is that the skin nerve branches in the femoral side is damaged, thus resulting in decreased sensation after surgery. As for the infrapatellar branch of saphenous nerve, when an incision is performed to the tibial tuberosity, the damage on the nerve is inevitable. Occasionally, some patients do not complain of decreased skin sensation after surgery, either because of the variability of innervation or because the lateral cutaneous nerve of the lower leg overlaps with the control area (Fig. 14.6).

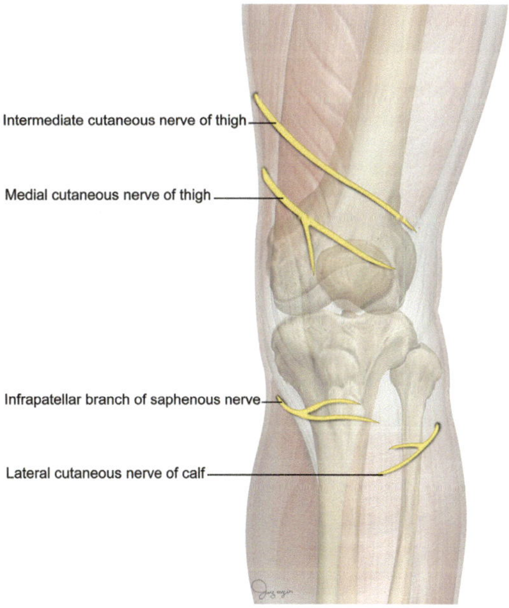

Fig. 14.6 Cutaneous nerve distribution around left knee joint

14.4.2 Drape and Tourniquet Use

The importance of drape in preventing postoperative infection cannot be overstated. Whole leg including surgical site should be sterilized thoroughly with betadine and alcohol using non-touch technique. The operating table must be wrapped with a tarpaulin to prevent possible contamination caused by liquid penetration. The skin should be fully covered with surgical drape so that the exposed area for surgery is not exposed to the air and does not interfere with bending and stretching the knee. Tourniquet is wrapped up to the proximal thigh to the maximum. Wrapping an auxiliary tool such as a cotton ball under the tourniquet is helpful in minimizing chafing. Wrapping a tourniquet minimizes bleeding, which helps to secure the surgical field of view for an accurate surgery. However, using a tourniquet may cause cardiovascular problems. Relative increase in cardiovascular blood flow causes a temporary increase in blood pressure, which in turn may lead to pulmonary edema and heart attack. For this reason, whether to use a tourniquet for a patient with cardiopulmonary disease or vascular disease should be cautious. Generally, the pressure is about twice the systolic blood pressure of the patient undergoing surgery, usually raised to 300–350 mmHg. However, for patients with large bodies, the pressure of 300 mmHg is insufficient, which may cause bleeding in the cancellous bone and the marrow cavity. However, even when the pressure of a tourniquet was less than 225 mmHg, the operation was effectively completed without postoperative complications [57]. This pressure is applied up to two hours, and if the surgery is prolonged, the tourniquet is briefly loosened and pressed again. Recently, several studies claimed that the use of tourniquet has no benefit on performing TKA [58–60].

14.4.3 Surgical Approach

The surgical approach affects the entire process of surgery from start to finish. During the surgical approach, sufficient visibility should be obtained.

In addition, surgical approach should ensure that the surgical procedure is carried out without damaging important anatomical structures. Since important nerves and blood vessels are located behind the knee, the anterior approaches for TKA are preferred.

14.4.3.1 Skin Incision

Skin incision should be made in a way that does not interfere with surgical procedure, while it does not cause problems concerning cosmetic and wound healing. As the skin of the knee is relatively thin, the joints are close to the skin. This increases the risk of deep infection, which requires much attention. For patients with thin and fragile skin, the incision should be made as long as possible to avoid applying excessive tension to the skin. Surgical scars are found in patients who had knee surgery before. Arthroscopic surgery scar is not much concern, however if there is a transverse incision scar, new incision should be performed tangentially. If there is a longitudinal incision scar, using the existing incision line as possible is recommended. However, if a completely new incision line is needed, a distance of at least 6 cm from old incision is required in principle. Considering that the blood flow coming from the medial side is more abundant and the blood flow from the lateral part is relatively poor, it is desirable to make an incision as more lateral side as possible (Fig. 14.7).

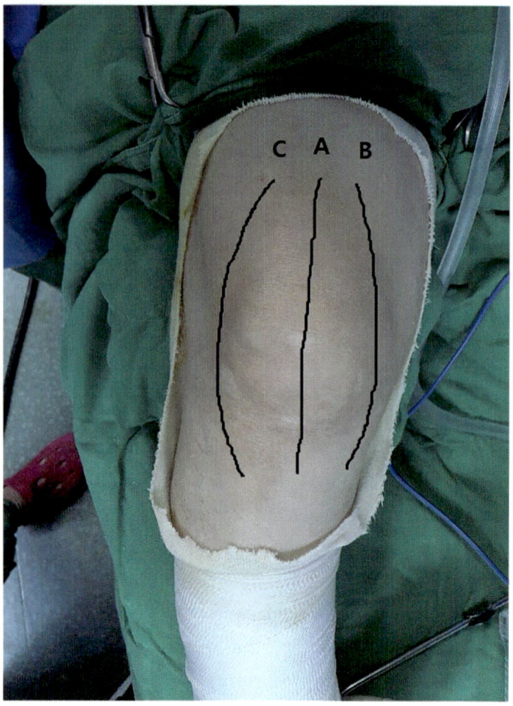

Fig. 14.7 Skin incision (**a**) midline (**b**) paramedial (**c**) anterolateral

In principle, the skin incision line during TKA is made vertically. The anterior skin incision is made straight midline, curvilinear medial or lateral para-patella according to location. Most preferred incision is straight midline incision. Midline incision is a method in which a straight incision is made passing through the center of the patella, from about 6–8 cm from the upper pole of the patella to about 1–3 cm below the patellar tendon attachment. The midline incision has the advantage that the incision can be easily extended up and down, if necessary. It is important that the incision ends in the medial than the tibial tuberosity at the distal part, which is beneficial for wound healing and minimizes dysfunction such as irritation caused by scarring. A medial para-patella incision is a method in which the start point and the end of an incision are similar to the midline incision, but the center of the incision lies in the medial side to the patella. Due to anatomical problems, it may cause wound healing problems and reoperation is difficult. For such reasons, this method is not often used nowadays. A lateral para-patella (anterolateral) incision is a method in which the start and end of the incision are similar to the midline incision, but the center of the incision lies in the lateral side of patella. Although this method has the advantage of being able to save the blood vessels supplying blood to the adjacent skin, the downside is that it is difficult to obtain a surgical visualization during surgery because arthrotomy is made in the lateral side. In general, this approach is useful for TKA in patients with severe valgus deformity.

14.4.3.2 Capsular Approaches

The standard approaches include a medial parapatellar approach, a subvastus approach, a midv-

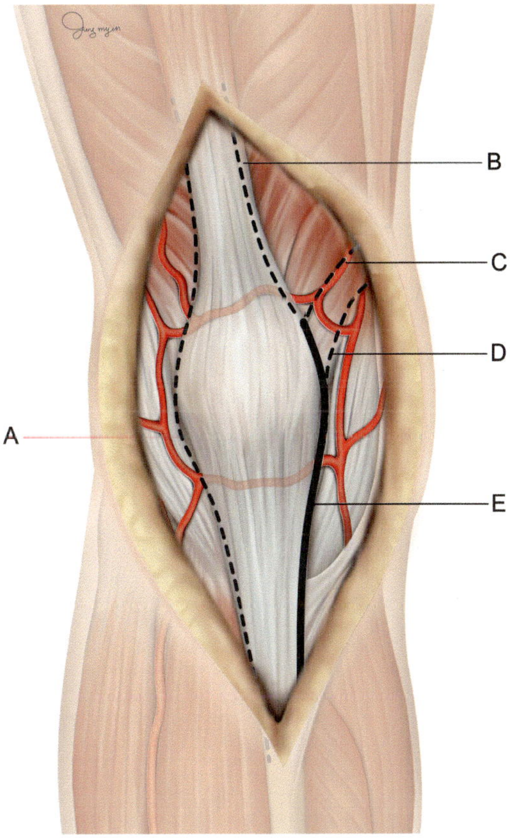

Fig. 14.8 The relationship between the distribution of blood vessels around the patella and joint incision method. (**A**) Anterolateral approach, (**B**) Medial parapatellar arthrotomy, (**C**) Midvastus arthrotomy, (**D**) Subvastus arthrotomy, (**E**) Quadriceps-sparing appraoch

astus approach, and an anterolateral approach (Fig. 14.8).

Medial Parapatellar Approach

The medial parapatellar approach is currently the most widely used. The advantage is that this method allows obtaining a surgical field of view more easily, the operation is not much difficult and it enables the extension of incision up and downwards. The incision for the area of the quadriceps tendon is made in the center or medial of this tendon or on the vastus medialis. As when incisions are made to the vastus medialis, problems such as bleeding, pain, and fibrosis of the muscles may arise, incisions are usually made in the medial 1/3 of the quadriceps tendon. The downside is that blood vessels from the medial side can be damaged and it may bring postoperative extension weakness.

Subvastus Approach

Subvastus approach is made along the medial side of the vastus medialis obliquus instead of making an incision on the quadriceps tendon, and then the entire extension mechanism is dislocated laterally. The skin incision is the same as the anterior midline incision, after that, an incision is made as the superficial fascia covering the vastus medialis and the incision reaches to the medial side of the vastus medialis. The vastus medialis can be elevated by blunt dissection from the intermuscular septum, which is approximately 10 cm above the adductor tubercle. Attention should be paid to avoid injury to the neurovascular contents of adductor canal. This method has several merits. There is no damage to the superior genicular artery going to the medial side of the patella. Furthermore, it might be helpful to the postoperative patella tracking because there is no damage to the extension mechanism. Curtin et al. [61] reported that with this approach, the extension mechanism was not impaired, thereby decreasing pain until 6 weeks after surgery. Tomek et al. [62] compared the subvastus approach to the medial parapatellar and found that in the group using the subvastus approach, there was less pain at rest on day 1 after surgery and at activity on day 3 after surgery, but still there was no meaningful difference in other factors.

Midvastus Approach

The midvastus muscle splitting arthrotomy is that the middle part of the vastus medialis is split in the direction of the muscle fibers at 4–5 cm of the superomedial part of the patella, and the joint incision is extended to the medial part of the patellar tendon. It is easier to evert the patella with midvastus approach than with the subvastus approach. This approach has the advantage of maintaining the extension mechanism as it preserves the nerves going to the quadriceps tendon of the upper patella and the vastus medialis, and the blood flow to the patella is preserved to some extent. White et al. [63] reported that this approach can be applied to obese patients or patients with severe deformity and even patients who have previously operated with this incision approach. Dalury et al. [64] reported that midvastus approach, compared to the medial parapatellar approach, has merits in that fewer lateral retinacular releases are required, and has advantages in terms of postoperative pain and earlier return to function for the first 6 months. However, there was no such difference after the first 6 months.

Anterolateral Approach

This approach opens the joint from the lateral part of the patella and is limitedly used in patients with valgus deformity. With an anterolateral incision of the skin, an incision is made from the lateral margin of the quadriceps tendon, along the patella and the lateral part of the patellar tendon, to the lateral part of the tibial tuberosity. This approach allows the blood circulation of the medial part to be preserved and correction to be made by directly reaching the deformity area. In addition, it enables less peeling of the skin and the gradual release of soft tissue in the lateral side. However, it is difficult to make eversion of the patella medially, not easy to obtain a good surgical view, and it might cause soft tissue defects in the lateral part. If necessary, the lateral arthrotomy can be used as a lateral release to help the patella tracking by leaving it opened.

Medial Trivector Retaining Approach

This approach aims to maintain the normal tracking of the patella by preserving the anatomic trivector arrangement of quadriceps. This approach is designed to retain the quadriceps muscle by cutting the medial vastus vertically at the medial part of the quadriceps tendon and by making an incision on the medial part of the patellar tendon and tibial tuberosity at the distal part. This approach is performed with the knee flexed 90°–110° so that the quadriceps muscle is under maximal tension and thinned out as much as possible during the incision. However, in fact, it is not often recommended as it weakens muscle strength by cutting the medial vastus, thus resulting in subluxation of the patella more often and blocks blood flow from the inside (Fig. 14.9).

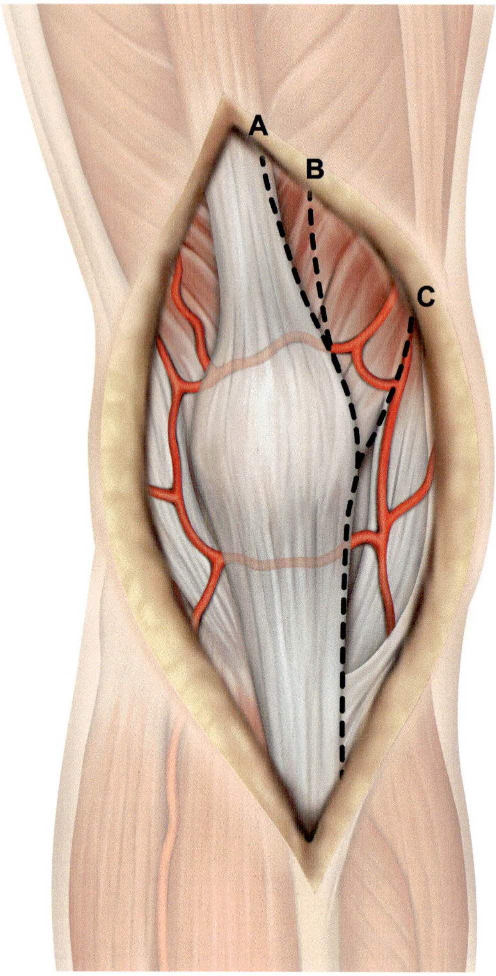

Fig. 14.9 Location relationship between Medial trivector retaining arthrotomy and other approach methods. (**a**) paramedial arthrotomy, (**b**) trivector retaining arthrotomy, (**c**) subvastus arthrotomy

14.4.3.3 Extensile Approach

In the case with ankylosed knee joint, there is always a risk of rupture of the extensor mechanism on performing TKA. If excessive force is applied to evert the patella or flex the knee for joint exposure in stiff knees, it may cause rupture of the patellar tendon and/or quadriceps tendon, or a patellar fracture. This tendency is particularly common in rheumatic patients or patients with severe osteopenia. Since injury to the knee extensor mechanism can seriously deteriorate the function of the knee joint, it must be avoided. Extensile approach is indicated when there is a risk of damage to extension mechanism during capsular approach. Extensile approaches include rectus snip, V–Y or Z-quadricepsplasty, tibial tubercle osteotomy.

Rectus Snip

This technique extends the proximal incision of the medial parapatellar approach to the proximal part, and then creates a 45° oblique incision laterally across the quadriceps tendon to the vastus lateralis. As the tibia is externally rotated and patella subluxated laterally, the joint is exposed without tension on the extensor mechanism. This technique has merits in that it is simple, prevents extensor lag and preserves the vastus medialis and the superior lateral genicular artery (Fig. 14.10a).

VY Quadricepsplasty, Quadriceps Turndown and Z-plasty

VY quadricepsplasty is a technique developed by Coonse and Adams that involves creating an inverted V-shaped incision with the proximal part of the quadriceps tendon as the apex and the distal part as the base. It allows the quadriceps tendon to be moved to the distal part, so it is useful for restoring the knee flexion movement when there has been contraction of the quadriceps tendon due to the limitation of flexion for a long time. While it has the advantage of securing a sufficient field of view as the patella can be turned down, the disadvantages include that blood supply to the patella is blocked, which increases the frequency of avascular necrosis of the patella and that the weakening of the quadriceps strength or the extension lag is inevitable. There is modification of the quadriceps turndown approach to preserve inferior lateral genicular artery. A medial parapatellar arthrotomy was performed, and second incision was made at an inclination of 45 degrees from the apex of the quadriceps tendon and extended distally and laterally through the vastus lateralis and the upper part of the iliotibial tract. This lateral incision must stop short of the inferior lateral geniculate artery (Fig. 14.10b).

Tibia Tubercle Osteotomy

This technique is useful for patients with severe contracture or fibrous ankylosis. Whiteside et al. [65] recommended elevating about 8–10 cm length fragment including the tibial tuberosity and the anterior tibial crest with anterolateral soft tissue attachment. It is desirable that the bone fragment be approximately 8–10 cm long with 2 cm in mediolateral (ML) width, in which the thickness would be about 1 cm from the anterior to the posterior, and the distal part be gradually beveled. During osteotomy, the soft tissue should be kept attached to the bone fragment in the lateral part in order to preserve blood supply as possible. If there is patella baja, improvement is expected by relocating the tibial tuberosity to the proximal part when fixating the tibial tuberosity. The advantages include that it offers great visualization, the position of the tibial tuberosity is adjustable, and it can be used to remove the tibial prosthesis during revision surgery. However, the disadvantages are that there is postoperative anterior knee pain and that it accompanies complications such as nonunion of osteotomy site, a fracture of the bone fragment, rupture of the patella tendon, or infection. It is recommended to use a wire for the revision TKA for less complication than to use a screw (Fig. 14.10c, d).

14.4.4 Soft Tissue Management Before Bone Resection

After joint exposure, the soft tissue in the knee joint must be properly managed to ensure a proper implementation of TKA such as bone resection and ligament balancing. Soft tissue management before bone resection includes removal of infrapatellar fat pad, resection of both menisci, removal of anterior cruciate ligament (ACL), and preliminary medial or lateral soft tissue release. The first soft tissue encountered after joint exposure is the infrapatellar fat pad. If TKA is performed with infrapatellar fat pad left, it has the advantage of preserving the blood supply at the anterior knee joint. On the other hand, leaving the fat pad blocks the surgical field and interferes with the surgical process.

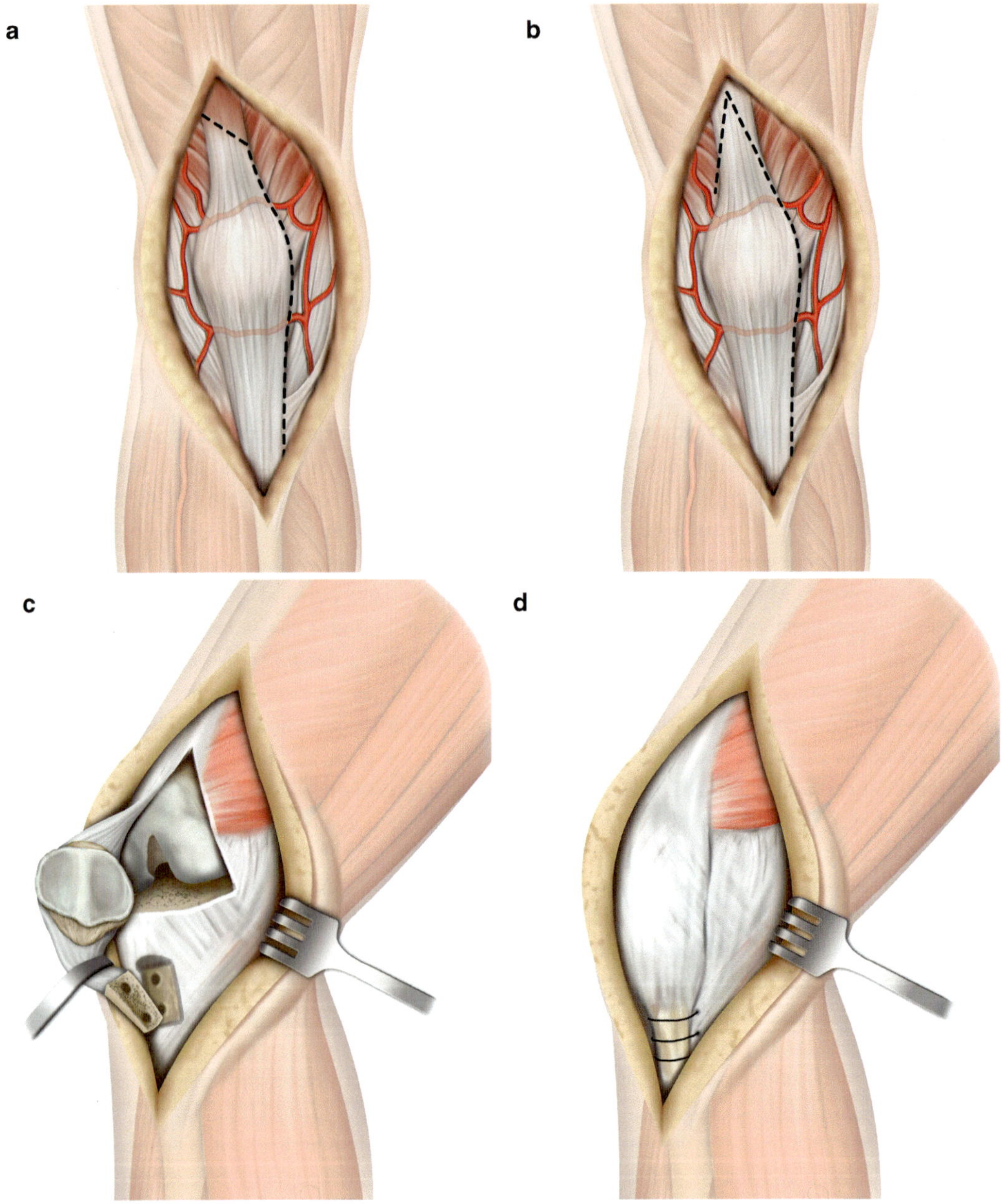

Fig. 14.10 Extensile approach. (**a**) Rectus snip, (**b**) VY quadricepsplasty, (**c, d**) Tibia tubercle osteotomy

Therefore, in order to obtain an appropriate visualization and prevent the fat pad impingement, it is inevitable to remove it to some extent and in particular, the anteromedial fat pad (Fig. 14.11). However, removing fat pad too much results in shortening of the patellar tendon, thereby leading to patella baja that might cause anterior knee pain. Preliminary medial or lateral soft tissue release should be performed just for the surgical exposure but not for full correction of deformity. If contacted medial or lateral soft tissues release fully during surgical exposure, it might induce ligamentous imbalance after bone resection. Therefore, preliminary soft tissue

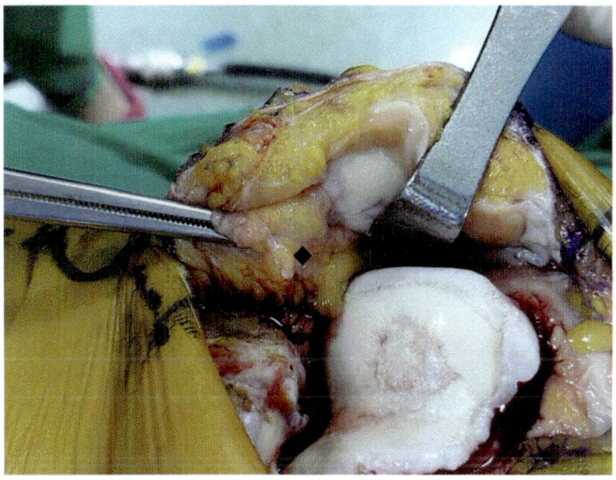

Fig. 14.11 Removing method of infrapatellar fat pad. Catching by Kocher forceps (♦) and excise appropriate amount for visualization

release should be performed only to a certain extent, and after implantation, a fine adjustment should be done to finally balance the ligaments. Ligament tissues should not cut transversely, but are released subperiosteally in a sleeved form. In modern designed TKA, the anterior cruciate ligament (ACL) is removed first. If CR type prosthesis is to be used, PCL should be carefully preserved. If the PCL shows a severe degenerative changes or has become thin and weak, PS type prosthesis should be considered to use. If PCL is too tight, recession is still possible, but it is desirable to make decision whether to use CR type or PS type after inserting the provisional prosthesis. During the resection of the ligament, the middle genicular artery is inevitably severed, therefore it is better to find the bleeding site and immediately cauterize it. Since the medial meniscus is firmly attached to the deep MCL, the peripheral margin is not easily distinguishable with naked eye. For this reason, if it is cut too much, the MCL may be weakened, while if it is cut too less, the remaining meniscal tissue impinges with prosthesis. As for the lateral meniscus too, if it is cut too less, remaining tissue impinges with the prosthesis, while if it is cut too much, the lateral inferior genicular artery may be injured, causing a serious loss of blood (Fig. 14.12). It is important to note that all the bleeding part should be cauterized.

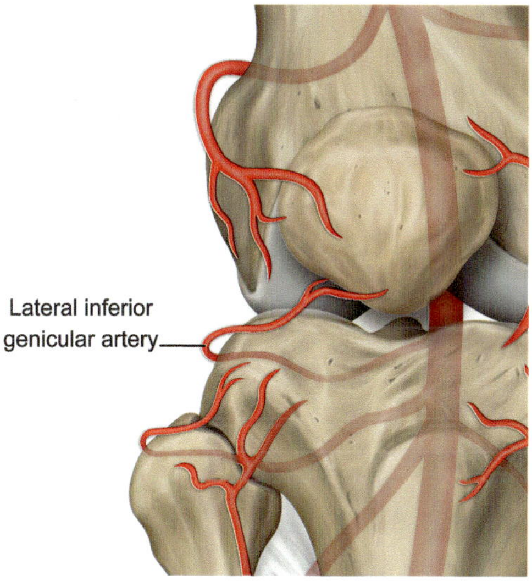

Fig. 14.12 Lateral inferior genicular artery

14.4.5 Principles of Bone Resection and Prosthesis Alignment

One of the most important factors in the longevity of a prosthesis in TKA is the alignment of the lower limb. In order to make an accurate restoration of the lower limb alignment, every effort to improve accuracy and reproducibility by using specialized surgical instruments should be made. Furthermore, it is necessary for understanding normal anatomy and biomechanics of the normal lower limb to enhance an accurate restoration of the lower limb alignment.

14.4.5.1 Theoretical Basis for Lower Limb Alignment

Lower Limb Alignment

The lower limb alignment should be considered based on the coronal, sagittal, and axial plane. The important concepts for the coronal alignment include the mechanical axis and the anatomical axis. The mechanical axis is a line connecting from center of the femoral head to center of the talus on the lower extremity scanogram with patients in full weight bearing, erect position. Normally, this line passes through center of the knee. Anatomical axis is the line passing center of the femoral and tibial shaft, respectively. The angle between the mechanical and anatomical axes in the femur is known to be approximately 60° and in the two axes coincides in the tibia. The center of body weight in an upright position is located in more medial than the femoral head, and the angle between the mechanical axis and the body weight axis is known to be about 3°. The tibial plateau is rather varus 3° to the mechanical axis, so the axis of the body weight forms a right angle to the tibia plateau. The axis of the body weight moves medially from the part where it forms about 3° angle form the tibia plateau, and this can vary depending on the length and shape of each person's pelvis, femur, and tibia.

In terms of the sagittal plane, the mechanical axis does not bear much significance as the center of weight-bearing axis greatly depends on the flexion angle of the ankle or knee. For this reason, making alignment in terms of the sagittal plane has not been paid much attention. The bony tibial plateau is known to form a posterior inclination angle of about 10° in sagittal plane. The posterior inclination angle of the tibia joint surface with meniscus is less than 10° and almost horizontal. This is because the posterior horn of the meniscus is thicker than the anterior horn, moderating the pure posterior inclination of the bone. The rotational alignment is associated with the medial and lateral balancing during flexion and is related to patellofemoral alignment (Fig. 14.13).

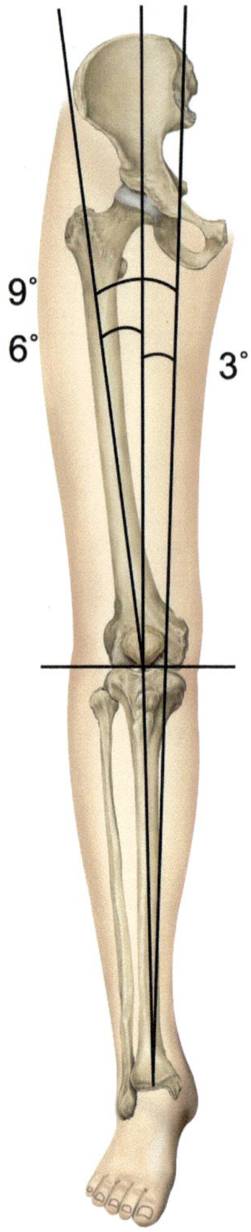

Fig. 14.13 Anatomical and mechanical alignment of lower extremities

Resection Method to Restore Lower Limb Alignment

There are classical and anatomical methods for performing bone resection in the coronal plane during TKA (Fig. 14.14a, b). The classical method is the most widely used method, in which the distal femur and the proximal tibia are cut perpendicular to the mechanical axis. As a result, the line connecting the center of the hip joint and the center of the ankle joint passes through the center of the knee joint. The classical method has the advantage in that it has excellent reproducibility. Classical method occasionally resulted in valgus alignment. However, valgus alignment should be avoided as it may cause gait disturbance. According to Bellemans et al. [66], constitutional varus with 3 degrees or more was found in 22% in males and 17% in females, and if bone resection is performed to fit with the mechanical axis, patients could complain of a significant discomfort, though it may be helpful for long-term survivorship. Therefore, a minor varus rather fits with biomechanics, thereby reducing discomfort. The anatomical method was introduced by Hungerford et al. [67], and since the tibial plateau is 3° varus with respect to the anatomical axis, the proximal tibia is cut to be 3° varus to the tibial long axis, and the distal femur is cut 3° valgus than the mechanical axis accordingly. Anatomical method has the advantage of cutting the proximal tibia parallel to the ground

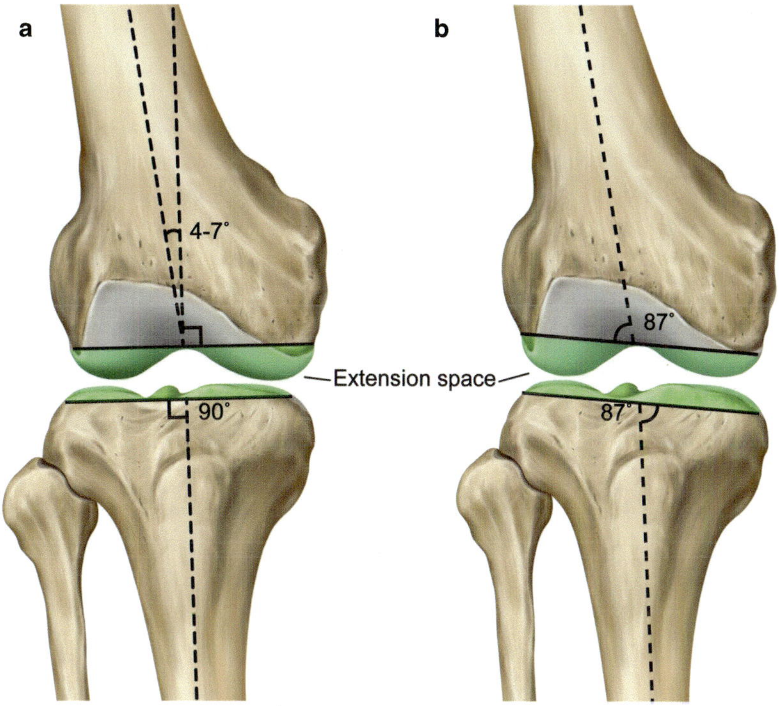

Fig. 14.14 Resection method. (**a**) traditional method, (**b**) anatomic method

to maintain a physiological joint function during gait. However, cutting 3° varus with respect to the tibia long axis reduces reproducibility. 3° varus resection of the proximal tibia is often resulted in more varus deformity with more than 3° and there is high risk of damage to the lateral collateral ligament since much of the lateral side of distal femur is resected with 3° valgus cut. If a tibial prosthesis is placed parallel to tibial plateau which has 3° varus to mechanical axis, it is highly likely that a more load concentrate to the medial side and wear can progress in the medial side. For these reasons, this method is not widely used at present.

Kinematic Alignment

Kinematic alignment refers to restoring of the alignment between the femur, tibia, and patella to the state before arthritis in terms of the coronal, sagittal, and axial planes. 20% of patients who had received TKA using traditional mechanical alignment methods resulted in unsatisfactory outcomes. Bone resection using kinematic alignment reduced pain, motion limitation, and instability, etc. compared to bone resection with the mechanical method [68]. Kinematic alignment TKA restores the natural pre-arthritic joint lines of the knee by performing distal femur and proximal tibia cut to restore the natural angle and level of the joint lines, which means the tibial component is aligned in natural varus. Bone resection based on the kinematic alignment also bears several problems. Without a patient specific templating system, the above-mentioned method cannot be used, and the kinematics may change after surgical removal of the meniscus, ACL, or PCL. The kinematics in unloading status differs from the weight-loaded state. Since, when balancing, the kinematic alignment is prioritized over the mechanical alignment, the mechanical alignment may change, resulting in negative outcome, such as the tibial component might result in early failure. One other problem is that there is no result of long-term follow-up examination. Howell et al. [68] reported that no fatal failure occurred in the 31-month long-term follow-up examination on 214 cases of surgery performed by the kinematic alignment method.

14.4.5.2 Theories of Surgical Technique

In the early development of surgical techniques of TKA, there were two distinct surgical techniques. It is a gap balancing technique and measured resection technique. With the recent development of surgical instruments and techniques, the two techniques have been used in combination. Gap balancing techniques are mainly used for PS type implants, and surgeons who prefer to use CR type implants mainly use measured resection techniques.

Measured Resection Technique

Measured resection technique is a method of resecting a bone in accordance with a predetermined angle and resection amount (Fig. 14.15). The method traditionally used in the CR type is to make the amount of the proximal tibia bone resection be equivalent to the thickness of the tibial prosthesis containing the PE insert. Distal femoral bone resection shall be generally performed to be 5–7° valgus to the anatomical axis, and the amount of distal femoral and posterior condyle bone resection shall be equivalent to the thickness of the prosthesis to maintain the joint surface. When resecting the anterior and posterior femoral bone, the rotation degree of the femoral component should be determined, and the bone resection should be performed in accordance with various anatomical indicators (transepicondylar axis, posterior condylar axis, anterior-posterior axis, tibial axis). This method has merit in that it is easy and convenient, but also has the drawback that the soft tissue may not be balanced after resection because the femur and the tibia bone resection is performed independently.

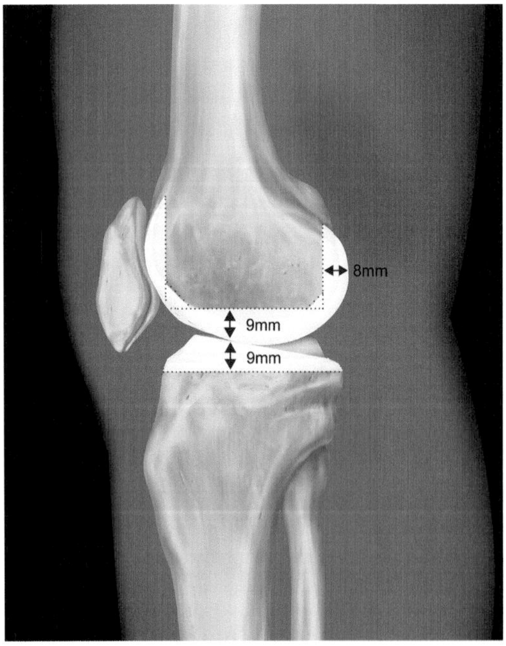

Fig. 14.15 Measured resection technique. Method of performing bone resection in accordance with a predetermined angle and amount of resected bone

Gap Technique

This is a method of determining the amount and angle of bone resection according to the balance of the flexion and extension gap. In this method, the femur and tibia bone resection is performed in relation to each other, and although depending on a surgeon, the resection order may differ, many surgeons perform tibia resection first. In this method, the proximal tibia is resected first and then the posterior femoral condyle is resected, then after aligning appropriate flexion spacing, the distal femur is resected to maintain the gap of the extension as much as the gap of the flexion. As an advantage, the condylar lift off may be reduced as it allows better balance in the ligaments. Another advantage is easy to obtain the gap balance between the flexion and extension. It also has the disadvantage that may occur in the rotational malalignment of the femoral component when the ligament is in an unbalanced state due to inaccurate tibial resection or remaining osteophytes. Further disadvantage is that bone resection may be performed excessively, and in certain cases, mid-flexion instability may occur because the ligament is balanced based on 90 degrees flexion and full extension. In addition, in case there is severe flexion contracture, more resection may occur in the distal femur, causing elevation of the joint line. Surgeons who prefer the gap technique claim that this method has excellent flexion stability, patella alignment, and reproducibility. However, it should be noted that the rotation degree of the femoral component might vary depending on the degree of ligament release and status of bone resection of the proximal tibia in coronal plane. If the proximal tibia is resected varus with respect to the mechanical axis, the femoral prosthesis will be inserted while being rotated internally, whereas if the proximal tibia is resected valgus, the femoral prosthesis will be inserted while being rotated externally. It is also affected by the condition of the collateral ligament. If the medial collateral ligament (MCL) is damaged or released, the medial flexion gap will be large and the femoral prosthesis will be inserted when being excessively rotated internally. Whereas if the lateral collateral ligament or the popliteus muscle is damaged and weakened, the lateral flexion gap will be large and the femoral prosthesis will be inserted when being rotated externally. In order to measure an accurate gap between femur and tibia, various devices such as a spacer block or tensor device are used.

Modified Gap Technique

This is a method in which the distal femur and the proximal tibia are resected based on a measured resection technique, and the rotational alignment of the femur, the balance of the mediolateral ligament, and the balance of the flexion-extension gap are performed using the gap technique. The distal femur and the proximal tibia are resected perpendicular to the mechanical axis with the predetermined thickness of a prosthesis. After removing the nearby osteophytes, then the soft tissue is released so that the tension of the varus and valgus becomes the same. At this time, mark the line that maintains the rectangular-shaped flexion and extension gap on the distal femur using tension devices. The rotation degree of the femoral bone resection area should be determined in knee 90° flexion, and after determining the anterior and posterior resection amount, the anterior-posterior referencing cutting guide should be placed on a marked line, then the resection is performed. The advantage of this modified gap technique is that it is simple because the balance of the soft tissue is achieved by forming a rectangular extension gap. After creating the extension gap, the flexion gap is freely determined by the rotation of the cutting guide and the anterior and posterior moves.

14.4.5.3 Preparation for Bone Resection and Fixation for Each Part

Since bone resection of the femur, the tibia and the patella is performed in relation to each other, it is hard to explain bone resection for each part separately, but in the following, surgical techniques for bone resection will be explained in the general surgical order of the femur, the tibia, and the patella.

Osteophytes Resection

Osteophytes in knee OA hinder accurate bone resection, ligament balancing, good motion, and secure implant fixation. It is advisable to remove the osteophyte before starting bone resection as possible, this step provides that the size and shape of the actual bone is accurately found and it reduces possibility of inaccurate attachment of the cutting guide due to the bony spur. If there are many protruding osteophytes around and they become the basis for bone resection, the bone will be resected less than the desired amount, which can be an obstacle when determining the gap between the flexion and extension and the size of the prosthesis. Since the osteophytes in the medial tibia and femur affect the postoperative pain as well as the postoperative ligament imbalance, it must be thoroughly removed. After all bone resection, the osteophytes remaining in the posterior part of the femoral posterior condyle must be removed too. The osteophytes remaining in the posterior femoral condyle not only cause pain but also can interfere with flexion by causing a collision with the PE insert. It is important to make sure to check if there is any remaining osteophytes or loose body on the preoperative radiograph. It is important to make sure to check whether a trial implant is in close contact with the resection surface and whether the flexion is not disturbed by the posterior condyle resection surface that is not covered by the osteophytes or trial implant. If there is any area not in close contact, trimming should be performed for such area where bone resection is insufficient by using a saw or rasp, and the osteophytes of the uncovered posterior condyle flexion surface should be removed.

Femur

The bone resection order for the femur may vary depending on the type of prosthesis and surgeons; nevertheless, the following steps shall include a description for bone resection in the order of the distal femur, anterior and posterior, and intercondylar bone resection, which is the most general order of the PS type.

Resection of Distal Femur

The insertion position of the rod in the marrow cavity in order to install the cutting guide in the femur should be determined. The insertion position should be within 10 mm anterior from the apex of intercondylar notch and slightly medial considering that bone resection of the distal femur tends to be valgus (Fig. 14.16). However, there may be individual differences, and in some cases, the insertion position is adjusted laterally if there is lateral bowing of the femur. When reaming, the reamer should naturally follow into the marrow cavity after piercing the cortical bone. In order to prevent fat embolism, the insertion position is sufficiently widened, but if it is too large, the valgus angle or the flexion-extension angle may become inaccurate, requiring much attention. It is also desirable to use a fluted-shape reamer as possible to prevent fat embolism and to suction and wash the marrow cavity before inserting the cutting rod. Prior to inserting a femoral prosthesis, bleeding from the marrow cavity can be reduced by blocking the intramedullary guide hole by bone plug (Fig. 14.17a, b).

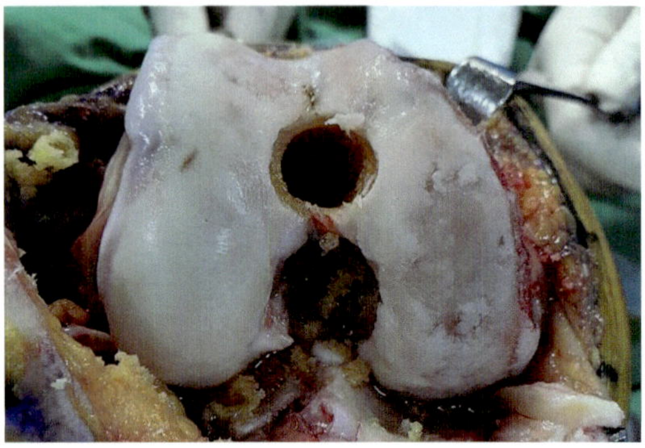

Fig. 14.16 Insertion position of cutting guide in the femoral marrow cavity. If located medially, resection shall be varus and if located laterally, resection shall be valgus

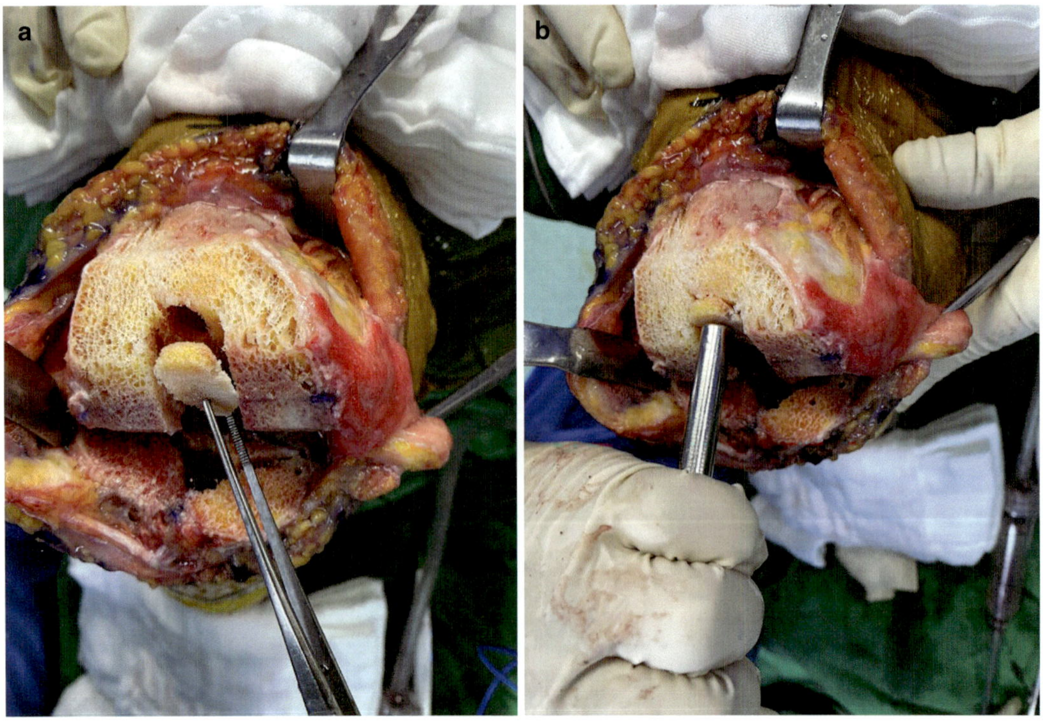

Fig. 14.17 Blocking of the guide hole in the femoral marrow cavity. (**a**) the autogenous bone plug harvested during bone resection is used, (**b**) put the bone block into the entry point and fix it with the impactor

In principle, distal femoral bone resection should be performed which coincides with the mechanical axis when viewed from the coronal plane. Bardakos et al. [69] reported that the angle between the femoral mechanical axis and the anatomical axis was 5.6 ± 0.5 degrees, but showed a wide range of 2–9° and 30–51% of patients were less than or more than 5–6°. They also claimed that the angle between the femoral anatomical axis and the mechanical axis is affected by gender, femoral neck-shaft angle and hip joint offset, and in male or, patients with small femoral neck-shaft angle and large hip joint offset, the femoral valgus resection angle should be larger. However, Kharwadkar et al. [70] reported that the angle between the femoral anatomical axis and the mechanical axis was 5.4 ± 0.6 degrees (range, 3.3–7.6 degrees) and showed the range of 5.2–5.6° in the 95% confidence interval, therefore, it is safe to uniformly cut the distal femur 5–6° valgus to the distal femoral anatomical axis. According to Deakin et al. [71], however, by comparing the group that received a uniformed bone resection with individual patients who received tailored bone resection, it was concluded that the uniformed bone resection is not an appropriate method. There are several methods to obtain an ideal mechanical alignment on resecting distal femur, which are a method of uniformly installing a cutting guide 5–6° valgus to the anatomical axis of the distal femur, a method of adjusting the valgus angle by predetermining the angle through preoperative radiographs or computed tomography, and a method of using a navigation device or robotics. In most cases, surgeons install a cutting guide on the rod in the marrow cavity 5–6° valgus, but in case the femoral curvature is severe, the neck-shaft angle is small, or the femoral neck offset is long, the femoral valgus resection angle is adjusted by measuring the angle between the femoral anatomical axis and the mechanical axis. On performing distal femoral resection, it is important to double check whether an extramedullary rod passes through the medial part 2–3 inches from the anterior superior iliac spine to increase the accuracy.

The amount of bone resection of the distal femur should generally correspond to the thickness of the distal part of a femoral prosthesis and is usually based on the thickness from the less affected femur. In order to make sure an accurate measurement of the bone resection amount, the distal cutting guide must be closely attached to the distal femur. Since the medial femoral condyle is more prominent distally than the lateral femoral condyle, the distal cutting guide only reaches the medial condyle, while failing to reach the lateral condyle in many cases. However, in case the varus deformity and the cartilage erosion of the femoral medial condyle are severe, the guide may reach both or may contact with lateral femoral condyle. If there is a flexion contracture of 15° or more, it is necessary to increase the extension gap by moving the distal cutting guide by one scale to the proximal part to increase the bone resection amount a little more. However, in order to avoid mid-flexion instability and changes in the dynamics of the knee joint due to joint line elevation, CR type and PS type should be limited to within 4 mm and 8 mm changes of joint line, respectively. During distal bone resection, the medial and lateral collateral ligaments should be protected. After resecting the distal femur, it is necessary to check whether the resection surface is flat, and if a notch is hard and cut small, it could bring about a seesaw effect mediolaterally, resulting in decrease in the stability of the femoral prosthesis; therefore, much attention should be paid.

Errors in distal femoral bone resection occur when a distal cutting guide is installed through rod insertion in the femoral marrow cavity and when bone resection is made using a saw blade. The femur normally has anterior bowing, the degree of which is affected by race, age, and bone density. Medial or lateral bowing of the femur may cause inaccurate insertion of the rod into the marrow cavity. It is important to be aware of various femoral anatomical characteristics in advance through preoperative radiographs. According to Reed et al. [72], there is a difference between proximal errors and distal errors when inserting a rod into the femoral marrow cavity. As for the proximal error, the wider the marrow cavity is and the thinner and shorter the rod used is, the more difficult the central position of the rod is in the femoral marrow cavity, thus errors tend to occur more. As for the distal errors, the greater the distance between the femoral intercondylar notch and the distal femoral articular surface passage point of the femoral anatomical axis, the more likely it is to occur. As mentioned above, the ideal insertion position of the rod in the marrow cavity is known to be anterior, central, or slightly medial to the top of intercondylar notch, but if located laterally, it is prone to valgus bony resection, while if located medially, it is prone to varus bony resection. Since errors often occur during the installation of the distal femoral cutting guide and during bone resection, experienced surgeons use various solutions to evaluate lower extremities alignment without relying entirely on the cutting guide. Using a navigation device or measuring and checking the amount of bone resection using a caliper will also be considered a good solution to avoid errors [73].

Anteroposterior Bone Resection of Femur

If the femoral rotation is inaccurate, the patella tracking deteriorates, causing the inclination or dislocation of the patella as well as anterior knee pain [74]. In addition, an inaccurate rotation affects the flexion gap, so if sufficient or excessive, it may cause wear of the PE insert, loosening of the prosthesis and instability of the knee joint, therefore, requiring much attention. The reference line of external rotation of femoral component includes the transepicondylar axis (TEA), the posterior condylar axis (PCA), the anteroposterior (AP) axis (Whiteside's line), and the transtibial axis (Fig. 14.18). The transepicondylar axis is a line connecting the medial and lateral epicondyle, and since it is where the medial and lateral collateral ligaments are attached, it is the basis for determining the amount of external rotation in that it accurately reflects the axis of flexion and extension movement. It is often used when there is valgus deformity or other anatomical indicators are not in a normal shape including revision surgery. The lateral epicondyle is the most protruding point where the lateral collateral ligament is attached and can be easily palpable. On

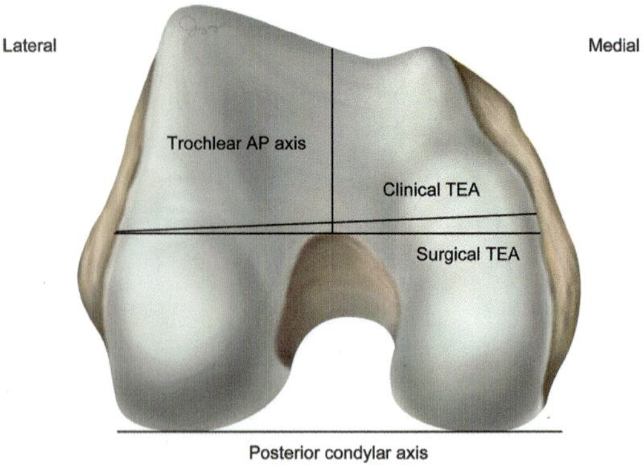

Fig. 14.18 The axis for rotation alignment of the femoral prosthesis. When other anatomical indicators are not in a normal shape, the surgical transepicondylar axis is the most preferred. TEA = transepicondylar axis

the other hand, the medial epicondyle, although protruding, is flat and covered with soft tissue, so it is often not easy to palpate it (Fig. 14.19a, b). Berger et al. [75] classified TEA into a clinical TEA which connects the most protruding point of the lateral epicondyle and the most protruding point of the medial epicondyle to which the superficial MCL is attached, and a surgical TEA which connects the most protruding point of the lateral epicondyle and the sulcus to which the deep MCL is attached. Here, the angle between the clinical TEA and PCA was defined as a condylar twist angle, and they reported that the angle was an average of 4.7° for males and 5.3° for females. The angle between the surgical TEA and the PCA was defined as the posterior condylar angle and the average angle was 3.5° for male and 0.3° for female. They also claimed that the surgical TEA was more accurate than the clinical TEA in TKA.

Based on a study that the TEA is externally rotated by an average of 3–4° to the PCA, the method of externally rotating 3° based on the PCA is most widely used as it is easy and simple. However, in the situation of hypoplasia or severely chondral loss of the femoral lateral condyle, the AP femoral cutting guide may be inserted internally rotated in this method. This phenomenon is common in genu valgum, and in this case, it is better to set the TEA or AP axis as a reference instead of PCA. 3° of external rotation base on the

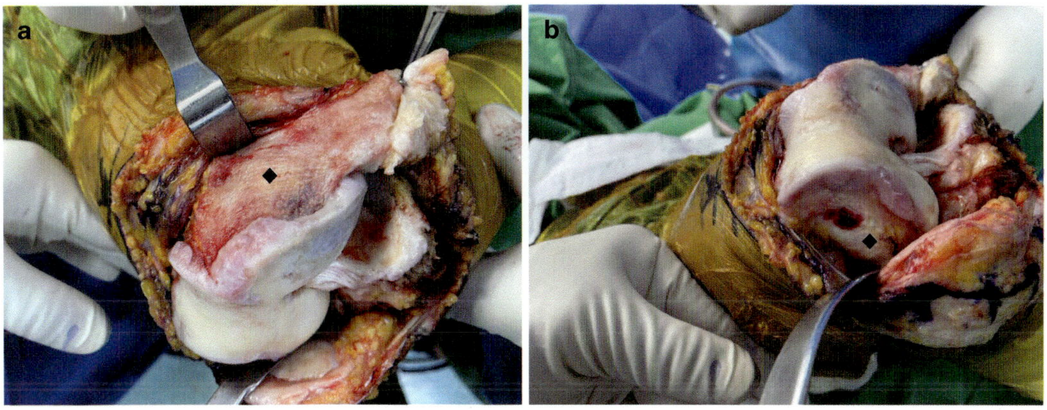

Fig. 14.19 The medial and lateral epicondyles have different morphologies. (**a**) the medial epicondyle epicondyle (◆) is covered with soft tissue and is relatively flat so difficult to find. (**b**) the lateral epicondyle (◆) is the protruding and attachment site of the lateral collateral ligament

PCA is insufficient, and especially when there is severe varus deformity of the knee joint or medial obliquity of the joint surface [76].

The AP axis is a line that extends from the center of the femoral intercondylar notch to the deepest point of the femoral trochlear groove, and when bone resection is performed perpendicular to this axis, it usually coincides with the TEA. However, there are wide variations depending on each individual, and the result may come out inaccurate if the femoral trochlear groove is destroyed by the patellar femoral arthritis, if there are many spurs in the intercondylar notch, or if there is condylar dysplasia [77]. The transtibial axis technique is a method of resecting the bone at a perpendicular angle to the long axis of the tibia, and it shares the same context as the gap technique. Transtibial axis technique is used after bone resection of the tibia is performed first, and then the flexion gap and the degree of external rotation of the femoral prosthesis are determined. Transtibial axis is useful in revision surgery, TKA in valgus deformity or TKA using a mobile bearing prosthesis.

In the step of determining the amount of external rotation and performing the AP femoral bone resection, the size of a femoral prosthesis should also be determined. Typically, the anterior and posterior (AP) size is more important than the medial and lateral (ML) size, but oversizing of a prosthesis is not desirable. The aspect (ML/AP) ratio differs for each individual and also varies depending on the type and size of the prosthesis. The AP placement and flexion gap of a femoral prosthesis is determined using anterior (AR) or posterior reference (PR) systems. AR system is to resect AP femoral bone based on anterior femoral cortex. AR system has merits to prevent anterior cortical notching but has disadvantages such as inconsistent flexion gap. PR system provides a consistent flexion gap but sometimes produces anterior femoral notching or overstuffing. If the AP length of a femoral prosthesis is the same as the AP length of a patient's femur condyle, the AP location of the femoral prosthesis and flexion gap will be the same regardless of which reference system is used, but a problem arises for the between size. In most cases, the anterior reference system is used, but if a mobile bearing prosthesis where maintenance of the flexion gap is important to prevent dislocation of the PE insert after surgery, the posterior reference system is preferred. When the anterior reference system is used and if the size of a prosthesis is between size, CR type is less effective in increasing the flexion gap due to the retained PCL, thus it is recommended to use a smaller size of prosthesis. As for the PS type, if the posterior cruciate ligament is removed, the flexion gap gets wider than the extension gap, thus it is recommended to use a larger sized femoral component.

Once the size and degree of external rotation of the femoral AP cutting guide is determined, bone resection is performed with the cutting guide being stably fixed to the distal femoral bone resection surface, and when performing, much care is required as errors in bone resection may occur due to differences in bone density and toggling of the saw blade. In general, bone resection is performed in the order of anterior, posterior, anterior chamfer, and posterior chamfer in order to make the bone and the cutting guide stably contact as many areas as possible during sawing. During the anterior bone resection, as the saw blade must proceed from the cancellous bone to the hard cortical bone, the cortical bone resection is likely to be inadequate and bone resection may be insufficient as the bone of the medial posterior edge is hard in the case of varus deformity. Due to an inadequate amount of bone resection in the aforementioned areas, the fitting of a femoral prosthesis might not be good, which requires much attention. When anterior bone resection is performed, the resected bony surface usually shows a bimodal curve with the lateral part higher and the medial part lower (grand piano sign), and this shape is also used to determine whether the bone has been properly resected. The amount of external rotation can be estimated by comparing the size of the posterior condyles after resection (Fig. 14.20). Generally, when external rotation is made 3° with respect to the PCA, the medial posterior condyle is resected 2–3 mm more than the lateral posterior condyle.

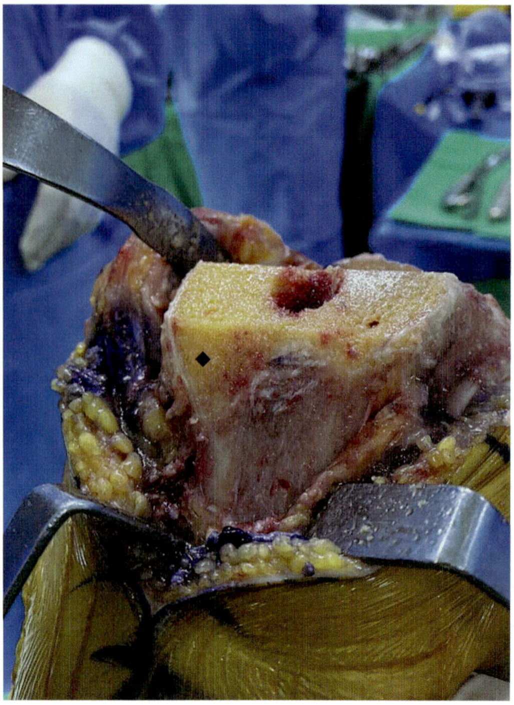

Fig. 14.20 Grand piano sign (♦) of the anterior bone resection area

Intercondylar Bone Resection

It is a step necessary to create a space for the post-cam mechanism when using the PS type, and care should be taken as it affects the medial and lateral displacement of a femoral prosthesis. In order to position the femoral prosthesis in the center of the resected surface more accurately, measure the area of the distal femoral bone resection surface with a caliper at the height of the femoral TEA, and then install the intercondylar cutting guide after marking the middle part of the measured area with a marking pen or electrocautery device.

Tibia

There are two proximal tibial resection methods: one is using the extramedullary (EM) guide, the other is using the intramedullary (IM) guide. The advantages of using the EM method are that it can be used even there is extra-articular deformity, reduces the frequency of fat embolism, and the proximal tibial cutting angle is adjustable in any side, such as the posterior slope or varus-valgus tilting, while the disadvantage is that it may be misaligned in obese patients. The IM method has the advantage that bone resection is relatively accurate in case of no bowing or offset to the tibial shaft but it cannot apply to extra-articular deformed tibia. The entry point is critical to alignment using IM guide. Templating to determine the proper entry point for the tibial guide on the tibial surface will minimize the risk of creating a varus tibial cut based on a medial entry point and a bowed tibia. A central entry hole often will cause the IM rod to impact against the tibial cortex, and placing the entry hole so that this does not happen alters the angle of the proximal guide. When using the EM method, the pinning point at the proximal part is not the center of the plateau, but the point where the mechanical axis of the tibia meets the plateau. Therefore, where the varus deformity is severe, the proximal pinning point moves laterally by such amount. The tibial crest 2 inches above the ankle joint is a reference point at the distal part, and this reference point slightly moves medially than the center of the ankle joint. The center of the ankle does not exactly correspond to the midpoint between the malleoli but instead is medial to this point (5–10 mm). This is because the lateral malleolus of the ankle joint is larger than the medial malleolus. Therefore, the center of the ankle joint and the center of the tibial axis do not fit into each other (Fig. 14.21a). In some cases, the second toe is used as a reference, but since the position of the second toe changes by the rotation of the foot, an accurate result cannot be obtained with this reference.

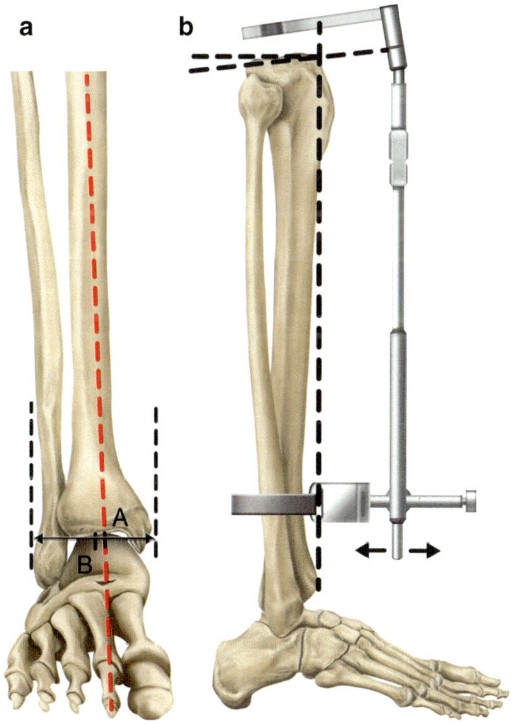

Fig. 14.21 Measuring of the tibial alignment. (**a**) center of the tibial axis (point A) is slightly more medial than center of the ankle joint (point B) in coronal plane, (**b**) tibial axis and posterior inclination angle on the sagittal plane

Severe varus deformity is accompanied by the rotational deformity of the proximal tibia. If the posterior tilt angle is given without considering the rotational deformity, the posterior tilt angle cannot be obtained as much as intended or the tibial alignment on the coronal surface is changed. According to Tsukeoka et al. [78], if 10° of external or internal rotational error occurred in the situation of 8 cm or more distance between bone-cutting guide and tibia can result in more than 3° of axial deviation in coronal plane. Therefore, it is important to make an accurate placement of tibial cutting guide and to make the distance between the guide and the bone short as much as possible.

With respect to the axis on the sagittal plane, a line connecting the fibular head and the lateral malleolus of the ankle joint is parallel to the tibial axis. The recommended angle for the posterior slope varies depending on each prosthesis (Fig. 14.21b). The recommended posterior inclination angle varies depending on each prosthesis, but typically, it is determined at between 3–7° but it is often performed at 0° on performing revision TKA. The posterior inclination of the tibial plateau is closely related to the knee flexion angle. According to Bellemans et al. [66], with 1° increase of the tibial posterior inclination angle, the range of flexion is also increased by 1.7°. Singh et al. [79] reported that in the PS type, if alignment in the coronal surface is well achieved, the maximum flexion could be obtained by creating an anatomical posterior tilt. The more knee flexion can be obtained by forming the posterior inclination angle to some extent, but excessive inclination angle is a risk factor that causes abrasion and fracture of the posterior part of PE insert. In particular, in the PS type, surgeon should pay much attention to the posterior inclination angle, and it has been known that when the posterior inclination angle is more than 7°, PE wear and post fracture occur more frequently.

Proximal Tibial Bone Resection

The depth of proximal tibial resection is determined such that enough bone is removed to accommodate the tibial component depending on implant type. Given the few additional millimeters of laxity produced following PCL excision, 1 cm of proximal tibia is excised to accommodate at least a 10-mm tibial component when a cruciate substituting knee is performed. The 10 mm of resection is typically measured using a stylus placed on the articular surface with the most residual cartilage; alternatively, the stylus can measure 2 mm of resection from the most eroded articular surface. The gap between flexion and extension widens or narrows depending on the amount of bone resection at the tibial side. If resection is performed too small, the gap between flexion and extension also is narrowed, making it difficult to operate, and since the thickness of PE becomes thin, PE wear may drastically increase. On the contrary, where proximal tibial bone is resected too much, small size of the prosthesis is chosen inevitably, which increases the load of force put on the prosthesis and decreases the mechanical strength of the trabecular bone resulting in weakened support for the prosthesis.

Determination of Size, Location, and Rotation

In determining the size for the tibia, it is desirable to have good medial-lateral coverage, but since the lateral plateau is about 2–3 mm smaller than the medial plateau, if the size is adjusted for the medial part, the overhang in the lateral side occurs. According to Martin et al. [80], effort for maximum coverage tibial resection surface increases malrotation of tibial prosthesis, and such malrotations were lessened using the asymmetrical tibial prosthesis. For deciding the tibial prosthesis rotation, there have been reported several methods with anatomical reference point; the method based on the line connecting the most medial and lateral parts of the tibial plateau; the method based on both posterior condyles of the tibial plateau; the method in which a reference is adjusted to the line connecting the two points of the attachment point of PCL for the back and the center of the plateau for the front; the method based on the point of the medial 1/3 of the tibial tuberosity; the method according to the line connecting the center of the PCL and the medial border of the patella tendon as well as the TEA of the femur [81]. In addition, the anterior cortical line can be also used as a reference for tibial rotational alignment. In PS type TKA, the rotational alignment is determined as occurring self-rotation of PE liner while flexion and extension of the knee with the trial implant inserted (free floating technique). There is no established theory for the axis of rotation; however, in general, the method of dividing the front part of the tibial tuberosity into 3 equal parts and using the medial 1/3 as a reference is widely used. In summary, it is desirable to try various methods stated above and consider the transverse axis of the proximal tibia, flex and extend the knee. However, tibial prosthesis should not be fixed with internal rotation state. Nicoll et al. [82] and Barrack et al. [83] said that internal rotation is closely related to abnormal tracking of the patella and postoperative pain. On the contrary, excessive external rotation deteriorates the patella tracking and causes changes in kinematics between the femur and the tibia, which may result in a post-cam collision in PS type.

Patella

It has been debated for a long time whether patellar resurfaced or not on implementing TKA. Resurfacing of the patella aims to reduce anterior pain and improve the patella-femur alignment. However, as complications from resurfacing of the patella increased, the number of surgeons performing resurfacing the patella gradually decreased. The basis for claiming patella resurfacing is that it reduces anterior knee pain, which increases satisfaction of patients, the overall function is improved, and the complications from resurfacing occur less. The basis for claiming patella non-resurfacing is shorter operation time, lower cost, and lower complication rate on the patella. In some cases, selective patellar resurfacing is performed in cases of severe arthritis of the patellar femoral joint, RA or other inflammatory arthritis or crystalline diseases, poor alignment of the patellar femoral joint, and non-anatomical patella and preoperative anterior knee pain. Many surgeons agree that if preoperative pain in the patella is more severe than mentioned above, resurfacing needs to be performed. Since the modulus of metal and cartilage is different, the joint surface of the patella is adjusted to fit the trochlea, which is called a "stress contouring" phenomenon. This phenomenon progresses gradually, and according to Keblish et al. [84], if the trochlea is anatomical, much remodeling is not required, but if it is not anatomical, a lot of remodeling is required; therefore, the trochlea of a femoral prosthesis and the form of the patella are important factors in determining whether to perform resurfacing. Even surgeons who prefer patella resurfacing do not tend to perform resurfacing for young and active patients with well-preserved articular cartilage or for patients whose patella is less than 15 mm in thickness or the bone stock is poor or patients with morbid obesity.

Patella Bone Resection

The purpose of patella resection is to restore thickness and the alignment of the patellofemoral joint. The amount of patella bone resection is usually 8–10 mm thickness, and it should be ensured that total thickness of patellar bone-prosthesis composite is the same or less than the patellar thickness before surgery. Greenfield et al. [85] reported that the frequency of performing lateral retinacular release was reduced from 55% to 12% by making the postoperative thickness the same or less than the thickness before surgery. Gerber et al. [86] reported that the thickness after surgery should not be thicker than before to reduce the frequency of the patellar tilt. If resurfaced patella is too thick, the pressure applied to the patella increases, causing anterior knee pain, premature wear, and loosening. Moreover, as the alignment between the patella and femur becomes unbalanced, ROM may decrease. According to Abolghasemian et al. [87], as the thickness of the patella increases, the joint movement drastically decreases. However, if it is too thin, although the alignment may become better, the strength of the quadriceps weakens and extensor disruption is easily caused, which brings about complications such as patella fracture. For this reason, many surgeons recommended that after the patella resection, the thickness of remaining bone should be at least 12 mm. Since the lateral part is thinner than the medial part, if the lateral and medial part is cut to the same thickness, it is resected asymmetrically. The medial part should be resected more to make the balance between medial and lateral part of patella (Fig. 14.22). Yao et al. [88] reported that the patella tracking becomes more appropriate if it is cut obliquely so that the medial part becomes thicker as in the shape of the patella.

Selection of Position and Size

Since the vertical ridge is located in the medial part, it is important to place a patellar prosthesis slightly medial to the center. However, Anglin et al. [89] reported that a patellar prosthesis should not be placed more than 2.5 mm to the medial part, this is because if it is positioned too medial, the lateral patella is exposed too much, thereby causing pain due to collision with the femur. In an anatomical shape of patella prosthesis, as the asymmetry is already reflected in a prosthesis, even if it is placed in the center, the ridge will be located in the medial part as is in the normal anatomy. If TKA is performed, about 50% experience patella baja. Patella baja increases compressive force on the patella-

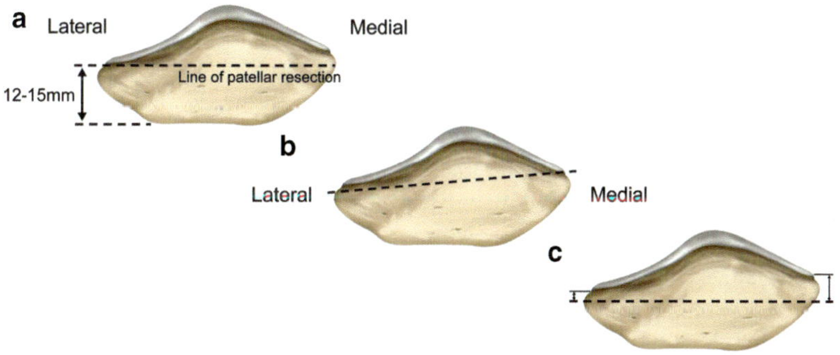

Fig. 14.22 Patella bone resection. (**a**) appropriate thickness of patella osteotomy, (**b**) if the medial and lateral side are cut to the same thickness, asymmetrical thickness may occur. (**c**) thickness of medial and lateral facet becomes symmetric by cutting medial side more

femur joint during initial flexion and decreases ROM. On the contrary, patella alta may cause instability of the patella. Therefore, it is desirable to place the patella prosthesis in the middle or slightly proximal site of the resected patella surface. If the patellar prosthesis is too large, it may cause the patella-femur impingement, while if it is too small, the stress put on the prosthesis increases as well as the lateral bone of the patella due to medially placed prosthesis is excessively exposed. In case the patellar prosthesis is oval-shaped or in an anatomical form, wrong placing of the patella worsens the patella tracking, thus, the rotation alignment must be adjusted. The axis of rotation is considered fit if the long axis of the patella is parallel to the femoral prosthesis. If the patella is not resurfaced, patelloplasty is recommended. This is a procedure that makes the shape of the patella and joint surface as normal as possible. In this procedure, osteophytes are removed, the joint surface is smoothened and the patellar rim is sometimes cauterized to block nerves.

14.4.6 Balancing

Knee function after TKA is closely related with ligamentous balancing. Knee ROM can be restricted by excessive collateral or PCL tension, and excessive laxity may lead to clinically unacceptable instability. Unbalanced TKA causes unexplained pain, recurrent joint effusion, and gait disturbance in the early postoperative period. Furthermore, it induces PE wear and implant loosening in the long term. Therefore, soft tissue balancing is essential to providing a stable, functional joint after TKA. Before release of any tightened soft tissue structure, all peripheral osteophytes should be removed from the femur and tibia. The removal of osteophytes alone may be enough to balance existing coronal or sagittal plane deformities. After bone preparation is completed, the flexion-extension or medial-lateral gaps should be evaluated for symmetry for equal height in flexion and extension or medial-lateral side. Basic principle for good balancing on performing TKA is to obtain a rectangular medial-lateral gap and an equal extension-flexion gap. However, this principle is difficult to realize in real clinical practice. In general, 1–2 mm of balanced varus-valgus motion in the prosthetic knee is a reasonable goal. Regardless of the type of deformity being corrected, stability should be checked after each stage of soft tissue release because over-release can lead to excessive coronal plane instability and require conversion to a constrained prosthesis. Ligamentous balancing in performing TKA with specific types of severe deformity will be described in the later section, and in this section, general principles regarding the ligamentous balancing in TKA will be described. Balancing procedures on performing TKA should be implemented in sagittal plane, coronal plane, and patella-femoral joint.

14.4.6.1 Extension-Flexion Gap Balancing

Factors affecting extension-flexion gap imbalance is the amount of distal femoral bone resection, AP size of a femoral prosthesis, PCL, and posterior joint capsule, etc. Depth of distal femoral bone resection relates to the extension gap. When extension gap is narrower than flexion gap, it can be solved with a more resection of distal femur bone or posterior capsular release or using larger size of femoral component that decreases flexion gap. Although bone resection of distal femur is a powerful solution for increasing extension gap, additional bone resection of 4 mm in the distal femur only increased the extension joint gap by a mean of 2 mm [90]. Excessive bone resection of distal femur has several disadvantages, such as joint line elevation, patella baja, and mid-flexion instability. Therefore, more than 4 mm resection from initial bone-cutting level in the distal femur is not recommended. Posterior capsular release is helpful for increasing extension gap (Fig. 14.23). Mitsuyasu et al. [91] reported that the extension gap increased by 2–3 mm with osteophyte removal and release of the deep medial collateral ligament or posteromedial capsule. However, where the flexion gap is slightly wider, it shows rather better flexion movement. Ismailidis et al. [92] reported that a controlled flexion gap increase of 2.5 mm may have a positive effect on postoperative flexion and patient

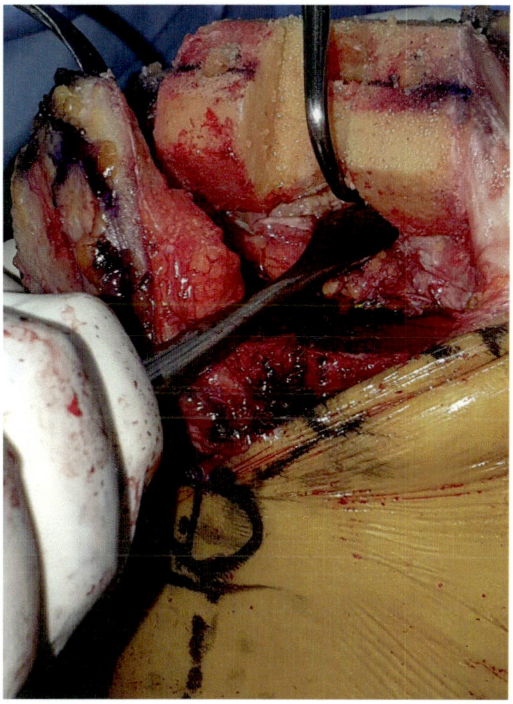

Fig. 14.23 Releasing posterior joint capsule for widening extension gap. Should be careful with posterior neurovascular injury

satisfaction after TKA. This is because the flexion gap narrows when the patella is located in a right place during the flexion gap test. Gejo et al. [93] reported that with the patella reduced, when the knee is bent 90 degrees, the flexion gap is reduced by 1.9 mm, and when the knee is bent 135 degrees, the gap is reduced by 5.5 mm.

When extension gap is wider than flexion gap, it can be solved with a less resection of distal femur bone or using a smaller size of femoral component or resection of PCL. However, if the distal femur is resected less, there is a risk such as patella alta or patellofemoral instability. If a smaller size of femoral component is used, a posterior condylar offset can be decreased, which might affect adversely in knee flexion motion. Mihalko et al. [94] reported that when PCL in cadaveric knees is removed, flexion gap at 90° flexion increased to 5.26 mm at rest and 6.4 mm under tension. Kayani et al. [95] reported that PCL resection in OA patients undergoing TKA increased the flexion gap in the medial (2.4 mm) and lateral (3.3 mm) compartments. Thus, PCL resection increased the flexion gap and useful solution for increasing gap. If CR type prosthesis is used, it needs a different approach. In the CR type, tight flexion gap can be solved by recession of the PCL. However, excessive recession is not recommended due to its low reproducibility and late flexion instability. Scott et al. [96] proposed the POLO (pull-out, lift off) test to determining the flexion gap in the CR type. According to POLO test, a good flexion gap should be that after inserting the trial prosthesis, with the knee bent 80–100 degrees, PE liner should not be pulled out or lifted off (Fig. 14.24).

However, a more bone resection of the tibia or change of PE thickness should be avoided in case of an imbalance between the extension and flexion gap because it effects on both the extension and flexion gap. Despite these measures, if there still remains instability due to imbalance, a constrained prosthesis should be used.

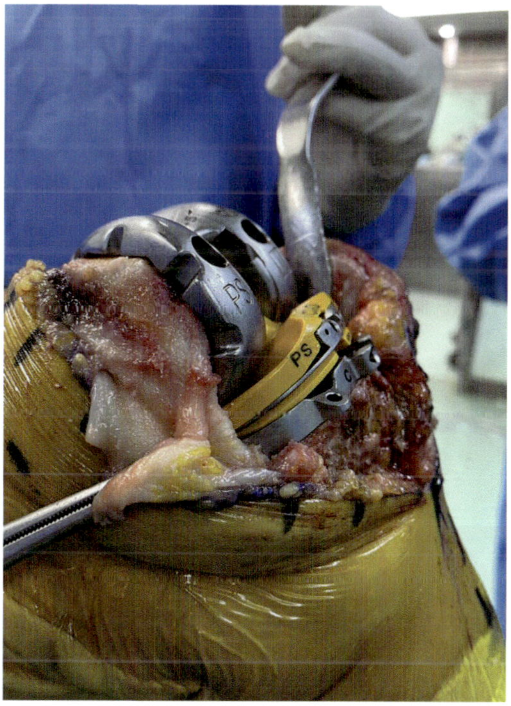

Fig. 14.24 In case the flexion gap is narrow, the front part of PE insert is lifted off

14.4.6.2 Medial-Lateral Balancing

Goal for ligament balancing in TKA is to obtain a rectangular space in coronal plane and an equal extension-flexion gap in sagittal plane. The main principle of equal gap is that when the leg is pulled in extension and flexion position after bone resection, the medial-lateral gap of the knee joint should be the same so that it does not form a trapezoid but a rectangular (Fig. 14.25). However, this goal hardly realizes in surgical theater. A perfect soft tissue balance is not always obtained during TKA because it can be obtained just in 7.7% of the knee undergoing TKAs [97]. Obsession for perfect soft tissue balance might lead to the catastrophic results. Over-release of contracted soft tissue can cause iatrogenic ligamentous rupture, increasing operation time that might relate to increase risk of infection. Therefore, understanding the medial-lateral ligament balance in normal knees helps to obtain stable ligament balance on performing TKA. Markolf et al. [98] reported that varus-valgus laxity was increased with knee flexion in normal cadaveric knees, which was 2 degrees in extension and 8 degrees in full flexion. Moreover, normal knee tends to be slightly more lax laterally than medially, especially in flexion. Tokuhara et al. [99] investigated to assess varus and valgus joint laxity of the normal living knee in 90 degrees flexion using MRI. Their result showed that the lateral joint gap opened by 6.7 ± 1.9 mm with varus stress whereas the medial joint gap opened by a mean of 2.1 ± 1.1 mm with valgus stress. They concluded that the tibiofemoral flexion gap in the normal knee is not rectangular and that the lateral joint gap is significantly lax. Even if a complete medial-lateral balance is not obtained, it does not affect clinical outcomes after TKA, but rather, clinical outcomes are better if there is some degrees of lateral laxity at the knee flexion position [100]. Okazaki et al. [101] reported that the widening of the lateral part is better than the widening of the medial part, which is caused by a compensatory mechanism by the dynamic stability of the long ligament. Although lateral laxity has good clinical results, it is controversial as to how much lateral laxity will be allowed. Matsuda et al. [102] allowed a lateral laxity of less than 2 degrees, Kuster et al. [103] allowed 4 degrees in knee flexion of 30 degrees, and Yoshihara et al. [104] allowed a lateral laxity of less than 5 degrees in knee extension and flexion of 90 degrees.

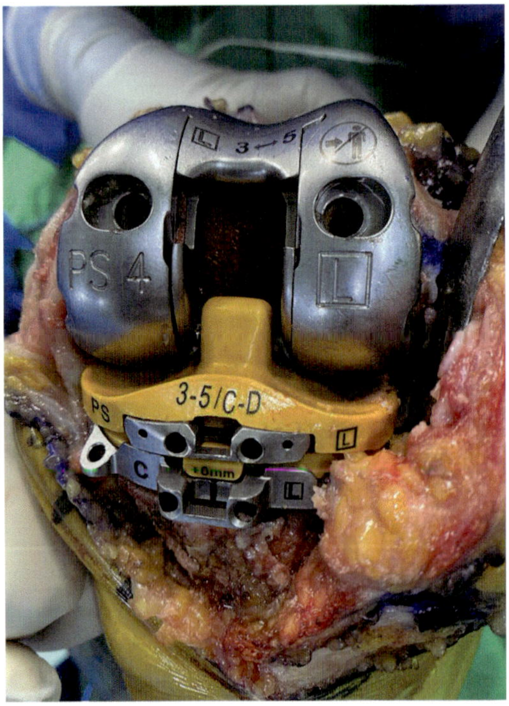

Fig. 14.25 By insufficient medial release, the medial side is tight and the lateral side is loose

14.4.6.3 Methods of Balancing

Medial Release

When correcting the varus deformity of knee, anatomic structures contributing to the deformity and the function of each structure according to the extension and flexion position of the joint should be understood. In other words, very careful not to cause valgus instability. Soft tissue structures contributing to varus deformity of the knee joint are superficial and deep MCL, pes anserinus, semimembranosus tendon, posteromedial joint capsule, and posterior oblique ligament. These structures play a different role in contributing to medial stability depending on the extension and flexion of the knee. Release of semimembranosus tendon and posteromedial capsule increases the medial laxity in extended position of the knee joint. Superficial MCL release is the most effective method for the correction of varus deformity in both extension and flexion. According to Whiteside [105], selective release of the superficial MCL can be useful when correcting the varus deformity. Medial tightness in flexion can help with correction by removing the anterior part of the superficial MCL whereas medial tightness in extension might help with release of posterior part of superficial MCL including posteromedial capsule and posterior oblique ligament. Medial soft tissue should be subperiosteally released from medial metaphysis of proximal tibia in a sleeve fashion. If soft tissue is subperiosteally released in a sleeve fashion, it will be healed into thick connective tissue, which will not interfere with function, but transverse cut of soft tissue structure will cause significant instability, so transverse cut should be avoided. The extent of medial soft tissue release generally depends on the degree of balance with the lateral structure, and during surgery, reevaluation of deformity correction should be performed at each stage of soft tissue release to avoid creating undesired instability due to over-release. However, if the superficial MCL released incompletely, the medial part becomes too tight, which may restrict movement or rather cause lateral instability. Although there is concern about medial instability after complete release of superficial MCL, if the superficial MCL is completely released from proximal tibia according to the rule such as a subperiosteal sleeve fashion, medial instability would not occur.

When correcting severe varus deformity, complete release of the medial soft tissue structures, including the superficial MCL, may be necessary, which may cause problems such as medial instability in knee flexion. There are several surgical techniques to avoid this. If CR type prosthesis is used in severe varus deformity, PCL itself inhibits deformity correction. In this case, conversion CR type to PS type prosthesis is helpful for deformity correction. Verdonk et al. [106] proposed that MCL could be extended by approximately 6–8 mm with puncturing using a knife No 11 several times. This method has the advantage of selectively releasing the medial soft tissue.

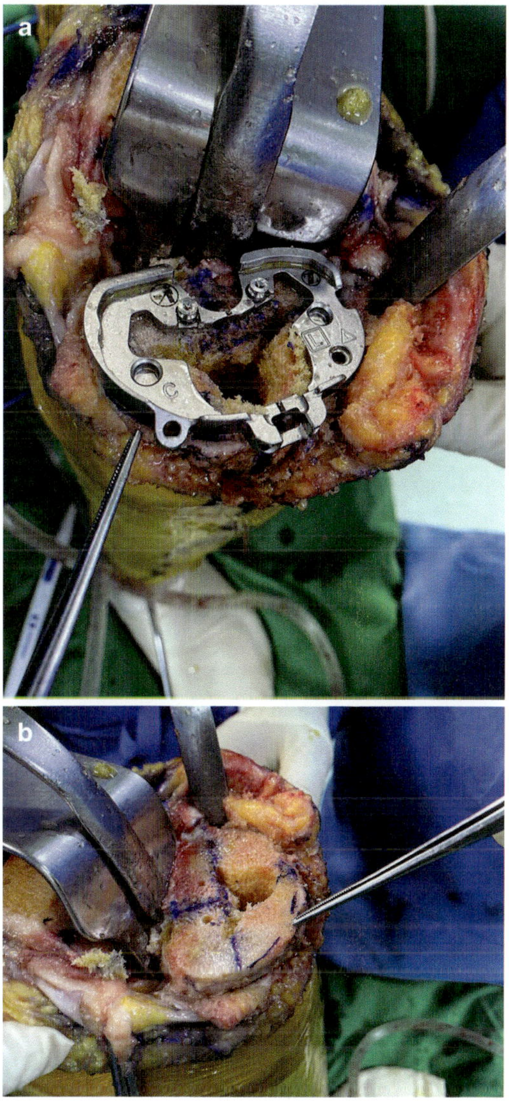

Fig. 14.26 Shift and resection method by Dixon. (**a**) tibial prosthesis moved laterally (**b**) amount of bone resected on the medial plateau

However, using a knife can cause the MCL to cut transversely, so another modification method is to use large bore needle such as 18G to make multiple punctures. Dixon et al. [107] proposed surgical technique called “shift & resect” as an alternative to medial release. This is a method of further resecting the medial side of tibial condyle and placing a little smaller tibial prosthesis on the lateral side of tibial plateau (Fig. 14.26a, b). This technique is useful for above 20 degrees varus deformed knees. Engh [108] introduced medial epicondylar osteotomy rather than performing complete release of the MCL. This is a method of detaching the medial epicondyle attached with the collateral ligament, of which detached bony fragment leave alone or fix with screws or suture. It has the advantage of not damaging to the soft tissue. It can be used for ankylosing joints, revision TKA, or extreme varus deformity.

Lateral Release

Valgus deformity of the knee is usually associated with lateral soft tissue contracture. The lateral soft tissue structures contributing to valgus deformity include the lateral collateral ligament, popliteus tendon, posterolateral capsule, iliotibial band, posterior joint capsule, biceps femoris, and lateral gastrocnemius tendon. When correcting the valgus deformity with lateral soft tissue release, it is necessary to distinguish between the structures involved in the extension and flexion of the knee joint. The iliotibial band and posterior joint capsule are responsible for stabilizing the lateral side in full extension state. The lateral collateral ligament is an effective lateral stabilizer in range of 0–90° flexion, and in the absence of this ligament, the popliteus tendon and posterolateral capsule play a role. In particular, the popliteus tendon contributes mainly to the lateral stability in knee flexion state, and the posterolateral capsule contributes to the lateral stability in near extension state.

Whiteside et al. [109] reported that lateral collateral ligament and popliteus tendon should be released when lateral structures are tense in both extension and flexion or only in flexion, and iliotibial band and posterior capsule should be released when lateral structures are tight in extension. When performing the valgus deformity correction, the joint capsule should be released at the tibial attachment and the iliotibial band be released at the Gerdy's tubercle. Clarke et al. [110] introduced pie-crusting techniques, in which, after inserting lamina spreader between joint space, multiple perforation or stabbing incision using No 11 blade was performed on the iliotibial band, lateral collateral ligament, and posterolateral joint capsule. Krackow et al. [111] reported that in some exceptional cases where a deformity cannot be corrected only by release, advancement can be done on the loose ligaments on the medial side. They proposed a new fixation method for advancement. Engh [108] introduced lateral epicondylar osteotomy with detaching the lateral epicondyle attached with the lateral collateral ligament and popliteus tendon for correction of severe valgus deformity. If balancing cannot be achieved with these methods, constrained prosthesis should be used.

14.4.6.4 Balance of Patellofemoral Joint

The balance of the patellofemoral joint is closely related to function, pain, and long-term survival of the prosthesis. There are several factors affecting patellofemoral malalignment, which are patient related, implant design related, and surgical technique-related factors. As for patient's related factors, condylar dysplasia of distal femur, valgus or rotational deformity of the knee joint, or tilting or dislocation of the patella are closely related to the patellofemoral malalignment after TKA. If the preoperative patellofemoral tracking is not good, the postoperative tracking is also bad [86, 112]. As for implant design related factors, the depth and shape of the trochlea of a femoral prosthesis and design of a patellar prosthesis should be considered. Recently, the patellar groove of a femoral prosthesis has been changed to be laterally tilted, deepened and the height of the lateral ridge was increased, and the direction of the track in which it descends slightly diagonally along the direction of the movement of the patella has also been changed. As for surgical technique-related factors, subvastus, midvastus, and medial-trivector retaining approach and release of the lateral patellofemoral ligament are beneficial for patellofemoral alignment. The size, rotation, and position of a prosthesis are also important. If a femoral component is oversized, lateral retinaculum is tensed and patellofemoral malalignment occur. Improper rotational alignment of the femur and the tibia may lead to malalignment of the patellofemoral joint. It is better to perform external rotation of both the femur and the tibia but excessive external rotation should be avoided because it accelerates PE wear and accompanies postoperative toe-in gait. The position of a prosthesis is also closely related to the patellofemoral alignment. It is better to place a femoral prosthesis to the center area or the lateral side of distal femoral cutting surface as possible. A tibial prosthesis should be placed on the lateral side of the tibial bone-cutting surface for better alignment. On the contrary, a patellar prosthesis should be placed to the medial side of patella bone-cutting surface. Use of thicker patella prosthesis than resected bone thickness might cause patellofemoral malalignment.

The patellofemoral alignment should be assessed intraoperatively after implant insertion and must be evaluated after tourniquet release. The evaluation methods are no thumb technique, towel clip technique, and one stitch technique. No thumb technique and towel clip technique are commonly used (Fig. 14.27).

The no thumb technique is a method of examining the patellofemoral tracking without applying any external force to the patella when the knee is bend after implant insertion. However, there is a concern that the incidence of lateral retinacular release may be increased because no thumb technique induces frequently overdiagnosis of the patella maltracking. The towel clip technique is a method in which the towel clip holds the incised quadriceps tendon at 8 cm above the patella, and then the patellofemoral tracking is evaluated with bending the knee to 60–90 degrees. Towel clip technique reduces the incidence of unnecessary lateral retinacular release because it can more strictly determine the patellofemoral maltracking. If the patella maltracking is found after implant insertion, the cause should be found and corrected. The lateral retinacular release is widely used for correction of patellofemoral maltracking. Care should be taken when attempting lateral retinacular release to avoid damaging the vessels supplying to the patella, such as superior lateral genicular artery. If blood vessels are damaged, postoperative hematoma occurs, causing persistent swelling and wound healing problems. In severe cases, the patella may be accompanied by complications such as avascular necrosis or fractures. Instead of lateral retinacular release, the lateral patellofemoral ligament can be released. When releasing, the thick lateral patellofemoral ligament in the middle part must be completely cut.

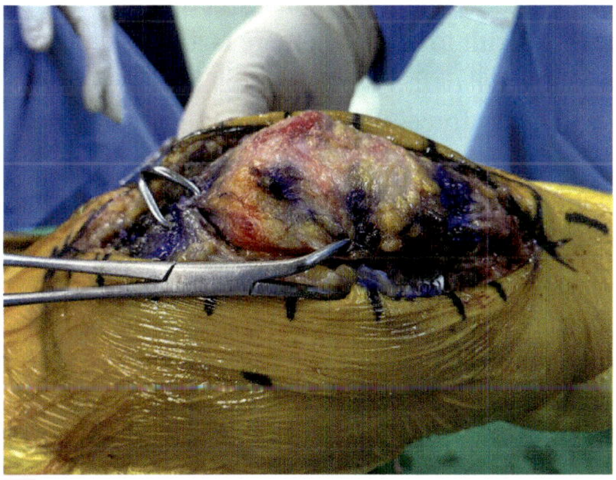

Fig. 14.27 Check-up the patella tracking with towel clip technique

14.4.7 Implant Fixation

Implants using TKA can be fixed with cementless or cemented method. The advantages of cementless fixation are bone stock preservation, cement debris protection, and the potential to achieve biologic fixation. The disadvantages of cementless fixation are expensive, limitation of use in osteoporotic bone, and delayed weight bearing. The advantages of cemented fixation are it provides firm fixation regardless of bone quality, early return to activity of daily life, reduces bleeding and acceptance of slightly inaccurate bone resection. The disadvantages of cemented fixation are late breakdown between bone and cement interface, cement debris induced inflammation. The use of cement in TKAs has been associated with excellent clinical outcomes and low rates of aseptic loosening at long-term follow-up, and it is the gold standard method of fixation in TKA.

The cementing techniques in TKA categorized into three groups such as preparation of the bone surface, cement choice and mixing, and cement implantation. During the preparation of the bone surface, washing or cleaning the entire bone surface using devices, such as pulsatile

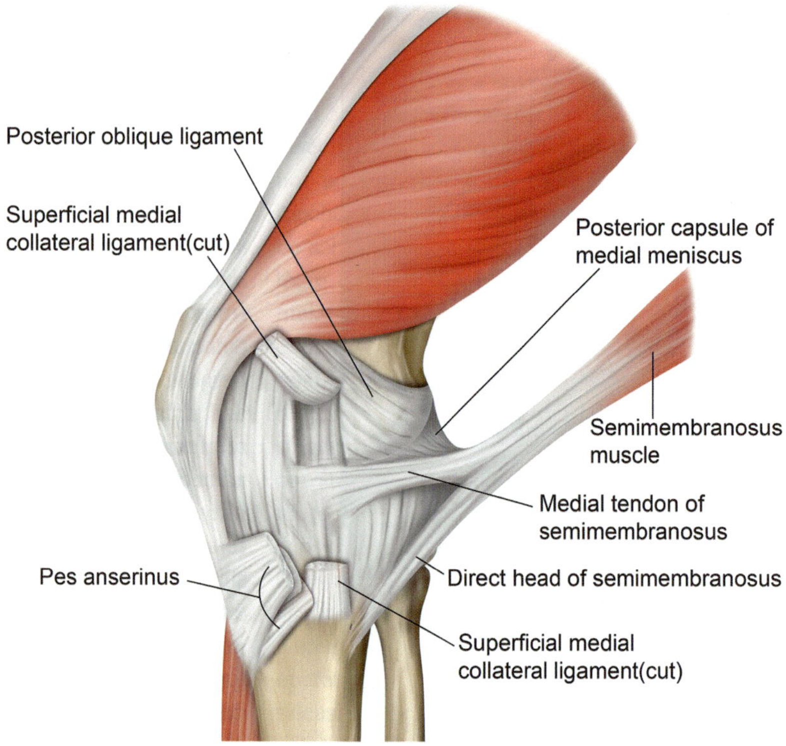

Fig. 14.33 Soft tissue structures around the knee joint that can cause varus deformity

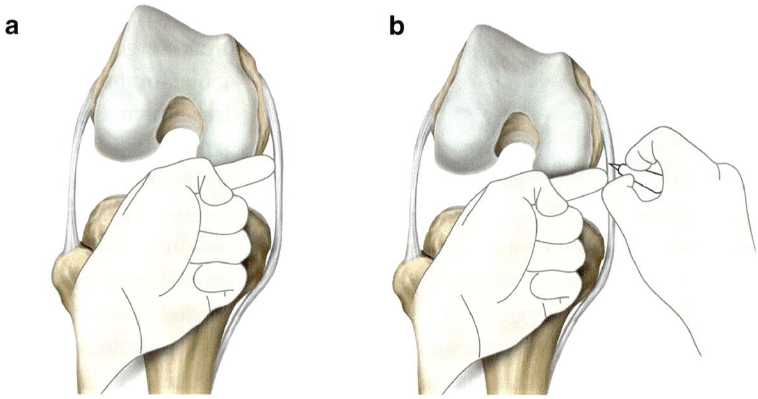

Fig. 14.34 Pie-crusting technique for medial release. (**a**) palpate the MCL and check the degree of tightness and the tightest point, (**b**) carefully puncture with a needle to release, and concurrently check the tension with the opposite finger. Care must be taken not to complete transect of MCL

will also be another solution. In severe varus deformity medial epicondylar osteotomy can be used for correction. For more detailed explanation, see Sect. 14.4.6.2.

14.5.2.3 Total Knee Arthroplasty in Valgus Deformity

Valgus deformity is not common in knee OA whereas it is occasionally observed in RA or traumatic arthritis. Although the criteria for classifying the degree of valgus deformity are not precisely established, the case where the anatomical femoro-tibial angle shows valgus more than 10 degrees is defined as valgus deformity. Valgus up to 10 degrees is classified as mild, 10–20, moderate, and more than 20 degrees, severe. As anatomic characteristics of the valgus deformity, the medial ligament becomes lax, while the lateral soft tissue is contracted, and hypoplasia of lateral femoral condyle or depression in the lateral tibial condyle occurs commonly. Therefore, in valgus deformity, it is necessary to release the contracted lateral soft tissue and realign it through soft tissue release or bone resection.

Structures that cause valgus deformity include iliotibial band, arcuate ligament, lateral collateral ligament, popliteus tendon, biceps femoris tendon, and the lateral and posterolateral joint capsule. There is a lot of controversy over which ligaments should be released first. After removal of lateral osteophyte, the lateral and posterolateral joint capsule and iliotibial band should be released first because they are the main ligaments that cause valgus deformity in the most cases. A pie-crusting technique can be used if necessary (Fig. 14.35). Then, it is released in order of popliteus tendon and lateral collateral ligament. Even if there is more than moderate valgus deformity, the deformity must be corrected by releasing the iliotibial band so that the primary correction of the deformity is achieved, and the peroneal nerve damage due to excessive traction is also prevented.

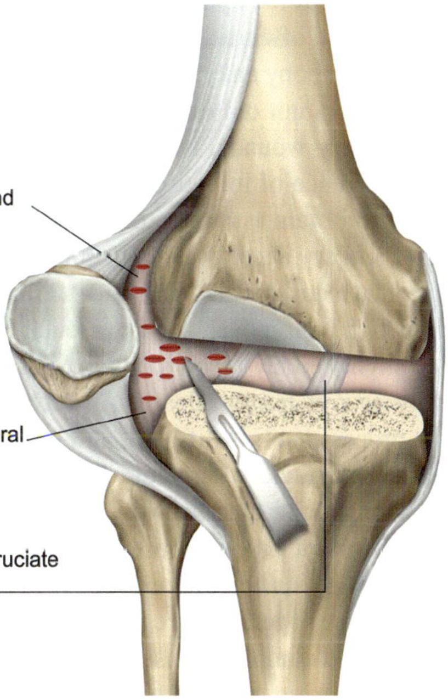

Fig. 14.35 Pie-crusting technique for lateral release. Make multiple punctures on iliotibial band and posterolateral capsule with needle or scalpel

In valgus deformity, erosion of the distal lateral condyle is often accompanied, so care should be taken not to resect too much of the distal femur. If genu recurvatum or medial laxity is accompanied, the joint line may be raised or too wide extension gap may be created, so the distal femoral resection should be minimized as much as possible. Since it is inappropriate to determine the rotation of the femur based on the PCA due to hypoplastic femoral condyle, the decision for femoral component rotation must be made based on the anteroposterior axis of the femur, the cut surface of the tibia and mediolateral ligamentous tension in the valgus deformity. When the valgus deformity is corrected, the elongation of the lateral soft tissue occurs. It may provoke peroneal nerve stretching injury. Especially, if the valgus deformity is accompanied by flexion contracture, the risk of paralysis is increased due to rapid correction of the deformity. To prevent this, the peroneal nerve is checked when correcting severe deformity, or some degree of flexion contracture after surgery is permitted. It is also recommended to gradually extend the knee joint after surgery. In severe valgus deformity, medial instability may accompany the lateral contracture. In this case, releasing the lateral side and simultaneous reinforcement of the medial side can be used. Such complicated surgical procedures might cause many problems. Therefore, some surgeons favor constrained prosthesis and minimal soft tissue resection. Easley et al. [125] reported that the use of constrained-type prosthesis in elderly patients with severe valgus deformity led to pain relief and improvement of function, and Griffin et al. [126] also used constraint-type prosthesis in elderly and inactive patients, thereby reducing complications of peroneal nerve palsy and instability. For more detailed explanation, see Sect. 14.4.6.2.

14.5.3 Total Knee Arthroplasty in Genu Recurvatum

Although the incidence of 5 degree or more genu recurvatum is relatively rare, if genu recurvatum is 15 degrees or more, it is advisable to consider

14.6.1 Postoperative Pain Management

The pain peaks at 2–3 days after TKA, and then declines, but it may usually persist for 3 months. Uncontrolled pain after TKA hinders patient from appropriate rehabilitation and negatively affects not only functional aspects such as motion limitation and gait disturbance but also patient's satisfaction. Therefore, postoperative pain management is necessary for successful rehabilitation and return to daily living. Various methods are being attempted for postoperative pain management. Postoperative pain is caused by tissue damage, nervous stimulus, and consequent activation of nerve-hormonal system. Bone and soft tissue damage from surgery causes secretion of transmitters like prostaglandin and bradykinin that further induces secretion of substance P1, a pain-causing substance. Once it stimulates nociceptor that exists near damaged tissue, the pain signal is transmitted via dorsal root ganglion and enters dorsal horn. Then, it enters spinothalamic tract in the spines and finally is transmitted to cerebral cortex to be recognized of pain. In addition, if the postoperative pain is not appropriately managed, stress reaction may stimulate catabolic hormones like cortisol, glucagon, growth hormone, catecholamine, causing hyperglycemia, muscular weakness, debilitated immune system, and stimulate sympathetic nervous system.

14.6.1.1 Preoperative Analgesic Regimens

Preoperative education can alleviate patients' fears about surgery, improve patients' satisfaction, and shorten hospitalization and rehabilitation periods through realistic explanations of the results of surgery. Educational contents should include overall surgical procedures, postoperative pain levels and patterns, methods of pain management, and rehabilitation protocols. Early drug administration before sensitization of the pain has been known to reduce sensitivity of neural tissue toward pain stimulus and block transmission of pain from peripheral nerve to spine and brain for maximum analgesia. The prerequisite of the drug used for preemptive analgesia should be easy to administer, fast to action, and free from side effects that may interfere with planned surgery. Most commonly used medications include COX-2 selective inhibitors, gabapentinoids, and acetaminophen, and usually administered 1–2 h before surgery begins. In some cases, glucocorticoids are used, which reduces postoperative inflammatory reactions, helps to suppress postoperative pain, and reduces the frequency of nausea and vomiting, and it has been reported that the incidence of infection is not particularly increased when used for a short time [129].

14.6.1.2 Intraoperative Analgesic Regimens

Regional anesthesia, such as spinal or epidural anesthesia, is recommended rather than general anesthesia if there are no specific contraindications, such as coagulopathy. Regional anesthesia reduces systolic pressure, reduces intraoperative bleeding, postoperative nausea and vomiting, and cardiovascular and pulmonary complications. It provides excellent pain relief and improves patient satisfaction. In addition, the epidural anesthesia also allows continuous infusion of painkillers via a catheter. However, as there is a risk of epidural hematoma and paraplegia, care should be taken not to initiate chemical prophylaxis for deep venous thrombosis up to 12 hours after removing the epidural catheter.

Peripheral nerve block is currently one of the most commonly used pain control techniques after TKA. It generally blocks femoral or sciatic nerve. Femoral nerve is located 1–2 cm exterior to femoral artery in inguinal ligament, and its block can prevent pain from upper-anterior leg and medial side of lower leg. Sciatic nerve block can be used simultaneously with femoral block, and sciatic nerve block can prevent pain from upper-posterior leg and posterior of lower leg. Disadvantage of peripheral nerve block is postoperative motor weakness. It prohibits early mobilization of patient. Meanwhile, adductor canal block was introduced to prevent the motor weakness from femoral or sciatic nerve block. Schnabel et al. [130] argued that adductor canal block can reduce pain after TKA. Recently, a procedure using ultrasound guided local anesthetic infiltration between the popliteal artery and the capsule of the knee (IPACK) is being performed to reduce pain in the back of the knee after TKA [131]. IPACK block has little risk of nerve or blood vessel injury and anesthetizes popliteal plexus and terminal branches of genicular nerves that innervate the posterior capsule of the knee joint, and is used with other peripheral nerve block methods.

Periarticular multimodal drug injection offers minimal risk of general side effect, but its effectiveness is still controversial. Many authors [132, 133] have argued that initial pain can be reduced by injecting local anesthesia to periarticular tissue before closing the surgical site. Chang and Cho [134] have reported that among methods for postoperative pain control, periarticular multimodal drug injection and peripheral nerve block are the most effective pain control methods for first 2 days after TKA.

14.6.1.3 Postoperative Analgesic Regimens

Patient controlled analgesia (PCA) is commonly used for postoperative pain control, which the patient administers appropriate dose of analgesic to oneself depending on the level of pain. However, disadvantage of PCA is that it is difficult to be administered while controlling the dosage. General dosage is 1 mg of morphine or 40 μg of fentanyl, but if it is less than appropriate, analgesic effect is insufficient, and if excessive, risk of side effect, such as nausea, vomiting, persists. Appropriate interval between the dosage is known to be 5–10 min.

Acetaminophen, NSAIDs, tramadol, and opioid are commonly used as analgesic after surgery. The first choice of analgesic is acetaminophen that is known to suppress synthesis of prostaglandin in central nervous system of which complication rate is relatively low. Acetaminophen has hepatotoxicity, and patients with liver disease must be cautious. NSAIDs inhibits COX pathway to inhibit synthesis of prostaglandin. COX pathways include COX-1 and COX-2, and COX-1 pathway is related to gastric mucosal protection mediated by prostaglandin E2 and coagulation by thromboxane. Once COX-1 inhibitor is used, it may cause gastrointestinal bleeding or bleeding tendency. COX-2 inhibitors include celecoxib, and when using COX-2 inhibitor, it does not have side effects like gastrointestinal bleeding but increases cardiovascular risk. Furthermore, one of the major side effects of NSAIDs is nephrotoxicity. Therefore, patient with poor renal function or chronic renal failure must be prescribed with caution. Tramadol works on central nervous system and binds to opioid receptor, suppressing serotonin and norepinephrine. It is effective in moderate postoperative pain management, with less risk of respiratory suppression, major organ toxicity, and reduced gastrointestinal motility. Opioid can be administered intravenous (IV), muscular (IM), and oral. It is generally administered IV initially, but later, oral. Oral opioid includes morphine, hydromorphone, oxycodone, hydrocodone, and codeine, with common side effects of nausea, vomiting, and constipation.

14.6.2 General Postoperative Management

14.6.2.1 Observation of General Status, Nerve, and Vascularity

After the surgery, the patient must be moved to recovery room to check vital signs and patient's consciousness and neurologic status. Once the consciousness of the patient is recovered, neurologic status must be checked, especially peroneal nerve. As peroneal nerve is located posterolateral side of the knee, it may be stretched due to correction of valgus deformity or be compressed or damaged due to wrong posture during the surgery, causing paralysis. If it is diagnosed to be paralyzed, it must be recalled if there has been any process that may have damaged peroneal nerve, and if the peroneal nerve damage is suspected, the patient must be inspected in the operating room again. Once the patient returns to ward, the patient is checked for vital signs again. Furthermore, it is crucial to maintain adequate blood circulation all the times by conducting postoperative evaluation. Appropriate management of blood may hasten recovery of the patient's general health and reduce medical complications.

14.6.2.2 Surgical Wound Management

The surgical site must be inspected 1 or 2 days after the surgery. If the patient has thin skin due to underlying disease or the suture is too tight, the suture site poses risk of skin necrosis. In addition, insufficient hemostasis may cause hematoma, which the surgical site must be inspected 1–2 days after the surgery. Afterwards, dressing change is recommended every 3–4 days. In each dressing, it must be thoroughly inspected of any skin necrosis, pus from incision or drainage, or inflammation. If there was wound problem during early postoperative period, more aggressive care must be taken to prevent deep infection and preserve the prosthesis. As hematoma occurs in all patients in early stage, it is crucial to discern if it is excessive. Excessive hematoma may cause pain and even compartment syndrome. It may also tense the skin and form blisters, hindering healing of the wound. If joint motion is limited due to constant bleeding or severe pain and swelling, it must be dealt with some precautions. Continuous passive movement (CPM) device, if it use, is first restricted, and if using thrombolytic agent, its cessation must be considered with caution. Bulla may form occasionally, and this is due to less vascular circulation from too much bandage compression or leg swelling. In such case, it is recovered once it is dried cleanly after loosening the bandage and popping the blister with needle or removing exudate.

14.6.2.3 Venous Thromboembolism Management

Venous thromboembolism (VTE) is one of the most common complications of TKA. In the western population, its occurrence ranges 41–85%, with pulmonary thromboembolism, 15–20%. Though Western population has higher risk of VTE, some research have reported similar incidence in Asian population comparing with west. Piovella et al. [135] have investigated occurrence of VTE in Asian peoples, using bilateral venography. After surveying 295 venography included in the analysis, overall frequency of deep vein thrombosis (DVT) was 41%, with proximal deep vein thrombosis, 10.2%. Preventive measures for DVT after TKA include lifestyle modification, mechanical and pharmacological measures. Early ambulation is very important for DVT prevention. As for early ambulation, the patient is induced of lower limb muscle contraction with ankle motion without any special equipment. Mechanical measures can be used safely without risk of bleeding and include compression stocking, and intermittent pneumatic compression device. Compression stocking also has its advantage in its safety and low price, but its effectiveness in its sole use has not been proven in high-risk DVT patients. The most effective mechanical measure is an intermittent pneumatic compression device that applies intermittent compression with a cuff to increase intravascular circulation and reduce DVT risk. Pharmacologic measures include warfarin, low molecular weight heparin (LWMH), fondaparinux, and rivaroxaban. Aspirin has been reported to be less effective in preventing VTE and provides more protection against heart attack and stroke than against DVT, which its sole use is not recommended. Warfarin is a vitamin K antagonist that shows anticoagulatory effect by inhibiting synthesis of coagulation factor II, VII, IX, and X, and when compared to non-warfarin, warfarin has reduced risk of VTE by 60% and proximal DVT by about 70%. However, oral dosage is possible, but non-oral administration is recommended for initial usage as its onset is slow. INR of 2–3 is recommended. LWMH is a fractionated heparin with molecular weight of 1000–10,000 Da. It shows high bioavailability compared to unfractionated heparin and longer half-life, allowing equal biological effect in patients with different body weight. Such characteristic allows oral dosage without monitoring.

14.6.2.4 Infection Prevention

Periprosthetic infections are a devastating complication. Incidence of deep infection after TKA is 0.5–2.0%. Every effort should be made for prevention of postoperative infection. Risk of infection must be minimized before, during, and after the surgery. Preoperative factors increasing risk of infection, such as malnutrition, DM, and obesity, should be treated or corrected. Any modifiable systemic factor that may affect infection must be resolved before the surgery. Preventive use of antibiotics just before the surgery is imperative to reduce the risk of infection. AlBuhairan et al. [136] reported that antibiotic prophylaxis should be routine in joint replacement but the choice of agent should be made on the basis of cost and local availability. Prophylactic antibiotics could be continued if there is risk of infection or reimplantation is performed due to infection. First generation cephalosporin is proposed as a drug of choice for prophylactic antibiotics. Meanwhile, in patients with history of MRSA infection, vancomycin is recommended. Smith et al. [137] have argued that prophylactic use of vancomycin can effectively reduce infection and infection by toxic resistant bacteria. However, Ponce et al. [138] argued spectrum of vancomycin is narrow, making its sole use less effective in prophylactic use than sole cefazolin treatment or combination of cefazolin and vancomycin. There is no consensus on the duration of postoperative antibiotics use and current study recommends use of prophylactic antibiotics for postoperative one day. Classen et al. [139] recommended prophylactic antibiotics use 30–40 min before surgery and to be no longer than 48 h after the surgery to reduce risk of urinary tract infection. Surgery must be simple and precise to shorten the surgical time. However, if the surgery has lasted too long, if the patient has recent history knee surgery, acupuncture or moxibustion, or intra-articular steroid infection, or if the patient has rheumatism or high risk of other infection, the antibiotics can be used for another 3–4 days or longer. Operating room environment should also be improved. The use of body exhaust suits, laminar flow rooms, and limit operating room traffic are important. A proper skin preparation, clean and meticulous wound closure are also helpful for decreasing infection rates. Blood transfusion increases risk of infection after TKA, therefore, rate of blood transfusion should be reduced as possible. In addition, proper management of indwelling urinary catheters and wound drainage also may decrease infection rates [140].

14.6.2.5 Rehabilitation

Rehabilitation aims to normalize physical and joint function and reduce any complication. Rehabilitation program is classified into 3 phases with goal for each phase of postoperative management. First week after the surgery is phase I, and the goal is to balance oneself by climbing out of the bed by oneself, walk by oneself with walker, and a complete full extension and 90-degree or more flexion. Phase II is 2–5 weeks after the surgery, with a goal of recovering motor and sensory of the operated leg, full function at home, and 0–110° ROM. In Phase III which is 6–8 weeks after the surgery, the goal is to be able to do house chores without help of orthosis and achieve 0–120° ROM. However, rehabilitation schedule varies depending on the individual capacity or situation, which must be planned by clinician. In most of arthroplasty, respiratory muscle exercise must be encouraged to prevent postoperative atelectasis, especially, if performed under general anesthesia, and inspirometer can be used for such exercise. In addition, to prevent DVT and muscle weakness, it is recommended to perform straight leg raise exercise or ankle pump during ambulation period (Fig. 14.37). Straight leg raise exercise is the most fundamental exercise that lifts the extended operated leg up and

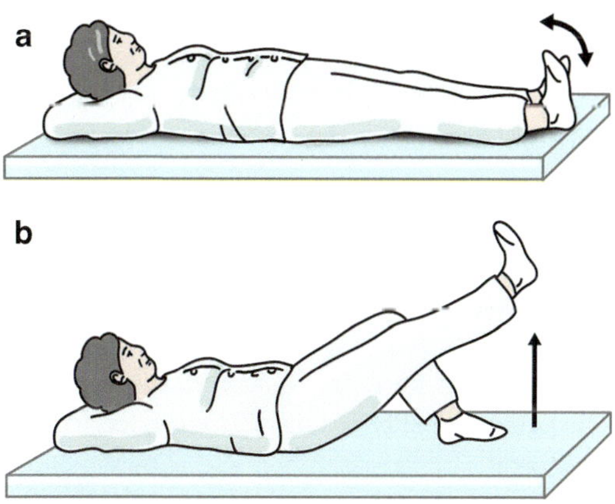

Fig. 14.37 Exercises to prevent DVT. (**a**) ankle pump, (**b**) straight leg raising exercise

down. Its effects can be maximized by slowly putting down the leg after holding its position in midair for about 10 s. Ankle pumping is to flick the ankle upward and downward, facilitating muscular strength growth and lower limb circulation to prevent DVT.

ROM exercise can be classified into active and passive exercise. Passive exercise can be started from the day of the surgery. CPM machine is the most commonly used device for passive ROM exercise. CPM executes joint exercise in an appropriate speed by a machine, allowing ROM exercise with less pain. Johnson et al. [141] have reported that the use of CPM is excellent in recovery of ROM in longer follow-up, while Colwell et al. [142] argued using CPM did not affect ROM but reduces pain and hospitalization period. When using CPM, it starts from 30° and the angle is increased until the patient can withstand it. If ROM is too limited, brisement can be performed under anesthesia. Yang et al. [143] have reported performing brisement in patients showing flexion less than 90° brought better outcome. Ambulation with walking aids is permitted at immediate postoperative period. If tolerable, waking aids can be discarded. However, careful attention should be paid to prevent fall accidents when the patient is walking.

14.6.3 Discharge Plan

Duration of hospital stay depends on health care system in each country, patient's physical status, and social environment. Generally, discharge is to be made about 7 days postoperatively if the patient shows no problem in the surgical site and is capable of more than 90 degrees knee ROM and walking in assist of walker. Before being discharged, the patient must be educated of knee rehabilitation, return to daily living activity, and precaution for knee and general health problem. The patient must be extensively educated to visit the hospital if the operation site shows redness or exudate.

14.7 Complications

Postoperative complications after TKA are the main cause for impediment of pain relief and functional recovery. Complications include systemic complications and knee related complications. The Knee Society had defined 22 standardized complications in TKA to improve the evaluation and reporting of results of arthroplasty (Table 14.3) [144].

14.7.1 Wound Complications

Among the local complications of TKA, wound complications can be the first red flag to healthy prognosis. Wound complications include wound drainage, delayed wound healing, hematoma, and skin necrosis, and the incidence rate is known to be quite high, with about 10–20% [145]. The most plausible explanation for such wound complications is partly due to the anatomy characteristics of its blood circulation (Fig. 14.38). Arterial supplies to the anterior soft tissue of the knee joint branches off to arterioles penetrating the subcutaneous fascia, forming a dermal plexus to supply blood to the skin. The superficial fascia must remain intact to the subcutaneous tissue so that the superficial arterial network can supply blood to the skin. Therefore, if a skin flap is made on the fascia, it may cause vascular disruption, resulting in skin necrosis [146].

To prevent wound complication, it is important to screen risk factors of wound complication, and risk factors include surgical technique-related factor and patient factor [147]. Risk factor for postoperative wound complication generally includes previous knee surgery history, skin scarring after trauma, smoking, steroid use, hypovolemia, DM, obesity, malnutrition, rheumatic arthritis, anemia, NSAIDs use, and old age [148]. Wound complications consist of 4 categories: (A) delayed wound healing or persistent drainage, (B) mild skin necrosis or superficial infection, (C) massive hematoma, and (D) extensive skin

Table 14.3 TKA complications and adverse events

Phase	Complication/Adverse events	Comments
Intraoperative/ Acute	Blood loss	Bleeding tolerance is low in patients with comorbid disease. Tranexamic acid application can be considered
	Wound complication	Detailed anamnesis (diabetes, hypertension, smoking, rheumatic arthritis, etc.) and physical exam should be done before surgery
	Thromboembolism	Thromboprophylaxis can reduce the prevalence of venous thromboembolism significantly. Symptomatic thromboembolic event requires intensive treatment during the first 3 months after TKA
	Neural deficit	Peroneal nerve injury is most common. Difficult to detect during operation
	Vascular injury	Intraoperative vascular injury requires tourniquet deflating and surgical repair
	MCL injury	Important for medial stabilization and intraoperative MCL injury requires operative treatment such as direct repair, reconstruction, constrained prosthesis use, and revision surgery
	Extensor mechanism injury	Disruption of the patellar tendon, quadriceps tendon, and patellar fracture are included. Operative treatment should be required
Intermediate/ Late	Periprosthetic joint infection	Debridement with retention of the prosthesis is required for early postoperative or acute hematogenous infection, and prosthesis removal with two-stage revision is required for late chronic infection with appropriate antibiotics treatment
	Patellofemoral dislocation	Advanced valgus alignment, previous high tibial osteotomy and malrotation of implants can be the cause of patellofemoral dislocation
	Tibiofemoral dislocation	Because of polyethylene damage or ligamentous incompetence. Re-dislocation is common if treated with closed reduction alone.
	Bearing surface wear	Symptomatic wearing of the bearing surface should be required revision operation
	Osteolysis	Expansile lytic lesion adjacent to one of the implants ≥1 cm in any one dimension or increasing in size on serial radiographs/CT scans
	Implant loosening	Loosening of implant is identified radiographically as a change in implant position or a progressive radiolucent line at the bone–cement or bone–implant interface
	Implant fracture or tibial insert dissociation	Implant design and malposition can be the cause of implant fracture or insert dissociation
	Periprosthetic fracture	Operative or nonoperative treatment would be selected by type of periprosthetic fracture. Revision TKA should be required for unstable implant.
	Instability	Symptomatic instability requires operative treatment such as gap balancing, thick insert change, and revision TKA
	Malalignment	Symptomatic malalignment confirmed radiographically with angular deformity in the coronal plane >10° from the mechanical axis
	Stiffness	If limited ROM continues despite CPM and manipulation, surgical release can be considered.

ROM range of motion, *CPM* continuous passive motion

necrosis [149]. It can cause superficial or deep infection in any case, and treatment for infection must be always considered [150]. If infection is suspected, early bacteria culture and more active, aggressive treatment is necessary, such as margin resection and antibiotics treatment.

14.7.1.1 Delayed Wound Healing or Persistent Drainage

Most of wound problem rarely progresses onto severe problem if treated early, but if the recovery is delayed or significant drainage persists, it is a red flag. Generally, wound must not show

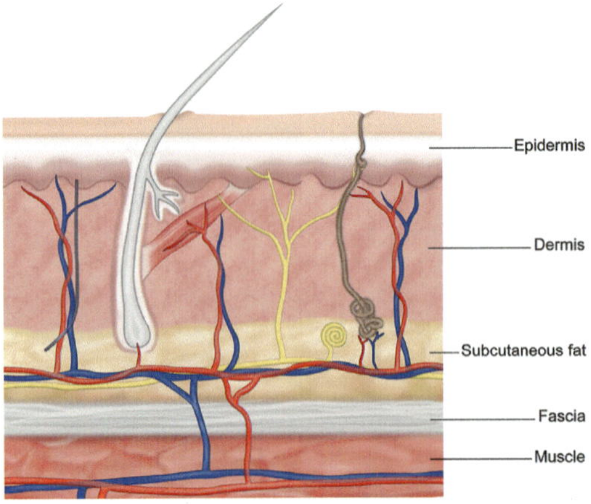

Fig. 14.38 Microvascular structure of soft tissue around knee

flare, tenderness, or pus. If the drainage persists, dressing must be performed frequently to dry the wound and create a sterile site so that it won't be contaminated [150]. After TKA, a persistent drainage is diagnosed if it lasts 72 h or longer with drainage larger than 2 cm × 2 cm gauze from the wound [151]. CPM or physical therapy is to be stopped briefly to rest the patient's knee and there is no need to prescribe antibiotics before bacteria culture or sensitivity test with joint aspiration. Such wound can be yet infected, and in case of deep infection, such use of antibiotics is not recommended as it can alter normal flora and sensitivity. Figure 14.39 shows treatment algorithm for acute wound problems after TKAs [152].

14.7.1.2 Mild Skin Necrosis or Superficial Infection

It ranges from pus formation around sutured site to cellulitis such as soft tissue infection, without any intra-articular infection. In general, debridement and dressing are sufficient for treatment of suture site infection. In superficial infection, bacteria culture must be performed. If it is suspected of deep infection, culture or biochemical test using joint aspiration must be considered. In such case, broad-spectrum antibiotics for anticipated infective organism must be started and may change depending on the culture result. The wound site should be immobilized and elevated until the drainage stops or the wound site shows improvement. However, skin necrosis may be worse than such superficial infection. If the necrosis is 3 cm or less, conservative treatments such as dressing are still available options, but if it does not respond to the treatment or necrosis is far beyond that size, debridement is required, removing all dead tissue thoroughly (Fig. 14.40). If the necrotized tissue involves intra-articular space and exposes prosthesis, muscular flap may be considered [153]. If it is only limited to superficial infection, it can be treated with debridement and simple suture, but suture after margin resection is decided based on size of the necrosis and elasticity of surrounding skin. If suture is difficult due to extensive necrosis or recurrent skin necrosis after re-suture, flap surgery may be needed. Depending on the case, local fasciocutaneous flap or gastrocnemius flap is reported to bring great outcomes [153].

14.7.1.3 Massive Hematoma

Massive hematoma can cause serious problems to the skin due to compression or toxicity of hemoglobin by-products. In addition, if these hematomas are contaminated and infected, it can be the optimal environment for bacteria to grow. If hemorrhage is too severe than expected during initial dressing of the wound after the surgery, or if the patient complains of more severe pain than expected postoperative pain, severe swelling, or discoloration in the wound area, it highly proposes presence of a hematoma [149]. In order to reduce subcutaneous hematoma and prevent leakage of synovial fluid, it is especially important to minimize the resection of the infrapatellar fat and to properly and delicately close lower incision around patellar tendon, as it is where most of the synovial drainage is placed [152]. Even though meticulous hemostasis before skin suture is performed, it must be reminded that hematoma can still occur. Use of tranexamic acid is helpful to reduce the postoperative bleeding and prevent hematoma. If a massive hematoma is diagnosed, reoperation is scheduled immediately to open the wound again, remove the hematoma, find bleeding site, and perform a thorough hemostasis.

14.7.1.4 Extensive Skin Necrosis

Despite the rarity of extensive necrosis inducing the prosthesis exposure, it is the most seri-

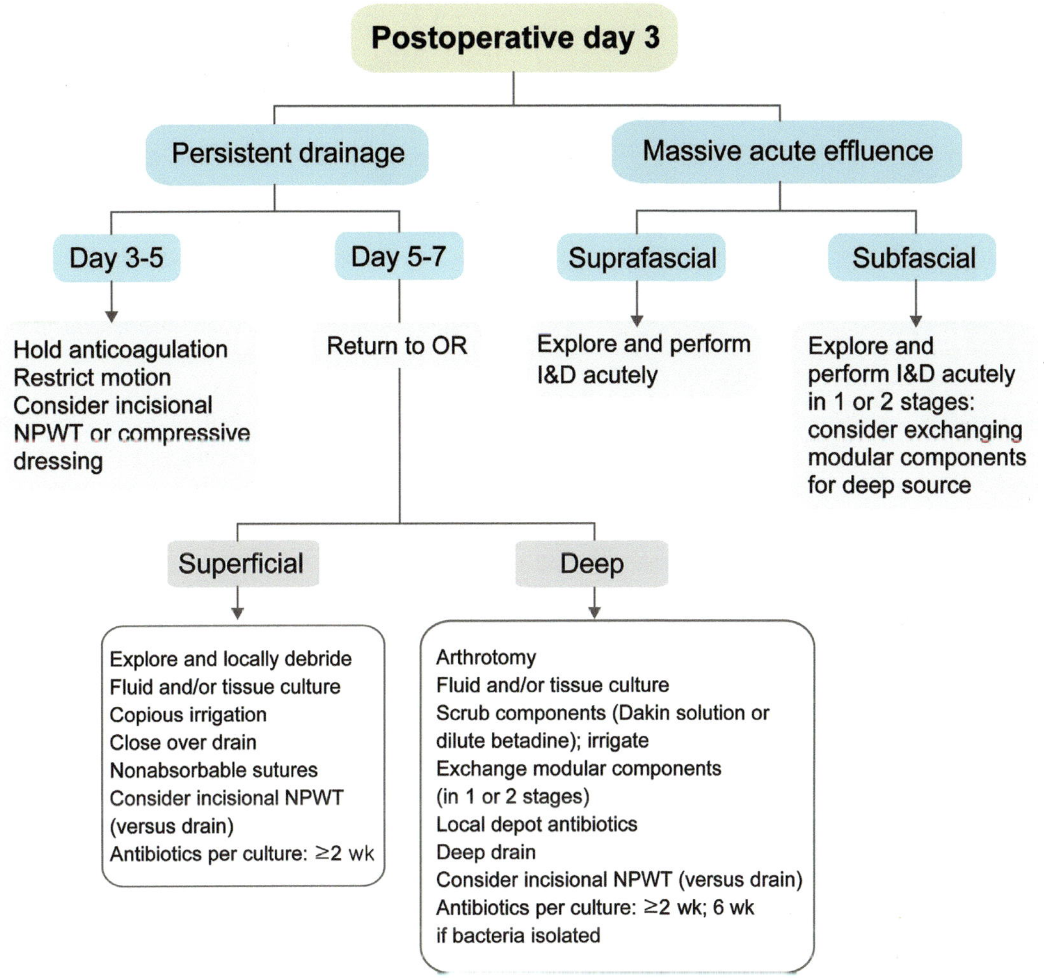

Fig. 14.39 Treatment algorithm for wound problems in acute postoperative stage. *I&D* incision and drainage, *NPWT* negative pressure wound therapy, *OR* operating room. (Reproduced from Simmons et al. 2017)

ous complication and is difficult to establish a specific treatment plan. In a worst case, removal of the prosthesis may be considered, but the first step in retaining the prosthesis is to open the incision and perform debridement. In most cases, it is impossible to re-suture the skin without tension, and flap reconstruction is generally required [154]. Type of the flap includes local, random pattern, and axial-type flap and gastrocnemius flap, fascia skin flap, and free flap. Success of the surgery depends on how viable these flaps are. Medial gastrocnemius is commonly used because medial head is longer and more viable than lateral head, and it is less likely to damage the peroneal nerve [155] (Fig. 14.41).

14.7.2 Periprosthetic Joint Infection (PJI)

PJI is a devastating complication that mostly needs reoperation and is the most common cause of revision TKA. Overall incidence of PJI has been known as 0.5–2% and in high-risk group or revision TKA, the incidence of infection increases further [156–158]. Early diagnosis and treatment is imperative for a favorable outcome. Infection must be treated with proper antibiotics. However, PJIs are difficult to treat without removing the prosthesis as bacteria continue to exist even after continuous use of antibiotics.

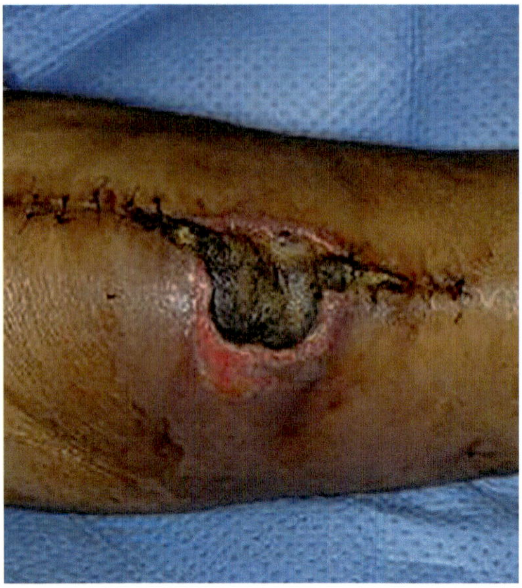

Fig. 14.40 Skin defects due to extensive necrosis are observed, and aggressive surgery such as flap is required

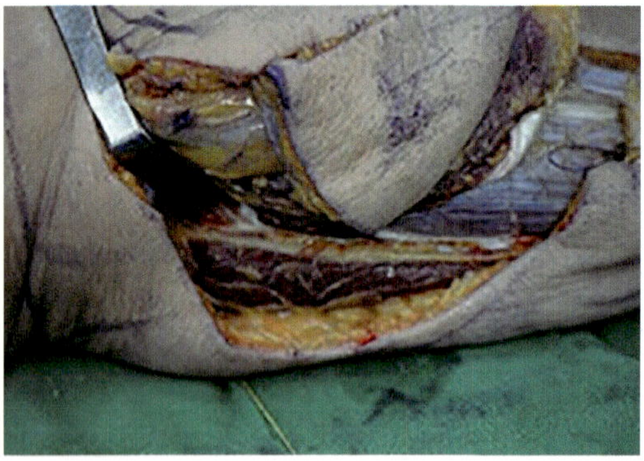

Fig. 14.41 Gastrocnemius flap using medial head of gastrocnemius

14.7.2.1 Classification

Traditionally, PJI was classified according to its onset, such as acute, subacute, and chronic [159]. However, classification according to disease onset does not help determine treatment plan. New classification based on clinical presentation helping determine treatment plan is proposed. Type 1 is positive intraoperative culture, which might represent contamination or true infection. Multiple specimens should be obtained for identifying true infection at the time of revision surgery. Diagnosis of infection is made only if the same pathogen is isolated from more than one specimen. This type can be treated with antibiotics alone, without further operation. Type 2 is early postoperative infection occurring within one month after TKA. Type 2 includes superficial and deep infection. Superficial suture infection usually can be treated with oral antibiotics. Deep infection needs operative treatment, such as debridement, implant retention. Type 3 is an acute hematogenous infection that has a sudden onset of acute septic symptoms in patients who had no symptoms after TKA. An acute hematogenous infection represents hematogenous seeding of organisms from distant site of infection. This type also needs operative debridement. Surgical treatment should be performed as soon as possible in early postoperative deep infection and acute hematogenous infection. Type 4 is a delayed chronic infection with inflammation persisting for more than a month, which accompanies often with no fever or leukocytosis, should be treated with removal of all implants [160] (Table 14.4).

Table 14.4 Classification of periprosthetic joint infection according to the time of occurrence and cause of infection

Type	Clinical Presentation	Definition	Treatment
I	Positive intraoperative culture	≥2 positive intraoperative cultures	A course of appropriate antibiotics
II	Early postoperative infection	Acute infection within 4 weeks after the operation	Debridement with retention of the prosthesis, intravenous antibiotics
III	Acute hematogenous infection	Acute onset of infection at the site of a previously well-functioning joint replacement	Debridement with retention of the prosthesis, intravenous antibiotics
IV	Late chronic infection	Chronic indolent infection, ≥4 weeks after the operation	Prosthesis removal with two-stage revision

14.7.2.2 Diagnosis

Diagnosis begins with a careful medical history taking and physical examination. Infection requires quick and accurate diagnosis. Any pain, swelling, redness, drainage that occurs irrelevant to the timing of surgery should be suspected of infection. Infection-related pain is suspected when unexpectedly severe pain persists after surgery or when pain occurs even at rest regardless of joint movement. However, if it is chronic, the pain may not be severe. Teller et al. [161] reported that sensitivity to the infection was 9% and specificity was 96% in presence of a fever of 37.5 degrees or higher, while sensitivity was 18% and specificity 100% in presence of a hot flash or redness in the joint.

If clinical symptoms suggest infection, hematologic test, microscopic inspection or culture of joint aspiration, or biopsy must be performed. In hematologic test, there may be an elevation in leukocyte count, erythrocyte sedimentation rate (ESR), or C-reactive protein (CRP), but this is not a confirmative finding and should be interpreted in comparison with other tests [162]. CRP is a more reliable indicator of acute inflammation than ESR or white blood cell (WBC) count [163]. It reaches its highest peak in 48–72 h after TKA and recovers to normal within 3 weeks [164]. However, there are cases where it gradually normalizes in 3 weeks or more due to the patient's age or preoperative medical conditions [165]. However, if CRP falls and rises again, a closer observation is needed [166].

Joint aspiration is a standard and mandatory test for diagnosing infection after TKA [167]. The sensitivity varies from 45 to 100% depending on the author, but the sensitivity can be increased with repeated tests [168]. Biochemical analysis is required along with visual inspection of the aspiration. Visual inspection includes volume, viscosity, color, and transparency. The normal properties of the aspiration are volume of about 4 cc, high viscosity, colorless or slightly straw-colored color with transparency. Biochemical tests mainly include WBC count, polymorphonuclear leukocyte (PMNL) or neutrophil ratio, bacterial culture, mucin clot, and glucose. Normal references are WBC <200/mm^3, neutrophils <25%, negative bacterial culture, film-like mucin clots, and glucose levels almost same as in hematological tests. However, after TKA, minor alterations may occur within normal range, but as there is no accurate analysis data, it is necessary to refer to normal synovial fluid findings before surgery. Infectious arthritis is diagnosed once synovial leukocyte count is 50,000/mm^3 or more, but 28,000/mm^3 or less, in immunocompromised patients. There may be various explanation for WBC count and PMNL ratio after TKA, but in general, infection is very likely in patients with the leukocyte count of 5000/mm^3 or more and PMNL ratio higher than 65%. Trampuz et al. [169] reported the sensitivity and specificity for diagnosis of PJI were high if ratio of synovial neutrophil is 65% or higher or synovial WBC count is 1700/mm^3 or higher. Mason et al. [170] reported that TKA patient with synovial WBC count of 2500/mm^3 or higher and PMNL ratio of 60% or higher is to be suspected of infection. Synovial WBC count of >1700/mm^3/μL (1100–3000/mm^3/μL) or synovial WBC ratio of 65% (64–80%) is a strong indicator of chronic infection. However, this guideline is yet to be established for synovial WBC count and ratio reference in acute infection occurring within 6 weeks after the surgery, making it difficult to employ such references in diagnosis of acute infection [171]. According to the 2013 Proceedings of the International Consensus on PJI [151, 172], in case of acute infection, the threshold of ESR in the joint fluid within postoperative 6 weeks is not determined, whereas the CRP was 100 mg/L or more and leukocyte count 10,000/mm^3, synovial PMNL ratio 90% was checked. In the case of chronic TKA infection, the ESR of 30 mm/hr or more, CRP 10 mg/L or more, synovial leukocyte count of 3000/mm^3 or more, and synovial PMNL ratio of 80% or more was checked in the joint fluid 6 weeks after surgery.

Even though a blood test, image study, or clinical sign confirms the infection, it is difficult to start treatment with appropriate antibiotics because causative organisms are not found. Bacteria culture should be timely appropriate and the specimen for culture should be acquired from an appropriate site [157]. Bacteria culture must be performed before using antibiotics due to suspected infection. When deep infection is suspected, culturing samples from exudate in superficial layer or sinus tract can result in polymicrobial contamination, which cannot be concluded as the causative pathogen of the deep infection. The most effective specimen is joint aspirates, or deep wound biopsy or curettage specimens. Gram staining is very useful for distinguishing whether the pathogen is Gram-positive or negative. Benston et al. [173] reported that Staphylococcus was most common (52.9%) in knee aspiration and bacterial culture tests performed in the operating room, followed by *E. coli* (5.9%). However, 41.2% of cases did not show any bacterial growth in the culture.

In plain radiography, no findings regarding PJI are available in early stage but can be only found in only advanced stages. Findings of advanced inflammation include bone absorption in bone cement, periosteal new bone formation, and gas formation in soft tissue [174]. Bone scans can be more helpful in early diagnosing infections after TKA than plain radiology and ultrasound. The indium labeled WBC scan has higher sensitivity and specificity than conventional bone scan, making it more useful when the results are arbitrary on physical, hematological, and radiographic studies [175]. In some cases, technetium and WBC scan are performed simultaneously to increase the diagnosis rate.

Table 14.5 Major criteria and minor criteria for diagnosing PJI

Diagnostic criteria for the periprosthetic joint infection (PJI)*	
Major Criteria	1. Pathogen isolated by periprosthetic culture from two separated samples 2. A sinus tract communicating with the joint
Minor Criteria	1. Elevated serum ESR AND CRP concentration 2. Elevated synovial fluid leukocyte count OR ++result on leukocyte esterase test strip 3. Elevated synovial fluid PMN% 4. Positive histological analysis of periprosthetic tissue 5. Pathogen isolated by culture in one sample

ESR erythrocyte sedimentation rate, *CRP* C-reactive protein, *PMN* polymorphonuclear neutrophil
*Diagnosis when one major criteria or three out of five minor criteria present

Diagnosis Algorithm

The clear diagnosis of PJI can be challenging because the definition is not standardized and is determined by the combination of criteria. However, as most of the criteria used for diagnosis of PJI use test results, they have limitations (such as false-positive tests) and there are some cases that need to be judged within the clinical context.

To standardize the definition of PJI, a number of diagnostic criteria such as the Musculoskeletal Infection Society (MSIS) criteria, the Infectious Disease Society of America (IDSA) guidelines, the International Consensus Meeting (ICM) criteria, European Bone and Joint Infection Society (EBJIS) criteria have been proposed [172, 176–179]. Among them, the MSIS diagnostic criteria remain widely accepted worldwide and have been endorsed at international consensus meetings [151, 180, 181] (Table 14.5).

Subsequently, a new evidence-based and validated criteria were developed in 2018 based on MSIS and ICM criteria [151, 177, 178, 180]. This new diagnostic criteria consists of major and minor criteria (Table 14.6) [178]. Major criteria include cases, in which there are two consecutive positive cultures of the same organism, or if there is a sinus tract exposed to the prosthesis, and if this is satisfied, it can be diagnosed with PJI. Minor criteria include serum CRP, D-dimer, ESR levels, non-synovial WBC, PMNL percentage, leukocyte esterase, alpha-defensin, and synovial CRP levels. When the reference value of each item exceeds the specified value, the score assigned is added to determine whether to diagnose with PJI. Parvizi et al. [178] also suggested some cases that may not be true infection even if the above criteria are satisfied and vice versa, which is nominated as a red flag sign. These include adverse local tissue reactions (ALTR), crystalline deposition arthropathy, inflammatory arthropathy flares, and infections due to slow growing organisms such as *Propionibacterium*

Table 14.6 New scoring based definition for periprosthetic joint infection (PJI). Proceed with caution in adverse local tissue reaction, crystal deposition disease, slow growing organisms

Major criteria (at least one)	Decision
Pathogen isolated by periprosthetic culture from two separated samples	Infected
A sinus tract communicating with the joint	

	Minor criteria		Score	Decision
Preoperative Diagnosis	Serum	Increased CRP or D-dimer	2	6 ≥ Infected 2–5 Possibly infected* 0–1 Not infected
		Increased ESR	1	
	Synovial	Increased synovial WBC count or LE	3	
		Positive alpha-defensin	3	
		Increased synovial PMN (%)	2	
		Increased synovial CRP	1	

	Inconclusive preop score or dry tab	Score	Decision
Intraoperative diagnosis	Preoperative score	–	6 ≥ Infected 4–5 Inconclusive[a] ≤3 Not infected
	Positive histology	3	
	Positive purulence	3	
	Single positive culture	2	

CRP C-reactive protein, *ESR* erythrocyte sedimentation rate, *WBC* white blood cell, *LE* leukocyte esterase, *PMN* polymorphonuclear neutrophil
*For patients with inconclusive minor criteria, operative criteria can also be used to fulfill definition for PJI
[a]Consider further molecular diagnostics such as next-generation sequencing

acnes, coagulase negative *Staphylococcus*, and others. The algorithm for diagnosing PJI has been summarized in Fig. 14.42 [181].

14.7.2.3 Treatment

The use of susceptible antibiotics and surgery is imperative for PJI treatment. Treatment methods for PJI include antibiotic suppression, debridement, antibiotics and implant retention, one-stage reimplantation, two-stage reimplantation, fusion and amputation. In some cases, the treatment is time-consuming and expensive because the infection can recur even after several surgeries. Even if the infection has eradicated, making a joint with good function is technically more difficult than non-infectious revision surgery, rendering its prognosis to be lower than that of non-infectious revision surgery. Therefore, in the treatment of infection, not only the problem of the knee itself, but also the patient's medical condition or comorbidity, social and economic conditions must be considered. The type of infection by onset, the timing of treatment, strain and antimicrobial susceptibility, the degree of loosening of the prosthesis, and presence of a draining sinus must be considered for treatment of PJI. Any form of surgery must be conducted to eradicate infection, and how well debridement is performed during surgery is closely related to the recurrence rate of infection. In order to maintain good function after surgery, reconstruction of bone defect, maintenance of extension and flexion gaps, and balancing of ligaments are important as in non-infectious revision surgery.

Principle of Antibiotics Administration

Fulkerson et al. [182] provided a general guideline for empiric antibiotic use for suspected PJI by the class of the infection and the findings of Gram staining. Acute hematogenous infections should initially be treated by a combination of cefazolin and gentamicin therapy until the final culture results are available. Acute and chronic postoperative infections with Gram-positive bacteria or failing to identify bacteria with Gram stain should be treated with vancomycin. Infections with Gram-negative bacteria should be treated with a third or fourth-generation cephalosporin. Infections with mixed Gram-positive and Gram-negative bacteria should be treated with a combination of vancomycin and a third or fourth-generation cephalosporin. If culture results and other confirmatory tests are not positive by the fourth postoperative day, termination of empiric

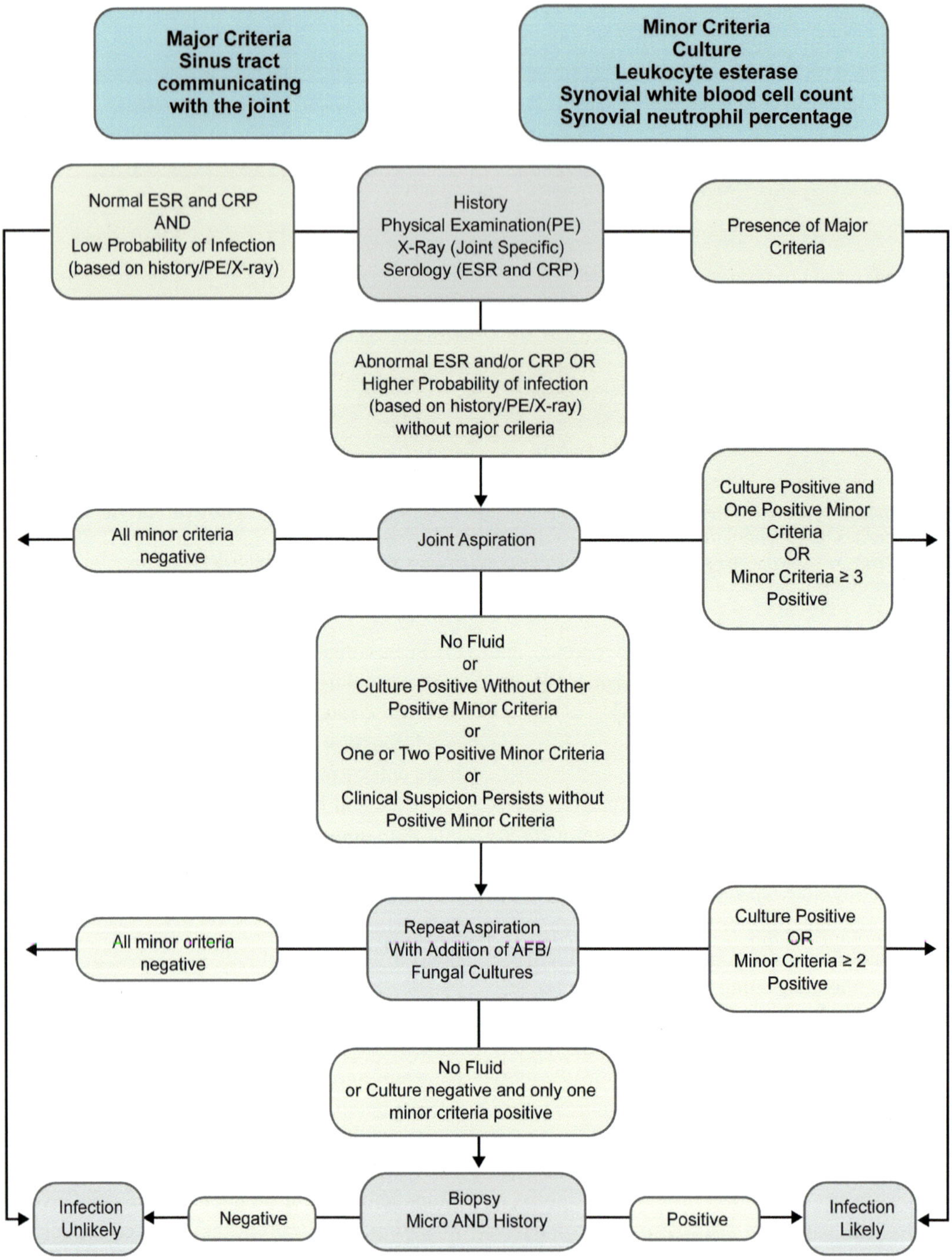

Fig. 14.42 Algorithm for diagnosis of PJI (Reproduced from Zmistowski et al. 2014)

antibiotic therapy should be considered. The general principle of antibiotic use is that if gram-positive bacteria are found in the smear before cultivation, vancomycin is recommended as it is highly likely to be methicillin resistant *Staphylococcus aureus* (MRSA) [183]. Although MRSA poses a formidable clinical threat, with persistently high morbidity and mortality, the choice of antibiotics should consider data regarding local infection control since *S. aureus* strains may have different prevalence (esp. for MRSA) and antibiotics sensitivity profiles for each region [182, 184]. In regions with low MRSA prevalence, parenteral agents including nafcillin, oxacillin, and cefazolin can be used in response to methicillin-sensitive *S. aureus* (MSSA), and ceftriaxone can be considered for oxacillin-susceptible staphylococcal PJIs [185, 186].

In the case of chronic infection caused by staphylococcus, etc., it should be considered that the bacteria create a biofilm on the surface of the prosthesis, thus making it unpassable with general concentration of antibiotics. This biofilm is supposed to form in 3 weeks after infection. Zimmerli et al. [187] recommended mixed administration of rifampin in chronic infections as rifampin facilitates passage of antibiotics through the biofilm. Quinolone is not recommended for Staphylococcus infections because Staphylococcus is more likely to develop a resistant strain. As infection by *Mycobacterium tuberculosis* takes too long to eradicate, anti-tuberculosis drugs should be prescribed for at least 1 year to 1 year and a half after revision surgery. In fungal infection, patients tend to have specific causes, that the patient may have history of malignant tumor, immunodepressant usage, or antibiotics overdose, or have implant (e.g., indwelling catheter). The fungal infection is mostly due to Candida, and though there is no established guideline of antifungal agent, amphotericin or fluconazole is commonly used. It is recommended to be used for at least 6 months up to 1 year with consistent follow-up of renal and hepatic function.

Antibiotic Suppression

If the patient is in poor health condition that cannot go through a surgery or refuses to have a surgery, antibiotics suppression is another treatment option for PJI. It can be used if the prosthesis shows no loosening, and the infectious strain shows minimal toxicity and responds to oral antibiotics. Though there is a report that continuous antibiotics administration has cured the infection, but it is only true for 10–25% of all the cases. It is just a temporary measure to alleviate symptom or stop debilitation of the symptoms. Duggal et al. [188] reported that after treating 74 infected patients with antibiotics in outpatient clinic, 58% of the patients recurred and 9% were re-hospitalized due to systemic problem.

Debridement, Antibiotics, and Implant Retention

This method is employed for acute postoperative or hematogenous infection without loosening of the prosthesis. Acute postoperative or hematogenous infections can be classified into superficial infections and deep infections, which are treated with antibiotics after debridement and implant retention. Debridement removes all fistulas including subcutaneous fat and joint capsule, resects skin margin in an elliptical shape, thoroughly cleans the wound. Appropriate antibiotics were prescribed. If there is no loosening of the prosthesis, prosthesis can be preserved. Debridement can be performed under arthroscopy or open method. Arthroscopic debridement resulted in high recurrence rate. Most surgeons preferred open debridement.

The outcomes of debridement and drainage show great differences between authors. It depends on mode of infection, duration of infection, infected organism, and surgical timing. Mirra et al. [189] and Chiu et al. [190] have reported relatively high success rates of 100% and 70% in acute postoperative infection, 71% and 50% in acute hematogenous infection, respectively. Gardner et al. [191] reported a reinfection rate of 57%, while Silva et al. [192] have reported a poor success rate of about 33%. Such difference is closely related to which strain was infected. In the case of MRSA, Bradbury et al. [193] reported a low success rate of 18% and argued that MRSA infection showed worse prognosis regardless of its onset, so that the prosthesis must be removed if infected by the strains with strong toxicity, even in acute infection. Deirmengian et al. [194] reported success rate of 35% in less toxic bacteria such as *Staphylococcus epidermidis* and streptococcus species and only 8% in *Staphylococcus aureus* with strong toxicity. It is also related to the timing of the surgery.

Comparing between within 2 weeks and thereafter in acute infection, Teeny et al. [195] reported that the success rate was high if the surgery was performed within 2 weeks, but 71% failed after 2 weeks. Hartman et al. [196] stated that chronic infections over 4 weeks have a high risk of failure and should not be operated with debridement.

Various methods have been introduced to increase success rate of the surgical method of preserving the original prosthesis. Mont et al. [197] have chosen a method of re-draping and re-wearing gloves when closing the surgical site after debridement. In addition, another surgical technique is to implant cement beads after debridement and remove those 1–2 weeks later via small incision. Estes et al. [198] reported success rate of about 90% by performing secondary debridement within 7 days of inserting cement beads after initial debridement. Tsumura et al. [199] reported the infection to be eradicated in 8 out of 10 cases except 2 cases of MRSA after continuous irrigation for 10–14 days after debridement until the culture is negative. Debridement is very vital in success of the surgery and it is crucial to remove infected tissue and pseudomembrane. Though the prosthesis is not removed, PE can be changed for easier debridement. However, if the implant-retention method fails, the prosthesis facilitates deeper invasion of bacteria and increases risk of recurrence.

One-Stage Reimplantation

In older and less active patients with susceptible acute infection, reimplantation can be sometimes performed immediately after removal of the prosthesis. This method has the advantage of reducing duration of the disease and time and cost by performing a single operation. However, while this method removes the prosthesis anyway, the success rate is lower than that of the two-stage reimplantation, which poses a limitation in its implementation. In comparative reviews by several authors, Hanssen et al. [156] reported that the success rate was 74% when the prosthesis was immediately replaced and antibiotic-impregnated cement was used and 72% when reimplantation using cement without antibiotics is performed within 3 weeks after removal. The success rate was 88% when using cement without antibiotics after 6 weeks and 91% when using antibiotic-impregnated cement after 6 weeks. Factors related to the success include onset of the symptoms within 4 weeks, Gram-positive bacteria susceptible to antibiotics, no osteomyelitis, well-fixated prosthesis, and young and healthy patient. Though it has higher recurrence rate than two-stage reimplantation, careful selection of patient and thorough debridement increase success rate of one-stage reimplantation up to 70–80%. For one-stage reimplantation, intravenous antibiotics injections are recommended for at least 6 weeks. There are various methods to reduce the recurrence rate. Buechel et al. [200] introduced a method of soaking the wound with povidone mixture for 30 min and injecting antibiotics intravenously before releasing tourniquet and closing the wound. Their method was able to eradicate infection in 91% of 22 patients in 10-year follow-up, and argued that the patient's health status was a very important factor.

Two-stage Reimplantation

Two-stage reimplantation is the gold standard treatment for PJI. The surgery is performed in 2 stages as it has significantly lower recurrence infection. In first surgery, a thorough debridement of necrotized tissue including pseudomembrane is performed along with removal of prosthesis and cement. In 4–6 weeks after antibiotic-impregnated cement spacer and/or bead insertion, second stage surgery is performed based on clinical symptom and blood test. Contraindication of the second stage reimplantation includes residual infection, extension mechanism disruption, and inability to withstand multiple surgery. The poor skin condition can be a relative contraindication as it raises risk of failure and must be treated with skin flap after consultation with plastic surgeon.

At first stage surgery, a meticulous and thorough debridement should be performed. If the joint motion was restricted, a more extensile capsular approach is recommended. If the prosthesis fixed firmly, maximum care must be exerted to its removal as it may not be easy and can accompany weakening and destruction of the bone. Thorough debridement of infected soft tissue and granulation tissue after removal of the prosthesis and cement is essential to prevent recurrence of inflammation and to obtain a good ROM. Debrided joint should be clean with copious saline or povidone mixed saline irrigation.

Antibiotic-impregnated cement insertion After the debridement, an antibiotic-impregnated cement is inserted. Role of antibiotic-impregnated cement maintains the length of the leg to ensure proper joint spacing during reoperation, facilitate reimplantation by minimizing contracture of soft tissue, increase the intra-articular concentration of antibiotics, eliminate dead space, and promote joint stability. Only antibiotics that are heat-stable and water-soluble are used, which includes gentamycin, cefazolin, tobramycin, and vancomycin. Infection by tuberculosis can be treated with streptomycin. It is recommended to use susceptible antibiotics, but it is more common practice to use multiple antibiotics simultaneously due to uncertainty of the causative bacteria and multiple infection. Antifungal agent is to be used for fungal infection. As for the dosage of antibiotics, up to 3.0–4.0 gm of vancomycin or 3.6 gm of tobramycin can be mixed in each pack of cement (40 mg). The use of such high concentrations of antibiotics does not seem to have a significant effect on the body. Factors affecting the release of antibiotics from the cement include type and dose of antibiotics, type and surface area of the cement. The time for the cement to release antibiotic properly after insertion varies from a day to 80 days after surgery, depending on the type of cement, type of antibiotic, and concentration of antibiotics. Palacos® is known to release antibiotics longer than any other cement, and high-dose tobramycin as well. Antibiotic-impregnated cement has cement bead type, static type, and articulating type. Cement bead is used to fill the dead space while static or articulating type cement is used in the space between femur and tibia. Selection of static type or articulating type depends on bone defect, soft tissue, necessity of joint movement, utility of the cement product, and operator's preference. Complication of antibiotic-impregnated cement includes instability, dislocation, prosthesis protrusion, overstuffing of joint spacing, and fracture.

Management between first stage and second stage surgery After the first stage surgery, patients with static type cement spacer are allowed of body weight loading only after wearing an orthosis, and if the patient has articulating cement spacer, joint exercise is also conducted. Intravenous antibiotics must be used for at least 4–6 weeks, and revision surgery is scheduled based on clinical symptom and hematologic findings. If the infection does not subside after 3 months, it is advisable to remove the cement and perform debridement again.

Follow-up of infection control and scheduling of second stage surgery In general, if the surgical scar has well healed, with no heat sensation or erythema at the surgical site and normal CRP and ESR, the infection is considered to have eradicated. Mont et al. [201] emphasized the use of bacterial culture and susceptibility tests with biopsy or articular puncture before the reimplantation. In their work, antibiotics were stopped for 4–6 weeks after 6 weeks of antibiotics administration, and if the culture was negative, reimplantation was performed; if the culture was positive, antibiotic therapy was performed again. Such treatment brought in better outcomes than reimplantation after 4–6 weeks.

Considerations before second stage surgery Before second stage surgery, it must be certain that the infection is eradicated. If there are no conclusive findings of infection after inspection during surgery, reimplantation is determined based on microscopic findings of the tissue. It is called the Mirra criteria [189], which Mirra collected synovial and capsular tissue debris from 5 different areas and used them to study what caused the failure of original prosthesis by examining the type and number of cells, the presence of metal particles, and PE. Infection was highly suspected when there were more than 5 PMNL in high-power field. Therefore, the theory states that reimplantation can be performed only when the number of WBCs is less than 5 at high-power field in frozen section sampled from five most dirty areas.

Second stage surgery The method of reimplantation is basically identical to that of non-infectious reimplantation. The inserted cement is carefully removed without damaging the remaining bone. After removing the cement, formation of a thin film can be identified. It is better to remove it as a whole, and if not possible, it is removed thoroughly using a curette. A thorough debridement of joint capsule and bone bed should be implemented to make clean joint. Bone defects management and ligaments reconstruction might be necessary after debridement. Constrained type implant may be used because bone defects and ligamentous imbalance during second stage surgery may be more severe than expected. Antibiotic after surgery is to be used for 5–7 days until the bacteria culture result come in, and henceforth, use of the antibiotic depends upon results of the culture. However, in reimplantation due to infection, there are many arguments that the use of the antibiotic for 4–6 weeks is recommended based on clinical and laboratory test results, as it is not a concept of prophylactic antibiotic treatment and a recurrence rate is reported to be about 10–15% even after the second stage surgery.

Outcome of two-stage reimplantation Two-stage reimplantation shows about 70–90% of success rate in eradicating infection, but it differs according to its strain. Kurd et al. [202] have reported 27% of reinfection even after two-stage reimplantation, and if infected by MRSA which is resistant to antibiotic, reinfection is 3.7 times higher than infection by other strains. Mittal et al. [203] reported 24% of reinfection after performing two-stage reimplantation in 37 cases of MRSA and MRSE infection, which the outcome was worse than outcome of infection eradication without considering strain. Fungal infection has shown very dismal outcome; Azzam et al. [204] have reported that 10 out of 19 patients with fungal infection still have required arthrodesis, resection arthroplasty, and amputation despite two-stage reimplantation. Therefore, one-stage reimplantation is not considered as an option in fungal infection, but two-stage reimplantation must be performed.

14.7.3 Instability After TKA

Instability is the second most common complication to cause revision TKAs. Although its' definition is still on debate, instability after TKA generally can be defined as patient's subjective feeling of the instability that can affect knee score and operator's sense of knee instability on physical examination. Some researchers propose that some degree of laxity is considered normal up to 2 mm medially and 3 mm laterally in extension, while in flexion, 3 mm medially and 4 mm laterally. Generally, patients with unstable TKA sense waddling while walking and experience dull pain around knee. Severe instability interferes walking, with joint swelling and dislocation if severe.

14.7.3.1 Classification

Classification of instability is described differently depending on the author. It may be classified depending on its direction: anteroposterior, varus-valgus, recurvatum, and global [205]. Anteroposterior instability is generally induced by flexion-extension mismatch. Anterior instability may occur in presence of weakened quadriceps or subluxation-dislocation of patella. Flexion instability is diagnosed if anteroposterior displacement of 5 mm or more or dislocation occurs. Flexion instability is also classified into symmetric instability and asymmetric instability, and the symptoms may not be so distinctive than extension instability. Generally, flexion instability is based on 90-degree flexion, but flexion instability at 30 and 45 degrees flexion induces instability in mid swing phase, creating inconvenience in stair gait, which can also be classified as mid-flexion phase instability [206]. Varus-valgus instability is determined by tension of collateral ligament, balancing the knee in extension [207]. It can be further classified into symmetric or asymmetric instability. Extension instability is identified if the widening is more than 2 mm to the medial and 3 mm to the lateral in stress test. Symmetric instability shows both medial and lateral instability commonly accompanied by genu recurvatum. Asymmetric instability is when instability exists in only lateral or medial (Fig. 14.43). Extension instability causes severe dysfunction and patient

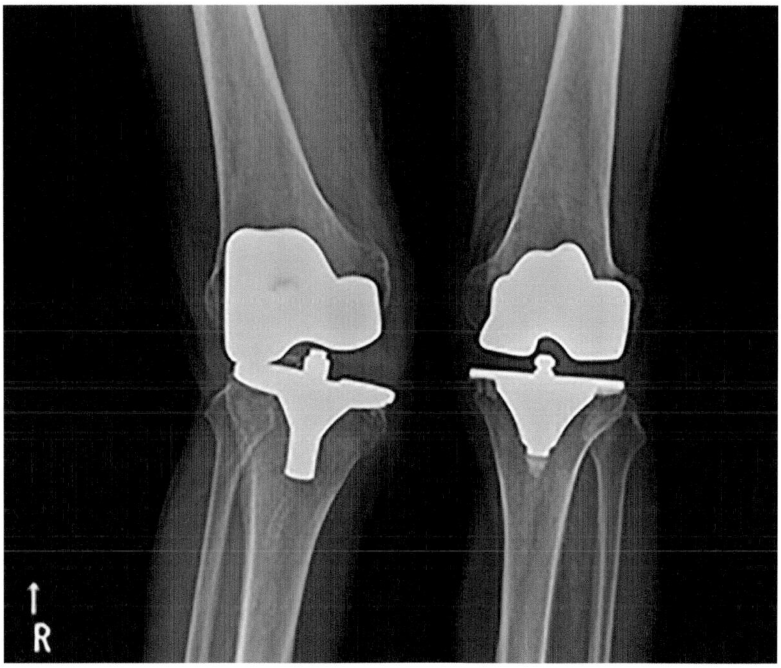

Fig. 14.43 Severe valgus instability is shown right side knee

feels even the mildest instability. Recurvatum is essentially when knee shows hyperextension of 0° or higher and often results from a weak quadriceps muscle and the necessity of walking with hyperextension. However, it has been reported that the hyperextension is made about 9.5° at average after TKA. Clinically, genu recurvatum is diagnosed when hyperextension is 5° or greater or patient or examiner does not sense endpoint during extension. Multidirectional (global) instability is when two or more of the mentioned instabilities occur simultaneously.

14.7.3.2 Cause of Instability

Instability after TKA is caused by complex causes. It mostly consists of patient factors, surgical factors, and postoperative factors. Most of instability is caused by wrongfully performed surgery, but it may also occur when muscular strength to support joint declines despite well-executed surgery, when the patient is too excessively active after surgery or gets hurt, or when complications such as infection, loosening, or wear occur [208–210].

If the patient has already had severe instability before surgery and its correction is inadequate, instability may occur. If there is deformity or stiffness to other lower limb joint or if the patient is pathologically obese, abnormal stress is repetitively forced onto knee joint, causing instability. CR type TKA performed in patients with RA can cause flexion instability due to weakening and loss of PCL. Subsidence of tibia prosthesis in osteoporosis patient can cause instability similar to instability from using a thin PE. High risk of instability exists in case of neurologic or musculoskeletal disease, soft tissue disease such as Ehlers-Danlos syndrome, weak quadriceps as a sequela of poliomyelitis, neuropathic arthritis [205, 211, 212].

Extension instability is further classified into symmetric instability and asymmetric instability. Both instabilities deteriorate with malalignment but disappear with correct alignment. Symmetric instability in extension occurs when excessive resection is made to distal femur or when prosthesis is too large, creating comparatively larger extension space. Excessive resection of distal femur is more complicated, requiring use of a block in femoral component to reduce extension gap. Asymmetric instability in extension usually occurs when collateral ligament is inadequately

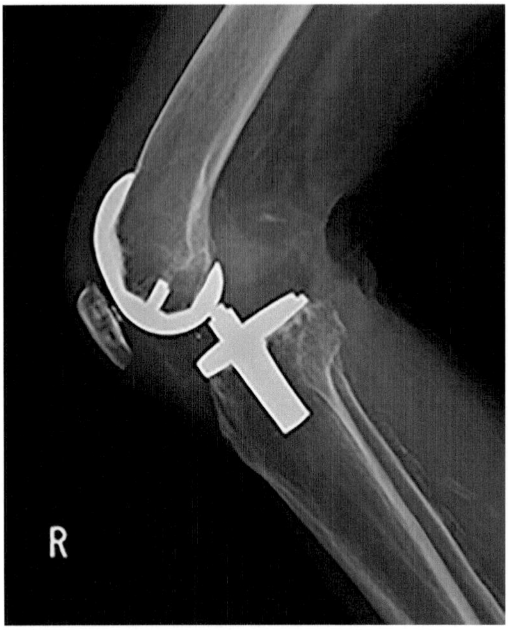

Fig. 14.44 In the case of CR type TKA when PCL is damaged or has little function due to severe degenerative lesions, PCL is weakened and function is lost, which causes posterior instability during flexion

or excessively released. Flexion instability is also classified into symmetric and asymmetric instability. Symmetric instability in flexion is when flexion gap is widened. Especially when performing PS type TKA, flexion gap becomes wider when resecting PCL. If the prosthesis is small, flexion instability occurs. Even in CR type TKA, the dysfunction of the ligament due to its damage or severe degeneration can contribute to flexion instability (Fig. 14.44) [213–215]. Increased posterior tibial slope can be the cause of symptomatic flexion instability. Asymmetric instability in flexion is caused by insufficient collateral ligament release or excessive release. Malrotation of the femoral prosthesis may cause asymmetric flexion instability. Mid-flexion instability occurs when there is instability at 30 and 45 degrees flexion, especially when the anterior fiber of MCL is weakened. When instability factors of the above are combined or an instability lasts for a long time, it progresses onto multidirectional (global) instability. Multidirectional instability occurs if both the extension and flexion gaps are wide. Dislocation can be seen as a more severe state of such instability. Patellofemoral instability is generally caused by malalignment of prosthesis or imbalance of patella retinaculum. Malalignment of the prosthesis is more closely related to rotational alignment of femoral/tibial prosthesis. Computerized tomography is crucial in its diagnosis [216–218].

14.7.3.3 Diagnosis

Thorough history taking is crucial. Detailed history taking of initial cause for TKA, diagnosis, preoperative joint deformity and ROM, surgical history before TKA, surgical technique, used prosthesis, postoperative rehabilitation or history of trauma is required. It is crucial to identify accurate etiology of the instability in the patient by performing physical examination [219]. Though instability of artificial joint due to damaged MCL or dysfunctional PCL can be easily identified. However, if symptoms of the instability are unclear, if patient only complains of symptoms such as catching, giving way or anterior knee pain, or if the knee shows repetitive hemarthrosis or hemorrhagic exudate, accurate diagnosis is difficult. Therefore, valgus-varus stability must be measured in extension, 30° and 90° flexion of the knee. Anteroposterior stress test must be performed in 90° flexion to assess flexion instability. Mid-flexion instability can be tested with external rotation-valgus stress test in flexion of 45–90°. Radiologic test includes knee AP, lateral, and patella axial view to confirm any position change of prosthesis and bone defect in anterior and posterior femur. In addition, it is to be performed to measure mechanical axis and anatomical axis with whole leg standing AP view. Patellar axial view is used to evaluate location of patella and its relative connection to trochlear groove of the femur. Radiologic finding with high risk of instability includes excessively resected posterior femoral condyle, inappropriate distal femoral resection, and interval between components showing a large difference between weight-bearing and non-weight bearing condition.

14.7.3.4 Prevention

In presence of neurologic or musculoskeletal disease or deformity or stiffness in other joint of lower limb, sufficient consideration and review should be undertaken before surgery. Such pathological factors are not contraindicated in TKA, but since the patient's condition may worsen than before surgery if postoperative instability appears, it is recommended to strictly apply the indications for the surgery in such patients. When selecting a prosthesis, it should be selected after considering degree of constraint such as constrained, semiconstrained, and unconstrained type. In the surgical technique, it is necessary to obtain a neutral alignment of the lower extremities and try to balance the extension and flexion during surgery.

Decision for implant choice is made by careful consideration of the degree of restriction of articulation, such as constrained, semiconstrained, or unconstrained. It is not recommended to use unconstrained prosthesis in patients with severe preoperative deformity or instability. In the case of severe deformity, the use of PS type is recommended because it is difficult to correct the deformity with CR type [94]. The use of PS type is also recommended because the PCL is weakened during surgery in severe knee OA, or in the case of RA, the PCL function cannot be expected over time [212]. In cases where ligament function cannot be restored by general methods such as chronically stiffed knees, neuropathic arthritis, or ligamentous instability cannot be restored intraoperatively, the quadriceps muscle strength that cannot overcome gravity, and the extension and flexion gap cannot be matched, hinged prosthesis as well as constrained prosthesis should be considered [220–222]. If the collateral ligament can be restored even with the constrained prosthesis, it is necessary to restore the collateral ligament as much as possible for stability and for long-term survival of the prosthesis [223]. Since the size of the prosthesis is closely related to the gap between flexion and extension, it is better to determine the implant size during surgery.

Lower extremity alignment and joint instability are closely related [205, 224], but if the ligament balance is inappropriate, malalignment may deteriorate instability. If femur and tibial prosthesis forms anterior slope in sagittal plane, it can induce genu recurvatum. If rotational alignment in axial plane is not accurate, it may cause instability during flexion and mid-flexion. Therefore, besides coronal alignment, it is important to correct not only sagittal and axial alignment. Extension and flexion gap balance is important in obtaining a stable joint. There are several methods for evaluating extension-flexion gap balance. It is precise to use a gapper or tensioner to check extension and flexion balance. The balance is achieved when the extension and flexion gaps are the same or when tension is equal while stress is applied. A trial prosthesis can also be used for assessment for extension and flexion balance. After inserting the trial prosthesis, if the anterior part of the tibia is lifted off or if the prosthesis pulled out during flexion, or there is a limitation in flexion, the flexion gap is narrow, whereas when tibia prosthesis is inserted without any resistance, the flexion gap is wide. In knee extension position, hyperextension implies the extension gap to be wide, whereas if the flexion contracture remains, it means a narrow extension gap. Simultaneous wide gap in flexion and extension causes multidirectional instability. In this case, metal augmentation to the tibial prosthesis or exchange to thicker PE might be helpful.

14.7.3.5 Treatment

Treatment of instability after TKAs varies depending on the type and degree of instability. If mild, conservative treatment is performed firstly. Mild instability is felt rarely, allowing the patients to live without much difficulty. If the leg waddles during the first walking after surgery, it is caused by muscular weakness, then rehabilitation exercise or orthosis must be provided. Mid-flexion instability is rarely felt by the patient. If the patient complains discomfort during stair gait, muscular strengthening training must be performed. If conservative treatment is failed, treatment may require revision surgery [207, 211]. If there is anteroposterior instability during flexion, the flexion gap must be narrowed. If severe, revision surgery can be performed with constrained prosthesis. In case of medial and lateral instability, orthosis is recommended for the first 6 weeks after the surgery because it helps the fibrous healing of the soft tissue. However, in most cases, revision surgery may be necessary due to high risk of recurrence. Constraint PE or rotating hinge-type constrained prosthesis is commonly used in revision surgery.

14.7.4 Stiffness After TKA

Limited ROM causes dysfunction and deteriorates the patient's satisfaction. Limited ROM can be classified into flexion contracture with incomplete extension (ankyloses in extension) and limited flexion with less flexion angle (ankyloses in flexion). Stiffness is not an uncommon complication that reported to occur in varying rate of 1.3–12% and serves as 5.6–30% of complication that requires revision surgery [225–229]. In order to prevent stiffness, appropriate selection of patient and prosthesis and precise surgical technique is crucial, and aggressive postoperative pain control and motivation to rehabilitation are also necessary.

14.7.4.1 Definition

Definition of stiffness after TKA is somewhat controversial. It can be defined as flexion contracture of 15 degrees or higher and/or maximum flexion of 75 degrees or less, depending on the author. It is otherwise variously defined as when ROM is 10–90 degrees, when flexion contracture is 20 degrees or higher with maximum flexion of 45 degrees or less, when maximum flexion is 85 degrees or less, or when maximum flexion angle is 70 degrees or less.

14.7.4.2 Cause

Factors affecting stiffness after TKAs include patient, surgical technique, chosen prosthesis, and postoperative pain management related factors. The most influential factor to postoperative stiffness is the ROM before surgery [230–232]. If the preoperative flexion is severely limited (if the flexion contracture is severe or the knee is stiff), regardless of how well the surgery is performed, the surgery would not provide the same outcome as a patient with normal ROM. In the case of patients with an ROM of less than 75 degrees, it is difficult to obtain a flexion angle of more than 110 degrees even after arthroplasty. Other patient factors include the type of disease, habit, depression, and low threshold for the pain.

One of the causes of flexion loss is flexion-extension gap imbalance. Use of thicker PE compensated for widened extension gap, narrowed flexion gap due to oversized or posteriorly placed femoral prosthesis can cause bilateral collateral ligament to limit flexion. Incorrect position of femoral prosthesis can cause limited flexion. If femoral prosthesis is placed internally rotated, flexion can be limited along with malalignment of patella. Elevation of joint line due to excessive resection of distal femur can induce excessive tension in soft tissue during knee flexion and cause limited flexion. Malalignment of the patellofemoral joint also reduces the ROM after surgery. Anterior overstuffness, which caused by insufficient resection of the patella, anterior positioning of the femur prosthesis, and use of the large femur prosthesis, can limit the flexion by causing excessive tension in the extension mechanism [233, 234]. Tibial bone should be resected with posterior slope in sagittal plane and tibial component should be positioned with a posterior slope. Posterior osteophytes incompletely removed during the surgery can also induce limited flexion [235]. Extension loss is more influenced by surgical technique than flexion loss. Permanent or excessive stiffness of knee flexor muscle can induce extension loss, but in most cases, it is because of insufficient release of soft tissues such as posterior joint capsule or insufficient resection of distal femur. Therefore, inserting trial prosthesis to observe alignment, knee joint must be extended frequently to assess the degree of extension.

ROM can differ depending on the design of the prosthesis. PS type prosthesis is known to have wider ROM than CR type. Though ROM may be assumed to be wider in mobile bearing joint compared to fixed bearing joint, no significant difference has been reported. In constrained prosthesis, extension, flexion, rotation, and varus-valgus have shown less motion, and high flex prosthesis has been introduced to supplement such disadvantage but there are still controversies whether high flexion design increases ROM or not.

Postoperative wound healing is closely related to ROM. If hematoma is excessive or wound healing is impeded at the early stage, the pain hinders rehabilitation, limits ROM, and restricts exercise, resulting in further exercise restriction. In addition, if the patient does not take rehabilitation sufficiently at the early stage of postoperative management, it may cause limitation of motion. Infection, arthrofibrosis, and reflex sympathetic dystrophy can be the cause of stiffness. Also, if ROM is limited after some time with excellent joint movement, infection, synovitis due to overuse, synovitis due to RA, and prosthesis damage should be considered.

14.7.4.3 Treatment

Conservative treatment is firstly performed and if the desired ROM is not achieved through conservative treatment, adhesiolysis or revision surgery should be considered. However, there is no guarantee of success if its cause is unknown. Aggressive physical therapy is necessary if flexion contracture of 15 degrees or less and flexion of more than 90 degrees are not achieved until 4–6 weeks after the surgery. Pariente et al. [236] and Daluga et al. [237] have revealed that flexion can be attempted during initial rehabilitation, and if flexion is 75 degrees or less after 6–12 weeks, brisement can be performed carefully under anesthesia for better outcome. Such treatment can reduce intra-articular adhesion and risk of permanent limitation in ROM. Adhesiolysis with arthroscope is the first step of surgical treatment. The procedure is optimal within 3–6 months after the surgery. It must be performed with care so that it may not damage the prosthesis. Diduch et al. [238] reported that arthroscopic adhesiolysis can achieve further ROM of 26 degrees, and Mont et al. [239] have argued that adhesiolysis has brought in great outcome in patients with limited ROM but no radiologically abnormal finding. However, if a patient has flexion contracture of 20 degrees or more and flexion less than 70 degrees, one must consider open adhesiolysis. Though open adhesiolysis can be performed over a year, limited ROM is difficult to be resolved if not ultimately corrected with revision surgery. Nelson et al. [232] reported that patient with flexion contracture of 15 degrees or more and flexion of less than 75 degrees showed improvement in ROM after revision surgery, but there was no difference in overall ROM between groups. Bellemans et al. [240] have proposed 4-stage treatment to correct flexion contracture: (1) mediolateral ligament balancing with resection of all osteophytes and overresection of the distal femur by 2 mm; (2) progressive posterior capsular release and gastrocnemius release; (3) additional resection of the distal femur up to a maximum of 4 mm; (4) hamstring tenotomy.

14.7.5 Periprosthetic Fracture After TKA

As more patients are receiving TKA due to a longer lifespan, prevalence of periprosthetic fracture is increasing. In periprosthetic fracture treatment, it is crucial to achieve bone union in adequate alignment without separation of the prosthesis and maintain ROM of the knee for 90 degrees or more. However, complications have been reported in 25–75% of the treatment for periprosthetic fractures. It is known that the results of conservative treatment are good in fractures without displacement, but in fractures with displacement, the result is poor due to the high incidence of complications. Since most of the patients are old and have osteoporosis, the bone quality is poor. Moreover, the size or amount of bone for internal fixation is insufficient due to prosthesis or bone cement. It proposes a great problem of treating the periprosthetic fracture while sparing function of prosthesis. Periprosthetic fracture includes femoral supracondylar fracture, proximal tibia fracture, and patella fracture, among them, femoral supracondylar fracture is more common and difficult to be treated.

14.7.5.1 Cause

Systemic cause includes osteopenia or any factors that can induce osteopenia (RA, long-term steroid use, neurologic defect, etc.) and local cause includes surgical cause and postoperative cause. Periprosthetic fracture during surgery occurs when a guide rod is inserted incorrectly

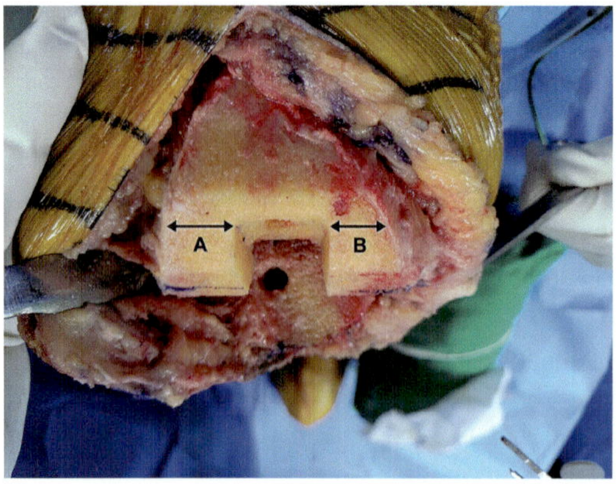

Fig. 14.45 The reason why medial condylar fractures occur more often than lateral condylar fractures in PS type TKAs. The bony cortex in medial (**b**) has thinner thickness than lateral (**a**)

in the femur, trial prosthesis is inserted with too small box cutting in PS type, or bone is weak due to excessive bone resection. Medial femoral condyle fracture is more common, it is because medial condyle width becomes relatively short at metaphysis and box cutting can make it smaller (Fig. 14.45).

Periprosthetic fracture after surgery is classified into factures with major trauma history such as fall or traffic accident and fractures due to repetitive stress and fatigue without major trauma. Anterior notching in the distal femur is one cause of postoperative fractures of the distal femur. Anterior notching is a stress riser because most fractures start from anterior notching at early recovery of the surgery, especially in patients with osteopenia. Lesh et al. [241] reported 18% decrease in bending strength and 39% decrease in torsional strength in presence of anterior notching. Zalzal et al. [242] reported notching with 3 mm or more in depth above the tip of femoral prosthesis has higher risk of fracture due to focused stress. Periprosthetic fracture around pin site used for navigation might be occurred, especially in patient with osteopenia. Excessively thick extension stem can induce endosteal thinning of reaming in which end of the stem may be stuck and induce fracture. If the tibial prosthesis is malpositioned or unskilled tibial tuberosity osteotomy can induce fracture at tibial side. Though patellar fracture can be caused by trauma, it is mostly due to stress fracture and sometimes asymptomatic (Fig. 14.46). Causes of fracture include excessive or insufficient patellar resection, bone necrosis due to excessive release of lateral patellar retinaculum, patella malalignment, and patellar maltracking. Design of the patella prosthesis is closely related to fracture. The incidence of fracture has been high with single hole at the center to fix patella prosthesis.

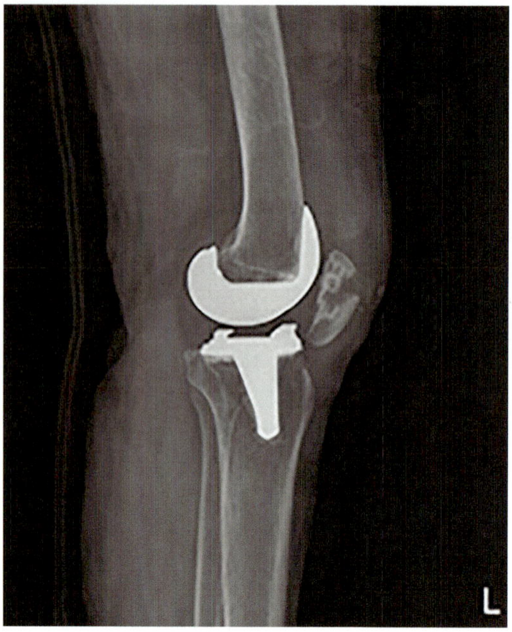

Fig. 14.46 Periprosthetic patella fracture

14.7.5.2 Classification

Femur

Rorabeck et al. [243] modified the classification based on Neer classification for its application to periprosthetic fractures (Fig. 14.47). Fractures without displacement are Type I, and fractures with displacement but stable prosthesis are Type II. Type II is further divided into A without comminution and B with comminution. In Type III, the prosthesis is unstable regardless of displacement. Su et al. [244] advocated a new, simple, but practical classification, taking into account that most fractures require surgery and the type of fixation used during surgery is important (Fig. 14.48). Su has classified fracture accord-

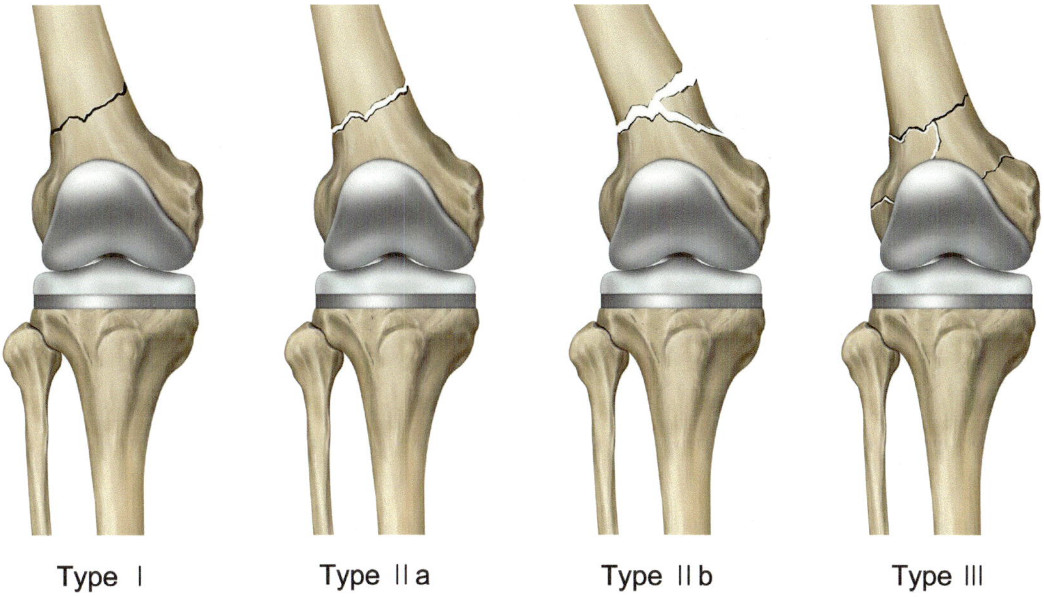

Fig. 14.47 Rorabeck classification in periprosthetic femoral fracture

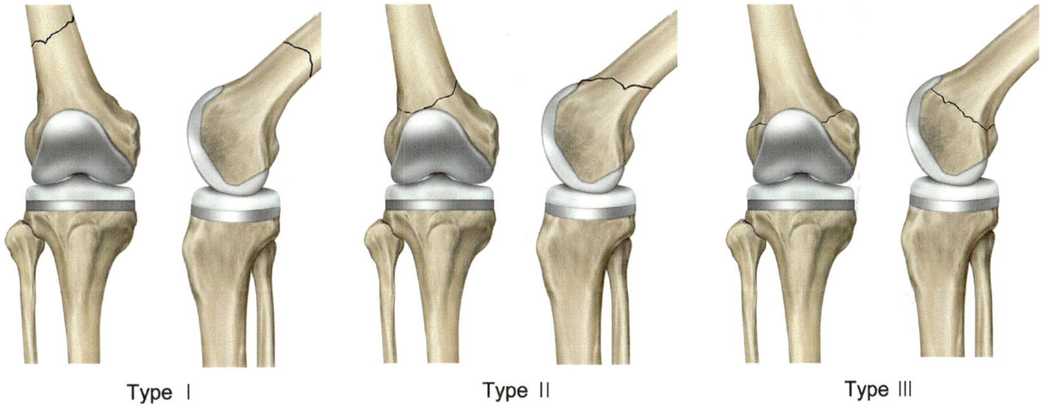

Fig. 14.48 Su classification in periprosthetic femoral fracture

ing to its location. If a fracture has occurred on the upper part of the prosthesis, Type I, if started around the prosthesis, Type II, and if within the prosthesis, Type III.

Tibia

Felix et al. [245] classified tibial periprosthetic fracture according to location of the fracture, loosening, and onset (Fig. 14.49). Depending on the fracture site, type I is a plateau fracture, type II is a fracture adjacent to prosthetic stem, type III is a fracture distal to stem, and type IV, a tibial tubercle fracture. The fracture onset is classified into intraoperative or postoperative fracture, and the classification according to the stability of the prosthesis is classified as A if it is stable, B if it is unstable, and C if it occurs during surgery.

Patella

Goldberg classification [246] is mostly used (Fig. 14.50); type 1 is a fracture that does not involve the prosthesis-cement composite and extensor mechanism, and type 2 is a fracture that involves the prosthesis-cement complex or the

Fig. 14.49 Felix classification in periprosthetic tibial fracture

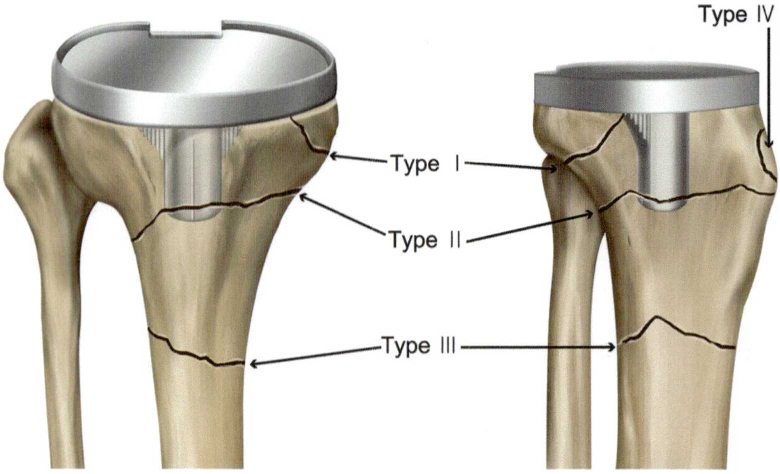

extensor mechanism. Type 3A is inferior pole fracture without patellar tendon rupture while type 3B is inferior pole fracture with patellar tendon rupture. Type 4 is fracture-dislocation.

14.7.5.3 Treatment

General Principle of Periprosthetic Fracture Treatment

Goal of treatment of periprosthetic fracture is to return the knee joint function back before fracture. Intraoperative fractures usually appear in split or bursting fractures. Treatment for fractures with stable prosthesis can be largely classified into conservative treatment and surgical treatment. If conservative treatment is performed, there is a high risk of complications such as stiffness or bedsores, moreover, treatment results are sometimes worse than surgical treatment. Fractures other than nondisplaced fractures or patella fractures usually require open reduction and internal fixation. Surgery is often preferred as it can restore alignment, allow early joint movement. If the prosthesis is unstable, revision arthroplasty combined with fracture treatment is required. In this case, advanced surgical techniques are required.

Treatment Depending on the Fracture Site

Distal femur fracture Rorabeck Type I with no displacements and no abnormalities with the prosthesis can be treated with cast immobilization. If the fracture is not linear, open reduction is often performed. In Rorabeck Type II with displacement and no abnormality of the prosthesis, conservative treatment can be performed after reduction by manual reduction or traction, but it is mostly treated with open reduction and internal fixation (Fig. 14.51). In Rorabeck Type III with displacement and unstable prosthesis, revision surgery can be performed with an internal fixation after open reduction. If the fracture is severely comminuted, tumor prosthesis can be used as a primary choice. Acceptable range of malalignment in the femoral side is within 10 degrees in the anteroposterior, varus-valgus, internal-external rotations, and the displacement is allowed 5 mm at the maximum. Various kinds of internal fixation devices can be used. Locking compression plate (LCP) is useful in fractures with osteopenia and has relatively excellent fixation power compared to other options. Intramedullary (IM) nails can also be performed on fractures, but the risk of nonunion and malunion is high. When using a metal plate, nonunion due to loss of fixation may occur. Autogenous or allogenic bone graft might be needed in comminuted fracture. Bone cement may be used if screw fixation is not applicable in severe osteoporotic bone. When using bone cement, it should be ensured that the cement does not get caught between the bone fragments and does not leak outside the cortical bone. It is possible to increase the fixation power when performing bone graft or fixing it with cement with

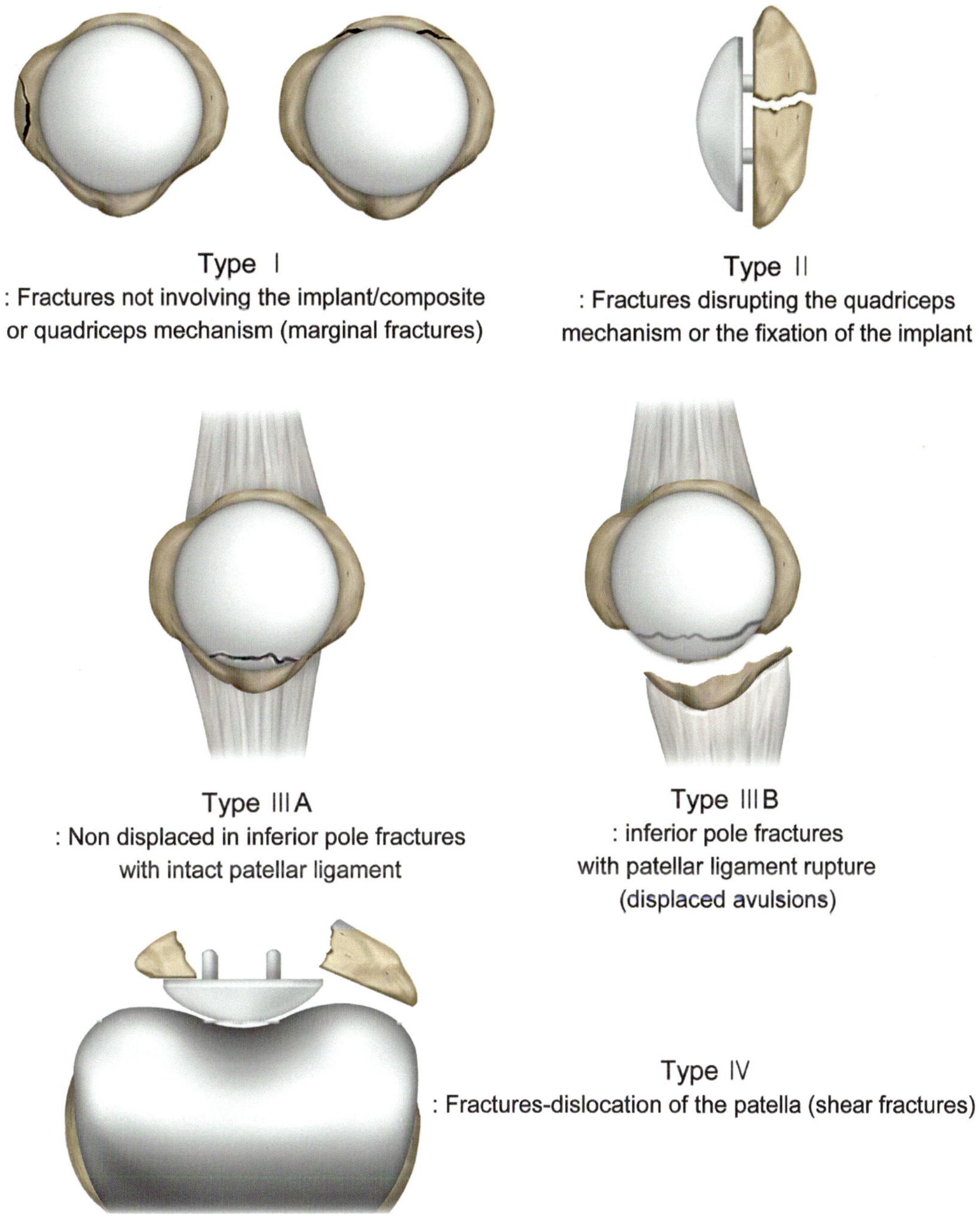

Fig. 14.50 Goldberg classification in periprosthetic patella fracture

a window in the condyle region [247] (Fig. 14.52). External fixation can also be used, but it has the disadvantage that the risk of infection is high and it is difficult to withstand the stress in osteopenia. If the prosthesis is unstable, revision arthroplasty is performed using a femoral prosthesis with a long stem. If the fracture is so severe that such prosthesis is impractical, allograft prosthesis composite (APC) or tumor prosthesis can be used.

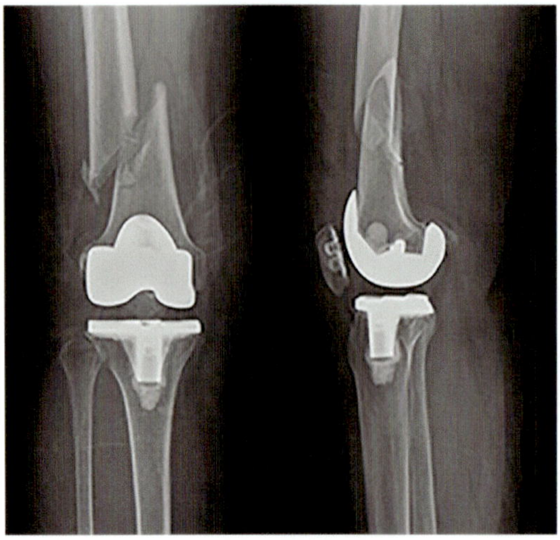

Fig. 14.51 Operative treatment is needed in periprosthetic femoral fracture. AP and lateral X-ray show Rorabeck type IIA fracture

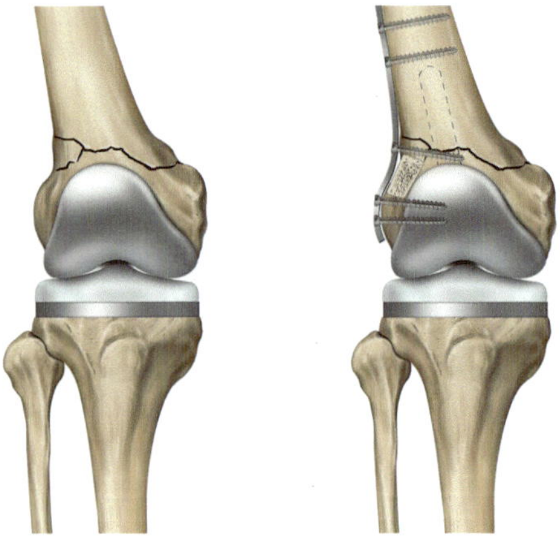

Fig. 14.52 Healy's method that managed the fractured site using cement or bone graft

Proximal tibial fracture Intraoperative fractures are usually vertical fractures and have no displacement. It can be treated using lag screw fixation or conservatively. If there is a displacement, the prosthesis with extension stem is inserted and the bone fragment is fixed with a screw. In Felix Type IV with tibial tuberosity fracture, conservative treatment is performed when displacement is not severe, and surgical treatment, if severely displaced. Fractures caused by high-velocity injury may be accompanied by nerve or vascular damage, and if so, emergency surgery is required.

Patella fracture Aim of treatment of periprosthetic patella fracture is to restore extensor mechanism. The treatment varies depending on comminution, remaining extension strength, stability of the prosthesis and whether patellar resurfaced or not. Conservative treatment is recommended when the displacement is less than 2 cm, extension mechanism is still intact, and there is no loosening of the prosthesis. If the displacement is more than 2 cm, if extension mechanism is severely damaged, or if prosthesis is unstable, a surgical treatment may be necessary. Even if the fracture gap is wide, the extension function can be restored to some extent if the medial and lateral ligaments are preserved. If the bone fragment is large, bone condition is good, and the prosthesis is stable, surgery is performed with a tension band wiring. If the bone fragment is small and bone quality is poor, removal of the small bone fragment and reinforcement of the extensor mechanism should be performed. If there is loosening of the prosthesis, the prosthesis can be removed and a partial or total patellectomy is performed, and then allogeneic tendon can be used to reinforce the extension function.

14.7.6 Rupture of the Extensor Mechanism After TKA

Rupture of the extensor mechanism in a normal knee joint is easily treatable and the results are relatively good. However, rupture of the extension mechanism after TKA is difficult to be treated and the postoperative result is also poor, which is considered a catastrophic complication. It is so catastrophic that the contraindications for TKA include incompetence of the extensor mechanism, because active extension of the knee joint is fundamentally necessary for the prosthesis to function properly. Therefore, the rupture of the extension mechanism must be restored [248]. Extensor mechanism of knee is composed of quadriceps tendon, patella, patellar tendon, and tibial tubercle. If any one of the components loses continuity, active extension of the knee joint becomes impossible [248]. After TKA, consequent postoperative pain and weak extension may be confused with the rupture of the extensor mechanism, and it is critical to assess active extension of the knee, and all the components must be assessed with physical examination [248]. It must be assessed if knee can be extended actively in a high sitting position away from the ground, or if the patient can maintain knee extension after the examiner removes support to the affected leg. In a simple lateral radiographic image, it is necessary to check whether the patella is at an abnormally high or low position, and the patella should be evaluated with axial images.

14.7.6.1 Disruption of Quadriceps Tendon

Disruption of quadriceps after TKA is very rare. Dobbs et al. [249] have reported incidence of 0.1% after primary TKA. As its incidence is low, it is difficult to identify predisposing factor, but patient with RA, obesity, steroid use, and DM has higher risk [250]. Excessive resection of patella, extensile approach such as quadriceps snip or V–Y advancement flap, excessive manipulation after the surgery, and history of trauma during rehabilitation can be the cause of quadriceps tendon disruption [251].

Since its treatment is difficult, it is most important to avoid the preceding factors of the above and prevent it with meticulous surgical techniques. Disruption of quadriceps tendon should be distinguished of partial and complete tear. A partial rupture is when a new extension defect is palpable, but the active extension of the knee joint is weak, but still possible. In contrast, a complete rupture is incapable of active extension of the knee joint. It has been reported that if active extension of the knee joint is possible due to partial rupture, favorable results can be obtained with only non-surgical treatment [248, 249, 252]. For non-surgical treatment, the knee should be immobilized at full extension for 4–6 weeks and then carefully started with passive joint movement [249, 253].

In the case of a complete rupture in which active knee extension is impossible, surgical treatment is required, but it is difficult to obtain favorable results with only primary repair of disrupted quadriceps. Dobbs et al. [249] reported rerupture in 4 out of 10 cases of completely ruptured quadriceps tendon treated with primary operative repair. Therefore, an additional reinforcement is required after repair of completely ruptured quadriceps tendon. It can be reinforced with a hamstring tendon or synthetic material such as Dacron tape or Marlex mesh. After the surgery, a sufficient period of immobilization must be taken with extended knee joint [253, 254]. It is also possible to reinforce with an allograft or to initially attempt reconstruction with only an allograft tendon. Achilles allograft or bone-patellar tendon-patellar-quadriceps tendon allograft can be used [248, 254]. Burnett et al. [255] reported favorable results by treating with allograft that includes all of the quadriceps (about 5 cm), patella, patella tendon, and tibial tuberosity (about 6–8 cm).

14.7.6.2 Patellar Tendon Rupture

The incidence of patellar tendon rupture after primary TKA is reported from 0.17% to 1.4% [256]. Patellar tendon rupture after TKA is uncommon but is a devastating complication [248, 257, 258]. As its incidence is low, it is difficult to clearly identify preceding factor, but excessive traction to the patella, chronic steroid use, trauma, multiple surgeries, impingement of tibia or patellar prosthesis, infection, and systemic diseases like DM and RA have been known for its cause [248, 257]. Patellar replacement is not related to the incidence of patellar tendon rupture. Boyd et al. [259] reported that 3 (0.8%) out of 396 cases in replacement group and 2 cases (0.4%) out of 495 cases in sparing group accompanied with patellar tendon rupture, which were no significant difference. However, in theory, replacement group, especially when asymmetric or excessive patellar resection has weakened insertion of patellar tendon, has higher risk of patellar tendon rupture.

Orthosis or cast fixation is preferred for cases with capability of active extension of the knee. However, if the active extension is lost, surgery is necessary [253]. Primary repair can be performed with suture or staple or suture anchor in case of patella tendon rupture with intact periosteum. However, any rupture or avulsion occurred during follow-up after surgery has bad prognosis with only primary reconstruction. Therefore, additional reconstruction is necessary. Re-rupture after primary repair is highly likely even though reinforcing the tendon with reconstruction and lengthy immobilization. As for reconstruction, autograft or allograft can be used. Cadambi and Engh [260] have reported reconstruction using autograft semitendinosus tendon. As another attempt, Jaureguito et al. [261] have used medial gastrocnemius flap, while Zanotti et al. [262] have reported their attempt of reconstruction using bone-patellar tendon-bone allograft to fix tibia with cortical screw and patella with interference fit and suture.

14.7.7 Wear and Osteolysis

PE wear and osteolysis were the main causes of late failure of TKA in the past, but PE wear is no longer the major cause of failure [263]. Since joint motion of the knee is performed by complex movements such as rolling, sliding, and rotational motions, PE wear occurs through mechanisms such as delamination, pitting, and fatigue failure [264]. It can also appear as a third-body wear by bone cement or bone fragments [264, 265]. PE wear is affected by property of PE, surgical techniques, and patient factors.

In terms of surgical technique, wear can be reduced only when proper alignment is made in the coronal, sagittal, and axial planes. Varus deformity more than 5 degrees in the coronal plane leads to PE wear. Excessive flexion of the femoral component, increase in the posterior inclination angle of the tibia prosthesis, hyperextension in the sagittal plane, and joint line elevation more than 5 mm can also induce wear. The PE insert is mainly concave shaped which increases the contact surface with the femoral component because flat shaped PE insert receives excessive stress per unit area, which can lead to wear. In the PS type TKA, wear or failure of the PE post may occur, and in the tibial component in which the locking device is unstable, backside wear may occur. In recent years, PE inserts have improved the position and design of the posts, and the locking mechanism for the tibial component is being made firmly. It is manufactured with a thickness of at least 6 mm to avoid excessive wear or failure [265]. Sterilization using gas plasma or ethylene oxide is performed since the mechanical properties are weakened when the PE insert is sterilized in the air by gamma radiation due to oxidation. Recently, highly cross-linked UHMWPE has been used to reduce wear, and it is reported to reduce wear by 67–80% compared to conventional PE. When gamma radiation is irradiated in a vacuum state, free radicals are generated in the PE chain and cross-linking occurs, resulting in a more stable structure, increasing resistance to wear. However, when the free radicals remain, they react with oxygen to cause oxidative denaturation, which is why heat treatment is performed to remove the free radicals. Annealing is a method of heating below the melting point, so the physical properties are less weakened, but free radicals remain, which may induce oxidation reactions. Recently, a second-generation highly cross-linked PE has been introduced to compensate for the shortcomings of heat treatment. By adding an antioxidant such as vitamin E after irradiation, it was attempted to reduce the oxidation reaction without loss of fatigue strength, which is a disadvantage of heat treatment. In vitro studies have shown that PE wear is reduced by 86%, but long-term clinical follow-up is needed. Patient factors affecting the wear are age, sex, activity level, and obesity.

Osteolysis is thought to be an immunological reaction by wear particles in which bone tissue around the prosthesis is absorbed [266]. When wear particle generated by fine motor, corrosion, and oxidation are phagocytized by macrophages, inflammatory mediators are released and osteoclast is activated to induce bone resorption. Since most patients are asymptomatic in osteolysis, it is confirmed through radiological examination. Though diagnosis is possible with a simple radiograph of the knee, it can be underdiagnosed by the shading of the prosthesis, which makes the location and extent of the bone loss should be evaluated through CT. If surgical treatment is required for wear, only PE implant can be replaced if the prosthesis is well aligned and stable. If osteolysis is accompanied, only curettage can be performed, but better results in case of bone graft are being reported. In some studies, the revision rate within 5 years is reported as 15–28% [267]. Careful judgment is thereby required if there are misalignment, stiffness, or instability of the prosthesis. If osteolysis is severe, revision surgery is required.

14.8 Summary

TKAs are one of the most successful procedures in all of medicine. The goal of TKA is to relieve knee pain, restore the function, and correct deformity. Appropriate patient selection is necessary to achieve this goal. TKAs are mostly indicated for end-stage arthritis not responding to conservative treatment or joint preserving procedures. However, neuropathic arthritis, severely ankylosed knee, and paralytic knee are relative contraindications, and infected arthritis is an absolute contraindication of TKA. In order to improve postoperative patient satisfaction and prevent complications, the patient's physical and mental health status besides knee condition should be carefully examined prior to surgery, in addition to selecting the appropriate surgical indications.

Materials used for prosthesis are metal and plastic. These materials should be biologically inert. Several types of prosthesis were developed to simulate the function of the native knee joint. The type of the prosthesis is divided into CR or PS type depending on PCL retention and fixed or mobile type depending on the method of PE insert fixation. There is no significant difference in clinical outcomes or long-term survival rates based on prosthesis types. Depending on the stability of the knee joint during surgery, more constraint PE insert may be required. Malalignment or inappropriate soft tissue balancing are factors that have a negative impact on postoperative outcomes. Therefore, the basic principle of performing TKA is to obtain proper soft tissue balancing and restoration of lower limb alignment. There are several ways to restore lower limb alignment, which include anatomical, mechanical, and kinematic alignment. Among them, mechanical alignment is the most widely used. Accurate bone resection is required to restore lower limb alignment, which is why various instruments and surgical techniques are used. Proper soft tissue balancing is also an important factor in the successful outcome of TKA. In order to achieve proper balance, it is necessary to understand the anatomy and function of various soft tissues around the knee including tendons and ligaments. In addition, soft tissue release must be carried out meticulously and gradually to avoid over-release. The prosthesis size is selected to fit the patient's joint size as much as possible, and the prosthesis is inserted by matching the coronal plane, sagittal plane, and rotational alignment. Fixation of the prosthesis is either cement or cementless type. The most widely used method for prosthesis fixation is cemented fixation.

Postoperative management is also important for patient satisfaction and clinical outcomes. Postoperative management includes pain management, DVT prophylaxis, surgical wound care, and infection prevention. Failure to control pain after surgery has a great effect on patient dissatisfaction and function loss. It is necessary to understand the cause and physiology of postoperative pain. Surgeon should appropriately utilize preemptive analgesics, regional anesthesia, peripheral nerve block, periarticular injection, and multimodal analgesics to decrease a postoperative pain. Symptomatic DVT or pulmonary thromboembolism is a serious complication after TKA. Considering the risk factors, nonpharmacologic measures and/or pharmacologic treatment should be considered to prevent the occurrence of DVT. Complications such as wound problem, periprosthetic deep infection, instability, periprosthetic fracture, extensor mechanism rupture, wear, and osteolysis may occur. The development of surgical techniques and materials has reduced complications after TKA, but PJI is still the most common cause of failed TKAs. PJI is a devastating complication of TKA. Prevention of PJI is important, but once it occurs, accurate diagnosis and prompt treatment are needed.

TKA is a successful surgical procedure for patients with knee OA. Successful outcomes require proper patient selection, preoperative planning, meticulous surgical techniques, and postoperative planned management. Surgeons should do their best to give patients the best results.

References

1. Ellis HB, Howard KJ, Khaleel MA, Bucholz R. Effect of psychopathology on patient-perceived outcomes of total knee arthroplasty within an indigent population. J Bone Joint Surg Am. 2012;94(12):e84. https://doi.org/10.2106/JBJS.K.00888.
2. Voskuijl T, Hageman M, Ring D. Higher Charlson Comorbidity Index Scores are associated with readmission after orthopaedic surgery. Clin Orthop Relat Res. 2014;472(5):1638–44. https://doi.org/10.1007/s11999-013-3394-8.
3. Foran JR, Mont MA, Rajadhyaksha AD, Jones LC, Etienne G, Hungerford DS. Total knee arthroplasty in obese patients: a comparison with a matched control group. J Arthroplast. 2004;19(7):817–24. https://doi.org/10.1016/j.arth.2004.03.017.
4. Dewan A, Bertolusso R, Karastinos A, Conditt M, Noble PC, Parsley BS. Implant durability and knee function after total knee arthroplasty in the morbidly obese patient. J Arthroplast. 2009;24(6 Suppl):89-94, e1–3. https://doi.org/10.1016/j.arth.2009.04.024.
5. Stundner O, Danninger T, Chiu YL, Sun X, Goodman SM, Russell LA, et al. Rheumatoid arthritis vs osteoarthritis in patients receiving total knee arthroplasty: perioperative outcomes. J Arthroplast. 2014;29(2):308–13. https://doi.org/10.1016/j.arth.2013.05.008.
6. Mont MA, Myers TH, Krackow KA, Hungerford DS. Total knee arthroplasty for corticosteroid associated avascular necrosis of the knee. Clin Orthop Relat Res. 1997;338:124–30. https://doi.org/10.1097/00003086-199705000-00019.
7. Baker D, Hastings R, Pruitt L. Study of fatigue resistance of chemical and radiation crosslinked medical grade ultrahigh molecular weight polyethylene. J Biomed Mater Res. 1999;46(4):573–81.
8. Bassett RW. Results of 1,000 Performance knees: cementless versus cemented fixation. J Arthroplast. 1998;13(4):409–13.
9. Mavrogenis A, Dimitriou R, Parvizi J, Babis GC. Biology of implant osseointegration. J Musculoskelet Neuronal Interact. 2009;9(2):61–71.
10. Levine BR, Della Valle AG, MacDonald S, Callaghan J, Meneghini RM. The modern total knee arthroplasty: what to make of all of these options? Instr Course Lect. 2020;69:151–66.
11. Jaeblon T. Polymethylmethacrylate: properties and contemporary uses in orthopaedics. JAAOS J Am Acad Orthop Surg. 2010;18(5):297–305.
12. Park SH, Silva M, Park JS, Ebramzadeh E, Schmalzried TP. Cement–cement interface strength: influence of time to apposition. J Biomed Mater Res. 2001;58(6):741–6.
13. Duffy GP, Berry DJ, Rand JA. Cement versus cementless fixation in total knee arthroplasty. Clin Orthop Relat Res. 1998;356:66–72.
14. Landon GC, Galante JO, Maley MM. Noncemented total knee arthroplasty. Clin Orthop Relat Res. 1986;205:49–57.
15. Mont MA, Pivec R, Issa K, Kapadia BH, Maheshwari A, Harwin SF. Long-term implant survivorship of cementless total knee arthroplasty: a systematic review of the literature and meta-analysis. J Knee Surg. 2014;27(05):369–76.
16. Niinomi M. Metallic biomaterials. J Artif Organs. 2008;11(3):105.
17. Navarro M, Michiardi A, Castano O, Planell J. Biomaterials in orthopaedics. J R Soc Interface. 2008;5(27):1137–58.
18. Zhuang L, Langer E. Effects of alloy additions on the fatigue properties of cast Co-Cr-Mo alloy used for surgical implants. J Mater Sci. 1990;25(1):683–9.
19. Song Y, Park C-H, Moriwaki T. Mirror finishing of Co–Cr–Mo alloy using elliptical vibration cutting. Precis Eng. 2010;34(4):784–9.
20. Nag S, Samuel S, Puthucode A, Banerjee R. Characterization of novel borides in Ti–Nb–Zr–Ta+ 2B metal-matrix composites. Mater Charact. 2009;60(2):106–13.
21. Levine BR, Sporer S, Poggie RA, Della Valle CJ, Jacobs JJ. Experimental and clinical performance of porous tantalum in orthopedic surgery. Biomaterials. 2006;27(27):4671–81.
22. Bal BS, Garino J, Ries M, Rahaman MN, editors. Ceramic materials in total joint arthroplasty. Seminars in Arthroplasty; 2006: Elsevier.
23. Bracco P, Bellare A, Bistolfi A, Affatato S. Ultra-high molecular weight polyethylene: influence of the chemical, physical and mechanical properties on the wear behavior. A review. Materials. 2017;10(7):791.
24. Song SJ, Park CH, Bae DK. What to know for selecting cruciate-retaining or posterior-stabilized total knee arthroplasty. Clin Orthop Surg. 2019;11(2):142.
25. Dennis DA, Komistek RD, Colwell CE Jr, Ranawat CS, Scott RD, Thornhill TS, et al. In vivo anteroposterior femorotibial translation of total knee arthroplasty: a multicenter analysis. Clin Orthop Relat Res. 1998;356:47–57.
26. Andriacchi TP, Galante JO. Retention of the posterior cruciate in total knee arthroplasty. J Arthroplast. 1988;3:S13–S9.
27. Montgomery RL, Goodman SB, Csongradi J. Late rupture of the posterior cruciate ligament after total knee replacement. Iowa Orthop J. 1993;13:167.
28. Schwartz AJ, Della Valle CJ, Rosenberg AG, Jacobs JJ, Berger RA, Galante JO. Cruciate-retaining TKA using a third-generation system with a four-pegged tibial component: a minimum 10 year followup note. Clin Orthop Relat Res. 2010;468(8):2160–7.

29. Bozic KJ, Kinder J, Menegini M, Zurakowski D, Rosenberg AG, Galante JO. Implant survivorship and complication rates after total knee arthroplasty with a third-generation cemented system: 5 to 8 years followup. Clin Orthop Relat Res (1976–2007). 2005;430:117–24.
30. Ritter MA, Berend ME, Meding JB, Keating EM, Faris PM, Crites BM. Long-term followup of anatomic graduated components posterior cruciate-retaining total knee replacement. Clin Orthop Relat Res. 2001;388:51–7.
31. Berger RA, Rosenberg AG, Barden RM, Sheinkop MB, Jacobs JJ, Galante JO. Long-term followup of the Miller-Galante total knee replacement. Clin Orthop Relat Res. 2001;388:58–67.
32. Stiehl JB, Komistek RD, Dennis DA, Paxson RD, Hoff WA. Fluoroscopic analysis of kinematics after posterior-cruciate-retaining knee arthroplasty. J Bone Joint Surg. 1995;77(6):884–9.
33. Bertin KC, Komistek RD, Dennis DA, Hoff WA, Anderson DT, Langer T. In vivo determination of posterior femoral rollback for subjects having a NexGen posterior cruciate–retaining total knee arthroplasty. J Arthroplast. 2002;17(8):1040–8.
34. Kleinbart FA, Bryk E, Evangelista J, Scott WN, Vigorita VJ. Histologic comparison of posterior cruciate ligaments from arthritic and age-matched knee specimens. J Arthroplast. 1996;11(6):726–31.
35. Parsley BS, Conditt MA, Bertolusso R, Noble PC. Posterior cruciate ligament substitution is not essential for excellent postoperative outcomes in total knee arthroplasty. J Arthroplast. 2006;21(6):127–31.
36. Easley ME, Insall JN, Scuderi GR, Bullek DD. Primary constrained condylar knee arthroplasty for the arthritic valgus knee. Clin Orthop Relat Res (1976–2007). 2000;380:58–64.
37. Shaw JA, Balcom W, Greer RB. Total knee arthroplasty using the kinematic rotating hinge prosthesis. Orthopedics. 1989;12(5):647–54.
38. Deehan DJ, Murray J, Birdsall PD, Holland JP, Pinder IM. The role of the rotating hinge prosthesis in the salvage arthroplasty setting. J Arthroplast. 2008;23(5):683–8.
39. Matsuda S, White SE, Williams VG II, McCarthy DS, Whiteside LA. Contact stress analysis in meniscal bearing total knee arthroplasty. J Arthroplast. 1998;13(6):699–706.
40. Kim Y-H, Kook H-K, Kim J-S. Comparison of fixed-bearing and mobile-bearing total knee arthroplasties. Clin Orthop Relat Res (1976–2007). 2001;392:101–15.
41. Price A, Rees J, Beard D, Juszczak E, Carter S, White S, et al. A mobile-bearing total knee prosthesis compared with a fixed-bearing prosthesis: a multicentre single-blind randomised controlled trial. J Bone Joint Surg. 2003;85(1):62–7.
42. Murphy M, Journeaux S, Russell T. High-flexion total knee arthroplasty: a systematic review. Int Orthop. 2009;33(4):887–93.
43. Lei T, Qian H, Hua L, de Abreu e Silva GM, Hu Y, Lei P. Is high flexion total knee arthroplasty a rewarding procedure? An updated meta-analysis of prospective randomized controlled trials. Arch Orthop Trauma Surg. 2020:1-11.
44. Malik A, Salas A, Ari JB, Ma Y, Della Valle AG. Range of motion and function are similar in patients undergoing TKA with posterior stabilised and high-flexion inserts. Int Orthop. 2010;34(7):965–72.
45. Kim Y-H, Choi Y, Kim J-S. Range of motion of standard and high-flexion posterior cruciate-retaining total knee prostheses*: a prospective randomized study. JBJS. 2009;91(8):1874–81.
46. Aglietti P, Insall JN, Walker PS, Trent P. A new patella prosthesis. Design and application. Clin Orthop Relat Res. 1975;107:175–87.
47. Longo UG, Ciuffreda M, Mannering N, D'Andrea V, Cimmino M, Denaro V. Patellar resurfacing in total knee arthroplasty: systematic review and meta-analysis. J Arthroplast. 2018;33(2):620–32.
48. Waterman BR, Belmont PJ Jr, Bader JO, Schoenfeld AJ. The total joint arthroplasty cardiac risk index for predicting perioperative myocardial infarction and cardiac arrest after primary total knee and hip arthroplasty. J Arthroplast. 2016;31(6):1170–4. https://doi.org/10.1016/j.arth.2015.12.013.
49. Leung YY, Allen JC, Ang LW, Yuan JM, Koh WP. Diabetes mellitus and the risk of total knee replacement among Chinese in Singapore, the Singapore Chinese Health Study. Sci Rep. 2017;7:40671. https://doi.org/10.1038/srep40671.
50. Kittle H, Ormseth A, Patetta MJ, Sood A, Gonzalez MH. Chronic corticosteroid use as a risk factor for perioperative complications in patients undergoing total joint arthroplasty. JAAOS Global Res Rev. 2020;4(7):e20.00001. https://doi.org/10.5435/JAAOSGlobal-D-20-00001.
51. Chio CC, Siu MK, Tai YT, Chen TG, Ho WP, Chen JT, et al. Renal insufficiency plays a crucial association factor in severe knee osteoarthritis-induced pain in patients with total knee replacement: a retrospective study. Medicine (Baltimore). 2020;99(6):e19125. https://doi.org/10.1097/MD.0000000000019125.
52. Pan X, Wang J, Lin Z, Dai W, Shi Z. Depression and anxiety are risk factors for postoperative pain-related symptoms and complications in patients undergoing primary total knee arthroplasty in the United States. J Arthroplast. 2019;34(10):2337–46.
53. Jenny JY, Bulaid Y, Boisrenoult P, Bonin N, Henky P, Tracol P, et al. Bleeding and thromboembolism risk of standard antithrombotic prophylaxis after hip or knee replacement within an enhanced recovery program. Orthop Traumatol Surg Res. 2020;106(8):1533–8. https://doi.org/10.1016/j.otsr.2020.02.026.
54. Mont MA, Jacobs JJ. AAOS clinical practice guideline: preventing venous thromboembolic disease in patients undergoing elective hip and knee

arthroplasty. JAAOS-J Am Acad Orthop Surg. 2011;19(12):777–8.
55. Hang G, Chen JY, Yew AKS, Pang H-N, Jin DTK, Chia S-L, et al. Effects of continuing use of aspirin on blood loss in patients who underwent unilateral total knee arthroplasty. J Orthop Surg. 2020;28(1):2309499019894390.
56. Goodman SM, Bass AR. Perioperative medical management for patients with RA, SPA, and SLE undergoing total hip and total knee replacement: a narrative review. BMC Rheumatol. 2018;2:2. https://doi.org/10.1186/s41927-018-0008-9.
57. Olivecrona C, Ponzer S, Hamberg P, Blomfeldt R. Lower tourniquet cuff pressure reduces postoperative wound complications after total knee arthroplasty: a randomized controlled study of 164 patients. J Bone Joint Surg Am. 2012;94(24):2216–21. https://doi.org/10.2106/JBJS.K.01492.
58. Abdel-Salam A, Eyres KS. Effects of tourniquet during total knee arthroplasty. A prospective randomised study. J Bone Joint Surg Br. 1995;77(2):250–3.
59. Tai TW, Chang CW, Lai KA, Lin CJ, Yang CY. Effects of tourniquet use on blood loss and soft-tissue damage in total knee arthroplasty: a randomized controlled trial. J Bone Joint Surg Am. 2012;94(24):2209–15. https://doi.org/10.2106/JBJS.K.00813.
60. Wakankar HM, Nicholl JE, Koka R, D'Arcy JC. The tourniquet in total knee arthroplasty. A prospective, randomised study. J Bone Joint Surg Br. 1999;81(1):30–3. https://doi.org/10.1302/0301-620x.81b1.8971.
61. Curtin B, Yakkanti M, Malkani A. Postoperative pain and contracture following total knee arthroplasty comparing parapatellar and subvastus approaches. J Arthroplast. 2014;29(1):33–6. https://doi.org/10.1016/j.arth.2013.03.021.
62. Tomek IM, Kantor SR, Cori LA, Scoville JM, Grove MR, Morgan TS, et al. Early patient outcomes after primary total knee arthroplasty with quadriceps-sparing subvastus and medial parapatellar techniques: a randomized, double-blind clinical trial. J Bone Joint Surg Am. 2014;96(11):907–15. https://doi.org/10.2106/JBJS.L.01578.
63. White RE Jr, Allman JK, Trauger JA, Dales BH. Clinical comparison of the midvastus and medial parapatellar surgical approaches. Clin Orthop Relat Res. 1999;367:117–22.
64. Dalury DF, Jiranek WA. A comparison of the midvastus and paramedian approaches for total knee arthroplasty. J Arthropl. 1999;14(1):33–7. https://doi.org/10.1016/S0883-5403(99)90199-7.
65. Whiteside LA, Ohl MD. Tibial tubercle osteotomy for exposure of the difficult total knee arthroplasty. Clin Orthop Relat Res. 1990;260:6–9.
66. Bellemans J, Robijns F, Duerinckx J, Banks S, Vandenneucker H. The influence of tibial slope on maximal flexion after total knee arthroplasty. Knee Surg Sports Traumatol Arthrosc. 2005;13(3):193–6. https://doi.org/10.1007/s00167-004-0557-x.
67. Romero J, Duronio JF, Sohrabi A, Alexander N, MacWilliams BA, Jones LC, et al. Varus and valgus flexion laxity of total knee alignment methods in loaded cadaveric knees. Clin Orthop Relat Res. 2002;394:243–53.
68. Howell SM, Howell SJ, Kuznik KT, Cohen J, Hull ML. Does a kinematically aligned total knee arthroplasty restore function without failure regardless of alignment category? Clin Orthop Relat Res. 2013;471(3):1000–7. https://doi.org/10.1007/s11999-012-2613-z.
69. Bardakos N, Cil A, Thompson B, Stocks G. Mechanical axis cannot be restored in total knee arthroplasty with a fixed valgus resection angle: a radiographic study. J Arthroplast. 2007;22(6):85–9.
70. Kharwadkar N, Kent RE, Sharara KH, Naique S. 5 degrees to 6 degrees of distal femoral cut for uncomplicated primary total knee arthroplasty: is it safe? Knee. 2006;13(1):57–60. https://doi.org/10.1016/j.knee.2005.07.001.
71. Deakin AH, Sarungi M. A comparison of variable angle versus fixed angle distal femoral resection in primary total knee arthroplasty. J Arthroplast. 2014;29(6):1133–7. https://doi.org/10.1016/j.arth.2013.11.009.
72. Reed SC, Gollish J. The accuracy of femoral intramedullary guides in total knee arthroplasty. J Arthroplast. 1997;12(6):677–82. https://doi.org/10.1016/s0883-5403(97)90141-8.
73. Bae DK, Song SJ, Park CH, Ko YW, Lee H. A comparison of the medium-term results of total knee arthroplasty using computer-assisted and conventional techniques to treat patients with extraarticular femoral deformities. J Arthroplast. 2017;32(1):71–8. https://doi.org/10.1016/j.arth.2016.06.030.
74. Meccia B, Komistek RD, Mahfouz M, Dennis D. Abnormal axial rotations in TKA contribute to reduced weightbearing flexion. Clin Orthop Relat Res. 2014;472(1):248–53. https://doi.org/10.1007/s11999-013-3105-5.
75. Berger RA, Rubash HE, Seel MJ, Thompson WH, Crossett LS. Determining the rotational alignment of the femoral component in total knee arthroplasty using the epicondylar axis. Clin Orthop Relat Res. 1993;286:40–7.
76. Tang WM, Zhu YH, Chiu KY. Axial alignment of the lower extremity in Chinese adults. J Bone Joint Surg Am. 2000;82(11):1603–8. https://doi.org/10.2106/00004623-200011000-00014.
77. Ozkurt B, Sen T, Cankaya D, Kendir S, Basarir K, Tabak Y. The medial and lateral epicondyle as a reliable landmark for intra-operative joint line determination in revision knee arthroplasty. Bone Joint Res. 2016;5(7):280–6. https://doi.org/10.1302/2046-3758.57.BJR-2016-0002.R1.
78. Tsukeoka T, Tsuneizumi Y, Lee TH. The effect of rotational fixation error of the tibial cutting guide and the distance between the guide and the bone on the tibial osteotomy in total knee arthroplasty.

J Arthroplast. 2013;28(7):1094–8. https://doi.org/10.1016/j.arth.2012.12.008.
79. Singh G, Tan JH, Sng BY, Awiszus F, Lohmann CH, Nathan SS. Restoring the anatomical tibial slope and limb axis may maximise post-operative flexion in posterior-stabilised total knee replacements. Bone Joint J. 2013;95-B(10):1354–8. https://doi.org/10.1302/0301-620X.95B10.31477.
80. Martin S, Saurez A, Ismaily S, Ashfaq K, Noble P, Incavo SJ. Maximizing tibial coverage is detrimental to proper rotational alignment. Clin Orthop Relat Res. 2014;472(1):121–5. https://doi.org/10.1007/s11999-013-3047-y.
81. Akagi R, Muramatsu Y, Mukoyama S, Sugiyama H, Yamaguchi S, Ohtori S, et al. Arthroscopic reduction and internal fixation of posterior cruciate ligament avulsion fracture using an adjustable-length loop device. Arthrosc Tech. 2020;9(12):e2001–e6. https://doi.org/10.1016/j.eats.2020.08.028.
82. Nicoll D, Rowley DI. Internal rotational error of the tibial component is a major cause of pain after total knee replacement. J Bone Joint Surg Br. 2010;92(9):1238–44. https://doi.org/10.1302/0301-620X.92B9.23516.
83. Barrack RL, Schrader T, Bertot AJ, Wolfe MW, Myers L. Component rotation and anterior knee pain after total knee arthroplasty. Clin Orthop Relat Res. 2001;392:46–55. https://doi.org/10.1097/00003086-200111000-00006.
84. Keblish PA. The lateral approach for total knee arthroplasty. J Knee Surg. 2003;16(1):62–8.
85. Greenfield MA, Insall JN, Case GC, Kelly MA. Instrumentation of the patellar osteotomy in total knee arthroplasty. The relationship of patellar thickness and lateral retinacular release. Am J Knee Surg. 1996;9(3):129–131; discussion 31.
86. Gerber BE, Maenza F. Shift and tilt of the bony patella in total knee replacement. Orthopade. 1998;27(9):629–36. https://doi.org/10.1007/PL00003538.
87. Abolghasemian M, Samiezadeh S, Sternheim A, Bougherara H, Barnes CL, Backstein DJ. Effect of patellar thickness on knee flexion in total knee arthroplasty: a biomechanical and experimental study. J Arthroplast. 2014;29(1):80–4. https://doi.org/10.1016/j.arth.2013.04.026.
88. Yao J, Yang B, Wang Y, Fan Y. Patella tracking calculation from patellofemoral positions at finite angles of knee flexion. Med Eng Phys. 2018;62:1–6. https://doi.org/10.1016/j.medengphy.2018.07.018.
89. Anglin C, Brimacombe JM, Wilson DR, Masri BA, Greidanus NV, Tonetti J, et al. Biomechanical consequences of patellar component medialization in total knee arthroplasty. J Arthroplast. 2010;25(5):793–802. https://doi.org/10.1016/j.arth.2009.04.023.
90. Minoda Y, Sugama R, Ohta Y, Ueyama H, Takemura S, Nakamura H. Four-millimeter additional bone resection in the distal femur does not result in an equivalent increase in the extension joint gap in total knee arthroplasty. J Arthroplast. 2021;36(3):958–62. https://doi.org/10.1016/j.arth.2020.09.002.
91. Mitsuyasu H, Matsuda S, Fukagawa S, Okazaki K, Tashiro Y, Kawahara S, et al. Enlarged post-operative posterior condyle tightens extension gap in total knee arthroplasty. J Bone Joint Surg. 2011;93(9):1210–6.
92. Ismailidis P, Kuster MS, Jost B, Giesinger K, Behrend H. Clinical outcome of increased flexion gap after total knee arthroplasty. Can controlled gap imbalance improve knee flexion? Knee Surg Sports Traumatol Arthrosc. 2017;25(6):1705–11. https://doi.org/10.1007/s00167-016-4009-1.
93. Gejo R, Morita Y, Matsushita I, Sugimori K, Kimura T. Joint gap changes with patellar tendon strain and patellar position during TKA. Clin Orthop Relat Res. 2008;466(4):946–51. https://doi.org/10.1007/s11999-008-0154-2.
94. Mihalko WM, Krackow KA. Posterior cruciate ligament effects on the flexion space in total knee arthroplasty. Clin Orthop Relat Res. 1999;360:243–50.
95. Kayani B, Konan S, Horriat S, Ibrahim MS, Haddad FS. Posterior cruciate ligament resection in total knee arthroplasty. Bone Joint J. 2019;101-B(10):1230–7. https://doi.org/10.1302/0301-620x.101b10.Bjj--2018-1428.R2.
96. Scott RD, Schai PA. Tibial osteotomy coincident with long stem total knee arthroplasty: a surgical technique. Am J Knee Surg. 2000;13(3):127–31.
97. Griffin FM, Insall JN, Scuderi GR. Accuracy of soft tissue balancing in total knee arthroplasty. J Arthroplast. 2000;15(8):970–3. https://doi.org/10.1054/arth.2000.6503.
98. Markolf KL, Mensch JS, Amstutz HC. Stiffness and laxity of the knee – the contributions of the supporting structures. A quantitative in vitro study. JBJS. 1976;58(5):583–94.
99. Tokuhara Y, Kadoya Y, Nakagawa S, Kobayashi A, Takaoka K. The flexion gap in normal knees: an MRI study. J Bone Joint Surg. 2004;86(8):1133–6.
100. Kobayashi T, Suzuki M, Sasho T, Nakagawa K, Tsuneizumi Y, Takahashi K. Lateral laxity in flexion increases the postoperative flexion angle in cruciate-retaining total knee arthroplasty. J Arthroplast. 2012;27(2):260–5.
101. Okazaki K, Miura H, Matsuda S, Takeuchi N, Mawatari T, Hashizume M, et al. Asymmetry of mediolateral laxity of the normal knee. J Orthop Sci. 2006;11(3):264–6. https://doi.org/10.1007/s00776-006-1009-x.
102. Matsuda Y, Ishii Y, Noguchi H, Ishii R. Varus-valgus balance and range of movement after total knee arthroplasty. J Bone Joint Surg Br. 2005;87(6):804–8. https://doi.org/10.1302/0301-620X.87B6.15256.
103. Kuster M, Bitschnau B, Votruba T. Influence of collateral ligament laxity on patient satisfaction after total knee arthroplasty: a comparative bilateral study. Arch Orthop Trauma Surg. 2004;124(6):415–7.
104. Yoshihara Y, Arai Y, Nakagawa S, Inoue H, Ueshima K, Fujiwara H, et al. Assessing coronal laxity in extension and flexion at a minimum of 10 years after

primary total knee arthroplasty. Knee Surg Sports Traumatol Arthrosc. 2016;24(8):2512–6.
105. Whiteside LA. Correction of ligament and bone defects in total arthroplasty of the severely valgus knee. Clin Orthop Relat Res. 1993;288:234–45.
106. Verdonk PC, Pernin J, Pinaroli A, Selmi TAS, Neyret P. Soft tissue balancing in varus total knee arthroplasty: an algorithmic approach. Knee Surg Sports Traumatol Arthrosc 2009;17(6):660-6.
107. Dixon MC, Parsch D, Brown RR, Scott RD. The correction of severe varus deformity in total knee arthroplasty by tibial component downsizing and resection of uncapped proximal medial bone. J Arthroplast. 2004;19(1):19–22. https://doi.org/10.1016/j.arth.2003.08.001.
108. Engh GA. Medial epicondylar osteotomy: a technique used with primary and revision total knee arthroplasty to improve surgical exposure and correct varus deformity. Instr Course Lect. 1999;48:153–6.
109. Whiteside LA. Selective ligament release in total knee arthroplasty of the knee in valgus. Clin Orthop Relat Res. 1999;367:130–40.
110. Clarke HD, Fuchs R, Scuderi GR, Scott WN, Insall JN. Clinical results in valgus total knee arthroplasty with the "pie crust" technique of lateral soft tissue releases. J Arthroplast. 2005;20(8):1010–4.
111. Krackow KA, Brooks RL. Optimization of knee ligament position for lateral extraarticular reconstruction. Am J Sports Med. 1983;11(5):293–302. https://doi.org/10.1177/036354658301100503.
112. Bindelglass DF, Cohen JL, Dorr LD. Patellar tilt and subluxation in total knee arthroplasty. Relationship to pain, fixation, and design. Clin Orthop Relat Res. 1993;286:103–9.
113. Bert JM, McShane M. Is it necessary to cement the tibial stem in cemented total knee arthroplasty? Clin Orthop Relat Res. 1998;356:73–8.
114. Huiskes R. Thermal injury of cancellous bone, following pressurized penetration of acrylic cement. Trans Orthop Res Soc. 1981;6:134.
115. Vanlommel J, Luyckx JP, Labey L, Innocenti B, De Corte R, Bellemans J. Cementing the tibial component in total knee arthroplasty: which technique is the best? J Arthroplast. 2011;26(3):492–6. https://doi.org/10.1016/j.arth.2010.01.107.
116. Vanlommel J, Luyckx JP, Labey L, Innocenti B, De Corte R, Bellemans J. Cementing the tibial component in total knee arthroplasty: which technique is the best? J Arthroplast. 2011;26(3):492–6. https://doi.org/10.1016/j.arth.2010.01.107.
117. Vaninbroukx M, Labey L, Innocenti B, Bellemans J. Cementing the femoral component in total knee arthroplasty: Which technique is the best? The Knee. 2009;16(4):265–8. https://doi.org/10.1016/j.knee.2008.11.015.
118. Brooks PJ, Walker PS, Scott RD. Tibial component fixation in deficient tibial bone stock. Clin Orthop Relat Res. 1984;184:302–8.
119. Ritter MA, Keating EM, Faris PM. Screw and cement fixation of large defects in total knee arthroplasty. A sequel. J Arthroplast. 1993;8(1):63–5. https://doi.org/10.1016/s0883-5403(06)80109-9.
120. Dorr LD, Ranawat CS, Sculco TA, McKaskill B, Orisek BS. Bone graft for tibial defects in total knee arthroplasty. Clin Orthop Relat Res. 1986;205:153–65.
121. Yoon JR, Seo IW, Shin YS. Correction to: use of autogenous onlay bone graft for uncontained tibial bone defects in primary total knee arthroplasty. BMC Musculoskelet Disord. 2018;19(1):31. https://doi.org/10.1186/s12891-018-1939-4.
122. Wang JW, Hsu CH, Huang CC, Lin PC, Chen WS. Reconstruction using femoral head allograft in revision total knee replacement: an experience in Asian patients. Bone Joint J. 2013;95-B(5):643–8. https://doi.org/10.1302/0301-620X.95B5.29915.
123. Samuelson KM. Bone grafting and noncemented revision arthroplasty of the knee. Clin Orthop Relat Res. 1988;226:93–101.
124. Murphy MT, Skinner TL, Cresswell AG, Crawford RW, Journeaux SF, Russell TG. The effect of knee flexion contracture following total knee arthroplasty on the energy cost of walking. J Arthroplast. 2014;29(1):85–9. https://doi.org/10.1016/j.arth.2013.04.039.
125. Easley ME, Insall JN, Scuderi GR, Bullek DD. Primary constrained condylar knee arthroplasty for the arthritic valgus knee. Clin Orthop Relat Res. 2000;380:58–64. https://doi.org/10.1097/00003086-200011000-00008.
126. Gerbino PG, Zurakowski D, Soto R, Griffin E, Reig TS, Micheli LJ. Long-term functional outcome after lateral patellar retinacular release in adolescents: an observational cohort study with minimum 5-year follow-up. J Pediatr Orthop. 2008;28(1):118–23. https://doi.org/10.1097/bpo.0b013e31815b4dcf.
127. Wang J-W, Wang C-J. Total knee arthroplasty for arthritis of the knee with extra-articular deformity. JBJS. 2002;84(10):1769–74.
128. Sculco PK, Kahlenberg CA, Fragomen AT, Rozbruch SR. Management of extra-articular deformity in the setting of total knee arthroplasty. JAAOS J Am Acad Orthop Surg. 2019;27(18):e819–e30.
129. Richardson AB, Bala A, Wellman SS, Attarian DE, Bolognesi MP, Grant SA. Perioperative dexamethasone administration does not increase the incidence of postoperative infection in total hip and knee arthroplasty: a retrospective analysis. J Arthroplast. 2016;31(8):1784–7.
130. Schnabel A, Reichl SU, Weibel S, Zahn PK, Kranke P, Pogatzki-Zahn E, et al. Adductor canal blocks for postoperative pain treatment in adults undergoing knee surgery. Cochrane Database Syst Rev. 2019;2019(10). https://doi.org/10.1002/14651858.CD012262.pub2.
131. Sankineani SR, Reddy ARC, Eachempati KK, Jangale A, Gurava Reddy AV. Comparison of

adductor canal block and IPACK block (interspace between the popliteal artery and the capsule of the posterior knee) with adductor canal block alone after total knee arthroplasty: a prospective control trial on pain and knee function in immediate post-operative period. Eur J Orthop Surg Traumatol Orthop Traumatol. 2018;28(7):1391–5. https://doi.org/10.1007/s00590-018-2218-7.
132. Vendittoli PA, Makinen P, Drolet P, Lavigne M, Fallaha M, Guertin MC, et al. A multimodal analgesia protocol for total knee arthroplasty. A randomized, controlled study. J Bone Joint Surg Am. 2006;88(2):282–9. https://doi.org/10.2106/JBJS.E.00173.
133. Busch CA, Shore BJ, Bhandari R, Ganapathy S, MacDonald SJ, Bourne RB, et al. Efficacy of periarticular multimodal drug injection in total knee arthroplasty. A randomized trial. J Bone Joint Surg Am. 2006;88(5):959–63. https://doi.org/10.2106/JBJS.E.00344.
134. Chang CB, Cho WS. Pain management protocols, peri-operative pain and patient satisfaction after total knee replacement: a multicentre study. J Bone Joint Surg Br. 2012;94(11):1511–6. https://doi.org/10.1302/0301-620X.94B11.29165.
135. Piovella F, Wang C-J, Lu H, Lee K, Lee LH, Lee WC, et al. Deep-vein thrombosis rates after major orthopedic surgery in Asia. An epidemiological study based on postoperative screening with centrally adjudicated bilateral venography. J Thrombosis Haemostasis. 2005;3(12):2664–70. https://doi.org/10.1111/j.1538-7836.2005.01621.x.
136. AlBuhairan B, Hind D, Hutchinson A. Antibiotic prophylaxis for wound infections in total joint arthroplasty: a systematic review. J Bone Joint Surg Br. 2008;90(7):915–9. https://doi.org/10.1302/0301-620X.90B7.20498.
137. Smith EB, Wynne R, Joshi A, Liu H, Good RP. Is it time to include vancomycin for routine perioperative antibiotic prophylaxis in total joint arthroplasty patients? J Arthroplast. 2012;27(8 Suppl):55–60. https://doi.org/10.1016/j.arth.2012.03.040.
138. Ponce B, Raines BT, Reed RD, Vick C, Richman J, Hawn M. Surgical site infection after arthroplasty: comparative effectiveness of prophylactic antibiotics: do surgical care improvement project guidelines need to be updated? J Bone Joint Surg Am. 2014;96(12):970–7. https://doi.org/10.2106/JBJS.M.00663.
139. Classen DC, Evans RS, Pestotnik SL, Horn SD, Menlove RL, Burke JP. The timing of prophylactic administration of antibiotics and the risk of surgical-wound infection. N Engl J Med. 1992;326(5):281–6. https://doi.org/10.1056/NEJM199201303260501.
140. Daines BK, Dennis DA, Amann S. Infection prevention in total knee arthroplasty. JAAOS J Am Acad Orthop Surg. 2015;23(6):356–64. https://doi.org/10.5435/jaaos-d-12-00170.
141. Johnson DP. The effect of continuous passive motion on wound-healing and joint mobility after knee arthroplasty. J Bone Joint Surg Am. 1990;72(3):421–6.
142. Colwell CW Jr, Morris BA. The influence of continuous passive motion on the results of total knee arthroplasty. Clin Orthop Relat Res. 1992;276:225–8.
143. Yang JM, Cha HG, Kim MK. Effects of manipulation of the thorax and intensity of the pressure biofeedback unit on the superficial cervical flexors muscle during craniocervical flexion exercise. J Phys Ther Sci. 2017;29(2):282–4. https://doi.org/10.1589/jpts.29.282.
144. Healy WL, Della Valle CJ, Iorio R, Berend KR, Cushner FD, Dalury DF, et al. Complications of total knee arthroplasty: standardized list and definitions of the Knee Society. Clin Orthop Relat Res. 2013;471(1):215–20.
145. Brockman BS, Maupin JJ, Thompson SF, Hollabaugh KM, Thakral R. Complication rates in total knee arthroplasty performed for osteoarthritis and post-traumatic arthritis: a comparison study. J Arthroplast. 2020;35(2):371–4. https://doi.org/10.1016/j.arth.2019.09.022.
146. Lazaro LE, Cross MB, Lorich DG. Vascular anatomy of the patella: implications for total knee arthroplasty surgical approaches. Knee. 2014;21(3):655–60. https://doi.org/10.1016/j.knee.2014.03.005.
147. Hou Y, Gao J, Chen J, Lin J, Ni L, Sun T, et al. The role of knee arthroscopy in managing common soft tissue complications after total knee arthroplasty: a retrospective case series study. J Orthop Surg Res. 2020;15(1):573. https://doi.org/10.1186/s13018-020-02112-8.
148. Vince K, Chivas D, Droll KP. Wound complications after total knee arthroplasty. J Arthroplast. 2007;22(4 Suppl 1):39–44. https://doi.org/10.1016/j.arth.2007.03.014.
149. Weiss AP, Krackow KA. Persistent wound drainage after primary total knee arthroplasty. J Arthroplast. 1993;8(3):285–9. https://doi.org/10.1016/s0883-5403(06)80091-4.
150. Dennis DA. Wound complications in total knee arthroplasty. Orthopedics. 1997;20(9):837–40.
151. Parvizi J, Gehrke T, Chen AF. Proceedings of the international consensus on periprosthetic joint infection. Bone Joint J. 2013;95-B(11):1450–2. https://doi.org/10.1302/0301-620X.95B11.33135.
152. Simons MJ, Amin NH, Scuderi GR. Acute wound complications after total knee arthroplasty: prevention and management. J Am Acad Orthop Surg. 2017;25(8):547–55. https://doi.org/10.5435/JAAOS-D-15-00402.
153. Bengtson S, Carlsson A, Relander M, Knutson K, Lidgren L. Treatment of the exposed knee prosthesis. Acta Orthop Scand. 1987;58(6):662–5. https://doi.org/10.3109/17453678709146510.
154. Markovich GD, Dorr LD, Klein NE, McPherson EJ, Vince KG. Muscle flaps in total knee arthroplasty. Clin Orthop Relat Res. 1995;321:122–30.
155. Sanders R, O'Neill T. The gastrocnemius myocutaneous flap used as a over for the exposed knee pros-

thesis. J Bone Joint Surg Br. 1981;63-B(3):383–6. https://doi.org/10.1302/0301-620X.63B3.7263750.
156. Hanssen AD, Rand JA. Evaluation and treatment of infection at the site of a total hip or knee arthroplasty. Instr Course Lect. 1999;48:111–22.
157. Segawa H, Tsukayama DT, Kyle RF, Becker DA, Gustilo RB. Infection after total knee arthroplasty. A retrospective study of the treatment of eighty-one infections. J Bone Joint Surg Am. 1999;81(10):1434–45. https://doi.org/10.2106/00004623-199910000-00008.
158. Peersman G, Laskin R, Davis J, Peterson M. Infection in total knee replacement: a retrospective review of 6489 total knee replacements. Clin Orthop Relat Res. 2001;392:15–23.
159. Gristina AG, Kolkin J. Current concepts review. Total joint replacement and sepsis. J Bone Joint Surg Am. 1983;65(1):128–34.
160. Tsukayama DT, Goldberg VM, Kyle R. Diagnosis and management of infection after total knee arthroplasty. J Bone Joint Surg Am. 2003;85-A(Suppl 1):S75–80. https://doi.org/10.2106/00004623-200300001-00014.
161. Teller RE, Christie MJ, Martin W, Nance EP, Haas DW. Sequential indium-labeled leukocyte and bone scans to diagnose prosthetic joint infection. Clin Orthop Relat Res. 2000;373:241–7. https://doi.org/10.1097/00003086-200004000-00029.
162. Duff GP, Lachiewicz PF, Kelley SS. Aspiration of the knee joint before revision arthroplasty. Clin Orthop Relat Res. 1996;331:132–9. https://doi.org/10.1097/00003086-199610000-00018.
163. Unkila-Kallio L, Kallio MJ, Eskola J, Peltola H. Serum C-reactive protein, erythrocyte sedimentation rate, and white blood cell count in acute hematogenous osteomyelitis of children. Pediatrics. 1994;93(1):59–62.
164. White J, Kelly M, Dunsmuir R. C-reactive protein level after total hip and total knee replacement. J Bone Joint Surg Br. 1998;80(5):909–11. https://doi.org/10.1302/0301-620x.80b5.8708.
165. Bilgen O, Atici T, Durak K, Karaeminogullari, Bilgen MS. C-reactive protein values and erythrocyte sedimentation rates after total hip and total knee arthroplasty. J Int Med Res. 2001;29(1):7–12. https://doi.org/10.1177/147323000102900102.
166. Laiho K, Maenpaa H, Kautiainen H, Kauppi M, Kaarela K, Lehto M, et al. Rise in serum C reactive protein after hip and knee arthroplasties in patients with rheumatoid arthritis. Ann Rheum Dis. 2001;60(3):275–7. https://doi.org/10.1136/ard.60.3.275.
167. Squire MW, Della Valle CJ, Parvizi J. Preoperative diagnosis of periprosthetic joint infection: role of aspiration. AJR Am J Roentgenol. 2011;196(4):875–9. https://doi.org/10.2214/AJR.10.5160.
168. Levitsky KA, Hozack WJ, Balderston RA, Rothman RH, Gluckman SJ, Maslack MM, et al. Evaluation of the painful prosthetic joint. Relative value of bone scan, sedimentation rate, and joint aspiration. J Arthroplast. 1991;6(3):237–44. https://doi.org/10.1016/s0883-5403(06)80170-1.
169. Trampuz A, Hanssen AD, Osmon DR, Mandrekar J, Steckelberg JM, Patel R. Synovial fluid leukocyte count and differential for the diagnosis of prosthetic knee infection. Am J Med. 2004;117(8):556–62. https://doi.org/10.1016/j.amjmed.2004.06.022.
170. Mason JB, Fehring TK, Odum SM, Griffin WL, Nussman DS. The value of white blood cell counts before revision total knee arthroplasty. J Arthroplast. 2003;18(8):1038–43. https://doi.org/10.1016/s0883-5403(03)00448-0.
171. Bedair H, Ting N, Jacovides C, Saxena A, Moric M, Parvizi J, et al. The Mark Coventry Award: diagnosis of early postoperative TKA infection using synovial fluid analysis. Clin Orthop Relat Res. 2011;469(1):34–40. https://doi.org/10.1007/s11999-010-1433-2.
172. Parvizi J, Gehrke T, International Consensus Group on Periprosthetic Joint I. Definition of periprosthetic joint infection. J Arthroplast. 2014;29(7):1331. https://doi.org/10.1016/j.arth.2014.03.009.
173. Bengston S, Knutson K, Lidgren L. Treatment of infected knee arthroplasty. Clin Orthop Relat Res. 1989;245:173–8.
174. Sartoris DJ. The role of radiology in orthopaedic sepsis. Orthop Rev. 1987;16(4):271–86.
175. Scher DM, Pak K, Lonner JH, Finkel JE, Zuckerman JD, Di Cesare PE. The predictive value of indium-111 leukocyte scans in the diagnosis of infected total hip, knee, or resection arthroplasties. J Arthroplast. 2000;15(3):295–300. https://doi.org/10.1016/s0883-5403(00)90555-2.
176. Parvizi J, Zmistowski B, Berbari EF, Bauer TW, Springer BD, Della Valle CJ, et al. New definition for periprosthetic joint infection: from the workgroup of the musculoskeletal infection society. Clin Orthop Relat Res. 2011;469(11):2992–4. https://doi.org/10.1007/s11999-011-2102-9.
177. Osmon DR, Berbari EF, Berendt AR, Lew D, Zimmerli W, Steckelberg JM, et al. Diagnosis and management of prosthetic joint infection: clinical practice guidelines by the Infectious Diseases Society of America. Clin Infect Dis. 2013;56(1):e1–e25. https://doi.org/10.1093/cid/cis803.
178. Parvizi J, Tan TL, Goswami K, Higuera C, Della Valle C, Chen AF, et al. The 2018 definition of periprosthetic hip and knee infection: an evidence-based and validated criteria. J Arthroplast. 2018;33(5):1309–14.e2.
179. McNally M, Sousa R, Wouthuyzen-Bakker M, Chen AF, Soriano A, Vogely HC, et al. The EBJIS definition of periprosthetic joint infection. Bone Joint J. 2021;103-B(1):18–25.https://doi.org/10.1302/0301--620X.103B1.BJJ-2020-1381.R1.
180. Parvizi J. New definition for periprosthetic joint infection. Am J Orthop (Belle Mead NJ). 2011;40(12):614–5.
181. Zmistowski B, Della Valle C, Bauer TW, Malizos KN, Alavi A, Bedair H, et al. Diagnosis of periprosthetic

joint infection. J Arthroplast. 2014;29(2 Suppl):77–83. https://doi.org/10.1016/j.arth.2013.09.040.
182. Fulkerson E, Valle CJ, Wise B, Walsh M, Preston C, Di Cesare PE. Antibiotic susceptibility of bacteria infecting total joint arthroplasty sites. J Bone Joint Surg Am. 2006;88(6):1231–7. https://doi.org/10.2106/JBJS.E.00004.
183. Obrebski M, Kicinski M, Bialecki J, Marczynski W, Walczak P. An analysis of complex, life-threatening infectious complications of hip and knee joint arthroplasty based on departmental data. Pol Orthop Traumatol. 2013;78:251–7.
184. Turner NA, Sharma-Kuinkel BK, Maskarinec SA, Eichenberger EM, Shah PP, Carugati M, et al. Methicillin-resistant *Staphylococcus aureus*: an overview of basic and clinical research. Nat Rev Microbiol. 2019;17(4):203–18. https://doi.org/10.1038/s41579-018-0147-4.
185. Bejon P, Berendt A, Atkins BL, Green N, Parry H, Masters S, et al. Two-stage revision for prosthetic joint infection: predictors of outcome and the role of reimplantation microbiology. J Antimicrob Chemother. 2010;65(3):569–75. https://doi.org/10.1093/jac/dkp469.
186. Tice AD, Hoaglund PA, Shoultz DA. Outcomes of osteomyelitis among patients treated with outpatient parenteral antimicrobial therapy. Am J Med. 2003;114(9):723–8. https://doi.org/10.1016/s0002-9343(03)00231-6.
187. Zimmerli W, Widmer AF, Blatter M, Frei R, Ochsner PE. Role of rifampin for treatment of orthopedic implant-related staphylococcal infections: a randomized controlled trial. Foreign-Body Infection (FBI) Study Group. JAMA. 1998;279(19):1537–41. https://doi.org/10.1001/jama.279.19.1537.
188. Duggal A, Barsoum W, Schmitt SK. Patients with prosthetic joint infection on IV antibiotics are at high risk for readmission. Clin Orthop Relat Res. 2009;467(7):1727–31. https://doi.org/10.1007/s11999-009-0825-7.
189. Mirra JM, Amstutz HC, Matos M, Gold R. The pathology of the joint tissues and its clinical relevance in prosthesis failure. Clin Orthop Relat Res. 1976;117:221–40.
190. Chiu FY, Chen CM. Surgical debridement and parenteral antibiotics in infected revision total knee arthroplasty. Clin Orthop Relat Res. 2007;461:130–5. https://doi.org/10.1097/BLO.0b013e318063e7f3.
191. Gardner J, Gioe TJ, Tatman P. Can this prosthesis be saved?: implant salvage attempts in infected primary TKA. Clin Orthop Relat Res. 2011;469(4):970–6. https://doi.org/10.1007/s11999-010-1417-2.
192. Silva M, Tharani R, Schmalzried TP. Results of direct exchange or debridement of the infected total knee arthroplasty. Clin Orthop Relat Res. 2002;404:125–31. https://doi.org/10.1097/00003086-200211000-00022.
193. Bradbury T, Fehring TK, Taunton M, Hanssen A, Azzam K, Parvizi J, et al. The fate of acute methicillin-resistant *Staphylococcus aureus* periprosthetic knee infections treated by open debridement and retention of components. J Arthroplast. 2009;24(6 Suppl):101–4. https://doi.org/10.1016/j.arth.2009.04.028.
194. Deirmengian C, Greenbaum J, Stern J, Braffman M, Lotke PA, Booth RE Jr, et al. Open debridement of acute gram-positive infections after total knee arthroplasty. Clin Orthop Relat Res. 2003;416:129–34. https://doi.org/10.1097/01.blo.0000092996.90435.35.
195. Teeny SM, Dorr L, Murata G, Conaty P. Treatment of infected total knee arthroplasty. Irrigation and debridement versus two-stage reimplantation. J Arthroplast. 1990;5(1):35–9. https://doi.org/10.1016/s0883-5403(06)80007-0.
196. Hartman MB, Fehring TK, Jordan L, Norton HJ. Periprosthetic knee sepsis. The role of irrigation and debridement. Clin Orthop Relat Res. 1991;273:113–8.
197. Mont MA, Waldman B, Banerjee C, Pacheco IH, Hungerford DS. Multiple irrigation, debridement, and retention of components in infected total knee arthroplasty. J Arthroplast. 1997;12(4):426–33. https://doi.org/10.1016/s0883-5403(97)90199-6.
198. Estes CS, Beauchamp CP, Clarke HD, Spangehl MJ. A two-stage retention debridement protocol for acute periprosthetic joint infections. Clin Orthop Relat Res. 2010;468(8):2029–38. https://doi.org/10.1007/s11999-010-1293-9.
199. Tsumura H, Ikeda S, Ono T, Itonaga I, Taira H, Torisu T. Synovectomy, debridement, and continuous irrigation for infected total knee arthroplasty. Int Orthop. 2005;29(2):113–6. https://doi.org/10.1007/s00264-004-0626-2.
200. Buechel FF, Femino FP, D'Alessio J. Primary exchange revision arthroplasty for infected total knee replacement: a long-term study. Am J Orthop (Belle Mead NJ) 2004;33(4):190–198; discussion 8.
201. Mont MA, Waldman BJ, Hungerford DS. Evaluation of preoperative cultures before second-stage reimplantation of a total knee prosthesis complicated by infection. A comparison-group study. J Bone Joint Surg Am. 2000;82(11):1552–7. https://doi.org/10.2106/00004623-200011000-00006.
202. Kurd MF, Ghanem E, Steinbrecher J, Parvizi J. Two-stage exchange knee arthroplasty: does resistance of the infecting organism influence the outcome? Clin Orthop Relat Res. 2010;468(8):2060–6. https://doi.org/10.1007/s11999-010-1296-6.
203. Mittal Y, Fehring TK, Hanssen A, Marculescu C, Odum SM, Osmon D. Two-stage reimplantation for periprosthetic knee infection involving resistant organisms. J Bone Joint Surg Am. 2007;89(6):1227–31. https://doi.org/10.2106/JBJS.E.01192.
204. Azzam K, Parvizi J, Jungkind D, Hanssen A, Fehring T, Springer B, et al. Microbiological, clinical, and surgical features of fungal prosthetic joint infections: a multi-institutional experience. J Bone Joint Surg Am. 2009;91(Suppl 6):142–9. https://doi.org/10.2106/JBJS.I.00574.

205. Vince KG, Abdeen A, Sugimori T. The unstable total knee arthroplasty: causes and cures. J Arthroplast. 2006;21(4 Suppl 1):44–9. https://doi.org/10.1016/j.arth.2006.02.101.
206. D'Lima DD, Patil S, Steklov N, Colwell CW Jr. An ABJS Best Paper: Dynamic intraoperative ligament balancing for total knee arthroplasty. Clin Orthop Relat Res. 2007;463:208–12.
207. Dennis DA, Berry DJ, Engh G, Fehring T, MacDonald SJ, Rosenberg AG, et al. Revision total knee arthroplasty. J Am Acad Orthop Surg. 2008;16(8):442–54. https://doi.org/10.5435/00124635-200808000-00003.
208. Blunn GW, Walker PS, Joshi A, Hardinge K. The dominance of cyclic sliding in producing wear in total knee replacements. Clin Orthop Relat Res. 1991;273:253–60.
209. Schroer WC, Berend KR, Lombardi AV, Barnes CL, Bolognesi MP, Berend ME, et al. Why are total knees failing today? Etiology of total knee revision in 2010 and 2011. J Arthroplast. 2013;28(8 Suppl):116–9. https://doi.org/10.1016/j.arth.2013.04.056.
210. Sharkey PF, Hozack WJ, Rothman RH, Shastri S, Jacoby SM. Insall Award paper. Why are total knee arthroplasties failing today? Clin Orthop Relat Res. 2002(404):7–13. https://doi.org/10.1097/00003086-200211000-00003.
211. Fehring TK, Valadie AL. Knee instability after total knee arthroplasty. Clin Orthop Relat Res. 1994;299:157–62.
212. Laskin RS, O'Flynn HM. The Insall Award. Total knee replacement with posterior cruciate ligament retention in rheumatoid arthritis Problems and complications. Clin Orthop Relat Res. 1997;345:24–8.
213. Pagnano MW, Hanssen AD, Lewallen DG, Stuart MJ. Flexion instability after primary posterior cruciate retaining total knee arthroplasty. Clin Orthop Relat Res. 1998;356:39–46. https://doi.org/10.1097/00003086-199811000-00008.
214. Saeki K, Mihalko WM, Patel V, Conway J, Naito M, Thrum H, et al. Stability after medial collateral ligament release in total knee arthroplasty. Clin Orthop Relat Res. 2001;392:184–9. https://doi.org/10.1097/00003086-200111000-00022.
215. Waslewski GL, Marson BM, Benjamin JB. Early, incapacitating instability of posterior cruciate ligament-retaining total knee arthroplasty. J Arthroplast. 1998;13(7):763–7. https://doi.org/10.1016/s0883-5403(98)90027-4.
216. Eisenhuth SA, Saleh KJ, Cui Q, Clark CR, Brown TE. Patellofemoral instability after total knee arthroplasty. Clin Orthop Relat Res. 2006;446:149–60. https://doi.org/10.1097/01.blo.0000214415.83593.db.
217. Kelly MA. Patellofemoral complications following total knee arthroplasty. Instr Course Lect. 2001;50:403–7.
218. Malo M, Vince KG. The unstable patella after total knee arthroplasty: etiology, prevention, and management. J Am Acad Orthop Surg. 2003;11(5):364–71. https://doi.org/10.5435/00124635-200309000-00009.
219. Victor J, Labey L, Wong P, Innocenti B, Bellemans J. The influence of muscle load on tibiofemoral knee kinematics. J Orthop Res. 2010;28(4):419–28. https://doi.org/10.1002/jor.21019.
220. Morgan H, Battista V, Leopold SS. Constraint in primary total knee arthroplasty. JAAOS J Am Acad Orthop Surg. 2005;13(8):515–24.
221. Naudie DD, Rorabeck CH. Managing instability in total knee arthroplasty with constrained and linked implants. Instr Course Lect. 2004;53:207–15.
222. Sculco TP. The role of constraint in total knee arthoplasty. J Arthroplast. 2006;21(4):54–6.
223. McPherson EJ, Portugal D. Revision total knee arthroplasty for excessive ligamentotaxis. J Arthroplast. 2007;22(8):1214–6.
224. Whiteside LA, Saeki K, Mihalko WM. Functional medical ligament balancing in total knee arthroplasty. Clin Orthop Relat Res. 2000;380:45–57. https://doi.org/10.1097/00003086-200011000-00007.
225. Christensen CP, Crawford JJ, Olin MD, Vail TP. Revision of the stiff total knee arthroplasty. J Arthroplast. 2002;17(4):409–15. https://doi.org/10.1054/arth.2002.32105.
226. Kim J, Nelson CL, Lotke PA. Stiffness after total knee arthroplasty. Prevalence of the complication and outcomes of revision. J Bone Joint Surg Am. 2004;86(7):1479–84.
227. Nicholls DW, Dorr LD. Revision surgery for stiff total knee arthroplasty. J Arthroplast. 1990;5(Suppl):S73–7. https://doi.org/10.1016/s0883-5403(08)80029-0.
228. Scranton PE Jr. Management of knee pain and stiffness after total knee arthroplasty. J Arthroplast. 2001;16(4):428–35. https://doi.org/10.1054/arth.2001.22250.
229. Yercan HS, Sugun TS, Bussiere C, Ait Si Selmi T, Davies A, Neyret P. Stiffness after total knee arthroplasty: prevalence, management and outcomes. Knee. 2006;13(2):111–7. https://doi.org/10.1016/j.knee.2005.10.001.
230. Harvey LA, Brosseau L, Herbert RD. Continuous passive motion following total knee arthroplasty in people with arthritis. Cochrane Database Syst Rev. 2010;3:CD004260. https://doi.org/10.1002/14651858.CD004260.pub2.
231. Malviya A, Lingard EA, Weir DJ, Deehan DJ. Predicting range of movement after knee replacement: the importance of posterior condylar offset and tibial slope. Knee Surg Sports Traumatol Arthrosc. 2009;17(5):491–8. https://doi.org/10.1007/s00167-008-0712-x.
232. Nelson CL, Kim J, Lotke PA. Stiffness after total knee arthroplasty. J Bone Joint Surg Am. 2005;87 Suppl 1(Pt 2):264–70. https://doi.org/10.2106/JBJS.E-00345.
233. Laskin RS, Rieger MA. The surgical technique for performing a total knee replacement arthroplasty. Orthop Clin North Am. 1989;20(1):31–48.

234. Lo CS, Wang SJ, Wu SS. Knee stiffness on extension caused by an oversized femoral component after total knee arthroplasty: a report of two cases and a review of the literature. J Arthroplast. 2003;18(6):804–8. https://doi.org/10.1016/s0883-5403(03)00331-0.
235. Gonzalez MH, Mekhail AO. The failed total knee arthroplasty: evaluation and etiology. J Am Acad Orthop Surg. 2004;12(6):436–46. https://doi.org/10.5435/00124635-200411000-00008.
236. Pariente GM, Lombardi AV Jr, Berend KR, Mallory TH, Adams JB. Manipulation with prolonged epidural analgesia for treatment of TKA complicated by arthrofibrosis. Surg Technol Int. 2006;15:221–4.
237. Daluga D, Lombardi AV Jr, Mallory TH, Vaughn BK. Knee manipulation following total knee arthroplasty: analysis of prognostic variables. J Arthroplast. 1991;6(2):119–28.
238. Diduch DR, Scuderi GR, Scott WN, Insall JN, Kelly MA. The efficacy of arthroscopy following total knee replacement. Arthroscopy. 1997;13(2):166–71. https://doi.org/10.1016/s0749-8063(97)90150-x.
239. Mont MA, Serna FK, Krackow KA, Hungerford DS. Exploration of radiographically normal total knee replacements for unexplained pain. Clin Orthop Relat Res. 1996;331:216–20. https://doi.org/10.1097/00003086-199610000-00030.
240. Bellemans J, Vandenneucker H, Victor J, Vanlauwe J. Flexion contracture in total knee arthroplasty. Clin Orthop Relat Res. 2006;452:78–82. https://doi.org/10.1097/01.blo.0000238791.36725.c5.
241. Lesh ML, Schneider DJ, Deol G, Davis B, Jacobs CR, Pellegrini VD Jr. The consequences of anterior femoral notching in total knee arthroplasty. A biomechanical study. J Bone Joint Surg Am. 2000;82(8):1096–101. https://doi.org/10.2106/00004623-200008000-00005.
242. Zalzal P, Backstein D, Gross AE, Papini M. Notching of the anterior femoral cortex during total knee arthroplasty characteristics that increase local stresses. J Arthroplast. 2006;21(5):737–43. https://doi.org/10.1016/j.arth.2005.08.020.
243. Rorabeck CH, Taylor JW. Periprosthetic fractures of the femur complicating total knee arthroplasty. Orthop Clin North Am. 1999;30(2):265–77. https://doi.org/10.1016/s0030-5898(05)70081-x.
244. Su ET, Kubiak EN, Dewal H, Hiebert R, Di Cesare PE. A proposed classification of supracondylar femur fractures above total knee arthroplasties. J Arthroplast. 2006;21(3):405–8. https://doi.org/10.1016/j.arth.2005.05.022.
245. Felix NA, Stuart MJ, Hanssen AD. Periprosthetic fractures of the tibia associated with total knee arthroplasty. Clin Orthop Relat Res. 1997;345:113–24.
246. Goldberg VM, Figgie HE 3rd, Inglis AE, Figgie MP, Sobel M, Kelly M, et al. Patellar fracture type and prognosis in condylar total knee arthroplasty. Clin Orthop Relat Res. 1988;236:115–22.
247. Healy WL, Siliski JM, Incavo SJ. Operative treatment of distal femoral fractures proximal to total knee replacements. J Bone Joint Surg Am. 1993;75(1):27–34. https://doi.org/10.2106/00004623-199301000-00005.
248. Bonnin M, Lustig S, Huten D. Extensor tendon ruptures after total knee arthroplasty. Orthop Traumatol Surg Res. 2016;102(1 Suppl):S21–31. https://doi.org/10.1016/j.otsr.2015.06.025.
249. Dobbs RE, Hanssen AD, Lewallen DG, Pagnano MW. Quadriceps tendon rupture after total knee arthroplasty. Prevalence, complications, and outcomes. J Bone Joint Surg Am. 2005;87(1):37–45. https://doi.org/10.2106/JBJS.D.01910.
250. Jujo Y, Yasui T, Nagase Y, Kadono Y, Oka H, Tanaka S. Patellar fracture after total knee arthroplasty for rheumatoid arthritis. J Arthroplast. 2013;28(1):40–3. https://doi.org/10.1016/j.arth.2012.04.022.
251. Yun AG, Rubash HE, Scott RD, Laskin RS. Quadriceps rupture associated with a proximal quadriceps release in total knee arthroplasty. A report of three cases. J Bone Joint Surg Am. 2003;85(9):1809–11. https://doi.org/10.2106/00004623-200309000-00024.
252. Schoderbek RJ Jr, Brown TE, Mulhall KJ, Mounasamy V, Iorio R, Krackow KA, et al. Extensor mechanism disruption after total knee arthroplasty. Clin Orthop Relat Res. 2006;446:176–85. https://doi.org/10.1097/01.blo.0000218726.06473.26.
253. Bates MD, Springer BD. Extensor mechanism disruption after total knee arthroplasty. J Am Acad Orthop Surg. 2015;23(2):95–106. https://doi.org/10.5435/JAAOS-D-13-00205.
254. Morrey MC, Barlow JD, Abdel MP, Hanssen AD. Synthetic mesh augmentation of acute and subacute quadriceps tendon repair. Orthopedics. 2016;39(1):e9–13. https://doi.org/10.3928/01477447-20151218-02.
255. Burnett RS, Berger RA, Della Valle CJ, Sporer SM, Jacobs JJ, Paprosky WG, et al. Extensor mechanism allograft reconstruction after total knee arthroplasty. J Bone Joint Surg Am. 2005;87 Suppl 1(Pt 2):175–94. https://doi.org/10.2106/JBJS.E.00442.
256. Schoderbek Jr RJ, Brown TE, Mulhall KJ, Mounasamy V, Iorio R, Krackow KA, et al. Extensor mechanism disruption after total knee arthroplasty. Clin Orthop Relat Res. 2006;446:176–85.
257. Andrikoula S, Tokis A, Vasiliadis HS, Georgoulis A. The extensor mechanism of the knee joint: an anatomical study. Knee Surg Sports Traumatol Arthrosc. 2006;14(3):214–20. https://doi.org/10.1007/s00167-005-0680-3.
258. Maffulli N, Spiezia F, La Verde L, Rosa MA, Franceschi F. The management of extensor mechanism disruption after total knee arthroplasty: a systematic review. Sports Med Arthrosc Rev. 2017;25(1):41–50. https://doi.org/10.1097/JSA.0000000000000139.
259. Boyd AD Jr, Ewald FC, Thomas WH, Poss R, Sledge CB. Long-term complications after total knee arthroplasty with or without resurfacing of the patella. J Bone Joint Surg Am. 1993;75(5):674–81. https://doi.org/10.2106/00004623-199305000-00006.

260. Cadambi A, Engh GA. Use of a semitendinosus tendon autogenous graft for rupture of the patellar ligament after total knee arthroplasty. A report of seven cases. J Bone Joint Surg Am. 1992;74(7):974–9.
261. Jaureguito JW, Dubois CM, Smith SR, Gottlieb LJ, Finn HA. Medial gastrocnemius transposition flap for the treatment of disruption of the extensor mechanism after total knee arthroplasty. J Bone Joint Surg Am. 1997;79(6):866–73. https://doi.org/10.2106/00004623-199706000-00010.
262. Zanotti RM, Freiberg AA, Matthews LS. Use of patellar allograft to reconstruct a patellar tendon-deficient knee after total joint arthroplasty. J Arthroplast. 1995;10(3):271–4. https://doi.org/10.1016/s0883-5403(05)80173-1.
263. Sharkey PF, Lichstein PM, Shen C, Tokarski AT, Parvizi J. Why are total knee arthroplasties failing today—has anything changed after 10 years? J Arthroplast. 2014;29(9):1774–8.
264. Fraser JF, Werner S, Jacofsky DJ. Wear and loosening in total knee arthroplasty: a quick review. J Knee Surg. 2015;28(02):139–44.
265. Chakravarty R, Elmallah RD, Cherian JJ, Kurtz SM, Mont MA. Polyethylene wear in knee arthroplasty. J Knee Surg. 2015;28(05):370–5.
266. Gallo J, Goodman SB, Konttinen YT, Wimmer MA, Holinka M. Osteolysis around total knee arthroplasty: a review of pathogenetic mechanisms. Acta Biomater. 2013;9(9):8046–58.
267. Pang H-N, Abd Razak HRB, Petis S, Naudie DD, MacDonald SJ. The role of isolated polyethylene exchange in total knee arthroplasty. EFORT Open Rev. 2017;2(3):66–71.

15 How to Make a Strategy for Knee Arthritis Treatment

Seung-Suk Seo and Sang-Myung Roh

Abstract

Osteoarthritis (OA) not only causes multiple problems such as pain, functional disability, and impaired quality of life to individual patients, but also causes social problems such as reduced general health status, working ability, and increased cost burden. Health care providers try various interventions for knee OA primarily aiming at improving pain and function and correcting modifiable risk factors. The clinical presentation of knee OA varies substantially among individuals and is influenced by many factors. Understanding specific OA patterns and related factors is the basis for strategic approaches to a broad category of OA patients. A personalized care plan may enhance adherence and positively influence treatment outcomes by giving patients realistic and positive expectations for treatment efficacy. In addition, establishing effective treatment strategies for OA is important as they may reduce both the individual and social burden of OA. Although it is important for health care providers to personalize the treatment pathways based on an individual patient profile, these must be based on the existing evidence. In this regard, there are evidence-based guidelines providing recommendations to guide the clinical management of knee OA. Implementation of clinical practice guidelines can reduce substantial variations in costs of care by reducing wide variations in care pathways while increasing patient outcomes. Every effort should be made for solving the barriers to the implementation of clinical practice guidelines. In addition, a coordinated, multidisciplinary team-based approach can provide care with clinical effectiveness and cost-effectiveness.

Keywords

Knee osteoarthritis · Phenotype · Personalized care · Evidence-based guideline · Clinical practice guideline · Barriers to implementation · Multidisciplinary approach · Strategic approach

15.1 Introduction

Osteoarthritis (OA) is a leading cause of disability worldwide [1, 2]. OA not only causes multiple problems such as pain, functional disability, and impaired quality of life to individual patients, but also causes social problems such as reduced general health status, working ability, and increased cost burden [3–5]. With population aging, increased life expectancy, and the increasing prevalence of obesity of the global population,

S.-S. Seo (✉) · S.-M. Roh
Department of Orthopedics, Haeundae Bumin Hospital, Busan, South Korea
e-mail: seoss@bumin.co.kr

S.-S. Seo (ed.), *A Strategic Approach to Knee Arthritis Treatment*,
https://doi.org/10.1007/978-981-16-4217-3_15

it is widely accepted that the burden of OA will continue to increase [6]. Therefore, establishing effective treatment strategies for OA is important as they may reduce both the individual and social burden of OA [7].

OA is characterized by complex pathogenesis and may manifest at different anatomic locations. Among them, knee OA is the most common site of pain that makes people seek health care providers [8]. Pain is the main target of OA treatment and multiple factors are related to the development of pain and its persistence [8–11]. As such related factors, painful stimuli to the periarticular structures and altered modulation of stimulus transmission act in concert with psychosocial and environmental influences [12, 13]. In addition, these factors and mechanisms often coexist in varying degrees among patients. Thus, patients with knee OA presents with varying degrees of joint pain and functional impairment. Target and individualized treatment in every clinical case are the base of the concept of personalized treatment. Identification of different disease phenotypes of OA and related factors is the basis for providing individualized therapeutic strategy to these broad category of OA patients [14].

The main goals of OA management are including pain relief, functional improvement, improvement of quality of life, and ultimately modification of the disease course. Given the current absence of effective disease-modifying treatments for knee OA, health care providers try complex therapeutic approaches primarily aiming at improving pain and function and correcting modifiable risk factors. However, the global results from the treatments are not satisfactory [15]. Clinical applications with non-targeted treatment induce low response rates, increased rate of adverse reaction and economic burden because knee OA is characterized with heterogeneous patient populations and disease progression [16].

To develop a realistic plan, it is important for health care providers to personalize the treatment pathways based on an individual patient's disease characteristics, further, these pathways must be based on the existing evidence-based medicine (EBM) [17]. In addition, these treatment pathways should be agreed upon with patients, considering their preferences, beliefs, and their bio-psycho-social context. An individualized therapeutic strategy may enhance adherence and positively influence treatment outcomes by giving patients realistic and positive expectations for treatment efficacy. Numerous therapeutic modalities have been proposed for knee OA treatment. So far, these therapeutic modalities remain based on the individualized assessment of the patient, taking into account patients' needs and preferences, or the subjective interpretation of the evidence by the clinician. For the proof of efficacy of these, careful analysis of the clinical evidence allows to prioritize these therapeutic modalities and guide clinicians into progressive and logical therapeutic steps [18]. For the purpose of these, several evidence-based guidelines providing recommendations to guide clinical management of knee OA have been proposed [18–20]. Knee OA is a multifactorial disorder with various clinical manifestation and different stage of disease progressing to a common end. Considering these characteristics of knee OA, traditional speciality-based therapy does not give patients therapeutic benefits. Therefore, a coordinated, multidisciplinary team-based approach can provide care with clinical effectiveness and cost-effectiveness [16].

In this chapter, we will explain the concept and effectiveness of the multidisciplinary team approach as a treatment strategy for knee OA, explain individual treatment methods for knee OA in accordance with the EBM, and describe the algorithmic treatment approach using internationally recommended guidelines. Finally, we will search the clinical phenotypes of knee OA and the proposed therapeutic modalities accordingly, and we will describe the outcomes and their influencing factors of pain and structural change trajectories of knee OA. This knowledge will help establish a strategic approach to knee OA treatment and provide personalized health care.

15.2 Changing Paradigm from a Discrete, Specialty-Based Service to Multidisciplinary Team Approach

The ongoing difficulty faced by health care providers is whether well-coordinated care plan with appropriate treatment to address multiple problems of patients with knee OA in a clear and well-managed fashion can be provided or not, under limited conditions. Care models consisting of discrete specialty-based services are difficult to address multiple problems, and have limitation on considering and reflecting the patient's preferences [16]. Inconsistent approaches by each professional may omit or delay referrals to appropriate experts, make patients exposed to multiple conflicting information, and necessary treatments may be omitted due to disconnection of information, conversely, there is a possibility of being exposed to duplicate treatments, and patients experience a sense of disconnection in overall care. Consequently, these fragmented care can potentially increase the cost burden as well as be less effective for patients [21]. On the contrary, the multidisciplinary team approach can provide comprehensive care tailored to the patients' needs and preferences [22]. In this approach, specialists and patients have a close working relationship and provide coordinated care and ongoing feedback on specific treatments, which are based on shared decision-making. A combination of health care professionals from multiple disciplines can effectively deliver coordinated information, meet the broad needs of patients, increase patient participation and promote favorable behaviors [23]. As a member of the care team, patients play an active role in the choice of treatment choice, and these shared decision-making provide both patient and provider satisfaction, by improving decision quality, patient engagement, confidence, patient knowledge, and more efficient use of their time during their office visit [24] (Fig. 15.1).

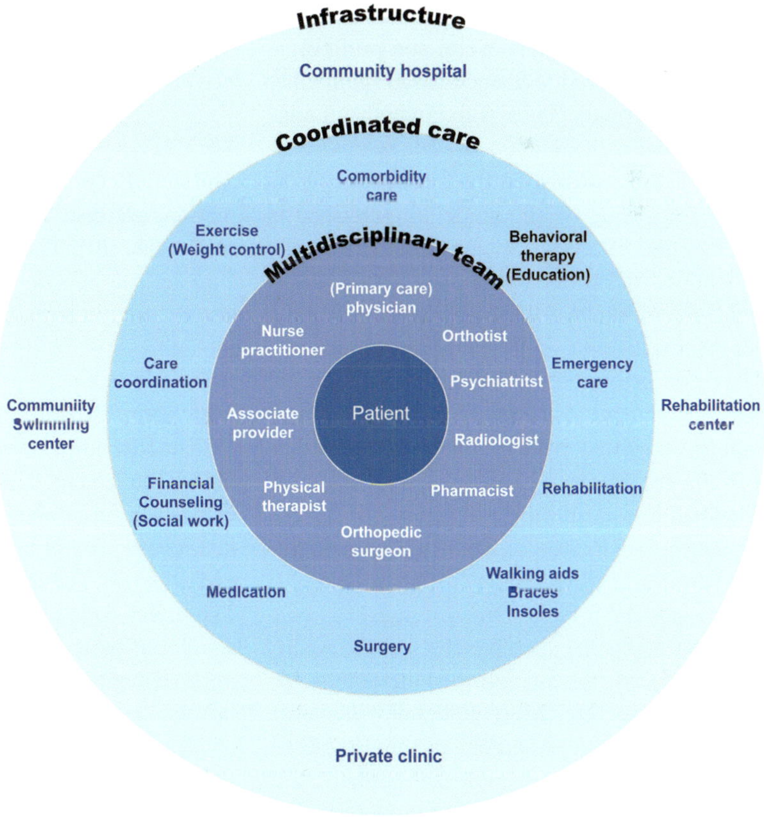

Fig. 15.1 Proposed model of a multidisciplinary team approach. A multidisciplinary team was formed and diagrammed according to the resources available in the author's institution, following the guidelines

Therefore, a specialized unit that organically combines professionals with multiple disciplines, patients, facilities, and supports systems can achieve more effective symptom control, more customized treatment planning, and better functional outcomes [25, 26]. Patients may avoid confusion caused by exposure to various opinions and information, safety issues such as overdosing occur due to overlapping care, cases in which necessary care is omitted can be avoided, and costs incurred in the overall service can also be reduced. Even if care is inevitable in different locations due to infrastructure problems, service continuity can be maintained and patients may feel themselves being supported through this unified treatment plan.

15.3 Clinical Practice Guideline (CPG) for Knee OA Treatment

Although a various combination of treatments is used for the treatment of knee OA, these must be based on a systematic appraisal of existing evidence. In this regard, several non-profit organizations published evidence-based guidelines providing recommendations to guide the clinical management of knee OA [17–20]. In this chapter, the authors addressed the management plan for OA, focusing on the guideline published in 2019 by the European Society for Clinical and Economic Aspects of Osteoporosis, Osteoarthritis and Musculoskeletal Diseases (ESCEO) [20]. For the recommendations or interpretation of evidence conflicting on the same type of treatment plan, the authors also described the recommendations suggested by the guidelines published over the last 3 years by the American College of Rheumatology/Arthritis Foundation (ACR) and Osteoarthritis Research Society International (OARSI) [17, 19, 20] (Table 15.1).

The guidelines have some differences in contents depending on expert panel selection, quality of evidence assessment, reviewed literatures, voting procedures, etc. Most guidelines, however, agree in their core treatment recommendations focusing on exercise, weight management, and education for knee OA [27]. The guidelines then either outline treatment recommendations for the management of knee OA by sequential/staged approach or by disease and/or comorbidity group followed by core treatments [17, 19, 20]. Management of knee OA consists of a combination of non-pharmacological interventions including a core set of initial measures/interventions and pharmacological interventions [20]. Surgical treatment is generally reserved for OA patients who do not respond to non-pharmacologic and pharmacologic treatment (Fig. 15.2).

15.3.1 Non-Pharmacological Treatment

Non-pharmacological interventions consist of modalities that can be used relatively safely compared to pharmacological interventions or surgery [28]. It includes a core set including information/education, weight loss if overweight, exercise program, and non-pharmacological background treatment such as knee braces, insoles, walking aids, thermal agents, mechanotherapy or manual therapy, bandage tape, hydrotherapy and aquatic exercises, and Tai Chi [20].

15.3.1.1 Core Set

The initial core set is based on education, information, exercise, and weight loss if overweight/obese [18, 29]. The treatments constituting the core set can be safely used in most patients and can be used in conjunction with other treatment modalities.

Education/Information

Patient education is an essential tool to optimize OA management. OA is a disease showing a chronic fashion, and education plays an important role in promoting adequate self-management and adherence to overall care plan [18, 20, 30]. The effect sizes of these programs are generally small, but in addition to the pain and functional improvements, there are other benefits that can be obtained by participating in programs, and above all, risks are minimal [19, 31]. All patients with OA should be thoroughly assessed with regard to their knowledge about the disease and

Table 15.1 Differences in the level of recommendations for the nonsurgical management of knee OA in knee OA clinical practice guidelines published within the last 3 years

	Strength of recommendation*		
Guideline publisher	ACR	ESCEO	OARSI
Core set	Strong recommendation	Strong recommendation	Strong recommendation
Paracetamol	Conditional recommendation (Short-term) Conditional recommendation (Long-term)	Weak recommendation (Short-term) Weak recommendation (Long-term)	Conditional recommendation *against* (Short-term) Conditional recommendation *against* (Long term)
Mind-body exercises	Strong recommendation (Tai-chi) Conditional recommendation (Yoga)	Strong recommendation (Tai-chi)	Strong recommendation (Tai-chi, Yoga)
Aquatic exercise	Strong recommendation	Strong recommendation	Conditional recommendation
SYSADOSs	Strong recommendation *against* (glucosamine, chondroitin sulfate)	Strong recommendation (pharmaceutical grade crystalline glucosamine sulfate and chondroitin sulfate) Weak recommendation (avocado soybean unsaponifiables, diacerein, combined glucosamine, and chondroitin sulfate)	Strong recommendation *against* (All SYSADOAs)
Topical NSAIDs	Strong recommendation	Strong recommendation	Strong recommendation Conditional recommendation (Widespread pain)
Oral NSAIDs	Strong recommendation	Strong recommendation	Conditional recommendation
Intra-articular hyaluronic acid	Conditional recommendation *against*	Weak recommendation	Conditional recommendation (Long-term pain relief (4–6 weeks))
Intra-articular corticosteroids	Strong recommendation	Weak recommendation	Conditional recommendation (Acute pain relief (1–2 weeks)) Conditional recommendation (Short-term pain relief (4–6 weeks))
Opioids	Conditional recommendation (Tramadol opioids)	Weak recommendation (Short-term weak opioids)	
	Conditional recommendation *against* (Non-tramadol opioids)	Weak recommendation (Classical oral or transdermal opioids)	Strong recommendation against (Oral or transdermal opioids)
Duloxetine	Conditional recommendation (*No recommendation* in previous guideline)	Weak recommendation	Conditional recommendation (*Appropriate* in previous guideline)

*The standards of strength of recommendation are different for each organization. *ACR* American College of Rheumatology/Arthritis Foundation, *ESCEO* European Society for Clinical and Economic Aspects of Osteoporosis, Osteoarthritis and Musculoskeletal Diseases, *OARSI* Osteoarthritis Research Society International

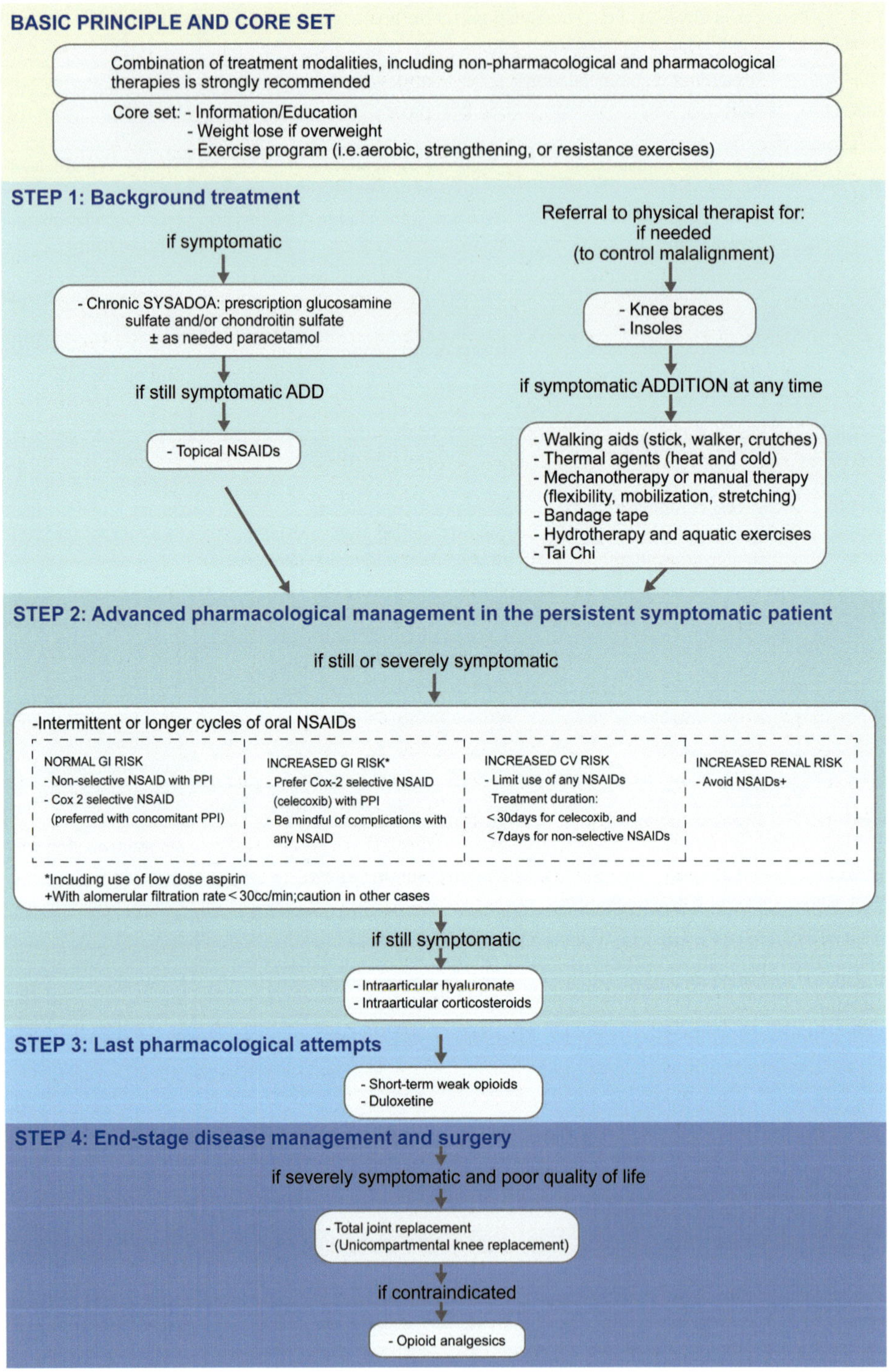

Fig. 15.2 Updated ESCEO stepwise treatment algorithm for knee osteoarthritis [20]. *COX-2* cyclooxygenase-2, *CS* chondroitin sulfate, *CV* cardiovascular, *GI* gastrointestinal, *GS* glucosamine sulfate, *IA* intra-articular, *NSAID* non-steroidal anti-inflammatory drug, *PPI* proton pump inhibitor, *SYSADOA* symptomatic slow-acting drugs in osteoarthritis, *OA* osteoarthritis

treatment alternatives, previous experiences with treatment, and expectations of current treatment. In addition, patients with OA should be fully informed about the etiology of OA, risk factors (especially the ones that are modifiable and specific to the patient) and expected prognosis [32]. Clear information about the treatment options along with their benefits, side effect profile, patient-specific impairments and preferences, costs of interventions and local availability should be discussed also. Creating realistic and positive expectations for treatment efficacy may enhance adherence, especially to therapies that require lifestyle changes, and has been shown to positively influence treatment outcomes [33, 34]. Self-management education is a complement to traditional patient education [35]. It can be performed as part of cognitive–behavioral therapy (CBT) session. It aims at teaching patients problem-solving skills and involves the concept of self-efficacy. This in turn gives patients confidence in their capacity to carry out a particular behavior necessary to reach a desired goal.

ACR strongly recommends self-efficacy and self-management programs as part of educational interventions [19]. This is a very comprehensive program, covering sessions such as skill-building (goal-setting, problem-solving, positive thinking), education about the disease and about medication effects and side effects, joint protection measures, and fitness and exercise goals and approaches. OARSI also includes education in core treatments, but it is said that there is insufficient basis for selecting detailed topics [17]. However, ESCEO and OARSI describes about its direction that education programs should provide necessary information about OA, learning self-care skills, and inducing behavioral change in a positive direction, including lifestyle changes [17, 18, 20]. The EULAR guideline describes in detail the operating principles of the information and education program [30]. These education programs can be held in person or online because a substantial part of the noncompliance with treatment, particularly when it comes to lifestyle changes, may occur due to the limited time that clinicians take to explain the purpose of the interventions and what the patient should expect in terms of pain relief. In this way, self-management education can occur through several ways such as face-to-face meetings, group sessions, the internet, and telephone-based sessions [28].

Exercise Program

ACR, ESCEO, and OARSI strongly recommend the need for structured exercise programs as core treatment regardless of age, severity of pain, degree of dysfunction, and comorbidity [19]. While patients and health care providers seek recommendations on the "best" exercise and the ideal dosage (duration, intensity, and frequency), current evidence is insufficient to recommend specific exercise prescriptions. Because the benefit of exercise on pain and function is evident, clinical guidelines give strong recommendations that all patients should be encouraged to consider some form of exercise as a central part of their treatment plan [17, 19]. In order to find a method that suits the individual in the broad menu of exercises and encourage them to carry out regular and ongoing exercises, we must address the problem of barriers to participating in the exercise. Barriers to the implementation of guidelines will be covered later. The effectiveness of an exercise program is enhanced when patient preferences and access to exercise programs are considered, as well as when they are supervised or coupled with self-efficacy, self-management, and weight loss programs. Overall, exercise programs are more effective if supervised, often by physical therapists and sometimes in a class setting, rather than when performed by the individual at home. They also tend to be more effective when combined with self-efficacy and self-management interventions or weight loss programs [19].

Weight Loss (if Overweight/Obese)

Although the characteristics of OA as an inflammatory disease are being revealed, maintaining ideal body weight is critical to preserve joint structures and improve symptoms as a mechanical factor [38–40]. ACR, ESCEO, and OARSI strongly recommend weight loss for overweight or obese patients in common [17, 19, 20]. Weight loss is an effective and safe core treatment that can be used effectively and safely in most knee OA patients, and it can be achieved by dietary control alone or along with an exercise program. Guidelines tried to suggest an appropriate goal of weight control, which is based on the results of research on the effect of weight loss in overweight and obese patients [41, 42]. In knee OA patients, a dose-response was observed between the amount of weight loss and symptom or functional improvement [41]. A difference was observed with only ≥5% of body weight change, but more than 10% was suggested as the goal of long-term weight control [40–42]. ACR emphasizes the role of weight management as one of the preventive strategies for OA in the absence of effective disease-modifying agents for OA [19]. Along with ACR, OARSI also emphasized the importance of dietary weight management in combination with exercise [17]. ESCEO has also emphasized the importance of weight loss from the prior version of the guideline published in 2014 [20]. However, in the elderly over 75 years of age, attention is paid to the paucity of data regarding the risk and benefit of the progress of the diet program [20].

15.3.1.2 Knee Braces/Insoles/Walking Aids/Thermal Agents/ Mechanotherapy or Manual Therapy/Bandage Tape/ Aquatic Exercises/Tai Chi

In the National Clinical Guideline Center (UK), patients with biomechanical joint pain or instability with OA should be considered for assessment for bracing/joint supports/insoles as an adjunct to their core treatment, and assistive devices (for example, walking sticks) and tap turners should be considered as adjuncts to core treatment for people with OA who have specific problems with activities of daily living [29].

ESCEO recommended that in Step 1 of background treatment and after adhering to the basic principle and core set, patients should be referred to a physical therapist or another specialist for assessment of whether correction for varus/valgus malalignment is needed [20]. Although evidence is insufficient, it is said that there is a theoretical rationale for the use of biomechanical interventions such as braces and insoles because varus or valgus malalignment is a risk factor for knee OA and its progression, and walking aids can provide security to patients. Thermal therapy, manual therapy, and taping may also have evidence of efficacy. Mechanotherapy or manual therapy is referred to as (flexibility, mobilization, stretching) in the treatment algorithm, but ESCEO says that there is actually no basis for differentiation between different exercise modalities, and is considered to be in the context of including all types of exercise. On the contrary. OARSI strongly recommends against braces (realigning patellofemoral, soft, varus/valgus unloading/realignment) for reasons of low-quality evidence or no efficacy [17]. Although insoles are conditionally recommended in all comorbidity subgroups, referring to the fact that OARSI basically recommends against using any interventions graded as Level 3, Level 4A, or Level 4B, it can be interpreted as generally not recommended [17]. Gait aids are conditionally recommended in all comorbidity subgroups [17]. Thermal therapy (hot or cold) is strongly recommended against for low-quality evidence [17]. Mechanotherapy/Manual therapy (massage) is strongly recommended against for reasons of lack of evidence [17]. Taping (Kinesio taping/strapping, patellar taping) is strongly recommended against because of its no efficacy [17].

In ACR, tibiofemoral knee braces are strongly recommended for patients with knee OA in whom disease in one or both knees are causing a sufficiently large impact on ambulation, joint stability, or pain to warrant use of an assistive device, and who are able to tolerate the associated inconvenience and burden associated with bracing [19]. A patellofemoral brace is conditionally recommended for patients with patellofemoral knee OA in whom disease in one or both knees is causing a sufficiently large impact on ambulation, joint stability, or pain to warrant the use of an assistive device. The reason is said to be due to the variability in results across published trials and the difficulty some patients will have in tolerating the inconvenience and burden of these braces [19]. Insole is conditionally recommended against for no clear efficacy [19]. In ACR guideline, for example, cane is strongly recommended for patients with knee OA in whom disease in one or more joints is causing a sufficiently large impact on ambulation, joint stability, or pain to warrant use of an assistive device [19]. ACR makes a conditional recommendation for thermal intervention for reasons of heterogeneity of modalities and short duration of benefit [19]. Manual therapy (lymphatic drainage, manual traction, massage, mobilization/manipulation, and passive range of motion) is conditionally recommended against for use alone for reasons of limited data and benefit and mentions that there are few studies related to exercise. The quality of evidence for kinesio-taping is poor but conditionally recommended for the advantage of permits range of motion compared to the brace fixed to the joint [19].

ACR, OARSI, and ESCEO all strongly recommend Tai Chi as one of the mind-body exercises that constitute the exercise of core treatments [17–20]. For mind-body exercise, ACR gives strong recommendations for Tai Chi, taking holistic effects such as strength, balance, and fall prevention, and for yoga, it may help improve OA symptoms, but conditional recommendations are given due to lack of data. In addition, other mind–body practices are not assessed for reasons of insufficient evidence, as well as a lack of standard definition [19]. OARSI recommends structured land-based exercise programs (Type 1—strengthening and/or cardio and/or balance training/neuromuscular exercise or Type 2—Mind-body Exercise including Tai Chi or Yoga) as core treatment [30]. ESCEO incorporated mind-body exercises including Tai Chi and Yoga into the core treatment, highlighting the importance of the holistic wellbeing of the individuals.

The ACR guideline includes aquatic exercise as a specific exercise program composition [17–20]. Unlike the aquatic exercise or Tai-Chi mentioned specifically in the prior guideline, the latest ESCEO recommendation says that there is insufficient ground to differentiate each exercise modalities, and in fact, accepts all types of exercise [19]. For aquatic exercise, OARSI gave appropriate ratings in the prior guideline because it was helpful for pain and function, but now conditional recommendations were given while excluding them from core treatments for realistic reasons for accessibility issues, financial burden [18, 20]. In addition, subdividing the comorbidity group, aquatic exercise is not recommended in patients with frailty due to potential risk of accidental injury.

15.3.2 Pharmacologic Treatment

Pharmacologic treatment can be used in combination with or after a trial of non-pharmacologic treatments, if satisfactory pain relief is not achieved with these measures alone.

15.3.2.1 Paracetamol (Acetaminophen)

Paracetamol (acetaminophen) is a widely used analgesic, but it has been reported to have minimal effect on OA-related pain [43]. In addition, reports of hepatotoxicity, acute liver failure, gastrointestinal, cardiovascular and renal adverse events following chronic widespread and unrestricted use of paracetamol raise concerns about their long-term use [44–46]. Despite this questionable efficacy and confirmed safety issues, opinions on the criteria for their use vary among institutions [17, 19, 20]. In the short-term use of paracetamol, ACR limits the indication to the case where the use of NSAIDs is limited, whereas ESCEO suggests a limited use as a short-term rescue analgesic. In the long-term use of paracetamol, ACR conditionally recommended its use on a regular basis if it is used under a specific dose while observing regular monitoring for hepatotoxicity, whereas ESCEO and OARSI avoid long-term use of paracetamol.

15.3.2.2 Symptomatic Slow-Acting Drugs for Osteoarthritis (SYSADOAs)

Symptomatic slow-acting drugs for osteoarthritis (SYSADOAs) is a class that includes glucosamine, chondroitin sulfate, avocado/soybean unsaponifiables (ASU), and diacerein [47]. Comparing to non-steroidal anti-inflammatory drugs (NSAIDs), the pharmacological effects of SYSADOAs are characterized by both a delay in the improvement of symptoms and a carry-over effect of that improvement. Nonetheless, one of the main proposed advantages of these medications over traditional medical therapies is their safety profile [48]. Among SYSADOAs, diacerein is associated with significantly more adverse events than placebo, particularly regarding the GI and renal and urinary systems. Therefore, the use of diacerein should be taken into account its benefit: risk profile according to individual patient characteristics. Currently, in the use of SYSADOAs, conflicting recommendations are provided for each guideline, and continuous consensus is required [17, 20, 49]. Background therapy with these products is recommended by ESCEO prior to the use of topical NSAIDs [20, 48, 50–52]. The ESCEO guidelines provide recommendations for the use of SYSADOAs, including strong recommendations for pharmaceutical grade crystalline glucosamine sulfate and chondroitin sulfate and weak recommendations for avocado soybean unsaponifiables and diacerein; they also make a weak recommendation against the use of combined glucosamine and chondroitin sulfate. The literature base evaluated by OARSI is the same as ESCEO, but they made negative recommendations for all glucosamine and chondroitin products (including pharmaceutical grade). ACR guidelines strongly recommend against the use of glucosamine and chondroitin sulfate for patients with knee OA [19].

15.3.2.3 Topical NSAIDs

Topical NSAIDs rather than oral NSAIDs are commonly used as first-line treatment for patients with mild knee OA. Topical NSAIDs can be used along with pharmacologic/non-pharmacologic measures and are a good treatment choice for long-term use with safety. Topical NSAIDs have similar efficacy and better safety profile compared to oral NSAIDs [19, 53]. The risk of gastrointestinal, renal, and cardiovascular toxicity is much lower with topical NSAIDs as compared with its oral formulation [54, 55]. The tolerability profile is also better with topical NSAIDs, with mild skin rashes being the most commonly reported side effect. ACR, ESCEO, and OARSI give strong recommendation to use of topical NSAIDs in knee OA. However, OARSI recommended the use of topical NSAIDs with careful monitoring in patients with widespread pain, because there is a possibility of exceeding total recommended doses [17]. The choice of topical agent may vary according to local availability and cost.

15.3.2.4 Oral NSAIDs

Oral NSAIDs remain the mainstay of the pharmacologic management of OA. Oral NSAIDs are usually the initial oral medication of choice used in the case of inadequate pain relief after using non-pharmacologic treatments and topical agents used in conjunction with core treatments at the prior stage of treatment [17, 19, 20]. The use of NSAIDs in most patients is limited by the increased risk of serious gastrointestinal (GI), cardiovascular (CV), and renal complications. All non-selective NSAIDs and COX-2 inhibitors have the potential for gastrointestinal and cardiovascular toxicity [56, 57]. In addition, all NSAIDs have shown an increased risk of acute kidney injury, which may be particularly high in the first 30 days after initiation of therapy [58]. In order to minimize toxicity, most guidelines recommend intermittent short- to mid-term use of all NSAIDs as required, in the minimal dose necessary to control symptoms, should be preferred over long-term fixed doses [17, 19, 20]. The selection of appropriate NSAID has been driven by assessment of benefit: risk balance, in terms of variability in GI and CV safety profile between individual drugs, and individual patient characteristics affecting risk of AEs. Regular monitoring for the development of potential adverse side effects is also required [20]. ESCEO and OARSI specifically suggest/recommend a selection of appropriate oral NSAIDs according to patient risk profile [17, 20]. In general, ESCEO and OARSI recommend the use of nonselective NSAIDs with proton pump inhibitor (PPI) or selective COX-2 inhibitors (with PPI) for patients with normal

GI risk or no comorbidity, and the use of selective COX-2 inhibitors with PPI for patients with increased GI risk is recommended. For patients with CV risk, ESCEO limits the use of any NSAIDs to <30 days for celecoxib, and <7 days for non-selective NSAIDs, and OARSI does not recommend the use of oral NSAIDs. For patients with renal risk, ESCEO recommends avoiding the use of NSAIDs.

15.3.2.5 Intra-Articular Hyaluronic Acid (IAHA)

Compared to intra-articular corticosteroids (IACS), the long-term safety profile of IAHA is superior to repeated IACS and the pain reduction was significantly better with HA supplementation after 12 weeks while the maximal benefit of IACS appeared more rapidly (within 2 weeks) [59, 60]. In addition, unlike the use of IACS, functional improvement is observed when using IAHA and has the effect of delaying the need for knee arthroplasty with an increase in the period during the repeated course of use [61, 62]. Furthermore, in some symptomatic mild knee OA patients, knee cartilage preservation of IAHA has also been reported [63, 64]. Although the apparent benefits of IAHA in knee OA were reported in prior systematic reviews, numerous trials, and meta-analyses, the efficacy of IAHA injections in patients with knee OA still remains controversial. Consistent with the contradictory results from different meta-analyses, available guidelines also have conflicting recommendations, despite being based on the same research evidence. In the 2019 ACR revised guideline, IAHA is conditionally recommended against patients with knee OA because the use of IAHA for knee OA failed to establish a benefit and harm associated with injection and can be used when other alternatives have been exhausted or failed to provide satisfactory benefit [19]. The 2019 ESCEO working group gives a weak recommendation to the use of IAHA in patients who have contraindications to NSAIDs, or those who is still symptomatic despite the use of NSAIDs [20]. The 2019 OARSI guidelines conditionally recommended IAHA for all patients at different stages of treatment depending on their comorbidity profiles. For example, in patients with knee OA who have no comorbidities, IAHA is recommended after failure to respond to core treatments, topical NSAIDs, and oral NSAIDs (including COX2 inhibitors).

15.3.2.6 Intra-articular Corticosteroids (IACS)

IACS is mainly used as a short-term treatment of severe knee pain with acute onset [17, 20, 65]. Although lack of evidence in functional improvement and benefits in a repeated course of use and long-term use have not been confirmed, IACS is more effective than IAHA in pain reduction in short-term use [66, 67]. When using IACS, the absence of concurrent infection in or around the joint and potential risk factors such as or allergy, coagulopathy/anticoagulant use, very poorly controlled diabetes, possible fracture, or uncooperative patients should be checked [68]. ACR gives a strong recommendation to use IACS and describes IACS as a treatment modality suitable for all patient groups. ESCEO suggests the same patient population as IAHA as a condition for using IACS but gives weak recommendations for the use of acute and short-term pain relief in consideration of its relatively more effectiveness compared to IAHA during the first few weeks of treatment and its efficacy may be higher in patients with more severe pain [20]. OARSI also conditionally recommends the use of IACS for knee OA for acute (1–2 weeks) and short-term (4–6 weeks) pain relief [17].

15.3.2.7 Opioids

Opioids are considered as among the most effective drug for the treatment of acute severe pain and chronic pain related to advanced medical illness. However, the long-term administration of opioids continues to be controversial in terms of effectiveness, safety, and abuse liability [69]. In addition, there are reports that opioids offer similar pain relief in OA patients even when compared to oral NSAIDs [70–73]. Nonetheless, there are circumstances in which tramadol or other opioids may be appropriate in the treatment of OA-related pain. In 2019 ACR, considering potential adverse effects, the use of opioids in the treatment process of OA is limited to specific circumstances, and if use is necessary, tramadol is conditionally recommended over non-tramadol opioids [19]. Tramadol rarely causes the adverse events of respiratory depression and physical dependence commonly associated with conventional opioid drugs, since its analgesic effects are through both weak opioid and non-opioid mechanisms [74]. The 2019 OARSI strongly recommended against the use of opioids for the devastating potential for chemical dependency and limited or no relevant benefit on OA symptoms [17]. ESCEO gives a weak recommendation to the use of short-term weak opioids as a last pharmacological attempt [20]. In addition, in the case of classical oral or transdermal opioids, ESCEO gives a weak recommendation for its use in patients whom surgery is contraindicated or unwilling to undergo surgery [20]. The use of opioids has the potential for non-serious AEs such as predominantly drowsiness, nausea, and constipation, involves well-established risks such as respiratory depression, dependence, and has the potential for abuse. Therefore, if the use of opioids is necessary, the lowest possible doses for the shortest possible length of time are recommended [19].

15.3.2.8 Duloxetine

Duloxetine is a balanced and potent reuptake inhibitor of serotonin (5-HT) and norepinephrine (NE) [75]. Duloxetine can be used in the management of chronic pain disease including OA and is associated with altered modulation of stimulus transmission such as central sensitization of nociceptive pathway [13, 76–78]. However, current studies do not provide a true gold standard diagnostic or acceptable and valid criterion for central sensitization. The ACR changed their opinion on the use of duloxetine from "no recommended (2012)" to "conditionally recommended (2019)" as a centrally acting agent with adequate evidence [19]. The ESCEO gives a weak recommendation to the use of duloxetine as an alternative to weak opioids in STEP 3 therapy and to the use of classical oral or transdermal opioids in end-stage knee OA patients for whom surgery is contraindicated [20]. The OARSI conditionally recommended the use of duloxetine in patients with widespread pain and/or depression [17]. Nausea was a common side effect, and fatigue, constipation, hyperhidrosis, somnolence, dizziness, diarrhea, insomnia, and dry mouth were also reported [79]. Nausea could be reduced through titration and administration of the medication with food [79, 80].

15.3.3 Surgical Treatment

Surgical treatment represented by total knee arthroplasty (TKA), unicompartmental knee arthroplasty (UKA), and osteotomy around the knee is generally reserved for refractory symptoms of knee OA. TKA is recommended for the first choice of surgery in severe end-stage knee OA. However, there is a lot of controversy in the isolated medical knee OA over which surgical method to choose. Pros and cons exist about the use of UKA versus TKA for isolated medial arthritis [81]. Moderate evidence supports no difference between UKA or valgus producing proximal tibial osteotomy in outcomes and complications in patients with isolated medial knee OA [81]. For optimal outcome and minimal risk of AEs on performing surgical treatment for knee OA, function-limiting pain, range of motion, functional instability, pattern of arthritis involvement, imaging, limb alignment, mechanical symptoms (meniscal tear of the loose body), age, health care systems (policy), and many other factors must be considered [82].

15.3.3.1 Total Knee Arthroplasty (TKA)

TKA is the definitive treatment/gold standard in patients with severe end-stage symptomatic knee OA who have failed to respond to nonpharmacologic and pharmacologic management, and who have significant impairment in their quality of life [83, 84]. TKA provides marked pain relief and functional improvement in patients with severe knee OA [85, 86]. While knee replacement is the only option in patients with advanced knee OA, it is important to individualize surgical decision making with each patient, including an informed discussion of the risks, benefits, and alternatives to surgery [82, 84]. Fifteen to twenty percent of patients are dissatisfied with their outcome, usually characterized by ongoing pain and poor function [87]. In addition, some patients who appear ready for a TKA may still improve with conservative therapy [86]. Following implantation, a 70-year-old patient has a 5% lifetime risk of requiring revision surgery, but this risk increases substantially with younger age groups [88]. The 10-year implant survival rate was 96.1%, and the 20-year implant survival rate was 89.7% [88].

15.3.3.2 Unicompartmental Knee Arthroplasty (UKA)

UKA can be used when the end-stage OA is limited to a single compartment such as medial, lateral, or patellofemoral compartment [89]. Historically, ideal candidates have been described as having isolated medial compartment disease, age greater than 60 years old, low levels of physical activity, weighing less than 82 kg, having a cumulative angular deformity of less than 15 degrees, both cruciate ligaments intact, a preoperative range of flexion of 90 degrees, a flexion contracture of less than 5 degrees, minimal pain at rest, and no radiographic or intraoperative evidence of chondrocalcinosis or patellofemoral OA [90]. However, many surgeons follow more liberal criteria when considering UKA, and many of the traditional criteria are being expanded [91]. The advantages of UKA compared to TKA include lower mortality, shorter length of stay, lower complication rate (including thromboembolism, myocardial infarction, and stroke), and a lower rate of re-admission, and greater cost-effectiveness [92, 93]. However, despite these advantages, UKA shows a lower implant survival rate and higher revision rate compared to TKA [91, 93–96]. Regardless, the absolute revision rates are relatively low, and UKA can be a good choice for carefully selected patients after a complete discussion of the risks and benefits of UKA versus TKA.

15.3.3.3 Osteotomy Around Knee

Osteotomy around the knee continues to be a viable surgical option for younger, more active patients with predominantly unicompartmental disease [97]. In most cases, HTO is implemented in the varus knee and DFO in the valgus knee. Among surgical procedures for knee OA, there is some evidence for pain relief and functional improvement of HTO for medial compartmental OA [98–100]. Other benefits of this procedure include preservation of knee anatomy, less restriction on function, and possible delay of need for arthroplasty [101]. Its use is restricted for people with unicompartmental knee OA (often varus malaligned) as the procedure induces a load transfer from the diseased compartment to the healthy compartment [100]. Comparing the ideal indications for UKA and HTO for medial knee OA, HTO allows improved activity for younger patients, whereas UKA is more suitable for older patients because of the shorter rehabilitation time and faster recovery period [102, 103]. Disadvantages of osteotomy include longer time to heal, possible nonunion may occur necessitating further surgery, incomplete pain relief, and increased complexity if later arthroplasty is needed [104, 105]. Moreover, TKA patients with a previous HTO are more likely to need an eventual revision of their TKA [106].

15.3.4 Clinical Practice Guidelines (CPG) for Knee OA Treatment: Barriers to Implementation and Its Solutions

A clinical decision is needed to select the appropriate treatment for the individual patient with knee OA. The judgment of clinical appropriateness should be based on EBM, and CPGs are a way to support the use of EBM in clinical practice. CPGs are statements that include recommendations intended to optimize patient care that is informed by a systematic review of evidence and an assessment of the benefits and harms of alternative care options [107]. The CPGs aim to guide clinicians in selecting the best care, taking into account the benefits and harms of treatment and the strength of the recommendations appraised [108]. Non-profit organizations or scientific communities, such as, ACR [19], OARSI

[17], ESCEO [20], NICE [29] and AAOS [109], have proposed numerous recommendations for OA treatment. These recommendations are similar in general consistency though there are subtle differences in the interested joints and the types of suggested treatments. Despite general consistency among recommendations, clinical practice does not reflect these recommendations [110]. In a national survey study performed in Norway, the degree of implementation of recommended care for OA is reported as under 50% [111]. Meiyappan et al. [112] performed a retrospective study to determine how closely orthopedic physicians adhered to the recommendations included in AAOS CPGs for nonoperative management of knee OA. This study showed that intraarticular injection with either corticosteroids or hyaluronic acid was the most common intervention (32%) despite inconclusive to a strong recommendation against their use, and concluded that adherence to the recommendations contained within the AAOS CPG for nonoperative treatment of knee OA was modest. Lack of adherence to CPGs for OA treatment is more prominent in non-pharmacologic treatment [113]. Three basic issues in influencing the uptake of evidence in clinical practice are quality of evidence, barriers and facilitators to changing practice, and effective dissemination and implementation strategies [114]. Among them, suboptimal uptake of GCPs in clinical practice due to a problem with dissemination and implementation rather than a lack of quality of evidence [27]. Therefore, the reasons for the gap between CPG recommendations and clinical practice should be investigated and solved for improving health care in knee OA treatment.

The reasons for low adherence to CPGs are likely multifactorial. Barriers to the implementation of CPGs exist within the patient, professional, health care team, health care organization, and socioeconomic environment [114]. Loyola-Sanchez et al. [115] reported three barriers for implementing the guideline to clinical practice in the Mexican health care system, which were individual (limitations of clinician skills, patient beliefs), organizational (insufficient time and inefficient referral process), and system (inadequate model care) related barriers. By involving patients in health care assessments, researchers may get more valid information on the most demanding tasks in everyday life for the patients [111]. Barriers to implementation of CPGs from the patient's perspective are negative experience with drugs, patients' limited comprehension of the disease process, and poor communication by the health care professional [116]. Selten et al. [117] reported that a lack of expertise of the health care provider, lack of evidence-based treatment, and suboptimal organization of care as three main barriers to the provision of non-pharmacological, non-surgical care for knee OA. As a solution to this, education focused on initiating and supporting lifestyle changes, promotion of interventions according to evidence-based recommendations, and improved organization of care were proposed. One of the problems faced by most general practitioners in the management of OA patients is time pressure and achieving adequate pain control, whereas more time with patients, collaboration with specialist colleagues, and improved communication tools were the most common needs identified to improve OA management. The composition of a multidisciplinary team, more time to see patients, and a coordinated care model can be tried to improve the dissemination of CPGs [118]. There are also areas that need improvement in the guidelines themselves. The contradiction between the guidelines and poor description for some treatment methods may cause uncertainty about the therapy and hinder appropriate decision-making. For this, a standard and appropriate methodology for developing OA CPG and further research are required [108]. Clinical algorithms helping the clinician to visualize the patient flow and timing of different treatment modalities are useful for osteoarthritis guideline dissemination. As the guidelines are revised, suggesting a treatment algorithm and adding considerations for comorbidities can be a way to help health care providers of guidelines quickly and easily set up a care plan [119]. Socioeconomic and political factors are also important. Eliminating unproven procedures and reducing needless costs is necessary for the improvement of the health care quality and reduction of the health care cost overall. In this regard, economic considerations are needed when developing a CPG. Financial incentives through pay for performance appear to be stronger drivers of adherence to CPGs than attitudes toward them or their general accessibility [120]. Optimizing the dissemination of CPGs requires improved reimbursement systems, and better promotion and educational initiatives for both patients and medical professionals. Further, a particular focus of education should include eliminating misinformation about OA [121].

15.4 Personalized Health Care (PHC) as Strategy for Knee OA Treatment

15.4.1 Identification of Clinical Phenotype of Knee OA and Its Application to PHC

Knee OA was once known as "wear and tear disease" simply, but is now considered a complex and "heterogenous disease" with various characteristics that include diversities in etiology, disease progression, clinical features, biochemical characteristics, and responses to treatments [122]. OA is mostly regarded as a final common pathway of joint destruction for multiple different pathophysiologic etiologies. Therefore, knee OA can be defined as a group of diseases, conditions, or subsets with a common endpoint. Moreover, OA is not a static disease, but a dynamic disease with discernable characteristics during the various stages of the disease [123]. The heterogeneity of knee OA makes the outcome from current therapies disappointing because it includes patients with various phenotypes at different stages of disease progression. Therefore, it is necessary to differentiate between discernable clinical and etiologic phenotypes, especially in the early stages of the disease, for adequate stratification of OA [124].

Phenotype is defined as any observable properties of a living organism that are produced by the interactions of the genotype and the environment. Further, a phenotype may be any observable characteristic or trait of a disease, such as morphology, development, biochemical or physiological properties, or behavior [125]. In clinical medicine, patients with common characteristics are often grouped together to guide therapy and improve management. Phenotyping is very useful for studying, diagnosing, and treating any disease, particularly those that are inflammatory and degenerative nature. Clinical phenotypes are the most common method of subgrouping for the purpose of providing a personalized medicine (PM) or personalized health care (PHC) for knee OA [126]. PHC is customizing a treatment as individualized as the disease, based on the patient's phenotype. PHC does not search for a novel therapy for patients, but stratify individuals into subpopulations that vary in their response to a therapeutic agent for their specific disease. Non-PHC (One-Size-Fits-All) approach may lead to drug toxicity, severe side effects, and increasing health care costs. The concept of PHC is 'the right drug, with the right dose at the right time to the right patient'. Thus, PHC offers improved medication selection and targeted therapy, reduced adverse effects, increased patient compliance, and improved cost-effectiveness [127].

Karsdal et al. [123] proposed a simplistic, conceptual idea that identification of phenotype helps PHC approach to knee OA treatment. They divided knee OA into three different subtypes (bone, cartilage, and inflamed synovium) based on the most actively involved joint tissue or the tissue with the prominent manifestations [128]. Patient phenotype 1: Traumatic OA, in the early disease course most likely involving a high level of protease activity destroying the cartilage subsequent to cartilage injury. These patients might benefit from a protease inhibitor treatment targeting cartilage lesions. Patient phenotype 2: Generalized OA, with high turnover of bone and progression of cartilage damage characterized by an intimate relationship between bone and cartilage in the pathogenesis of OA. These patients may benefit from an anti-resorptive treatment inhibiting bone resorption and subchondral bone turnover. Patient phenotype 3: Episodic subacute and acute inflammatory events progressively worsen the disease. Specific anti-inflammatory therapies might be helpful because macrophages in inflamed synovium play a role in this process. Thus, these three different phenotypes of OA would require different therapeutic approaches and one treatment may be successful in one patient population or may fail in another. As result, targeting a specific disease phenotype with the appropriate treatment would be expected to result in far higher response rates [123].

15.4.2 Pain and Structural Change Trajectories in Knee OA: A Guidance to PHC

Knee OA is structurally characterized by progressive hyaline articular cartilage destruction accompanied by changes in subchondral bone and synovium. Knee OA patients may experience arthritic symptoms such as pain and functional limitation with structural deterioration. Structural deterioration and symptoms are thought to gradually and consistently worsen over time [129]. Symptoms and structural changes in knee OA are interconnected but do not match up one-to-one in individual patients. Dieppe et al. [130] reported there was no correlation between radiographic and clinical changes and concluded that radiographic change may not be a good surrogate for clinical outcome in established OA. Peters et al. [131] reported that generally pain and disability in knee OA were worsened over the 7 years, but 29% of those initially reporting knee pain respectively had improved. They concluded that OA does not invariably deteriorate but social as well as biological factors were associated with greater deterioration for knee OA. Felson et al. [132] showed that only 4.1% of OA patients without symptomatic OA and up to 13.7% with incident OA progress over a 1-year period and concluded that structural progression fits a pattern of inertia, in which knees with recently developed OA are more likely to develop X-ray progression than knees that have been stable. These studies of symptomatic and structural progression suggest that knee OA may have diverse disease trajectories over time. The ability to characterize and predict OA progression could improve the design and efficacy of studies investigating treatment and prevention strategies. Further, it could facilitate the development of novel treatments, which may be effective for fast, but not slow progressors, or vice versa [133]. Therefore, factors that trigger the transition from stable disease to progression should be sought. As result, it is essential to identify the drivers of disease progression in order to develop effective interventions [134].

Knee pain is a major cause of OA patients seeking medical care. The pain caused by knee OA is not always constant but varies depending on the patient's characteristics and the disease progression. Many studies of pain progression suggest that knee OA may have diverse pain trajectories over time [14, 134–138]. A better understanding of the characteristics and trajectories of pain caused by knee OA will reduce unnecessary treatment, reduce the adverse reaction, and provide cost-effective treatment. Moreover, such understandings would offer important insights into disease prognosis and would help make treatment plans. Nicolls et al. [135] studied pain trajectory groups from the knee OA population in UK and USA at 18-month intervals for up to 6 years. They reported study population are grouped to mild, non-progressive (35%), progressive (28%), moderate (22%), improving (12%), and severe, non-improving (3%). They concluded that pain trajectories of knee OA are not slowly progressive but it has mild, non-progressive, or improving symptom trajectories. Collins at al [134]. conducted a multi-center, longitudinal study of subjects from the Osteoarthritis Initiative (OAI) to describe pain trajectories and risk factors assessing pain annually for 6 years. They found 5 distinct pain trajectories, such as no pain (11%), mild pain (35%), low moderate pain (32%), high moderate pain (17%), and severe pain (6%). None of the trajectories exhibited substantial worsening. Higher KL grade, obesity, depression, medical comorbidities, female sex, non-white race, lower education, and younger age were associated with trajectories characterized by greater pain. They concluded knee OA is characterized by persistent rather than inexorably worsening symptoms. Bastick et al. [137] conducted to define knee pain trajectories in early symptomatic knee OA using 5 years of data from the CHECK study. They identified 6 distinct pain trajectories such as constant mild pain (26.3%), moderate regression (29.4%), major regression (3.3%), severe progression (4.9%), moderate progression (25.5%) and constant severe (10.5%). They reported that higher BMI, lower level of education, greater comorbidity, higher activity limitation scores, and joint space tenderness were more often associated with trajectories characterized by more pain at first presentation and pain progression. Trouvin et al. [139] studied daily pain trajectory in knee OA patients over 1 month period and identified relationships with patients' characteristics. The results showed that daily pain trajectory was stable in 59.5% of patients but unstable in 40.5% of patients. Factors associated with stable daily pain trajectory were a more recent disease, morning stiffness ≥15 min, and flare-up. Previtali et al. [14] conducted a systematic review to analyze pain trajectories in order to identify the predictors of specific pain trajectories in patients with knee OA and to provide a characterization of patients with different pain progression. Their result showed that daily knee OA pain trajectories were unstable in almost half of the patients but in the mid-term, knee OA had a steady pain trajectory in 85% of the patients, 8% experienced pain reduction, while 7% experienced pain worsening. They also reported that factors related to severe/worsening pain were low education, comorbidities, and depression. However, age, alcohol, smoking, pain coping strategies, and medications were not related to pain evolution, and conflicting/no evidence was found for all joint-related factors, such as baseline radiographic severity. These studies show that there are distinct pain trajectories in knee OA. In the past, knee OA symptoms have been known to worsen over time, but in recent studies, some pain symptoms in knee OA are mild, non-progressive, and sometimes improved. Like this favorable prognosis, preventing unnecessary costs and harms associated with over-diagnosis and over-management are very important. From these studies, a clinician must differentiate those patients who require a more specific approach in the management of early symptomatic knee OA from those for whom a 'wait-and-see' policy seems justifiable [137]. A better understanding of pain trajectories will be one of the treatment strategies to provide PHC in knee OA patients.

Knee OA is characterized by a slow, progressive structural damage in hyaline cartilage. The mean estimated annual joint space narrowing rate measured in simple radiography was 0.13 ± 0.15 mm/year [140]. In knee OA treatment, it has been focused on treatment to improve symptoms so far, but interest in disease-modifying osteoarthritis drugs (DMOAD), which improves damage to the joint structure, is currently increasing. Considering the treatment of knee OA with DMOADs, it is helpful to understand the trajectory of structural damage to the articular cartilage. Knee OA does not always deteriorate structural damage. Felson et al. [132] reported that for knees that have been experiencing radiographic deterioration at least in terms of joint space narrowing, there is likely to be further worsening defined as further narrowing for 12 and 24 months afterward. On the contrary, for knees with a disease that has been stable, it is likely that they will remain stable. Bartlett et al. [141] studied to identify common patterns of joint space narrowing over 2 years period. They reported that most (70%) people with OA demonstrated no significant joint space narrowing (JSN) over 2 years; 20% showed slow progression, 7% had moderate, and 2% had rapid JSN. Progressors tended to have less joint space widening at study entry and were older and heavier; rapid progressors were more likely to be men. Halilaj et al. [133] studied to predict knee OA progression over 8 years. The results showed that JSN was progressive in 29% but non-progressive in 71%. JSN over the course of 8 years was not accompanied by worsening of pain. Thus, understanding of structural change trajectory helps the development of DMOAD therapy and clinical study.

15.4.3 Phenotypes in Knee OA as Background for PHC

Identification of knee OA phenotypes allows targeted treatments for specific subgroups and provides more effective treatments to the patients [142]. In the past, knee OA was classified as generalized vs joint-specific OA or secondary vs primary OA or incident vs progressive OA, etc. However, recent medical developments have led to attempts to determine phenotype by classifying knee OA genetically, biochemically, radiologically epidemiologically, and clinically [143]. Karsdal et al. [123] reported a review article to suggest factors related to OA progression, which might be helpful to identify OA phenotype and develop PHC. Those factors were low-grade autoimmunity, inflammation, genetic, hormonal, metabolic, and mechano-transduction. As such, different approaches to phenotype identification in the knee OA population have been advocated. However, Felson et al. [23] suggested that phenotype research should be focused on those subgroups that could influence the treatment plan and management of the disease. Furthermore, identification of clinically relevant phenotypes may offer a specific targeted treatment and provide the most beneficial effects on the patients. Deveza et al. [144] conducted a systematic review to examine what OA characteristics are relevant for phenotyping and their relevance for outcomes. They found that pain sensitization, psychological distress, radiographic severity, body mass index (BMI), muscle strength, inflammation, and comorbidities are associated with clinically distinct phenotypes and poor clinical outcomes. Gender, obesity and other metabolic abnormalities, the pattern of cartilage damage, and inflammation are associated with distinct structural phenotypes and poor structural outcomes. They recommended that patient's and disease's characteristics (possibly reflecting different disease stages) should be considered to phenotype knee OA patients.

Herrero-Beaumont et al. [145] reported that OA developed pathophysiologically with the interactions of genetic alterations, sex hormone deficit, aging with mechanical factors, systemic inflammation associated metabolic syndrome, and these interactions could give defined OA phenotypes with specific therapeutic targets. They proposed 4 clinical phenotypes – biomechanical, osteoporotic, metabolic, and inflammatory, and suggested therapeutic approaches. Patients with a biomechanical phenotype may benefit from non-pharmacology therapy (i.e., load-modifying approaches), hyaluronic acid, etc. Patients with osteoporosis phenotype potentially may be particularly responsive to bone active drugs (estrogen therapy, etc.). Patients with metabolic phenotype may potentially benefit from anti-lipidemic drugs, caloric restriction, etc. Patients with inflammatory phenotype may respond to NSAIDs, methotrexate, biologics, etc.

Knoop et al. [36] conducted a cross-sectional study to identify phenotypes of knee OA patients using 4 clinically relevant patient characteristics, and to compare clinical outcomes of these phenotypes. They used data from knee OA patients of the Osteoarthritis Initiative (OAI). They choose 4 clinically relevant patient characteristics, which were radiographic severity of OA, muscle strength, body mass index (BMI), and depression. They identified 5 phenotypes of knee OA patients which were minimal joint disease phenotype, strong muscle phenotype, non-obese and weak muscle phenotype, obese and weak muscle phenotype, and depressive phenotype. Among them, depressive phenotype and obese and weak muscle phenotype showed higher pain levels and more severe activity limitations than the other 3 phenotypes. Further, van der Esch et al. [37] conducted a cross-sectional study to identify and validate previously established five phenotypes of knee OA based on similarities in clinical patient characteristics. Study design was similar to the above-mentioned study (Knoop et al.) except patient population, which was from the Amsterdam OA cohort. They identified five phenotypes of knee OA patients that were minimal joint disease phenotype, strong muscle strength phenotype, severe radiographic OA phenotype, obese phenotype, and depressive mood phenotype. The findings are mostly similar to the above-mentioned study (Knoop et al.). Among the identified five phenotypes, minimal joint disease, strong muscle strength, and depressive mood phenotypes were similar in both studies. In the Amsterdam

OA cohort study, non-obese and weak muscle strength phenotype was renamed into severe radiographic OA phenotype and obese and weak muscle strength phenotype into obese phenotype. Because the more prominent finding of radiographic OA and BMI characteristics were found in the Amsterdam OA cohort study. Both studies theoretically proposed a targeted therapeutic approach to the treatment of knee OA based on the identified five phenotypes of knee OA. Minimal joint disease phenotype may not be in need of specific treatment. Self-management approach including an educational program, pain coping skill training, and home-based exercises might be helpful. Strong muscle strength phenotypes are not likely to benefit from exercise therapy but appropriate education and pain medication might be a targeted approach. Although there is controversy about whether degradation of the joint structure can be indications for surgery, severe radiographic OA phenotype might be indications for orthopedic surgery if pain and activity limitations are severe. In addition, patients with severe radiographic OA could have beneficial effects from muscle strengthening exercises. Patients of obese phenotype may need both weight loss including dietary changes and exercise therapy focused on muscle strengthening. Because of the slight increase in depressive mood in obese phenotype, this should be considered in the treatment plan. Patients of the depressive mood phenotype may need the use of antidepressants, in addition to combination therapy of OA including an educational program, a cognitive–behavioral therapy, and an exercise therapy (Table 15.2).

Dell'Isola et al. [146] conducted a systematic review to identify clinical phenotypes in knee OA. They identified six clinical phenotypes: (1) chronic pain in which central mechanisms (e.g. central sensitization) are prominent; (2) inflammatory (high levels of inflammatory biomarkers); (3) metabolic syndrome (high prevalence of obesity, diabetes, and other metabolic disturbances); (4) bone and cartilage metabolism (alteration in local tissue metabolism); (5) mechanical overload characterized primarily by varus malalignment and medial compartment disease, and (6) minimal joint disease characterized as minor clinical symptoms with slow progression over time. The same research group [147] further investigated to classify patients with knee OA into pre-defined groups characterized by specific variables that can be linked to different disease mechanisms, and compare these phenotypes for demographic and health outcomes, and identify whether the group of complex knee OA patients who met the criteria for more than one phenotype exist. They used from the OAI database FNIH. Patients meeting the criteria for more than one phenotype were classified separately into a 'complex KOA' group. From this study, eight hypothesized phenotypes were classified into, which were minimal joint disease phenotype (MJD) (25%), chronic pain phenotype (CP) (11%), malaligned biomechanical phenotype (MB) (11%), inflammatory phenotype (I) (5%), metabolic disorders phenotype (MD) (4%), bone and cartilage metabolism (BCM) (12%), complex knee OA (17%), and non-classification (16%). Phenotype allocation including complex knee OA was successful for 84.1% of cases with an overlap of 20%. Disease duration was shorter in the MJD while the CP phenotype included a larger number of women (81%). MJD phenotype had minimal or no change in symptoms severity, showed a low prevalence of comorbidities (e.g., depression, diabetes) that combined with the slow radiographic progression. This phenotype may need a core set program such as education, weight loss, and exercise program. CP phenotype demonstrated the highest levels of pain, disability, and the lowest muscle strength. Central sensitization and hypersensitivity, as well as depression, might be associated with CP phenotype that may need treatment different from those targeted toward joint pain. A cognitive–behavioral intervention and pain education may be helpful and may optimize the results of other traditional treatments such as exercise therapy and joint replacement. MB phenotype has high levels of muscle strength, high prevalence of malalignment, lower BMI, and low prevalence of other comorbidities and are characterized by disrupted biomechanics. Therefore, treatments focusing on restoration of optimal load distribution in the knee such as laterally wedged insoles and knee braces rather than drug treatment may be more effective. I phenotype shows a higher prevalence

Knee osteoarthritis (OA) is known as a heterogeneous disease with multiple etiologies. Although international guidelines recommend a combination of pharmacologic and non-pharmacologic treatment for symptomatic knee OA, this therapeutic approach is One-Size-Fit-All method that does not take into account heterogeneity of OA. Several attempts have been made to classify heterogeneous knee OA into homogenous subgroups with the aim of providing PHC that improves therapeutic efficacy. However, the identification of clinical phenotypes has some limitations. There is no clear definition of clinical phenotypes in the published literatures. Therefore, a clear and shared definition of knee OA phenotypes would help to better direct future research in the field. Moreover, clinical phenotypes identified in the literatures may not be able to explain fully heterogeneity of the whole knee OA population. Future research may yet lead to the identification of different disease mechanisms suggesting the existence of new phenotypes. For the robustness of clinical phenotype, predefined clinical phenotype should be tested in randomized controlled trials and be proved its clinical effectiveness before being applied in clinical practice.

15.5 Conclusion

The strategic approach of knee OA is a process of efforts to provide the right treatment to the right person at the right time. In a situation where a gradual increase in the OA population is predicted, it is necessary to develop personalized treatment strategies to effectively manage broad categories of patients with different problems. In this respect, understandings the characteristics of OA and its phenotype are the basis for providing individualized therapeutic strategies to these broad categories of OA patients. As the understanding of the overall OA increases, there will be fewer conflicts of interpretation of evidence among guidelines. Implementing evidence-based guidelines can help to select treatment methods in consideration of the best evidence available and safety and can improve outcomes. To achieve this, efforts are needed to remove barriers that exist in health care providers and patients. The more widely accepted and used these guidelines, the more helpful it will be to develop better treatment strategies through consensus.

References

1. Diseases GBD, Injuries C. Global burden of 369 diseases and injuries in 204 countries and territories, 1990–2019: a systematic analysis for the Global Burden of Disease Study 2019. Lancet. 2020;396(10258):1204–22. https://doi.org/10.1016/S0140-6736(20)30925-9.
2. Bijlsma JW, Berenbaum F, Lafeber FP. Osteoarthritis: an update with relevance for clinical practice. Lancet. 2011;377(9783):2115–26. https://doi.org/10.1016/S0140-6736(11)60243-2.
3. Pincus T, Mitchell JM, Burkhauser RV. Substantial work disability and earnings losses in individuals less than age 65 with osteoarthritis: comparisons with rheumatoid arthritis. J Clin Epidemiol. 1989;42(5):449–57. https://doi.org/10.1016/0895-4356(89)90135-2.
4. Hawley DJ, Wolfe F. Pain, disability, and pain/disability relationships in seven rheumatic disorders: a study of 1,522 patients. J Rheumatol. 1991;18(10):1552–7.
5. Arden N, Nevitt MC. Osteoarthritis: epidemiology. Best Pract Res Clin Rheumatol. 2006;20(1):3–25. https://doi.org/10.1016/j.berh.2005.09.007.
6. Safiri S, Kolahi AA, Smith E, Hill C, Bettampadi D, Mansournia MA, et al. Global, regional and national burden of osteoarthritis 1990–2017: a systematic analysis of the Global Burden of Disease Study 2017. Ann Rheum Dis. 2020;79(6):819–28. https://doi.org/10.1136/annrheumdis-2019-216515.
7. Moe RH, Uhlig T, Kjeken I, Hagen KB, Kvien TK, Grotle M. Multidisciplinary and multifaceted outpatient management of patients with osteoarthritis: protocol for a randomised, controlled trial. BMC Musculoskelet Disord. 2010;11:253. https://doi.org/10.1186/1471-2474-11-253.
8. Peat G, McCarney R, Croft P. Knee pain and osteoarthritis in older adults: a review of community burden and current use of primary health care. Ann Rheum Dis. 2001;60(2):91–7. https://doi.org/10.1136/ard.60.2.91.
9. Nguyen US, Zhang Y, Zhu Y, Niu J, Zhang B, Felson DT. Increasing prevalence of knee pain and symptomatic knee osteoarthritis: survey and cohort data. Ann Intern Med. 2011;155(11):725–32. https://doi.org/10.7326/0003-4819-155-11-201112060-00004.
10. Castaneda S, Roman-Blas JA, Largo R, Herrero-Beaumont G. Osteoarthritis: a progressive disease with changing phenotypes. Rheumatology (Oxford). 2014;53(1):1–3. https://doi.org/10.1093/rheumatology/ket247.

11. Sofat N, Ejindu V, Kiely P. What makes osteoarthritis painful? The evidence for local and central pain processing. Rheumatology (Oxford). 2011;50(12):2157–65. https://doi.org/10.1093/rheumatology/ker283.
12. Neogi T. The epidemiology and impact of pain in osteoarthritis. Osteoarthr Cartil. 2013;21(9):1145–53. https://doi.org/10.1016/j.joca.2013.03.018.
13. Kidd B. Mechanisms of pain in osteoarthritis. HSS J. 2012;8(1):26–8. https://doi.org/10.1007/s11420-011-9263-7.
14. Previtali D, Andriolo L, Di Laura FG, Boffa A, Candrian C, Zaffagnini S, et al. Pain Trajectories in Knee Osteoarthritis—a systematic review and best evidence synthesis on pain predictors. J Clin Med. 2020;9(9):2828.
15. Hunter DJ, Bierma-Zeinstra S. Osteoarthritis. Lancet. 2019;393(10182):1745–59. https://doi.org/10.1016/S0140-6736(19)30417-9.
16. Jayakumar P, Moore MLG, Bozic KJ. Team approach: a multidisciplinary approach to the management of hip and knee osteoarthritis. JBJS Rev. 2019;7(6):e10. https://doi.org/10.2106/JBJS.RVW.18.00133.
17. Bannuru RR, Osani MC, Vaysbrot EE, Arden NK, Bennell K, Bierma-Zeinstra SMA, et al. OARSI guidelines for the non-surgical management of knee, hip, and polyarticular osteoarthritis. Osteoarthr Cartil. 2019;27(11):1578–89. https://doi.org/10.1016/j.joca.2019.06.011.
18. Bruyere O, Cooper C, Pelletier JP, Branco J, Luisa Brandi M, Guillemin F, et al. An algorithm recommendation for the management of knee osteoarthritis in Europe and internationally: a report from a task force of the European Society for Clinical and Economic Aspects of Osteoporosis and Osteoarthritis (ESCEO). Semin Arthritis Rheum. 2014;44(3):253–63. https://doi.org/10.1016/j.semarthrit.2014.05.014.
19. Kolasinski SL, Neogi T, Hochberg MC, Oatis C, Guyatt G, Block J, et al. 2019 American College of Rheumatology/arthritis foundation guideline for the management of osteoarthritis of the hand, hip, and knee. Arthritis Rheumatol. 2020;72(2):220–33. https://doi.org/10.1002/art.41142.
20. Bruyere O, Honvo G, Veronese N, Arden NK, Branco J, Curtis EM, et al. An updated algorithm recommendation for the management of knee osteoarthritis from the European Society for Clinical and Economic Aspects of Osteoporosis, Osteoarthritis and Musculoskeletal Diseases (ESCEO). Semin Arthritis Rheum. 2019;49(3):337–50. https://doi.org/10.1016/j.semarthrit.2019.04.008.
21. Porter ME. Value-based health care delivery. Ann Surg. 2008;248(4):503–9. https://doi.org/10.1097/SLA.0b013e31818a43af.
22. Singer SJ, Burgers J, Friedberg M, Rosenthal MB, Leape L, Schneider E. Defining and measuring integrated patient care: promoting the next frontier in health care delivery. Med Care Res Rev. 2011;68(1):112–27. https://doi.org/10.1177/1077558710371485.
23. Allen KD, Choong PF, Davis AM, Dowsey MM, Dziedzic KS, Emery C, et al. Osteoarthritis: models for appropriate care across the disease continuum. Best Pract Res Clin Rheumatol. 2016;30(3):503–35. https://doi.org/10.1016/j.berh.2016.09.003.
24. Bozic KJ, Belkora J, Chan V, Youm J, Zhou T, Dupaix J, et al. Shared decision making in patients with osteoarthritis of the hip and knee: results of a randomized controlled trial. J Bone Joint Surg Am. 2013;95(18):1633–9. https://doi.org/10.2106/JBJS.M.00004.
25. Cosgrove JL, Nicholas JJ, Barmak J, Brewer C, Mientus JM, McConnell RL, et al. Team treatment. Does a specialized unit improve team performance? Am J Phys Med Rehabil. 1988;67(6):253–60.
26. Ahlmen M, Sullivan M, Bjelle A. Team versus non-team outpatient care in rheumatoid arthritis. A comprehensive outcome evaluation including an overall health measure. Arthritis Rheum. 1988;31(4):471–9. https://doi.org/10.1002/art.1780310403.
27. Nelson AE, Allen KD, Golightly YM, Goode AP, Jordan JM. A systematic review of recommendations and guidelines for the management of osteoarthritis: the chronic osteoarthritis management initiative of the U.S. bone and joint initiative. Semin Arthritis Rheum. 2014;43(6):701–12. https://doi.org/10.1016/j.semarthrit.2013.11.012.
28. McAlindon TE, Bannuru RR, Sullivan MC, Arden NK, Berenbaum F, Bierma-Zeinstra SM, et al. OARSI guidelines for the non-surgical management of knee osteoarthritis. Osteoarthr Cartil. 2014;22(3):363–88. https://doi.org/10.1016/j.joca.2014.01.003.
29. National Clinical Guideline Centre. National Institute for Health and Clinical Excellence: Guidance. Osteoarthritis: Care and Management in Adults. London: National Institute for Health and Care Excellence (UK). 2014.
30. Fernandes L, Hagen KB, Bijlsma JW, Andreassen O, Christensen P, Conaghan PG, et al. EULAR recommendations for the non-pharmacological core management of hip and knee osteoarthritis. Ann Rheum Dis. 2013;72(7):1125–35. https://doi.org/10.1136/annrheumdis-2012-202745.
31. Kroon FP, van der Burg LR, Buchbinder R, Osborne RH, Johnston RV, Pitt V. Self-management education programmes for osteoarthritis. Cochrane Database Syst Rev. 2014;1:CD008963. https://doi.org/10.1002/14651858.CD008963.pub2.
32. French SD, Bennell KL, Nicolson PJ, Hodges PW, Dobson FL, Hinman RS. What do people with knee or hip osteoarthritis need to know? An international consensus list of essential statements for osteoarthritis. Arthritis Care Res (Hoboken). 2015;67(6):809–16. https://doi.org/10.1002/acr.22518.
33. Hammer NM, Bieler T, Beyer N, Midtgaard J. The impact of self-efficacy on physical activity maintenance in patients with hip osteoarthritis – a mixed methods study. Disabil Rehabil.

2016;38(17):1691–704. https://doi.org/10.3109/09638288.2015.1107642.
34. Damush TM, Perkins SM, Mikesky AE, Roberts M, O'Dea J. Motivational factors influencing older adults diagnosed with knee osteoarthritis to join and maintain an exercise program. J Aging Phys Act. 2005;13(1):45–60. https://doi.org/10.1123/japa.13.1.45.
35. Bodenheimer T, Lorig K, Holman H, Grumbach K. Patient self-management of chronic disease in primary care. JAMA. 2002;288(19):2469–75. https://doi.org/10.1001/jama.288.19.2469.
36. Knoop J, van der Leeden M, Thorstensson CA, Roorda LD, Lems WF, Knol DL, et al. Identification of phenotypes with different clinical outcomes in knee osteoarthritis: data from the Osteoarthritis Initiative. Arthritis Care Res. 2011;63(11):1535–42.
37. Van der Esch M, Knoop J, Van der Leeden M, Roorda L, Lems W, Knol D, et al. Clinical phenotypes in patients with knee osteoarthritis: a study in the Amsterdam osteoarthritis cohort. Osteoarthr Cartil. 2015;23(4):544–9.
38. Gomez R, Conde J, Scotece M, Gomez-Reino JJ, Lago F, Gualillo O. What's new in our understanding of the role of adipokines in rheumatic diseases? Nat Rev Rheumatol. 2011;7(9):528–36. https://doi.org/10.1038/nrrheum.2011.107.
39. de Boer TN, van Spil WE, Huisman AM, Polak AA, Bijlsma JW, Lafeber FP, et al. Serum adipokines in osteoarthritis; comparison with controls and relationship with local parameters of synovial inflammation and cartilage damage. Osteoarthr Cartil. 2012;20(8):846–53. https://doi.org/10.1016/j.joca.2012.05.002.
40. McAlindon TE, Wilson PW, Aliabadi P, Weissman B, Felson DT. Level of physical activity and the risk of radiographic and symptomatic knee osteoarthritis in the elderly: the Framingham study. Am J Med. 1999;106(2):151–7. https://doi.org/10.1016/s0002-9343(98)00413-6.
41. Messier SP, Resnik AE, Beavers DP, Mihalko SL, Miller GD, Nicklas BJ, et al. Intentional weight loss in overweight and obese patients with knee osteoarthritis: Is more better? Arthritis Care Res. 2018;70(11):1569–75. https://doi.org/10.1002/acr.23608.
42. Christensen R, Bartels EM, Astrup A, Bliddal H. Effect of weight reduction in obese patients diagnosed with knee osteoarthritis: a systematic review and meta-analysis. Ann Rheum Dis. 2007;66(4):433–9. https://doi.org/10.1136/ard.2006.065904.
43. Bannuru RR, Schmid CH, Kent DM, Vaysbrot EE, Wong JB, McAlindon TE. Comparative effectiveness of pharmacologic interventions for knee osteoarthritis: a systematic review and network meta-analysis. Ann Intern Med. 2015;162(1):46–54. https://doi.org/10.7326/M14-1231.
44. Conaghan PG, Arden N, Avouac B, Migliore A, Rizzoli R. Safety of paracetamol in osteoarthritis: what does the literature say? Drugs Aging. 2019;36(1):7–14. https://doi.org/10.1007/s40266-019-00658-9.
45. Gulmez SE, Larrey D, Pageaux GP, Bernuau J, Bissoli F, Horsmans Y, et al. Liver transplant associated with paracetamol overdose: results from the seven-country SALT study. Br J Clin Pharmacol. 2015;80(3):599–606. https://doi.org/10.1111/bcp.12635.
46. Craig DG, Bates CM, Davidson JS, Martin KG, Hayes PC, Simpson KJ. Staggered overdose pattern and delay to hospital presentation are associated with adverse outcomes following paracetamol-induced hepatotoxicity. Br J Clin Pharmacol. 2012;73(2):285–94. https://doi.org/10.1111/j.1365-2125.2011.04067.x.
47. Henrotin Y, Marty M, Mobasheri A. What is the current status of chondroitin sulfate and glucosamine for the treatment of knee osteoarthritis? Maturitas. 2014;78(3):184–7. https://doi.org/10.1016/j.maturitas.2014.04.015.
48. Schneider H, Maheu E, Cucherat M. Symptom-modifying effect of chondroitin sulfate in knee osteoarthritis: a meta-analysis of randomized placebo-controlled trials performed with structum((R)). Open Rheumatol J. 2012;6:183–9. https://doi.org/10.2174/1874312901206010183.
49. Verges J, Monfort J, Abarca B, Carné X, Giménez S, Möller I, et al. An expert consensus on the appropriate use of oral sysadoas for the treatment of the osteoarthritic patient in primary health care: a delphi study. Osteoarthr Cartil. 2020;28:S450–S1. https://doi.org/10.1016/j.joca.2020.02.704.
50. Zegels B, Crozes P, Uebelhart D, Bruyere O, Reginster JY. Equivalence of a single dose (1200 mg) compared to a three-time a day dose (400 mg) of chondroitin 4&6 sulfate in patients with knee osteoarthritis. Results of a randomized double blind placebo controlled study. Osteoarthr Cartil. 2013;21(1):22–7. https://doi.org/10.1016/j.joca.2012.09.017.
51. Reginster JY, Dudler J, Blicharski T, Pavelka K. Pharmaceutical-grade Chondroitin sulfate is as effective as celecoxib and superior to placebo in symptomatic knee osteoarthritis: the ChONdroitin versus CElecoxib versus Placebo Trial (CONCEPT). Ann Rheum Dis. 2017;76(9):1537–43. https://doi.org/10.1136/annrheumdis-2016-210860.
52. Kahan A, Uebelhart D, De Vathaire F, Delmas PD, Reginster JY. Long-term effects of chondroitins 4 and 6 sulfate on knee osteoarthritis: the study on osteoarthritis progression prevention, a two-year, randomized, double-blind, placebo-controlled trial. Arthritis Rheum. 2009;60(2):524–33. https://doi.org/10.1002/art.24255.
53. Derry S, Moore RA, Rabbie R. Topical NSAIDs for chronic musculoskeletal pain in adults. Cochrane Database Syst Rev. 2012;9:CD007400. https://doi.org/10.1002/14651858.CD007400.pub2.

54. Bennell KL, Hunter DJ, Hinman RS. Management of osteoarthritis of the knee. BMJ. 2012;345:e4934. https://doi.org/10.1136/bmj.e4934.
55. Zhang W, Nuki G, Moskowitz RW, Abramson S, Altman RD, Arden NK, et al. OARSI recommendations for the management of hip and knee osteoarthritis: part III: Changes in evidence following systematic cumulative update of research published through January 2009. Osteoarthr Cartil. 2010;18(4):476–99. https://doi.org/10.1016/j.joca.2010.01.013.
56. Coxib, traditional NTC, Bhala N, Emberson J, Merhi A, Abramson S, et al. Vascular and upper gastrointestinal effects of non-steroidal anti-inflammatory drugs: meta-analyses of individual participant data from randomised trials. Lancet. 2013;382(9894):769–79. https://doi.org/10.1016/S0140-6736(13)60900-9.
57. Cooper C, Chapurlat R, Al-Daghri N, Herrero-Beaumont G, Bruyère O, Rannou F, et al. Safety of oral non-selective non-steroidal anti-inflammatory drugs in osteoarthritis: what does the literature say? Drugs Aging. 2019;36(1):15–24. https://doi.org/10.1007/s40266-019-00660-1.
58. Ungprasert P, Cheungpasitporn W, Crowson CS, Matteson EL. Individual non-steroidal anti-inflammatory drugs and risk of acute kidney injury: a systematic review and meta-analysis of observational studies. Eur J Intern Med. 2015;26(4):285–91. https://doi.org/10.1016/j.ejim.2015.03.008.
59. Strand V, McIntyre LF, Beach WR, Miller LE, Block JE. Safety and efficacy of US-approved viscosupplements for knee osteoarthritis: a systematic review and meta-analysis of randomized, saline-controlled trials. J Pain Res. 2015;8:217–28. https://doi.org/10.2147/JPR.S83076.
60. Caborn D, Rush J, Lanzer W, Parenti D, Murray C, Group SS. A randomized, single-blind comparison of the efficacy and tolerability of hylan GF 20 and triamcinolone hexacetonide in patients with osteoarthritis of the knee. J Rheumatol. 2004;31(2):333–43.
61. Ong KL, Anderson AF, Niazi F, Fierlinger AL, Kurtz SM, Altman RD. Hyaluronic acid injections in medicare knee osteoarthritis patients are associated with longer time to knee arthroplasty. J Arthroplast. 2016;31(8):1667–73.
62. Altman R, Lim S, Steen RG, Dasa V. Hyaluronic acid injections are associated with delay of total knee replacement surgery in patients with knee osteoarthritis: evidence from a large US health claims database. PLoS One. 2015;10(12):e0145776.
63. Jubb R, Piva S, Beinat L, Dacre J, Gishen P. A one-year, randomised, placebo (saline) controlled clinical trial of 500–730 kDa sodium hyaluronate (Hyalgan) on the radiological change in osteoarthritis of the knee. Int J Clin Pract. 2003;57(6):467.
64. Wang Y, Hall S, Hanna F, Wluka AE, Grant G, Marks P, et al. Effects of Hylan GF 20 supplementation on cartilage preservation detected by magnetic resonance imaging in osteoarthritis of the knee: a two-year single-blind clinical trial. BMC Musculoskelet Disord. 2011;12(1):195.
65. Bannuru RR, Natov NS, Obadan IE, Price LL, Schmid CH, McAlindon TE. Therapeutic trajectory of hyaluronic acid versus corticosteroids in the treatment of knee osteoarthritis: a systematic review and meta-analysis. Arthritis Care Res. 2009;61(12):1704–11.
66. Bellamy N, Campbell J, Welch V, Gee TL, Bourne R, Wells GA. Intraarticular corticosteroid for treatment of osteoarthritis of the knee. Cochrane Database Syst Rev. 2006;2
67. McAlindon TE, LaValley MP, Harvey WF, Price LL, Driban JB, Zhang M, et al. Effect of intra-articular triamcinolone vs saline on knee cartilage volume and pain in patients with knee osteoarthritis: a randomized clinical trial. JAMA. 2017;317(19):1967–75. https://doi.org/10.1001/jama.2017.5283.
68. Schumacher HR, Chen LX. Injectable corticosteroids in treatment of arthritis of the knee. Am J Med. 2005;118(11):1208–14.
69. Rosenblum A, Marsch LA, Joseph H, Portenoy RK. Opioids and the treatment of chronic pain: controversies, current status, and future directions. Exp Clin Psychopharmacol. 2008;16(5):405–16. https://doi.org/10.1037/a0013628.
70. Smith SR, Deshpande BR, Collins JE, Katz JN, Losina E. Comparative pain reduction of oral non-steroidal anti-inflammatory drugs and opioids for knee osteoarthritis: systematic analytic review. Osteoarthr Cartil. 2016;24(6):962–72. https://doi.org/10.1016/j.joca.2016.01.135.
71. Stewart M, Cibere J, Sayre EC, Kopec JA. Efficacy of commonly prescribed analgesics in the management of osteoarthritis: a systematic review and meta-analysis. Rheumatol Int. 2018;38(11):1985–97. https://doi.org/10.1007/s00296-018-4132-z.
72. Krebs EE, Gravely A, Nugent S, Jensen AC, DeRonne B, Goldsmith ES, et al. Effect of opioid vs nonopioid medications on pain-related function in patients with chronic back pain or hip or knee osteoarthritis pain: the SPACE randomized clinical trial. JAMA. 2018;319(9):872–82. https://doi.org/10.1001/jama.2018.0899.
73. da Costa BR, Nuesch E, Kasteler R, Husni E, Welch V, Rutjes AW, et al. Oral or transdermal opioids for osteoarthritis of the knee or hip. Cochrane Database Syst Rev. 2014;9:CD003115. https://doi.org/10.1002/14651858.CD003115.pub4.
74. Zeng C, Zhang W, Doherty M, Persson MSM, Mallen C, Swain S, et al. Initial analgesic prescriptions for osteoarthritis in the United Kingdom, 2000–2016. Rheumatology (Oxford). 2021;60(1):147–59. https://doi.org/10.1093/rheumatology/keaa244.
75. Shelton RC. Serotonin and norepinephrine reuptake inhibitors. Handb Exp Pharmacol. 2019;250:145–80. https://doi.org/10.1007/164_2018_164.
76. Arendt-Nielsen L, Nie H, Laursen MB, Laursen BS, Madeleine P, Simonsen OH, et al. Sensitization in patients with painful knee osteoarthritis. Pain.

2010;149(3):573–81. https://doi.org/10.1016/j.pain.2010.04.003.
77. Wang G, Bi L, Li X, Li Z, Zhao D, Chen J, et al. Maintenance of effect of duloxetine in Chinese patients with pain due to osteoarthritis: 13-week open-label extension data. BMC Musculoskelet Disord. 2019;20(1):174. https://doi.org/10.1186/s12891-019-2527-y.
78. Lluch E, Torres R, Nijs J, Van Oosterwijck J. Evidence for central sensitization in patients with osteoarthritis pain: a systematic literature review. Eur J Pain. 2014;18(10):1367–75. https://doi.org/10.1002/j.1532-2149.2014.499.x.
79. Wang ZY, Shi SY, Li SJ, Chen F, Chen H, Lin HZ, et al. Efficacy and safety of duloxetine on osteoarthritis knee pain: a meta-analysis of randomized controlled trials. Pain Med. 2015;16(7):1373–85. https://doi.org/10.1111/pme.12800.
80. Whitmyer VG, Dunner DL, Kornstein SG, Meyers AL, Mallinckrodt CH, Wohlreich MM, et al. A comparison of initial duloxetine dosing strategies in patients with major depressive disorder. J Clin Psychiatry. 2007;68(12):1921–30. https://doi.org/10.4088/jcp.v68n1213.
81. McGrory BJ, Weber KL, Jevsevar DS, Sevarino K. Surgical management of osteoarthritis of the knee: evidence-based guideline. JAAOS-J Am Acad Orthopaedic Surgeons. 2016;24(8):e87–93.
82. Manner PA, Tubb CC, Levine BR. AAOS appropriate use criteria: surgical management of osteoarthritis of the knee. J Am Acad Orthop Surg. 2018;26(9):e194–e7. https://doi.org/10.5435/JAAOS-D-17-00425.
83. Mandl LA. Determining who should be referred for total hip and knee replacements. Nat Rev Rheumatol. 2013;9(6):351–7. https://doi.org/10.1038/nrrheum.2013.27.
84. Dieppe P, Lim K, Lohmander S. Who should have knee joint replacement surgery for osteoarthritis? Int J Rheum Dis. 2011;14(2):175–80. https://doi.org/10.1111/j.1756-185X.2011.01611.x.
85. Buckwalter JA, Lohmander S. Operative treatment of osteoarthrosis. Current practice and future development. J Bone Joint Surg Am. 1994;76(9):1405–18. https://doi.org/10.2106/00004623-199409000-00019.
86. Skou ST, Roos EM, Laursen MB, Rathleff MS, Arendt-Nielsen L, Simonsen O, et al. A randomized, controlled trial of total knee replacement. N Engl J Med. 2015;373(17):1597–606. https://doi.org/10.1056/NEJMoa1505467.
87. Beswick AD, Wylde V, Gooberman-Hill R, Blom A, Dieppe P. What proportion of patients report long-term pain after total hip or knee replacement for osteoarthritis? A systematic review of prospective studies in unselected patients. BMJ Open. 2012;2(1):e000435. https://doi.org/10.1136/bmjopen-2011-000435.
88. Bayliss LE, Culliford D, Monk AP, Glyn-Jones S, Prieto-Alhambra D, Judge A, et al. The effect of patient age at intervention on risk of implant revision after total replacement of the hip or knee: a population-based cohort study. Lancet. 2017;389(10077):1424–30. https://doi.org/10.1016/S0140-6736(17)30059-4.
89. Griffin T, Rowden N, Morgan D, Atkinson R, Woodruff P, Maddern G. Unicompartmental knee arthroplasty for the treatment of unicompartmental osteoarthritis: a systematic study. ANZ J Surg. 2007;77(4):214–21. https://doi.org/10.1111/j.1445-2197.2007.04021.x.
90. Kozinn SC, Scott R. Unicondylar knee arthroplasty. J Bone Joint Surg Am. 1989;71(1):145–50.
91. Campi S, Tibrewal S, Cuthbert R, Tibrewal SB. Unicompartmental knee replacement – current perspectives. J Clin Orthop Trauma. 2018;9(1):17–23. https://doi.org/10.1016/j.jcot.2017.11.013.
92. Burn E, Liddle AD, Hamilton TW, Judge A, Pandit HG, Murray DW, et al. Cost-effectiveness of unicompartmental compared with total knee replacement: a population-based study using data from the National Joint Registry for England and Wales. BMJ Open. 2018;8(4):e020977. https://doi.org/10.1136/bmjopen-2017-020977.
93. Liddle AD, Judge A, Pandit H, Murray DW. Adverse outcomes after total and unicompartmental knee replacement in 101,330 matched patients: a study of data from the National Joint Registry for England and Wales. Lancet. 2014;384(9952):1437–45. https://doi.org/10.1016/S0140-6736(14)60419-0.
94. Mohammad HR, Strickland L, Hamilton TW, Murray DW. Long-term outcomes of over 8,000 medial Oxford Phase 3 Unicompartmental Knees-a systematic review. Acta Orthop. 2018;89(1):101–7. https://doi.org/10.1080/17453674.2017.1367577.
95. Niinimaki T, Eskelinen A, Makela K, Ohtonen P, Puhto AP, Remes V. Unicompartmental knee arthroplasty survivorship is lower than TKA survivorship: a 27-year Finnish registry study. Clin Orthop Relat Res. 2014;472(5):1496–501. https://doi.org/10.1007/s11999-013-3347-2.
96. Chawla H, van der List JP, Christ AB, Sobrero MR, Zuiderbaan HA, Pearle AD. Annual revision rates of partial versus total knee arthroplasty: a comparative meta-analysis. Knee. 2017;24(2):179–90. https://doi.org/10.1016/j.knee.2016.11.006.
97. Kim JH, Kim HJ, Lee DH. Survival of opening versus closing wedge high tibial osteotomy: a meta-analysis. Sci Rep. 2017;7(1):7296. https://doi.org/10.1038/s41598-017-07856-8.
98. Brouwer RW, van Raaij TM, Bierma-Zeinstra SM, Verhagen AP, Jakma TS, Verhaar JA. Osteotomy for treating knee osteoarthritis. Cochrane Database Syst Rev. 2007;3:CD004019. https://doi.org/10.1002/14651858.CD004019.pub3.
99. Brouwer RW, Huizinga MR, Duivenvoorden T, van Raaij TM, Verhagen AP, Bierma-Zeinstra SM, et al. Osteotomy for treating knee osteoarthritis. Cochrane Database Syst Rev. 2014;12:CD004019. https://doi.org/10.1002/14651858.CD004019.pub4.
100. Delva ML, Samuel LT, Roth A, Yalcin S, Kamath AF. Contemporary knee osteotomy in the united

states: high tibial osteotomy and distal femoral osteotomy have comparable complication rates despite differing demographic profiles. J Knee Surg. 2019; https://doi.org/10.1055/s-0039-3400742.
101. Kunze KN, Beletsky A, Hannon CP, LaPrade RF, Yanke AB, Cole BJ, et al. Return to work and sport after proximal tibial osteotomy and the effects of opening versus closing wedge techniques on adverse outcomes: a systematic review and meta-analysis. Am J Sports Med. 2020;48(9):2295–304. https://doi.org/10.1177/0363546519881638.
102. Dettoni F, Bonasia DE, Castoldi F, Bruzzone M, Blonna D, Rossi R. High tibial osteotomy versus unicompartmental knee arthroplasty for medial compartment arthrosis of the knee: a review of the literature. Iowa Orthop J. 2010;30:131–40.
103. Santoso MB, Wu L. Unicompartmental knee arthroplasty, is it superior to high tibial osteotomy in treating unicompartmental osteoarthritis? A meta-analysis and systemic review. J Orthop Surg Res. 2017;12(1):50. https://doi.org/10.1186/s13018-017-0552-9.
104. Vena G, D'Adamio S, Amendola A. Complications of osteotomies about the knee. Sports Med Arthrosc Rev. 2013;21(2):113–20. https://doi.org/10.1097/JSA.0b013e3182900720.
105. Cotter EJ, Gowd AK, Bohl DD, Getgood A, Cole BJ, Frank RM. Medical comorbidities and functional dependent living are independent risk factors for short-term complications following osteotomy procedures about the knee. Cartilage. 2020;11(4):423–30. https://doi.org/10.1177/1947603518798889.
106. Seo SS, Nha KW, Kim TY, Shin YS. Survival of total knee arthroplasty after high tibial osteotomy versus primary total knee arthroplasty: A meta-analysis. Medicine (Baltimore). 2019;98(30):e16609. https://doi.org/10.1097/MD.0000000000016609.
107. https://www.aafp.org/family-physician/patient-care/clinical-recommendations/cpg-manual.html. 2019.
108. Ferreira de Meneses S, Rannou F, Hunter DJ. Osteoarthritis guidelines: Barriers to implementation and solutions. Ann Phys Rehabil Med. 2016;59(3):170–3. https://doi.org/10.1016/j.rehab.2016.01.007.
109. Jevsevar DS, Brown GA, Jones DL, Matzkin EG, Manner PA, Mooar P, et al. The American academy of orthopaedic surgeons evidence-based guideline on: treatment of osteoarthritis of the knee, 2nd edn. JBJS. 2013;95(20):1885–6.
110. Brand C. Translating evidence into practice for people with osteoarthritis of the hip and knee. Clin Rheumatol. 2007;26(9):1411–20. https://doi.org/10.1007/s10067-007-0633-y.
111. Grønhaug G, Hagfors J, Borch I, Østerås N, Hagen KB. Perceived quality of health care services among people with osteoarthritis–results from a nationwide survey. Patient Prefer Adherence. 2015;9:1255.
112. Meiyappan KP, Cote MP, Bozic KJ, Halawi MJ. Adherence to the American Academy of Orthopaedic Surgeons clinical practice guidelines for nonoperative management of knee osteoarthritis. J Arthroplast. 2020;35(2):347–52.
113. DeHaan MN, Guzman J, Bayley MT, Bell MJ. Knee osteoarthritis clinical practice guidelines – how are we doing? J Rheumatol. 2007;34(10):2099–105.
114. Grol R, Grimshaw J. From best evidence to best practice: effective implementation of change in patients' care. Lancet. 2003;362(9391):1225–30.
115. Loyola-Sanchez A, Richardson J, Pelaez-Ballestas I, Sánchez JG, González MA, Sánchez-Cruz J, et al. Barriers to implementing the "2008 Mexican Clinical Practice Guideline recommendations for the management of hip and knee osteoarthritis" in primary healthcare practice. Reumatologia Clinica. 2014;10(6):364–72.
116. Spitaels D, Vankrunkelsven P, Desfosses J, Luyten F, Verschueren S, Van Assche D, et al. Barriers for guideline adherence in knee osteoarthritis care: a qualitative study from the patients' perspective. J Eval Clin Pract. 2017;23(1):165–72.
117. Selten EMH, Vriezekolk JE, Nijhof MW, Schers HJ, van der Meulen-Dilling RG, van der Laan WH, et al. Barriers impeding the use of non-pharmacological, non-surgical care in hip and knee osteoarthritis: the views of general practitioners, physical therapists, and medical specialists. JCR J Clin Rheumatol. 2017;23(8):405–10. https://doi.org/10.1097/rhu.0000000000000562.
118. Kingsbury SR, Conaghan PG. Current osteoarthritis treatment, prescribing influences and barriers to implementation in primary care. Prim Health Care Res Dev. 2012;13(4):373–81.
119. Meneses SR, Goode A, Nelson A, Lin J, Jordan J, Allen K, et al. Clinical algorithms to aid osteoarthritis guideline dissemination. Osteoarthr Cartil. 2016;24(9):1487–99.
120. Hunter DJ, Neogi T, Hochberg MC. Quality of osteoarthritis management and the need for reform in the US. Arthritis Care Res. 2011;63(1):31–8.
121. Wallis JA, Ackerman IN, Brusco NK, Kemp JL, Sherwood J, Young K, et al. Barriers and enablers to uptake of a contemporary guideline-based management program for hip and knee osteoarthritis: a qualitative study. Osteoarthritis Cartilage Open. 2020;2(4):100095.
122. Driban JB, Sitler MR, Barbe MF, Balasubramanian E. Is osteoarthritis a heterogeneous disease that can be stratified into subsets? Clin Rheumatol. 2010;29(2):123.
123. Karsdal M, Christiansen C, Ladel C, Henriksen K, Kraus V, Bay-Jensen A. Osteoarthritis–a case for personalized health care? Osteoarthr Cartil. 2014;22(1):7–16.
124. Castañeda S, Roman-Blas JA, Largo R, Herrero-Beaumont G. Osteoarthritis: a progressive disease with changing phenotypes. Oxford: Oxford University Press; 2014.
125. Wikipedia C. "Phenotype – Wikipedia, The Free Encyclopedia". https://enwikipedia.org/w/indexphp?title=Phenotype&oldid=1000590055. 2021.

126. Mobasheri A, Saarakkala S, Finnilä M, Karsdal MA, Bay-Jensen A-C, van Spil WE. Recent advances in understanding the phenotypes of osteoarthritis. F1000Research. 2019;8.
127. Mathur S, Sutton J. Personalized medicine could transform healthcare. Biomed Reports. 2017;7(1):3–5.
128. Karsdal M, Bay-Jensen A, Henriksen K, Christiansen C. The pathogenesis of osteoarthritis involves bone, cartilage and synovial inflammation: may estrogen be a magic bullet? Menopause Int. 2012;18(4): 139–46.
129. Dieppe PA, Lohmander LS. Pathogenesis and management of pain in osteoarthritis. Lancet. 2005;365(9463):965–73.
130. Dieppe PA, Cushnaghan J, Shepstone L. The Bristol 'OA500'study: progression of osteoarthritis (OA) over 3 years and the relationship between clinical and radiographic changes at the knee joint. Osteoarthr Cartil. 1997;5(2):87–97.
131. Peters TJ, Sanders C, Dieppe P, Donovan J. Factors associated with change in pain and disability over time: a community-based prospective observational study of hip and knee osteoarthritis. Br J Gen Pract. 2005;55(512):205–11.
132. Felson D, Niu J, Sack B, Aliabadi P, McCullough C, Nevitt MC. Progression of osteoarthritis as a state of inertia. Ann Rheum Dis. 2013;72(6):924–9.
133. Halilaj E, Le Y, Hicks JL, Hastie TJ, Delp SL. Modeling and predicting osteoarthritis progression: data from the osteoarthritis initiative. Osteoarthr Cartil. 2018;26(12):1643–50.
134. Collins JE, Katz JN, Dervan EE, Losina E. Trajectories and risk profiles of pain in persons with radiographic, symptomatic knee osteoarthritis: data from the osteoarthritis initiative. Osteoarthr Cartil. 2014;22(5):622–30.
135. Nicholls E, Thomas E, Van der Windt D, Croft P, Peat G. Pain trajectory groups in persons with, or at high risk of, knee osteoarthritis: findings from the Knee Clinical Assessment Study and the Osteoarthritis Initiative. Osteoarthr Cartil. 2014;22(12):2041–50.
136. Wesseling J, Bastick AN, Ten Wolde S, Kloppenburg M, Lafeber FP, Bierma-Zeinstra SM, et al. Identifying trajectories of pain severity in early symptomatic knee osteoarthritis: a 5-year followup of the Cohort Hip and Cohort Knee (CHECK) Study. J Rheumatol. 2015;42(8):1470–7.
137. Bastick AN, Wesseling J, Damen J, Verkleij SP, Emans PJ, Bindels PJ, et al. Defining knee pain trajectories in early symptomatic knee osteoarthritis in primary care: 5-year results from a nationwide prospective cohort study (CHECK). Br J Gen Pract. 2016;66(642):e32–e9.
138. Dai Z, Lu N, Niu J, Felson DT, Zhang Y. Dietary fiber intake in relation to knee pain trajectory. Arthritis Care Res. 2017;69(9):1331–9.
139. Trouvin A-P, Marty M, Goupille P, Perrot S. Determinants of daily pain trajectories and relationship with pain acceptability in hip and knee osteoarthritis. A national prospective cohort study on 886 patients. Joint Bone Spine. 2019;86(2):245–50.
140. Emrani PS, Katz JN, Kessler CL, Reichmann WM, Wright EA, McAlindon TE, et al. Joint space narrowing and Kellgren–Lawrence progression in knee osteoarthritis: an analytic literature synthesis. Osteoarthr Cartil. 2008;16(8):873–82.
141. Bartlett SJ, Ling SM, Mayo NE, Scott SC, Bingham CO III. Identifying common trajectories of joint space narrowing over two years in knee osteoarthritis. Arthritis Care Res. 2011;63(12):1722–8. https://doi.org/10.1002/acr.20614.
142. Karsdal M, Michaelis M, Ladel C, Siebuhr A, Bihlet A, Andersen J, et al. Disease-modifying treatments for osteoarthritis (DMOADs) of the knee and hip: lessons learned from failures and opportunities for the future. Osteoarthr Cartil. 2016;24(12):2013–21.
143. Felson DT. Identifying different osteoarthritis phenotypes through epidemiology. Osteoarthr Cartil. 2010;18(5):601–4.
144. Deveza L, Melo L, Yamato T, Mills K, Hunter D. Knee osteoarthritis phenotypes and their relevance for outcomes: a systematic review of the literature. Osteoarthr Cartil. 2017;25:S57–S8.
145. Herrero-Beaumont G, Roman-Blas JA, Bruyère O, Cooper C, Kanis J, Maggi S, et al. Clinical settings in knee osteoarthritis: pathophysiology guides treatment. Maturitas. 2017;96:54–7.
146. Dell'Isola A, Allan R, Smith S, Marreiros S, Steultjens M. Identification of clinical phenotypes in knee osteoarthritis: a systematic review of the literature. BMC Musculoskelet Disord. 2016;17(1):1–12.
147. Dell'Isola A, Steultjens M. Classification of patients with knee osteoarthritis in clinical phenotypes: data from the osteoarthritis initiative. PLoS One. 2018;13(1):e0191045.

Index

A
Abrasion arthroplasty, 218
Absolute contraindications, 182
Acetaminophen, 144, 145, 152, 153, 155, 156, 161
ACR, 368, 369, 371–377, 380
Action mechanism, 183, 188, 200
Acute pseudoseptic reaction, 175, 182
Adductor tubercle, 7, 9
Adhesiolysis, 321, 345
Adipose-derived mesenchymal stromal cells (AD-MSCs), 201–202
Advanced age, 143, 162, 164
Adverse events, 172, 181–182, 187, 188
Aerobic exercise, 125, 126, 128, 130, 133, 138
Age, 55–58, 60, 274, 299, 325, 330, 333, 334
Ahlback scoring system, 92
Alignment, 113–115, 281, 285, 293–296, 299, 303, 310, 311, 315, 320, 322, 342–344
All cemented fixation, 277
Allograft prosthesis composite (APC), 305
All-PE type patella, 282
All-poly tibial component, 254
Aluminium vanadium titanium alloy (Ti 6Al-4V), 278
American Society of Anesthesiologists (ASA) classification, 275
Anabolism, 81, 85
Anaerobic exercise, 126, 128, 130, 133
Anakinra, 195
Anatomical alignment of lower extremities, 294
Anatomical axis, 285, 293, 294, 296, 299, 300, 342
Anatomical axis of the femur and the tibia, 25, 26
Anatomic resection method, 295, 302
Angle of incidence, 178, 179
Ankle pump, 327, 328
Ankylosed knee, 290, 320–322
Ankylosing spondylitis, 116–118
Anterior cruciate ligament, 2, 16–19
Anterior cut type, 267
Anterior-posterior axis, 296
Anterolateral, 175, 176
  approach, 289, 290
  and posteromedial bundle, 19
Anteromedial, 175
Anteromedial and posterolateral bundle, 16, 18
Antero-posterior axis, 2, 19, 27
Anteroposterior bone resection of femur, 300–302
Antibiotics, 277, 327, 329–340
Antibiotic suppression, 335, 337
Anticoagulation, 143, 163
Anti-rheumatic drug, 284–285
Anti-thrombotic drug, 284
Apoptosis, 81, 82, 86
Arrhythmia, 283
Arthroplasty, 251–269
Arthroscopy, 213, 214, 221
Articular branches of the femoral nerve, 6
Articular cartilage, 35–52, 63–65, 70
Aseptic technique, 181–182
Asymmetric instability, 340–342
Athlete, 65, 68, 70–74
Atrophy
  of subcutaneous fat, 182
  of subcutaneous muscle, 182
Autologous chondrocyte implantation, 218
Autologous matrix-induced chondrogenesis, 219
Autologous protein solution (APS), 171, 194, 199, 200
Avocado soybean unsaponifiables, 148–150

B
Backflow technique, 175
Balance training, 125, 130
Balancing, 291, 294, 296, 308, 310, 339, 340, 345
Barriers to implementation, 365, 377, 378
Basic fibroblast growth factor (bFGF), 81, 84
Basic function examination, 111, 114
Bearing
  dislocation, 254, 263–265
  fixed, mobile, 278–281, 293, 301, 323, 329, 342, 344
  surfaces, 279–281
  surface wear, 329
Biceps femoris, 1, 4, 11–13, 16, 24
  direct arm, the anterior arm, and the lateral aponeurotic expansion, 12, 13
Biologic treatment, 171–205
Biomaterials, 277–279

S.-S. Seo (ed.), *A Strategic Approach to Knee Arthritis Treatment*,
https://doi.org/10.1007/978-981-16-4217-3

Biplane, 225, 241
Blind (palpation guided or landmark guided) technique, 175, 176
Blood
  loss, 284, 329
  supply, 285–287, 291, 328
  supply around knee joint, 286
Bone
  cement, 312–314, 329, 334, 345
  defect, 277, 282, 285, 312–317, 322, 335, 339, 340, 342
  graft, 312, 314, 315, 323
  marrow lesion, 99, 102, 105, 108
  marrow mesenchymal stem cells, 219
  resection, 278, 285, 291–293, 295–302, 305–308, 311–314, 316, 317, 319–323
  scintigraphy, 115
Bone marrow aspirate concentrate (BMAC), 194, 196–198, 200, 204
Bone marrow-derived mesenchymal stromal cells (BM-MSCs), 201, 202
Bursitis, 107

C
Calcified cartilage, 83, 85, 89
Capsular approaches, 288–290
Cardiovascular disease, 275, 283
Cartilage, 79–89, 214–220, 222
Cartilage abnormality, 93–94, 101
Cartilage oligomeric matrix protein (COMP), 111, 115
Cartistem, 202
Catabolism, 81, 85
Cavitary defect, 314
Cellular therapy, 194, 196–197, 204
Cement, 277, 278, 282, 311–315, 329, 338–340, 345
Cemented fixation, 277, 311, 315
Cementless fixation, 277, 278, 311
Center of rotation of angulation (CORA), 227
Ceramics, 278, 279
Charlson comorbidity index, 275
Chief complaint, 113
Choice of needle, 181–182
Chondral defects, 214
Chondrocyte(s), 35–40, 42–45, 49–52, 79, 81–83
Chondroitin sulfate, 144, 148–150, 156, 157
Chondrolysis, 187
Chondromalacia, 81, 83
Chondroplasty, 213, 214, 217–220
Chondrotoxic effect, 186
Chronic renal disease, 283–284
Classification, 143, 144, 275, 276, 312, 315, 332, 340–341
Clinical phenotype, 366, 379, 382–384, 386
Clinical practice guideline, 365, 368, 369, 377
Clinical results, 251, 254, 256, 260, 262, 265, 269
Cobalt chrome alloy, 278
Cold therapy, 135
Collagen, 36–47, 49, 51–52
Common peroneal nerve, 1, 16, 21, 22, 24
  deep peroneal nerve, 24
  recurrent peroneal nerve, 24
  superficial peroneal nerve, 24
Comorbid medical illness, 274–275
Competitive, 75
Complications, 251, 253, 263–265, 267, 269, 274, 282, 283, 291, 304, 325–329, 331, 339, 340, 344
Composition, 183, 198, 204
Computed tomography (CT), 97–98, 105
Conformity, 254
Confounding factor, 66, 70
The constrained condylar knee (CCK) type implants, 280, 316
Constrained prosthesis, 280, 281, 306, 307, 310, 316, 319, 320, 329, 343, 344
Constraint PE, 344
Contained defect, 312, 313
Continuous passive motion (CPM), 329
Contraindications, 182, 184, 187–189, 191, 251–253, 264–266, 277, 324, 338
Conversion to TKA, 256, 264
Correction goals, 232
Corticosteroid-induced osteoporosis, 187
Corticosteroids, 144, 148, 159, 162, 172, 182–187, 191
C-reactive protein, 111, 115, 117
Creep phenomenon, 42
Cruciate retaining (CR) type, 279–281
Cruciate sacrificing (CS) type, 279, 280
Crystal-induced inflammatory arthropathy, 111, 118
Cutaneous nerve distribution, 287
Cyclooxygenase-2 (COX-2), 79, 82
Cytokine, 82, 83, 85
Cytokine antagonist, 194–196, 204

D
Debridement, 329–332, 335, 337–340
Deep medial collateral ligament (DMCL), 7, 10
Deep vein thrombosis (DVT)
Deformity, 277, 280, 281, 285, 288, 290, 292, 295, 299, 300, 303, 306, 308, 315–320, 322, 323, 329, 341–343
Deformity (extra-articular), 302, 323
Defunctionalization of nociceptive fibers, 193
Degeneration, 81, 82
Delayed wound healing, 328–330
Density, 55, 56
Descending branch of the lateral femoral circumflex artery, 21
Dgemric (delayed gadolinium enhanced MRI of cartilage), 99
Diabetes mellitus (DM), 283
Diacerein, 148–150, 157
Diagnosis, 111–120, 311, 331–336, 342
Diet, 55, 56, 60
Differential diagnosis, 111–120
Discharge plan, 323, 328
Discoid meniscus, 46–47
Disease modifying osteoarthritis drugs, 150

Disruption of quadriceps tendon, 289, 291, 311, 320
Distal femoral osteotomy, 376, 377
Distal femur fracture, 295, 298
Distal femur osteotomy (DFO), 225, 227, 238, 241, 243
Dose, 183–185, 188, 190, 193, 195, 197, 201–203
Double level osteotomy (DLO), 229, 243, 244
Drape, 287
Dugdale method, 233, 234
Duloxetine, 150, 151, 155–157
Duration, 183–185, 193, 199, 204

E

Echogenicity, 178
Economic condition, 274, 335
Effects, 143, 144, 146–151, 158–160, 162, 163
Efficacy, 172, 175, 182, 184, 186, 187, 190–193, 196–199, 201–205
Elderly patients, 143, 161, 162, 164, 165
Elite, 65, 70–75
Endocrine disease, 283–284
ESCEO, 368–376, 378
Ethnic characteristics, 55, 56
Etiology, 55–61
Evidence-based medicine, 366
Exercise, 55, 56, 58, 63–68, 75, 76, 123–126, 128–135, 138
Exercise dosing, 130–134
Extensile approach, 290–292, 321
Extension-flexion gap balancing, 306–307
Extension gap, 281, 297, 299, 301, 306, 307, 316, 320, 343, 344
Extension instability, 280, 340, 341
Extension mechanism, 289, 291, 320, 321, 338, 344
Extensive skin necrosis, 330–331
Extensor mechanism injury, 329
Extra articular deformity, 302, 323
Extracellular matrix, 35, 36, 42–44, 51
Extramedullary (EM) guide, 299, 302, 322
Extrinsic factors, 55, 56

F

Fabellofibular ligament, 4, 11, 13, 15
Factors affecting the response, 186
Factors related to accuracy rate, 177, 178
Fascia lata, 11
Feedback, 124, 130, 131, 134
Felix classification, 348
Female, 70, 72–74
Femoral artery, 21, 24
Femoral roll back, 279, 280, 282
Femur, 225–229, 238, 240–244, 277, 279–281, 287, 294, 297, 298, 304, 306, 310, 319, 322, 323, 339, 341, 344, 345
FGFR-3, 195
Fibrillation, 81, 83, 84, 86, 87, 89
Fibrin clot, 219
Fibrocartilage, 35, 47, 218–220
Fibula styloid, 4, 13
Fin, 254
Fixed bearing, 251, 254, 256, 260, 261, 263–265
Flat-on-flat, 254
Flexion contracture, 277, 285, 296, 299, 316–316, 320, 343–345
Flexion instability, 281, 296, 306, 307, 322, 341–343
Flushing, 187
Football, 71–76
Free floating technique, 304

G

Gamma radiation, 352
Gap technique, 296, 297, 301
Gastrocnemius flap, 330–332
Gastrocnemius tubercle, 9
Gastrointestinal ulcer, 143
Gender, 55, 56, 58
General population, 65–71, 73–75
Gene therapy, 172, 182, 194, 196, 202–204
Genetics, 55, 56, 59
Genicular artery
  descending genicular artery, 21
  inferior lateral and medial genicular arteries, 13, 24
  middle genicular artery, 20, 21
  superior lateral and medial genicular arteries, 21
Genu recurvatum, 319, 320, 322, 340, 341, 343
Gerdy's tubercle, 3, 11, 13
Glucosamine, 144, 148–150, 154–157
Glycoprotein, 36, 38, 42, 49
Gout, 113, 115–119
Grand piano sign, 302
Growth factor, 191, 192, 194–200, 202–205

H

Heart failure, 283
Heat therapy, 124, 135
Heavy physical work, 55, 56, 58
Hemiarthroplasty, 251
High flexion design, 282, 344
High frequency line transducer, 178
High tibial/tibia osteotomy (HTO), 225, 226, 229, 320, 322, 329, 376
Hip, 65–68, 700–74
Hip–knee–ankle (HKA) angle, 24, 25, 232
History taking, 111–113
Human lymphocyte antigen (HLA)-B27 gene, 117
Human serum albumin, 194–195, 201, 204
Human umbilical cord blood-derived mesenchymal stem cells (hUCB-MSCs), 202
Humphrey ligament, 47, 48
Hunter's canal, 21
Hyaline cartilage, 84, 218, 220
Hyaluronic acid, 172, 173, 187–189, 191
Hyaluronic acid-corticosteroid combination, 191
Hybrid fixation, 277
Hypertension, 143, 159, 161–163, 274, 282, 283, 329
Hypertonic dextrose (prolotherapy, proliferative therapy), 182, 192–193, 204

I

Iliopatellar band, 12, 13
Iliotibial band (ITB), 3, 11–13, 16
Image guided technique, 175, 204
Imaging, 91, 97–99, 102, 105, 107, 108
Impaired renal function, 143, 163
Implant designs, 251, 252, 262, 263, 266, 267, 281–282, 310, 329
Implant fixation, 277–278, 297, 311–312
Implant fracture or tibial insert dissociation, 329
Implant loosening, 306, 313, 314, 329
Implant options, 277–282
Implant retention, 332, 335, 337–338
Indications, 188–190, 251–253, 264–266, 274–277, 343
Individual approach, 143
Infection prevention, 326–327
Infectious arthritis, 111, 118, 120, 187, 189
Infiltration between the popliteal artery and the capsule of the knee (IPACK), 325
Inflammation, 56, 59
Injection site pain, 182, 189, 203
Inlay type, 267, 269
Innervation, 285–287
In-plane needle placement method, 180, 181
Inspection, 111, 113
Instability, 276, 277, 281, 285, 296, 299, 306, 308, 340–343
Instability after TKA, 340–343
Insulin, 81, 82
Insulin-like growth factor-1 (IGF-1), 81, 82
Intercondylar bone resection, 298, 302–304
Intercondylar eminence, 2, 3
Intercondylar fossa, 2, 16, 19
Intercondylar notch, 1, 2
Interleukin-1(IL-1), 81, 82, 85
Interleukin (IL)-1β antagonist, 195
Intermeniscal ligament, 45, 47, 48
International cartilage repair society (ICRS), 102, 103
International guidelines, 143, 151, 152
Intra-articular injection, 171–205
  approach, 175–177
  site, 175–177
  technique, 175–177
Intraarticular loose body, 92, 96, 97
Intra-articular therapeutic agents, 182
Intramedullary (IM) guide, 302
Intrameniscal signal intensity, 104–107
Intraoperative analgesic, 324–325
Intrasubstance degeneration, 105
Intrinsic factors, 55, 56
Isometric exercise, 129–131

J

Joint, 79–85
  degeneration, 56
  effusion, 97, 99, 105–106
  fluid analysis, 111, 115, 116

K

Kellgren and Lawrence score, 79
Kellgren-Lawrence class, 92, 93
Kinematic alignment, 295
Kinematics, 279, 295, 304
Knee, 63–76, 143–146, 148–158, 160, 213–222, 273–345
  brace, 125, 136
  injury, 55–57, 63, 66, 74
  osteoarthritis (OA), 116, 123–126, 128–131, 134–138

L

Laboratory finding, 112, 115
Laser chondroplasty, 219
Lateral bifurcate ridge, 16
Lateral closing wedge osteotomy, 226
Lateral collateral ligament (LCL), 1, 2, 4, 11, 13, 14, 24
Lateral compartmental arthritis, 264
Lateral inferior genicular artery, 286, 293
Lateral intercondylar posterior ridge, 16
Lateral intercondylar ridge (resident's ridge), 16
Lateral mid-patellar, 175, 177
Lateral release, 290, 310, 319
Lateral suprapatellar bursa, 175, 177, 178
Lavage, debridement, 213, 214, 220, 221
Leisure, 65–68
Life style, 55, 56, 60
Ligament laxity, 55, 56
Ligament rupture, 97, 106
Load transmission, 35, 51
Local factors, 55, 56
Local swelling, 182
Longitudinal ridge, 4
Long-term corticosteroids user, 283
Loose body, 214, 221, 222
Loosening, 274–276, 282, 305, 311, 326, 329, 335, 337, 341
Lower limb alignment, 293–294, 320
Lubrication, 35, 36, 38, 42, 45, 51
Lug, 258

M

Magnetic resonance imaging (MRI), 97–102, 104–107
Malalignment, 55–58, 97, 281, 296, 310, 311, 329, 341–344
Male, 68, 70–75
Massive hematoma, 328, 330
Matrix metalloprotease (MMP), 80–82, 85
Matrix metalloproteinase, 40, 41
Max heartrate, 133
Measured resection technique, 296, 297
Mechanical alignment of lower extremities, 294
Mechanical axis, 226, 227, 229, 231–233, 235, 239, 240, 242, 243, 293, 294, 297, 299, 303, 317, 323, 329, 342
Mechanical axis of the femur and the tibia, 24–26

Mechanical lateral distal femoral angle (mLDFA), 227, 228
Mechanical medial proximal tibial angle (mMPTA), 227
Mechanism of action, 143, 144, 163
Medial and lateral facet, 27
Medial and lateral femoral condyle, 1, 2, 16, 27
Medial and lateral femoral epicondyle, 13
Medial and lateral head of the gastrocnemius, 7, 10, 13, 16, 24
Medial and lateral sural cutaneous nerve, 24
Medial and lateral tibial plateau, 2, 24, 28
Medial and tibial spine, 3, 16, 25
Medial collateral ligament (MCL), 293, 297, 306, 308, 309, 317, 318, 329, 342
  injury, 329
Medial compartmental arthritis, 264
Medial-lateral balancing, 308
Medial mid-patellar, 175–176
Medial parapatellar approach, 288–291
Medial patellofemoral ligament (MPFL), 7–9
Medial release, 308, 309, 317, 318
Medial retinaculum, 7, 21
Medial trivector retaining approach, 290, 310
Medial trivector retaining arthrotomy, 290
Medical evaluation, 282–284
Meniscal-bearing, 254
Meniscal lesion, 102, 104
Meniscal tear, 102, 104
Meniscectomy, 75
Meniscus, 35–52, 213–216, 220, 221
Menisectomy, 213–217, 220–222
Menopause, 56, 58
Mental status, 274
Mesenchymal stromal (or stem) cells (MSCs), 194, 196, 200–202
Metal augmentation, 312, 314, 315, 343
Metal-backed patella, 282
Metal-backed tibal component, 254–256
Method of checking lower limb alignment during surgery, 233
Methods of balancing, 308–310
Methylprednisolone, 183–185, 187
Microvascular structure of soft tissue around knee, 330
Mid-flexion instability, 296, 299, 306, 342, 343
Midvastus approach, 289–290
Mikulicz line, 226
Mild skin necrosis, 328, 330
Miniaci method, 233, 240
Minimally invasive surgery, 255–257
Mobile bearing, 251, 254, 259, 260, 263–265
Mobile bearing design, 281
Modified gap technique, 297
Modularity, 254
Motor control, 130
Multidisciplinary approach, 365–367, 378, 385
Multiple drilling, 214
Muscle weakness, 55–56
Myopathy, 187
Myxoid degeneration, 105

N
Neer classification, 346
Neural deficit, 329
Nitric oxide (NO), 81, 82
Non-cellular therapy, 182, 194–197, 204
Noncollagenous protein, 32, 44, 45
Non-contained defect, 312, 313
Non-operative treatment, 143, 144, 152
Non-pharmacologic management, 123–138
Non-steroidal Anti-inflammatory Drugs (NSAIDs), 144, 147, 153, 156, 157, 163, 164, 275, 283, 284, 325, 328
Non-touch technique, 287

O
OA Research Society International (OARSI), 102, 368, 369, 371–377
Obesity, 55, 56, 59, 143, 148, 158, 159, 275, 305, 327, 328
Oblique popliteal ligament (OPL), 10
Obturator nerve, 1, 21, 24
Odd facet, 4, 5, 27
One-stage reimplantation, 335, 338, 340
Onlay type, 267, 269
Onset, 183
Open medial HTO, 226
Open wedge osteotomy, 225, 230
Opioids, 144–146, 148, 152, 157, 163, 164
Oral agents, 162
Osteoarthritis, 55, 56, 58, 63–76, 79–89, 143–146, 148–150, 152, 154, 156–158, 160, 161, 213, 214, 222, 251, 253, 264–266, 276, 365, 368–370, 373, 378, 380–382, 384–386
Osteoblasts, 81
Osteochondral autograft, 218
Osteolysis, 329
Osteophyte(s), 66–69, 72, 73, 79, 84, 85, 92–99, 102, 105, 107, 213, 214, 217, 218, 221, 222, 276, 296, 297, 306, 315–317, 319, 344, 345
Osteophytes resection, 297–298
Osteotomy, 225–244, 291, 292, 305, 310, 318, 320–323, 329
Other compartment disease, 252, 253, 263, 265, 269
Outcome, 274, 275, 280, 284, 295, 311, 313, 323, 330, 337, 339, 340, 344, 345
Out-of-plane needle placement method, 180, 181

P
Pain (management), 323, 324, 344
Pain control, 125, 135
Palpation, 111, 114
Paramedial arthrotomy, 290
Patella
  bone resection, 305
  fracture, 280, 282, 305, 345

Patella (*cont.*)
  osteotomy, 305
  tendon, 3–7, 21, 24
  tracking, 289, 290, 300, 304–306, 311
Patellar clunk syndrome, 281
Patellar tendon, 288–290, 292, 321, 323, 329, 330
Patellar tendon rupture, 280
Patellofemoral and patellomeniscal ligaments, 7–9, 11
Patellofemoral arthritis, 264–266
Patellofemoral arthroplasty, 251, 265–269
Patellofemoral dislocation, 329
Patellofemoral joint reaction force (PFJRF), 28, 31
Patient characteristics, 143, 150, 157
Patient information, 111, 112
Patient optimization, 282–285
Patient selection, 274–277
Peg, 260
Periarticular multimodal drug injection, 325
Perioperative management, 275, 283
Peripheral nerve block, 324, 325
Periprosthetic femoral fracture, 279, 280, 282, 297
Periprosthetic fracture, 277, 329, 345
Periprosthetic joint infection (PJI), 329, 331–340
Periprosthetic patella fracture, 282
Periprosthetic tibial fracture, 277
Persistent drainage, 328–330
Personalized healthcare, 365, 366, 379, 386
Pes anserinus
  gracilis, 7, 9
  sartorius, 7, 9
  semitendinosus, 7, 9
Pharmacodynamics, 183
Pharmacokinetics, 172, 183, 184, 191, 195
pharmacokinetics of synovial joint, 172
Pharmacologic treatment, 143–145, 165
Physical activity, 63–68, 70, 74–76
Physical education teacher, 74
Physical examination, 111, 112
Physical therapy, 123, 138
Pie-crusting technique, 310, 317–319
Platelet-rich plasma (PRP), 194, 196, 198–200, 204, 205
Polydeoxyribonucleotide (PDRN), 182, 191–192
Polyethylene (PE), 278–280, 329
Polyethylene insert wear, 251, 258
Polymethylmethacrylate (PMMA), 277
Popliteal artery, 16, 19–21
Popliteomeniscal fascicle, 46
Popliteous muscle, 297, 310, 319, 320
Popliteus, 2, 10, 24, 27, 28
  arcuate ligament, 11, 13, 15
  fossa, 16, 17
  popliteofibula ligament, 4, 13–15
Position of the needle, 175
Posterior condylar axis, 296, 300
Posterior cruciate ligament, 2, 3, 19, 28
Posterior distal femoral angle (PDFA), 26
Posterior intercondylar fossa, 19
Posterior oblique ligaments (POL), 9, 10
  superficial, central and articular arm, 9, 10
Posterior stabilized (PS) type, 279–281
Posterior tibial slope, 231, 232, 234, 235
Postinjection flare, 187
Postoperative analgesic, 325
Postoperative management, 282, 323, 324, 345
Postoperative pain management, 324, 325, 344
Post-traumatic osteoarthritis, 160
Preoperative analgesic, 324
Preoperative examination, 274, 275, 285
Preoperative preparation, 282–284
Preparation for bone resection and fixation for each part, 297–306
Prevention, 323, 326–327, 342–343
Principle of antibiotics administration, 335–337
Procedural precaution, 184, 192
Professional (athlete), 70, 73–75
Proprioception, 123, 130, 131
Prostaglandin E2 (PGE2), 82, 85
Prosthesis alignment, 293–306
Proteoglycan, 36–45, 49, 80–83, 87
Proximal tibial bone resection, 303–304
Proximal tibial fracture, 302, 304
Proximal tibiofibular joint, 4
Pseudogout, 118, 119
Psoriatic arthritis, 116–118
Psychiatric comorbidities, 284
Pulse sequence protocol, 99

Q
Q-angle, 26
Quadriceps, 128–131, 133, 137
  retinaculum, 11
  tendon, 281, 289–291, 311, 320, 321, 329
  turn down, 291

R
Radiofrequency, 220
Radiography, 91–93, 98, 102, 105, 107, 108
Radiologic (osteoarthritis), 66, 71, 73, 74
Range of motion, 123, 125, 126, 128, 135, 136, 138
Range of motion (ROM), 329
Recreational, 66, 67, 70, 71, 75
Rectus femoris, 4, 6, 7
Rectus snip, 291, 292, 321
Recurrent branch of the anterior tibial artery, 21
Rehabilitation, 274, 316, 323, 324, 327–328, 343–345
Reimplantation, 327, 335, 338–340
Reinforcing the implant fixation, 254, 259
Reiter's syndrome, 116–118
Relative contraindications, 182
Removing method of infrapatellar fat pad, 293
Resection method, 294, 295, 302, 309
Resection of distal femur, 298–300, 306, 307, 316, 341, 344
Resurfacing type, 267
Reverberation artifact, 179, 180
Rheumatoid arthritis, 113, 115–120

rhFGF18, 195
Risk factors, 55–61
Rollback movement, 27
Rolling and sliding, 28
Rorabeck classification, 347
Rotating hinged prosthesis (RH prosthesis), 281
Rotating hinge-type constrained prosthesis, 344
Rotational alignment of the femur, 297, 310
Rotation alignment, 300, 306
Round-on-round, 254, 255, 261, 268
RPE scale, 133
Running, 64–66, 69, 70, 75
Rupture of the extensor mechanism, 350–353

S
Salvage pathway, 191
Saphenous nerve
  infrapatella branch, 21, 22
  sartorial branch, 21
Sclerosis, 79, 85, 89
Screw-home movement, 27, 28, 30
Secondary osteonecrosis, 111, 119, 120
Selection of patellar components, 282
Selective muscle training, 129
Semimembranosus, 10, 16
Side effects, 143, 146, 148, 158, 159
Size-dependent sieving effect, 173
Skin
  defects, 290
  hypopigmentation, 182
  incision, 288
  preparation, 181–182
Smoking, 56, 60
Soccer, 68–75
Social condition, 274
Socio economic burden, 80
Sodium MRI, 99
Soft tissue management, 291–293
Spacer block, 297
Spondyloarthropathies, 111, 117, 120
Spontaneous osteonecrosis, 111, 119
Sport activity, 63, 68, 69
Sports, 55, 56, 58, 59
Sprifermin (recombinant human fibroblast growth factor 18; rhFGF18), 195
Stem, 312, 314, 315
Stiffness, 277, 329, 341, 342, 344, 345
Straight leg raising exercise, 327
Strategic approach, 365, 366, 386
Stretching, 123, 128, 129
Stromal vascular fraction (SVF), 194, 196, 197, 200, 204
Subchondral attrition, 107
Subchondral bone, 83–85, 87, 94–95, 97, 99, 101–103, 105, 218, 219
Subchondral cysts, 85
Subchondral sclerosis, 91–96, 99, 107
Subcutaneous lipoatrophy, 187
Subluxation, 91, 93, 95, 97, 102
Subvastus approach, 288, 289
Subvastus arthrotomy, 289, 290
Superficial infection, 328, 330, 332, 337
Superficial medial collateral ligaments (SMCL), 7–10
Superficial zone, 83
Superolateral patellar, 175, 177
Superomedial patellar, 175, 176
Surgical approach, 287–291
Surgical techniques, 251, 260, 264, 268, 273, 282, 285–293, 296, 309, 310, 328, 338, 343, 344
Surgical wound management, 326
Symmetric instability, 340–342
Symptomatic (osteoarthritis), 66–68, 72, 74
Symptomatic rapid acting drugs for osteoarthritis, 144, 145
Symptomatic slow acting drugs for osteoarthritis, 144, 148
Synovectomy, adhesiolysis, 214
Synovial fluid, 35, 42, 52
Synovial membrane, 79, 82–84, 88
Synovitis, 96–97, 99, 105, 106
Synovium, 84, 85
Systemic factors, 55, 56

T
Takeuchi type, 237
Taping, 124, 125, 137, 138
TCA/Krebs cycle, 126, 127
TENS, 136
Tensor device, 297
Thermal chondroplasty, 219, 220
Thromboembolism, 326, 329
Tibia, 225–236, 238, 240, 243, 244, 291, 292, 302
Tibia bone varus angle (TBVA), 231
Tibial alignment, 303
Tibial axis, 296, 300, 301, 303
Tibial insertional ligament, 47
Tibial nerve, 16, 21, 24
Tibial tubercle osteotomy, 229
Tibial tuberosity, 3, 4, 6, 7, 11, 26
Tibia tubercle osteotomy, 292
Tibiofemoral dislocation, 329
Tidemark, 39, 43, 44
TissueGene-C, 202, 203
T2 mapping, 99, 100
Topical agents, 144
Total knee arthroplasty, 273–351, 376
  after osteotomy, 322–323
  in ankylosed knee, 320–322
  in bone defect, 312–313
  in flexion contracture, 315–316
  in genu recurvatum, 319–320
  in valgus deformity, 318–319
Tourniquet, 287, 311, 329, 338
Towel clip technique, 311
Trabecular metal augments, 312, 314
Tracked-bearing, 254
Traditional resection method, 294, 302

Trajectory
pain, 380, 381
structural change, 366, 380, 381
acetaminophen, 373
analgesics, 373, 376
aquatic exercise(s), 368, 369, 372, 373
bandage taping, 368, 372
brace(s), 368, 372, 373, 383
cognitive-behavioral therapy, 371, 383, 384
COX-2 inhibitors, 369, 376
diclofenac,
education, 368, 371, 378–381, 383–385
exercise, 368, 369, 371–373, 383, 384
information, 367, 368, 371, 378, 379
insole(s), 368, 372, 373, 383, 385
intra-articular injection(s), 369, 370, 375
corticosteroid(s), 369, 375, 378
hyaluronic acid, 369, 375, 378, 382
manual therapy, 368, 372, 373
mechanotherapy, 368, 372
nonsteroidal anti-inflammatory drugs, 370, 374
oral, 369, 371, 372, 374–376
topical, 369, 374, 375
opioid(s), 369, 375, 376
SYSADOA(s), 369, 370, 373, 374
avocado/soybean unsaponifiable(s), 369, 373, 374
chondroitin, 369, 370, 373, 374
diacerein, 369, 374
glucosamine, 369, 370, 373, 374
Tai-chi, 369, 373
thermal agent(s), 368, 372
tramadol, 369, 375, 376
walking aid(s), 368, 372
weight loss, 368, 371, 372, 383, 384
Trans-capsaicin, 193, 204
Transepicondylar axis (TEA), 24, 26, 296, 300
Transfibular lateral closing wedge HTO, 226
Transforming growth factor- ß (TGF-ß), 82
Transtibial axis, 300, 301
Transverse axis, 2, 28
Transverse ridge, 4, 5
Trauma, 63, 64, 66
Treatment, 274–276, 283, 312, 322, 329–331, 333, 335, 339, 343, 345
T1rho mapping, 99
Triamcinolone, 183–185, 187
Trigonometric data, 234
Trivector retaining arthrotomy, 290
Trochlear groove, 1, 2, 27, 31
Tumor necrosis factor-α (TNF-α), 81, 82, 85
Tumor necrotizing factor (TNF) antagonist, 194–196, 200
Two-stage reimplantation, 335, 338–340
Type II collagen, 80, 81

U
Ultra-high molecular weight polyethylene (UHMWPE), 278, 279
Ultrasound-guided injection, 176–181, 186, 204
Ultrasound guided injection technique, 178–181
Unicompartmental, 251–269
Unicompartmental arthroplasty, 376, 377
Unicondylar knee arthroplasty (UKA), 230
Uniplane, 225, 241

V
Valgus deformity, 225–227, 229, 238, 239, 277, 288, 290, 301, 310, 312, 318–320, 323, 325
Varus deformity, 225–227, 229–232, 238, 243, 295, 299, 301–303, 308–310, 312, 316–318, 323
Varus-valgus constrained (VVC), 280–281
Varus-valgus constrained prosthesis, 280–281
Varus-valgus stress X-ray, 229
Vascular endothelial growth factor (VEGF), 84, 85
Vascular injury, 329
Vastus intermedius, 4, 6, 7, 9
Vastus lateralis, 4, 6, 7, 21
Vastus medialis, 4, 21
Vastus medialis longus (VML), 6
Vastus medialis obliquus (VMO), 6, 7, 9
Venous thromboembolism (VTE), 326, 329
Venous thromboembolism management, 326
Vertical median bridge, 4, 5
Viscosupplementation, 188, 190, 204
Vitamin E, 279
VY quadricepsplasty, 291, 292

W
Walker, 136
Wear, 274, 275, 278–282, 295, 300, 303–306, 310, 317, 329, 338, 339, 341
Wedged insole, 137
Weight-bearing line, 226, 228, 233, 234, 240
Weight bearing scanography method, 226, 228, 229, 233, 234, 237, 239–241, 243
Weight loss, 123–126, 131, 133, 138
Whiteside's line, 300
Wnt genes, 193
Wnt receptors, 193, 204
Wound complications, 273, 328–329
Wrisberg ligament, 47, 48

Y
Young patients, 143, 158

Z
Zirconium, 278, 279
Zones of articular cartilage
calcified cartilage zone, 37–39, 44
deep/radial zone, 38–39
middle/transitional zone, 38
superficial zone, 36–42, 44
Z-plasty, 291

Printed by Printforce, the Netherlands